Owen
81

Current Practice of Clinical Electroencephalography

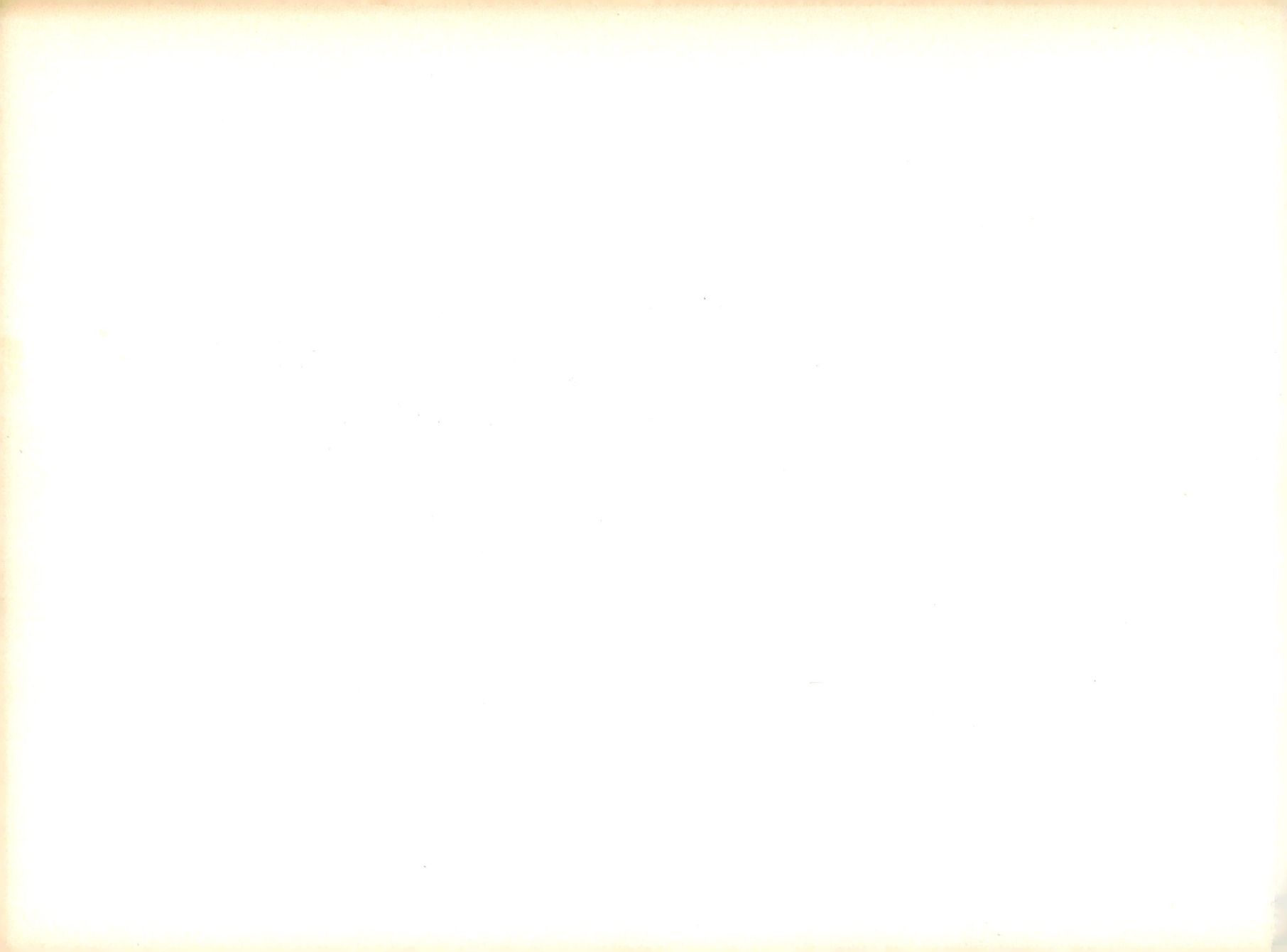

Current Practice of Clinical Electroencephalography

Editors

Donald W. Klass, M.D.
*Professor of Neurology
Mayo Medical School
and Head, Section of Electroencephalography
Department of Neurology
Mayo Foundation and Mayo Clinic
Rochester, Minnesota*

David D. Daly, M.D., Ph.D.
*Professor of Neurology
Southwestern Medical School
University of Texas
Health Science Center at Dallas
Dallas, Texas*

Raven Press ▪ New York

Raven Press, 1140 Avenue of the Americas, New York, New York 10036

© 1979 by Raven Press Books, Ltd. All rights reserved. This book is protected by copyright. No part of it may be reproduced, stored in a retrieval system, or transmitted, in any form or by any means, electronic, mechanical, photocopying, recording, or otherwise, without the prior written permission of the publisher.

Made in the United States of America

Library of Congress Cataloging in Publication Data
Main entry under title:

Current practice of clinical electroencephalography.

   Includes bibliographical references and index.
   1. Electroencephalography. 2. Brain—Diseases—
Diagnosis. I. Klass, Donald W. II. Daly, David D.
[DNLM: 1. Electroencephalography. WL150 C976]
RC386.6.E43C87   616.8'04'754   75-32088
ISBN 0-98004-088-5

Second Printing, February, 1980

Dedication

We dedicate this book to the memory of our friend and colleague, Dr. Michael G. Saunders, who died suddenly while preparation of this book was in progress. During his lifetime, Mike had given generously of his time and skilled effort to advance the field of electroencephalography in North America. We continue to miss him greatly.

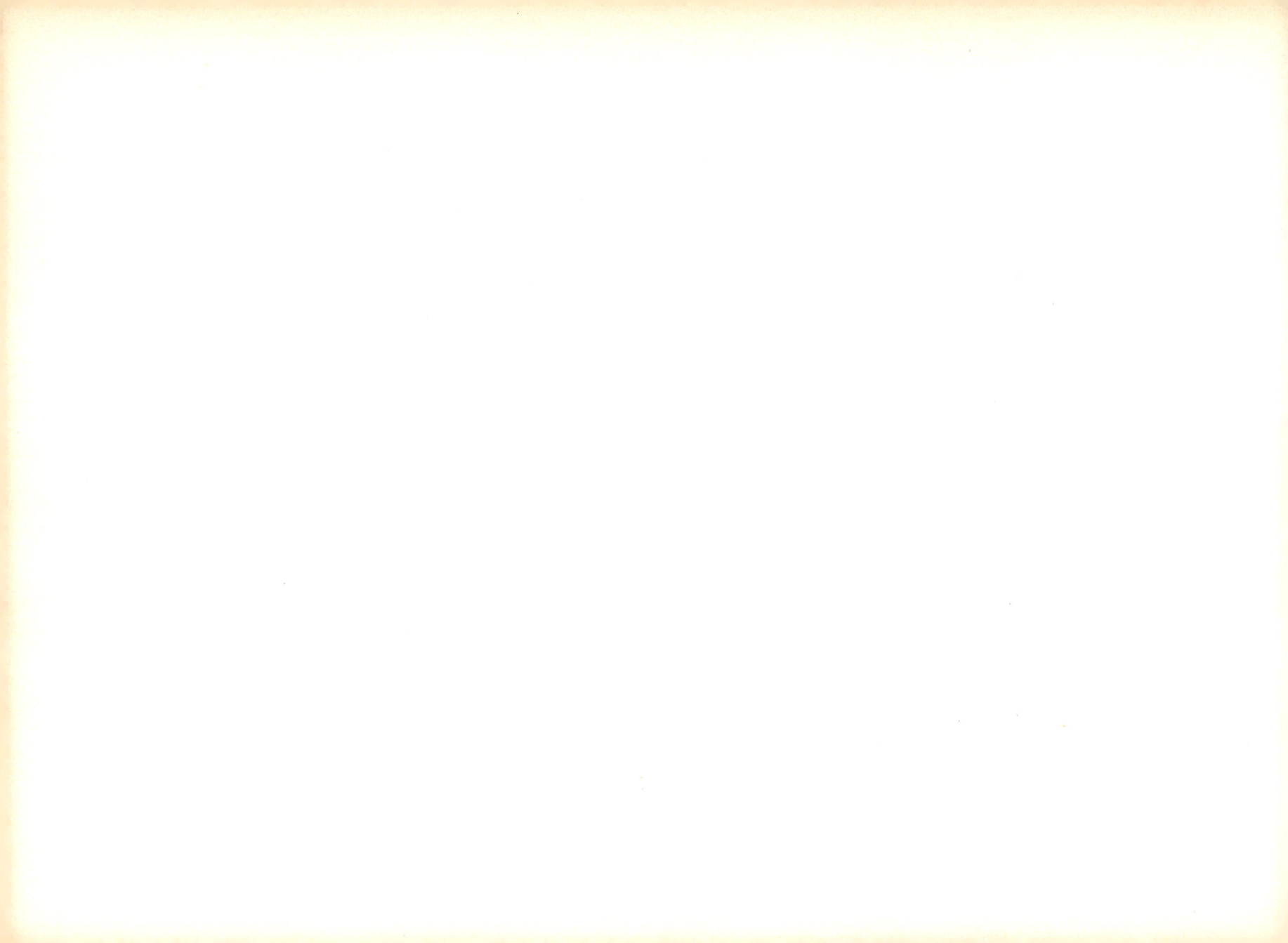

Preface

Half a century after the first publication by Hans Berger, *On the Electroencephalogram of Man,* electroencephalography has become a diagnostic tool used extensively throughout the world. The increasing requirements for accurate diagnostic service have led to the establishment of increasingly large numbers of EEG laboratories. Furthermore, the nature of EEG practice continues to evolve as knowledge and experience accumulate and as indications for its use change. In this text, the current state of clinical EEG practice is assessed by some of its foremost practitioners in North America.

The impetus for assembling this text came originally from audience response to the annual continuation courses on EEG that have been sponsored by the American Electroencephalographic Society since 1966. All the principal contributors to this book have served on the faculty of those courses.

The chapters of this book represent a synthesis of information that the authors consider important for understanding the current applications of EEG to clinical medical practice. An overview of the field is presented with a selective rather than an all-inclusive compilation of references.

We hope that this text will provide a convenient means of updating information for the EEG practitioner. It should serve as a useful review for those who are seeking to meet the standards for competence in clinical EEG set by the American Board of Qualifications in Electroencephalography. It should also serve as a useful adjunct for trainees. However, we have not designed the book to serve as an encyclopedic text or to supplant other methods of teaching. We recognize that the best method of teaching the fundamentals of clinical EEG involves close interaction between an experienced instructor and a small group of students who review together a large number of diverse tracings. To learn visual analysis and clinical interpretation of EEG adequately requires many months of increasingly independent experience in a good laboratory under competent supervision.

The contributors to this book have attempted not merely to summarize but to evaluate significant current information. While they emphasize areas of consensus, they also discuss significant topics that are at present controversial or about which current knowledge is insufficient. Edited transcripts of selected discussions at the courses have been included to illustrate topics of continuing controversy or general agreement. We hope that the reader will benefit from exposure to individual differences in approach to problems confronting the electroencephalographer. For this reason, the editors have not acted as censors.

Although the contributors to this book are members of the American EEG Society and some are also members of the American Board of Qualifications in Electroencephalography, Inc., neither of these organizations should be held responsible for the views expressed herein. The only official policy statements are the Guidelines in EEG of the American EEG Society that are included as an Appendix.

Donald W. Klass, M.D.
David D. Daly, M.D. Ph.D.

Contents

1. Standards of Practice in Clinical Electroencephalography 1
   Robert J. Ellingson

2. Minimum Technical Requirements for Performing Clinical Electroencephalography: Illustrative Examples of Principles on Which some of the Technical Guidelines of the American EEG Society are Based. 7
   Michael G. Saunders

3. Basis for Visual Analysis: Polarity Convention, Principles of Localization, and Electrical Fields 27
   Robert L. Maulsby

4. Artifacts: Activity of Noncerebral Origin in the EEG 37
   Michael G. Saunders

5. An Orderly Approach to Visual Analysis: The Parameters of the Normal EEG in Adults and Children 69
   Peter Kellaway

6. EEGs of Premature and Full-Term Newborns 149
   Robert J. Ellingson

7. Optimal Display of EEG Activity 179
   Charles E. Henry

8. Use of the EEG for Diagnosis and Evaluation of Epileptic Seizures and Nonepileptic Episodic Disorders 221
   David D. Daly

CONTENTS

9 Activation Procedures and Special Electrodes 269
   Reginald G. Bickford

10 Use of the EEG for Evaluation of Focal Intracranial Lesions 307
   Eli S. Goldensohn

11 The EEG in Evaluation of Disorders Affecting the Brain Diffusely 343
   Michael G. Saunders and Barbara F. Westmoreland

12 EEG in the Evaluation of Headaches 381
   Barbara F. Westmoreland

13 Evaluation of Psychiatric Disorders and the Effects of Psychotherapeutic and Psychotomimetic Agents 395
   Morton D. Low

14 EEG Patterns of Uncertain Diagnostic Significance 411
   Robert L. Maulsby

15 Neurophysiologic Substrates of EEG Activity 421
   Eli S. Goldensohn

16 Event-Related Potentials and Their Clinical Applications 441
   Morton D. Low

17 Newer Methods of Recording and Analyzing EEGs 451
   Reginald G. Bickford

   Appendix 481

   Discussions 499

   Subject Index 523

Contributors

Reginald G. Bickford
Department of Neurosciences
University of California
La Jolla, California 92037

David D. Daly
Department of Neurology
Southwestern Medical School
University of Texas Health
Science Center of Dallas
Dallas, Texas 75235

Robert J. Ellingson
Departments of Neurology and Psychiatry
University of Nebraska
College of Medicine
Omaha, Nebraska 68105

Eli S. Goldensohn
Department of Neurology
College of Physicians and Surgeons
Columbia University
New York, New York 10032

Charles E. Henry
EEG Laboratory
Cleveland Clinic Center
Cleveland, Ohio 44106

Peter Kellaway
Division of Neurophysiology
Department of Neurology
Baylor College of Medicine
Texas Medical Center
Houston, Texas 77030

Donald W. Klass
Section of Electroencephalography
Department of Neurology
Mayo Foundation and Mayo Clinic
Rochester, Minnesota 55901

John R. Knott
Professor-Emeritus
Neurology and Psychiatry
University of Iowa
Iowa City, Iowa 52242
and Department of Neurology
Tufts University
School of Medicine
Boston, Massachusetts 02111

Morton D. Low
Department of Medicine (Neurology) and Physiology
University of British Columbia
and Department of Electroencephalography
Vancouver General Hospital
Vancouver, B.C., Canada

Robert L. Maulsby
Department of Neurology
Wayne State University
School of Medicine
and Harper Hospital EEG Laboratory
Detroit, Michigan 48201

Michael G. Saunders (deceased)
Formerly Section of Electroencephalography
Computer Department
and Department of Physiology
Faculty of Medicine
University of Manitoba
Winnipeg, Canada

Barbara F. Westmoreland
Section of Electroencephalography
Department of Neurology
Mayo Medical School and
Mayo Graduate School of Medicine
Rochester, Minnesota 55901

Chapter 1

Standards of Practice in Clinical Electroencephalography

Robert J. Ellingson

University of Nebraska Medical Center, Omaha, Nebraska 68105

Qualifications of Electroencephalographers 2
Qualifications of EEG Technologists and Technicians 3
Equipment 3
Telephone Transmission of EEGs 3
References 4

In any branch of clinical medicine the most important factors determining the difference between first rate, just adequate, and substandard services are the knowledge and care of its practitioners. Knowledge in turn depends upon training plus experience. In the case of electroencephalography these criteria must be applied not only to the electroencephalographer who establishes procedures, supervises the laboratory, and interprets the recordings, but also to the technologist who is responsible for obtaining quality recordings.

As in any other new field there were at first no formal training programs either for electroencephalographers or for technicians, much less any standards for the direction and content of such programs or for the qualifications of teachers of electroencephalography.

In the 1930s and 1940s the pioneers who broke the ground in the field of electroencephalography taught their students and trained their technicians in their own laboratories, usually on an individual basis and for however long seemed necessary. Their students later established their own laboratories, trained their technicians, and some of them eventually taught students of their own. And so it went. All this largely took place within colleges of medicine and a few other large medical centers. Although electroencephalography is now much more widely practiced, it is for the most part still taught by the same more or less informal methods.

The establishment of formal training programs and training standards has taken much longer in electroencephalography than in many other subspecialty fields of medicine that sprang up during the first half of the century. The American EEG Society's Guidelines in EEG is an effort to fill a long recognized gap and to establish standards for training and practice in electroencephalography. The American Medical Association has recently accepted EEG technology as an allied health profession, set up a Joint Committee on Accreditation of Educational Programs in Electroencephalographic Technology, and promulgated standards for such programs. No similarly formal standards have as yet been established for electroencephalographers themselves.

The five sets of guidelines issued to date by the American EEG Society are reprinted as an appendix to this text. The reader is urged to consult them, especially Guidelines No. 3 (Revised 1976) and 5, in conjunction with this chapter.

First, be it clearly understood that the guidelines by and large describe minimal, not optimal or ideal, standards of electroencephalographic practice at the time they were written. It is reemphasized that, as stated in the introduction of Guidelines No. 3, "If the standards set forth cannot be met, it would be well to consider *not* operating an EEG laboratory." Bad electroencephalography is much worse than no electroencephalography; it often misleads rather than assists the referring physician.

QUALIFICATIONS OF ELECTROENCEPHALOGRAPHERS

The requirement of 1 year of specific training in EEG during or after medical specialty training is an absolute minimum in preparation for the independent practice of electroencephalography. The 6-months training cited in sections B2 and 3 of Guidelines No. 3 (1971) is no longer considered even minimally adequate (cf. Guidelines No. 3, Revised 1976). The intricacies of EEG recording and interpretation problems are too numerous and too great to master in the 3 to 6 months provided in most specialty training programs; such training is intended rather to educate the specialist to understand EEG reports and to utilize the information intelligently in diagnosis.

EEG specialty training should be obtained in medical centers with specific training programs headed by electroencephalographers certified by the American Board of Qualification in Electroencephalography (ABQEEG). Even after a full year of training it is advisable to begin practice in association with a more experienced electroencephalographer. Such experience should include opportunity for frequent interaction in the laboratory. Criticism, argument, and other forms of mutual interaction make for growth and increasing breadth of knowledge. Experience in isolation may merely result in the consolidation of errors.

The minimum requirement cited in the 1971 Guidelines No. 3 of 1 full year of training plus 1 year of additional experience in EEG for the heads of teaching laboratories is also no longer considered adequate. The additional requirement of certification by ABQEEG for heads of teaching and other major laboratories should be considered mandatory.

QUALIFICATIONS OF EEG TECHNOLOGISTS AND TECHNICIANS

When Guidelines No. 3 was first published in 1971, the qualification for chief technologists was set at eligibility for taking Part II of the examinations of the American Board of Registration in EEG Technology (ABRET). The reason that the requirements were not set higher was that there was not then a sufficient number of Registered EEG Technologists (REEGTs) in the country to fill the available positions. A sufficient number of technologists have now been certified by ABRET so that it should soon no longer be necessary to compromise on this qualification. Certainly only REEGTs should be appointed chief technologists of large metropolitan hospitals and university medical centers. Only REEGTs should train student technicians under the supervision of a qualified electroencephalographer.

Among the requirements of the AMA Joint Committee for designation as an EEG technician is successful completion of a 6-month formal training course in EEG technology and for designation as an EEG technologist is the successful completion of 1 year of formal training. Opinion within the American Society of EEG Technologists and the American EEG Society has tended more and more toward considering less than 1 year of formal training inadequate, although this trend in attitude was not incorporated into Guidelines No. 3 (1976). It is predicted that 1 year of training will soon become the minimum. Two-year training programs are already coming into existence—1 year of general college level experience, preferably including courses in biology and related subjects, followed by 1 year of specific training in EEG technology, including both didactic courses and practicum experience in the EEG laboratory, leading to an Associate degree. The establishment of such training programs in schools of allied health professions in major universities is to be encouraged and promoted.

EQUIPMENT

Guidelines No. 3 recommends that "Equipment should meet the latest equipment standards of the American EEG Society or the International Federation of Societies for EEG and Clinical Neurophysiology" (IFSECN). The most recently published comprehensive statement on standards is the Report of the Committee on EEG Instrumentation Standards of IFSECN presented at the Ninth International Congress of EEG and Clinical Neurophysiology in 1977 (1).

TELEPHONE TRANSMISSION OF EEGs

A topic not dealt with in Guidelines No. 3 is telephonically transmitted EEG. A separate Guidelines (No. 5) dealing with this subject was published in 1976. Equipment standards for telephonic transmission are described in the IFSECN committee report (1). [See also (5), Chapter 17.]

Given that equipment adequate for the transmission of high quality EEGs is available,[1] the principal question is, under what circumstances should such equipment be used? Obviously, there is no point in telephonic transmission when a qualified electroencephalographer is available locally. Only when it is impossible to bring the patient to a fully staffed and equipped laboratory, or when the cost of doing so is prohibitive, is telephonic transmission justified. In evaluating

---

[1] An important addendum was appended to Guidelines No. 5 by the Council of the American EEG Society after the first 1,000 copies had been distributed: "At the present time, telephone transmission of EEG cannot be used for determination of electrocerebral silence in the diagnosis of brain death because of the inherent and unpredictable electrical noise present in telephone networks. Should technical advances permit this to occur, the American EEG Society will formally review its Guidelines at that time." See also (5).

what constitutes prohibitive costs, it must be noted that telephonically transmitted EEGs are much more expensive than ordinary EEGs. Two sets of recording equipment are required, one at each end of the telephone line, and both must be amortized;[2] recording paper cost is doubled; telephone transmission equipment must also be amortized; telephone line time must be paid for; and during the period of actual recording two qualified technicians are required with continuous two-way voice communication between them.

Thus the technical cost of a telephonically transmitted EEG is more than double that of a standard EEG. Consequently, unless the cost of bringing the patient to the primary EEG laboratory is significantly more than double the cost of a standard EEG or the patient is unmovable, telephonic transmission should not be considered. But how much more costly? A precise answer cannot be given to this question; one can only reply, a good deal more. However good the telephonically transmitted EEG may be, it can be no better than, and is as yet usually not as good as, an EEG recorded by standard procedures in the primary laboratory by a technician who is in direct communication with the interpreting electroencephalographer.

Guidelines No. 5 states, "Under no circumstances should the technologist at the transmitting laboratory be less qualified than one who works independently under a laboratory director who is based outside of a hospital. Indeed, the responsibilities falling upon the EEG technologist staffing a telephone transmitting laboratory are greater than those of a technologist working under relatively direct supervision in a hospital or office laboratory." In actual practice, however, the laboratory at the transmitting end is usually less adequate than the primary (or receiving) laboratory. It is likely to be in a remote location with a smaller (usually much smaller) recording load, and consequently almost always with a less experienced, and often part-time, technician. Recognition of important events (artifacts, seizures) is likely to be less prompt and less efficient.

The obvious conclusion of these considerations is that telephonically transmitted electroencephalography as an alternative to traditional methods is difficult to justify, save where population density is low and distances great. There are not many such places in the eastern half of the United States. They are undoubtedly more common in the West and Canada.

The development of networks of satellite laboratories, some or all of which are located within reasonable driving distance of established hospital and office laboratories, is a practice especially to be deplored.

Finally, in his presidential report on EEG telephone transmission to the Western EEG Society, Bennett (2) makes an important point. The electroencephalographer has an obligation to meet and interact with the physicians who refer patients to the sending laboratory on some regular basis, and not be "just a name sitting in an office 100 miles away." A hospital staff appointment at the sending site can be among the mechanisms for developing appropriate relationships.

REFERENCES

1. Barlow, J. S., Kamp, A., Morton, H. B., Ripoche, A., Shipton, H., and Tchavdarov, D. B. (1978): EEG instrumentation standards (revised 1977): Report of the Committee on EEG Instrumentation Standards of the International Federation of Societies for Electroencephalography and Clinical Neurophysiology. *Electroencephalogr. Clin. Neurophysiol.*, 45:144–150.

---

[2] If in order to save money full write-out capacity is not provided at both sending and receiving ends with technicians following the recording as it unfolds at both ends, efficiency is greatly decreased and the adequacy of the recording tends to fall below acceptable standards. However, with further technical improvements the recommendation for full write-out capacity at both ends of the line may be modified (see Guidelines No. 5, section 3).

2. Bennett, D. R. (1976): Presidential report on EEG telephone transmission. Western EEG Society. Unpublished.
3. Chatrian, G. E., Chastain, J., Martin, M. J., Henry, C. E., and Knott, J. R. (1974): Recommended job descriptions for electroencephalographic technologists. *American EEG Society Guidelines in EEG,* No. 4.
4. Ellingson, R. J., Walter, R. D., Knott, J. R., Henry, C. E., Klass, D. W., and Saunders, M. G. (1971); and Mattson, R. H., Tharp, B. R., Prichard, J. W., and Klass, D. W. (Revised 1976): Standards of practice in clinical electroencephalography. *American EEG Sociey Guidelines in EEG,* No. 3.
5. Frost, J. D., Jr., and Barlow, J. S. (1976): Telephone transmission of EEGs—practical aspects. *Handbook Electroencephalogr. Clin. Neurophysiol.,* 3B:20–23.
6. Saunders, M. G., Hughes, J. R., Klass, D. W., Maulsby, R. L., and Reiher, J. (1971): Minimum technical requirements for performing clinical electroencephalography. *American EEG Society Guidelines in EEG,* No. 2.
7. Silverman, D., Masland, R. L., Saunders, M. G., Schwab, R. S., and Henry, C. E. (1971): Minimal technical standards for EEG recording in suspected cerebral death. *American EEG Society Guidelines in EEG,* No. 1.
8. Wilder, B. J., Bennett, D. R., Seaba, P. J., Barlow, J. S., Everts, W. H., Brittenham, D. M., Rodin, E. A., Martin, M. J., Lettich, H., Henry, C. E., Billinger, T. W., and Knott, J. R. (1976): Provisional recommendations for telephone transmission of EEGs. *American EEG Society Guidelines in EEG,* No. 5.

Chapter 2

Minimum Technical Requirements for Performing Clinical Electroencephalography: Illustrative Examples of Principles on Which Some of the Technical Guidelines of the American EEG Society Are Based

Michael G. Saunders*

Formerly, Section of Electroencephalography; Department of Physiology and Computer Department, Faculty of Medicine, University of Manitoba, Winnipeg, Canada

These comments and examples were originally based on "Minimum Technical Requirements for Performing Clinical Electroencephalography," Guidelines #2 of the American Electroencephalographic Society, and they have been modified to conform to the 1976 revision of the *Guidelines* reprinted as the Appendix in this volume.

1.1[1] Sixteen channels of simultaneous recording of the electroencephalogram (EEG) are encouraged. In no event should less than 8 channels be used.

In Fig. 1 (A,B,C, and D) the abnormalities in C4, P4, O2, T4 and T6 areas are not all recorded simultaneously but separately in different time sequence. It is difficult to be certain of the distribution

---

* Deceased April 4, 1975. This material was posthumously assembled and edited by John R. Knott, Ph.D. to bring the text into conformation with the 1976 revision of the original *Guidelines*.

[1] All numbered paragraph designations in this chapter refer to that section of AEEGS Guidelines which has the same title as this chapter. *(See Appendix.)*

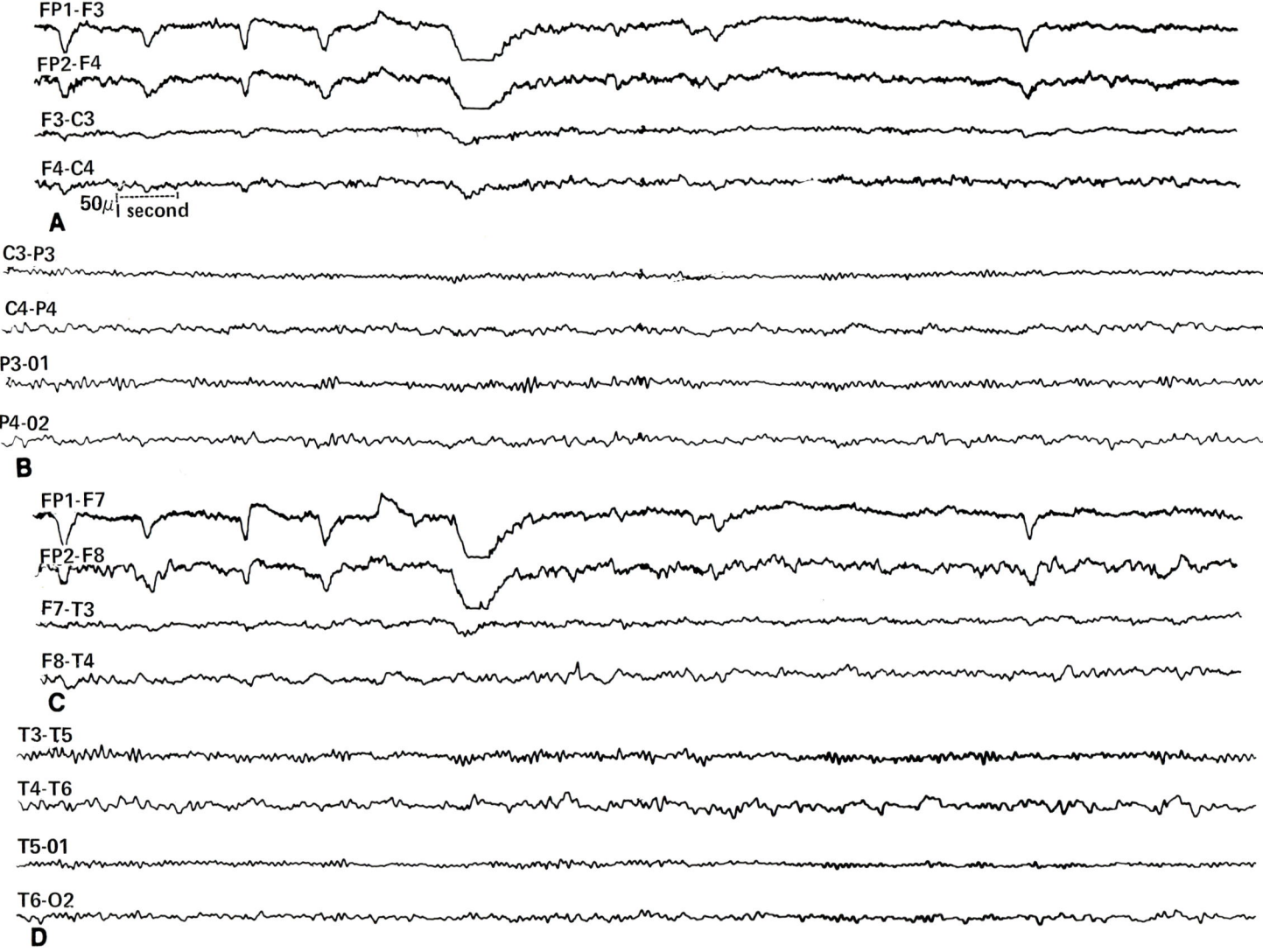

of the EEG abnormality over the head from these four separate 4-channel records.

In Fig. 2 (A and B) with 8 channels of recording, the left and right parasagittal EEG activity can be easily compared. Similarly temporal lobe activity can be seen. In this record the distribution of the abnormality in the right central, parietal, and temporal areas is quite obvious.

In Fig. 3 with 16 channels of simultaneous recording, the distribution of the EEG abnormality in the areas supplied by the right middle cerebral artery is obvious. Other montages can make this pattern of distribution even more obvious.

2.1 The full 21 electrodes and placements recommended by the International Federation of Societies for EEG and Clinical Neurophysiology should be used (except in premature infants with small heads). These placements include: frontal-polar, frontal, central, parietal, and occipital areas, the inferior frontal or anterior temporal area, the middle and posterior temporal areas, the auricular (ear) or mastoid region (all bilaterally), and midline regions in the frontal, central (vertex), and parietal area. Except in intensive care units where other electrical equipment is attached to the patient, a grounding electrode should be added but not connected to any other electrode.

Figure 4 shows the electrodes of the International 10–20 System. With less than the 21 electrodes, areas of cortex will not be covered. It is important ". . . to insure that EEG activity having a small area of representation on the scalp is recorded, and to analyze accurately the distribution of more diffuse activity. Occasionally, additional electrodes placed between those representing the standard placements are needed in order to record very localized activity" *(Appendix).* The 10–20 System is becoming the standard throughout the world. It is simple, logical, and based on definable anatomical landmarks. Other electrode placement positions such as those described by Gibbs are still in common use, particularly in the United States. Some of these are imprecise and not based on measurement from well-defined anatomical landmarks.

2.2 Interelectrode impedances should be checked as a routine prerecording procedure. Ordinarily, electrode impedance should not exceed 5 k Ω.

In Fig. 5, a diminution of alpha activity is seen in the right posterior temporal and occipital areas. Low amplitude delta activity is present. The cause of this local abnormality requires more analysis. In this case neither electrode T6 nor electrode O2 was connected to the inputs of the EEG. The patterns recorded were from the C_z reference and the ground electrode. This mistake would be noted immediately on checking electrode resistances.

3.1 Both scalp-to-scalp (bipolar) and referential montages should be used.

In Fig. 6, the four different montages were recorded simultaneously on a 16-channel instrument. The activity of each of the scalp electrodes was identical for that area. The use of bipolar or different reference montages modifies the recorded patterns markedly. Each type of montage has its specific advantages and disadvantages. Each should be used to get the maximum amount of information from the EEG.

FIG. 1. Four channel bipolar recording of parasagittal **(A,B)** and temporal **(C,D)** chains, recorded at different times. It is necessary to mentally synthesize these separate data to localize.

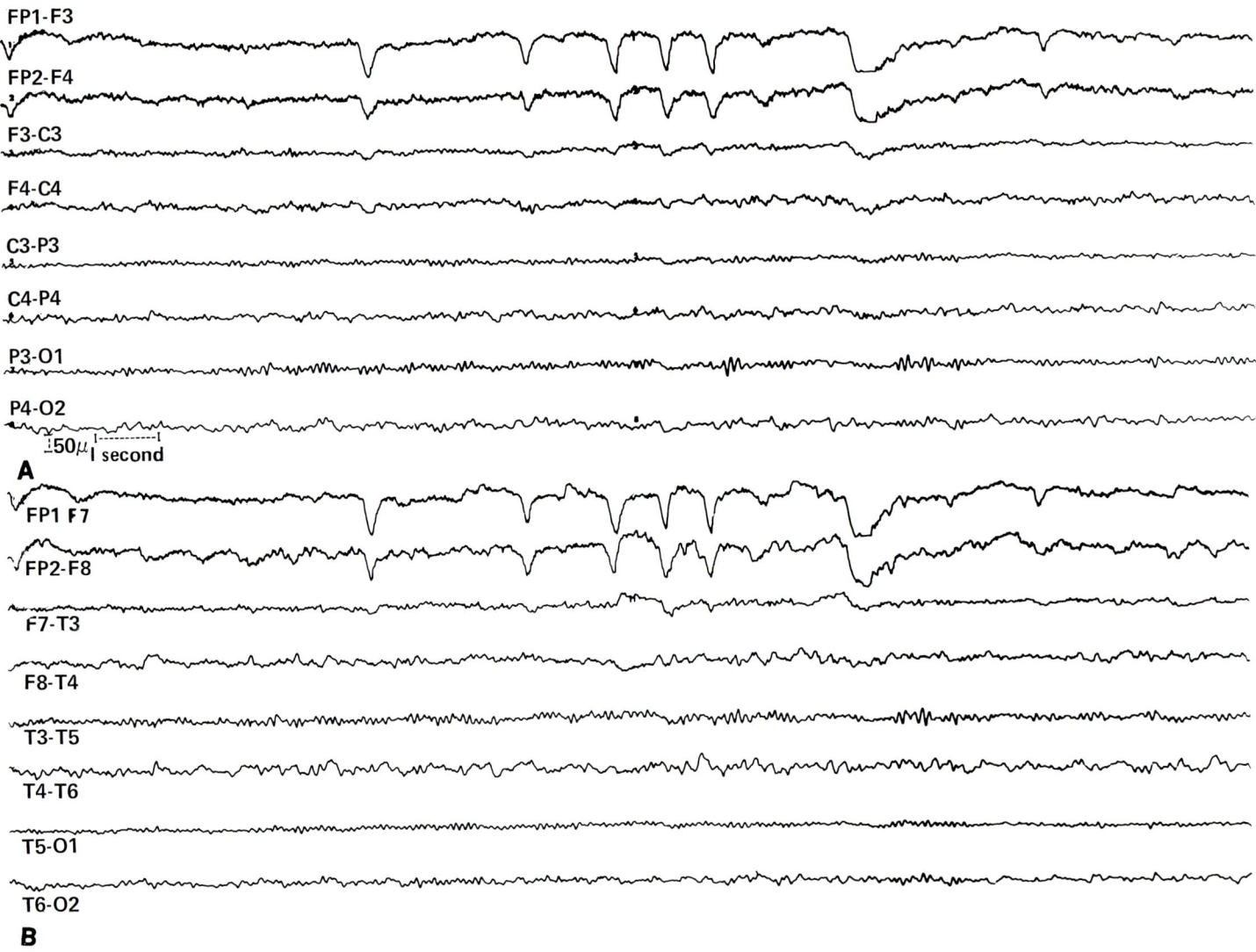

FIG. 2. Eight channel recording, similar to Fig. 1. Synthesis still necessary.

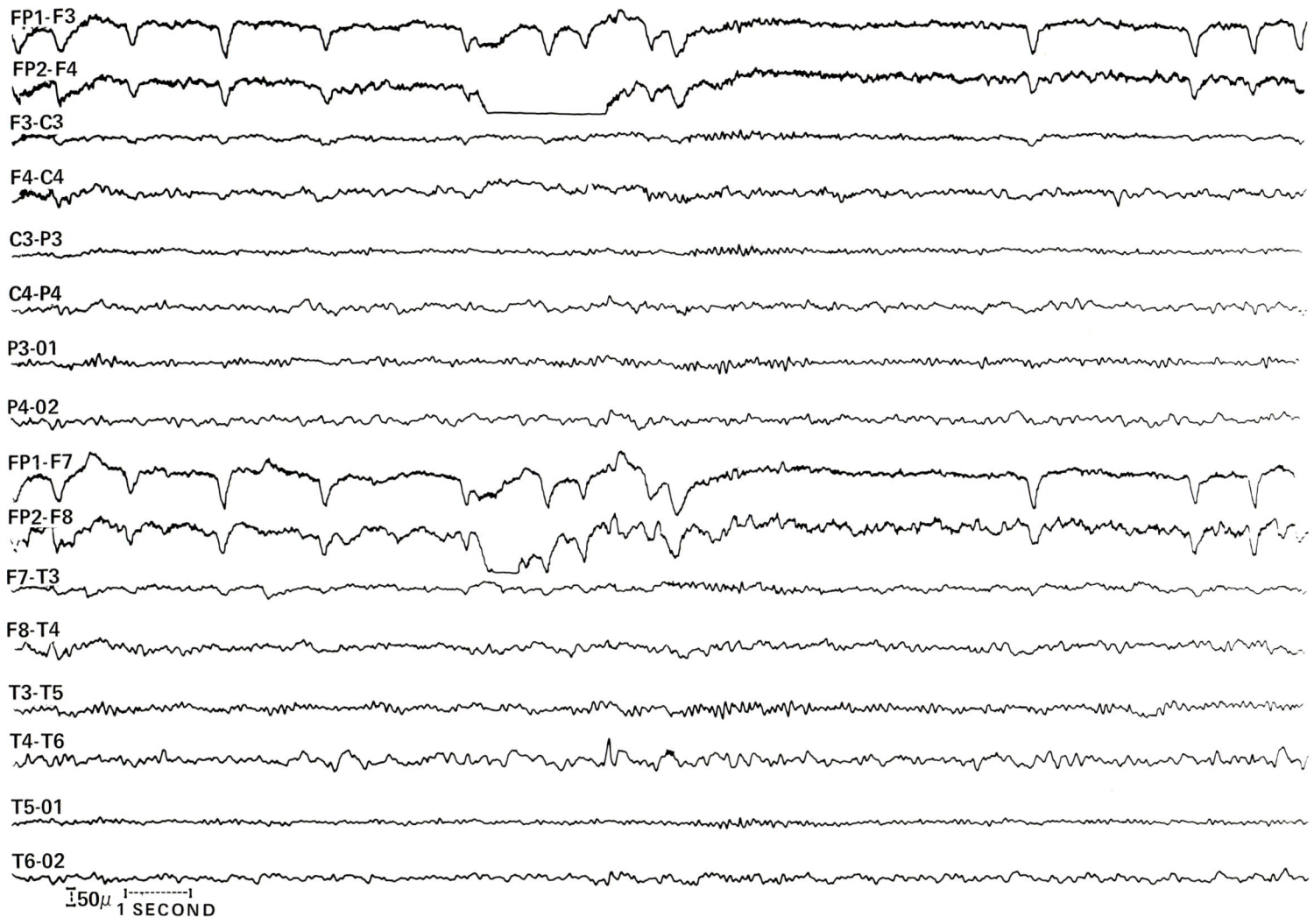

FIG. 3. Sixteen channel recording. Simultaneous view of EEG activity of all channels.

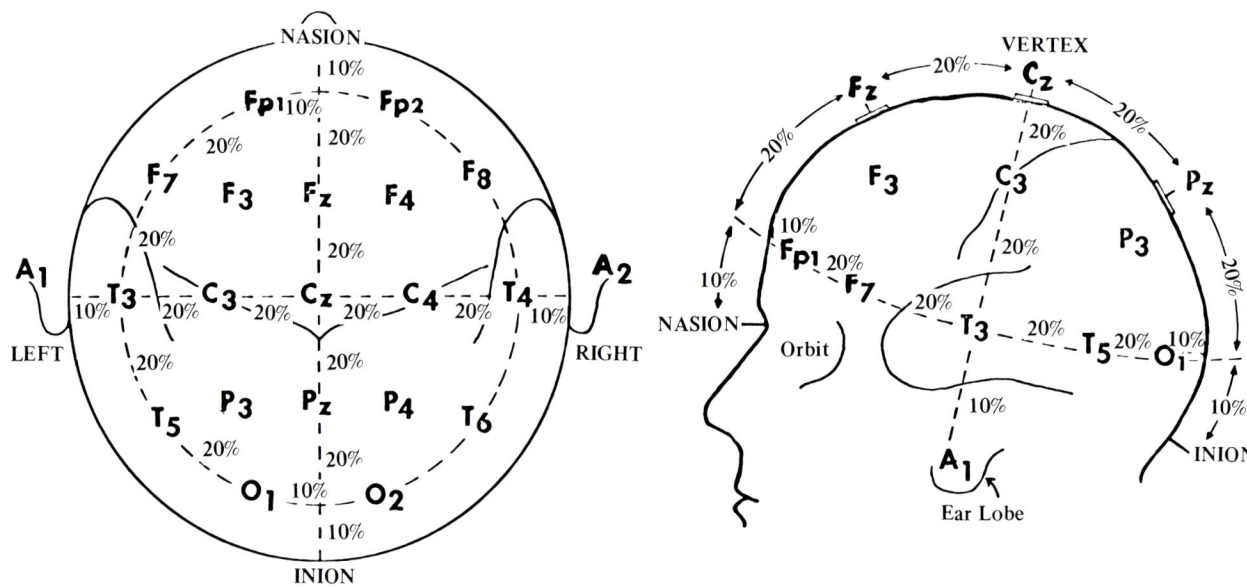

FIG. 4. The "ten-twenty" electrode placements. Note that circumferential spacing is based on hemicircumference.

3.2 The electrode connections for each channel should be clearly indicated at the beginning of each montage.

Without any identification, it is impossible to analyze the strip of EEG in Fig. 7. Are the signal marks photic stimulation? If so, then channels 12 to 15 are probably recording from the occiput. But why the subtle differences between channels 12, 13 and 14, 15, and which other regions of the head are included?

3.4 The patterns of electrode connections or montages should be made as simple as possible. They should run in lines, and the interelectrode distances should be kept equal.

Montages of the type shown on the left of Fig. 8 have been used routinely in some EEG laboratories. Most of the interelectrode distances are equal—but sorting out which activity comes from where is very difficult.

The referential montage on the right is much simpler. The frontal activity is at the top of the EEG record, central and temporal in the middle, and posterior activity at the bottom. However, the interelectrode distances for the parasagittal electrodes are much greater than for the temporal electrodes. Allowance for differences in amplitude caused by this have to be made, although voltages can be computed. An anteroposterior scalp-to-scalp montage such as Fp2-F4-

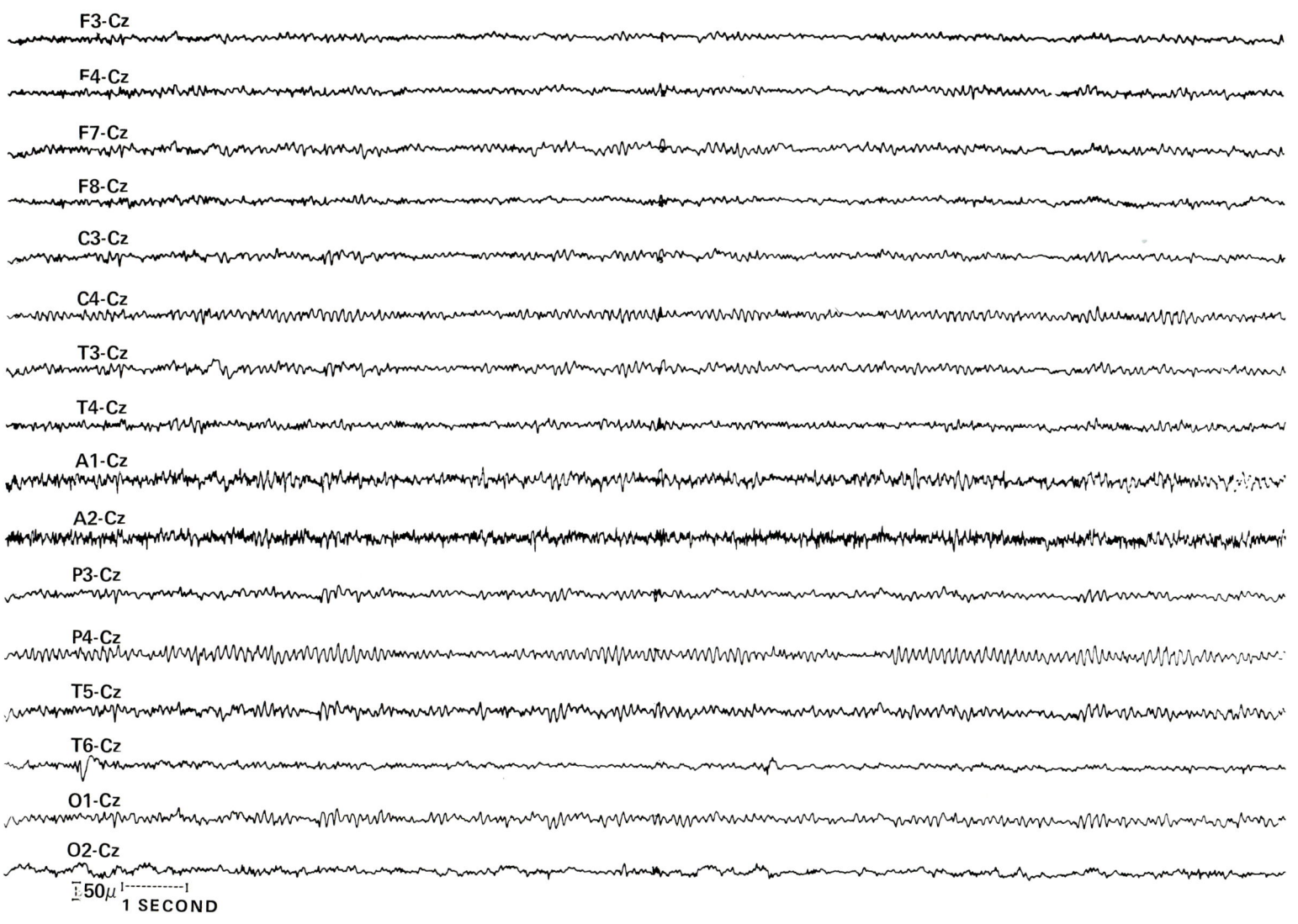

FIG. 5. Impedances of channels 4, 14, and 16 are exceedingly high and produce artificial amplitude asymmetries.

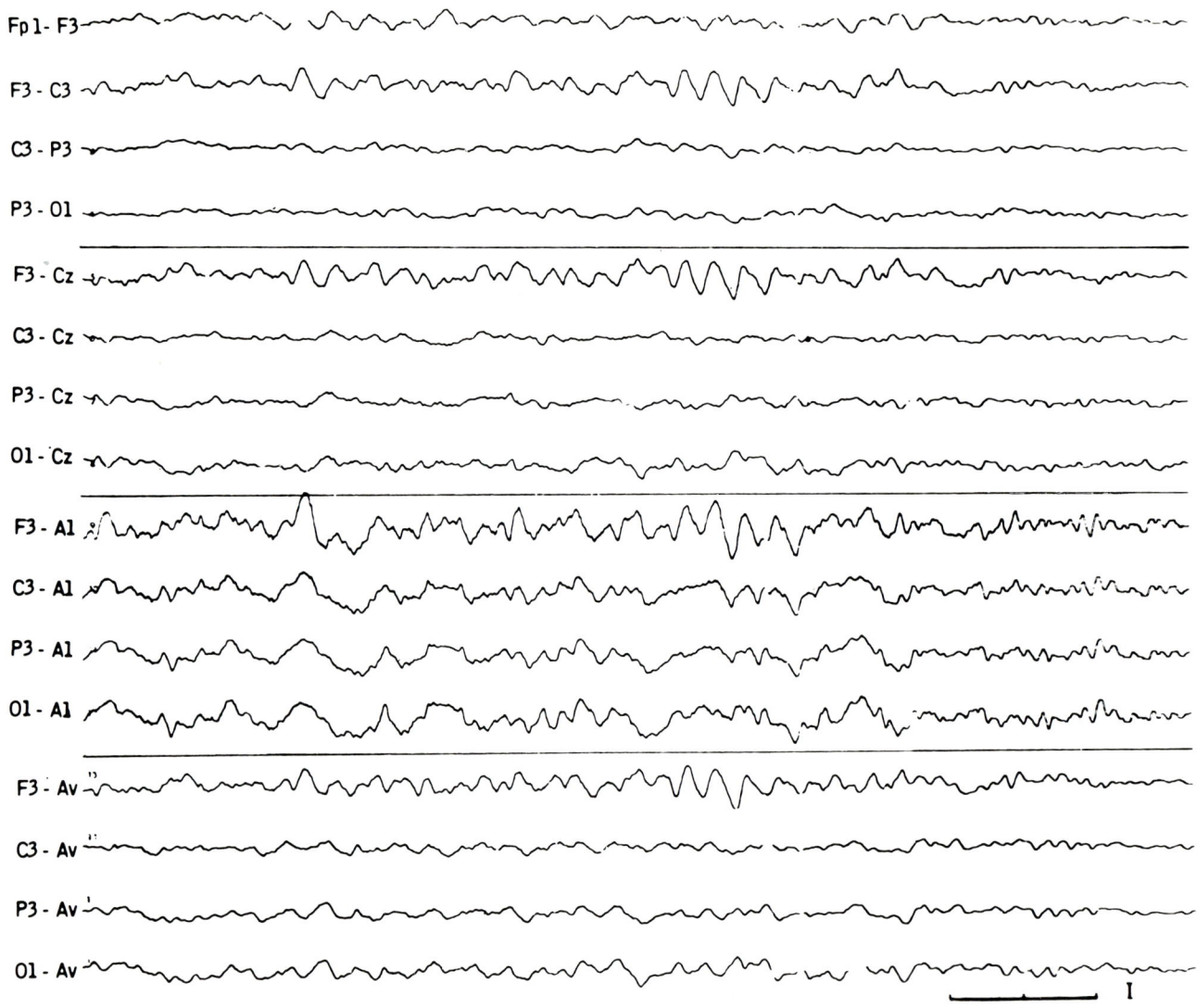

FIG. 6. Comparison of bipolar and three different referential montages, all sampling the same areas. Not all references are "equal."

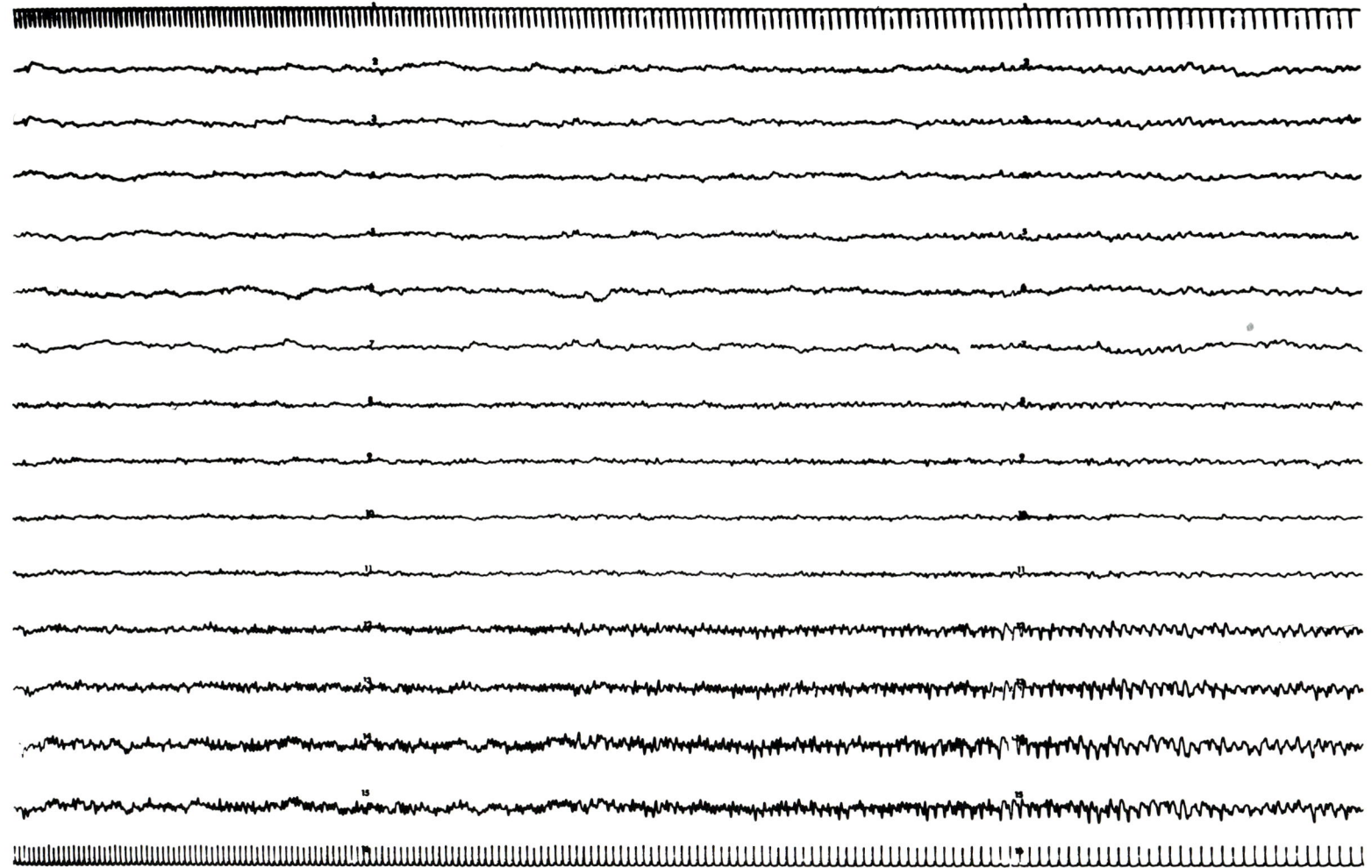

FIG. 7. Failure to label derivations renders this illustration useless.

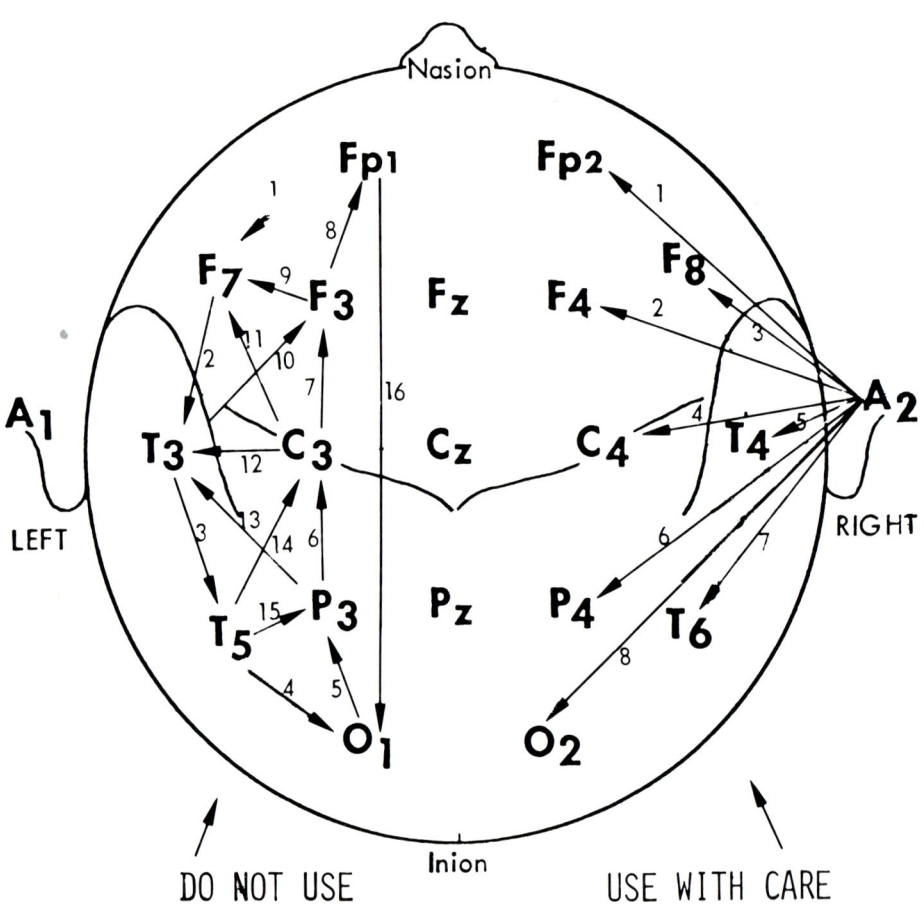

FIG. 8. Useless vs useful montages *(see text)*.

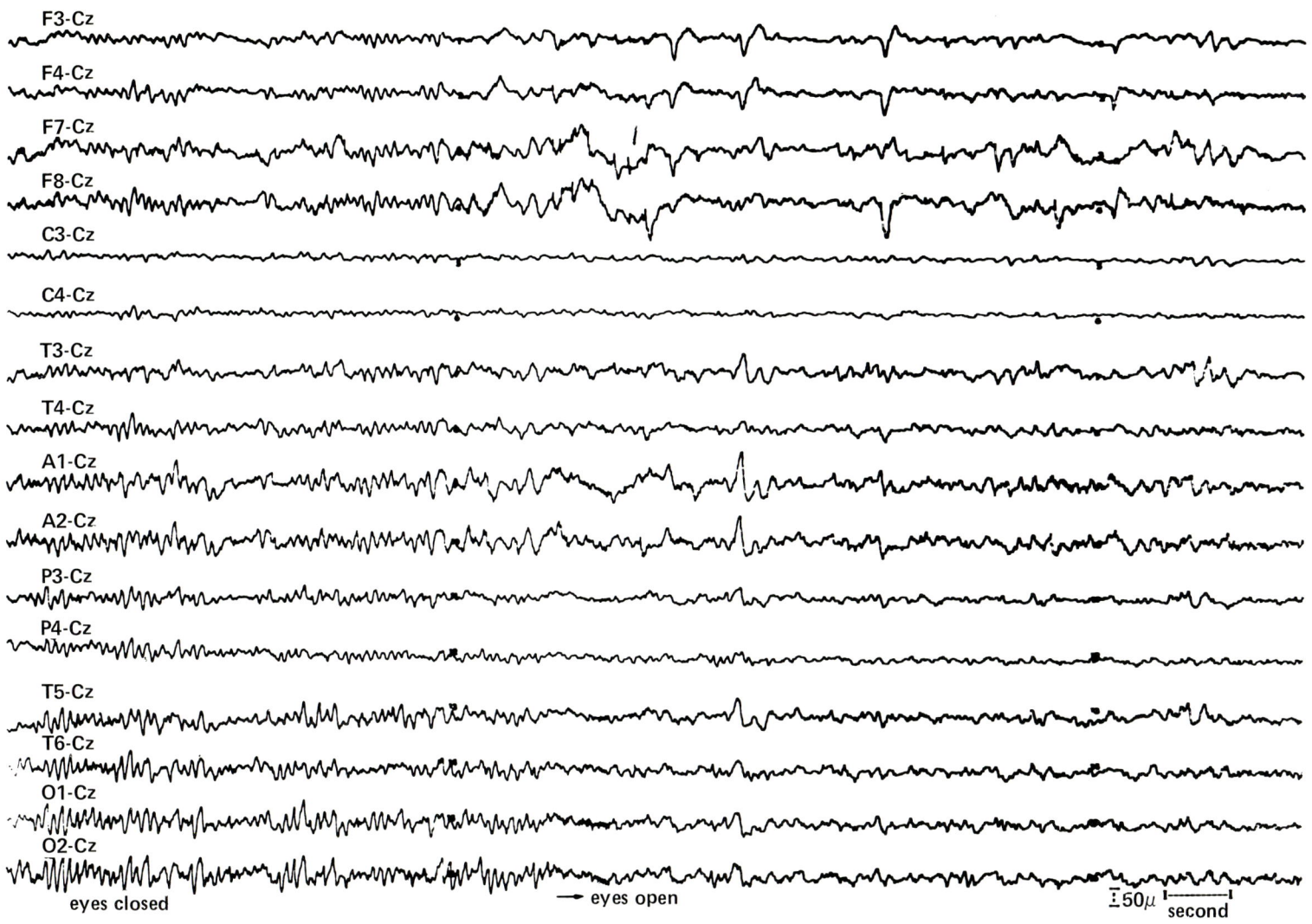

FIG. 9. Example of test of reactivity of EEG to eye-opening, a simple form of stimulation.

C4-P4-O1 uses equal interelectrode spacing; so would Fp2-F8-T4-T6-O2.

4.1 The recording should include periods when the eyes are open and when they are closed.

Patterns hidden by alpha activity appear with the eyes open, and there is blocking of theta activity (Fig. 9). These findings are of significance in interpreting the record and they would be lost without recording during both eye-open and eye-closed periods.

5.1 Calibration should be recorded at the beginning and end of every EEG recording. At the outset, all channels should be adjusted to respond equally and correctly to the calibration signal.

Aligning the pens (Fig. 10) is too often neglected. Even use of lined paper can lead one into a false assumption of alignment sometimes. Remember also the effects of the high and low frequency filters on the calibration signal. One can learn much about a technologist and laboratory by examining the calibration signals on routine records.

5.2 When instrument settings (sensitivities, frequency filters, paper speed) are changed during the recording, the settings should be clearly identified on the record at the time of change. The final calibration(s) should include *each* sensitivity and filter setting used in the recording and should include calibration voltages appropriate to the sensitivities used.

In Fig. 11 three different records use the same montage and are from the same patient. They could be interpreted quite differently. The paper speeds are 15, 30, and 60 mm/sec, but this has not been marked. When paper speed is known, frequency of EEG activity can be determined. Thus, all three records would be similarly interpreted.

5.3 The sensitivity of the EEG equipment for routine recording should be in the range of 5 to 10 μV/mm of pen deflection.

In Fig. 12 sensitivity is set at 10 μV/mm. Low amplitude slow activity in C4-P4, F8-T4, and T4-T6 suggests the probability of abnormality in these areas. Failure to increase sensitivity leads to an unnecessary degree of uncertainty in the interpretation.

In Fig. 13 sensitivity is now set at 7 μV/mm. The distribution of abnormality in the central, temporal, and parietal areas is now much more evident, and the information is more readily demonstrated.

In Fig. 14 sensitivity is set at 5 μV/mm. The distribution of the abnormalities is obvious; one can have little uncertainty about its presence and particularly about the distribution over the area supplied by the middle cerebral artery.

5.5 Except for specific and identifiable reasons, recording of the lower frequencies should be such that 1-Hz activity is not attenuated by more than 30% of the activity in the alpha range (8 to 13 Hz). Recording of the higher frequencies should be such that 50-Hz activity is not attenuated by more than 30% of the activity in the alpha range.

FIG. 10. Use of calibration signals. At vertical line, channel 7 is misaligned and needs correcting. Last 4 signals show inequality of sensitivity controls (channels 1 through 3), of high frequency filters and 60-Hz filter (channels 4 through 6) and of low frequency filters (time constants) (channels 7, 8, and 9). Remaining channels show "standard" sensitivity, high frequency, and low frequency controls.

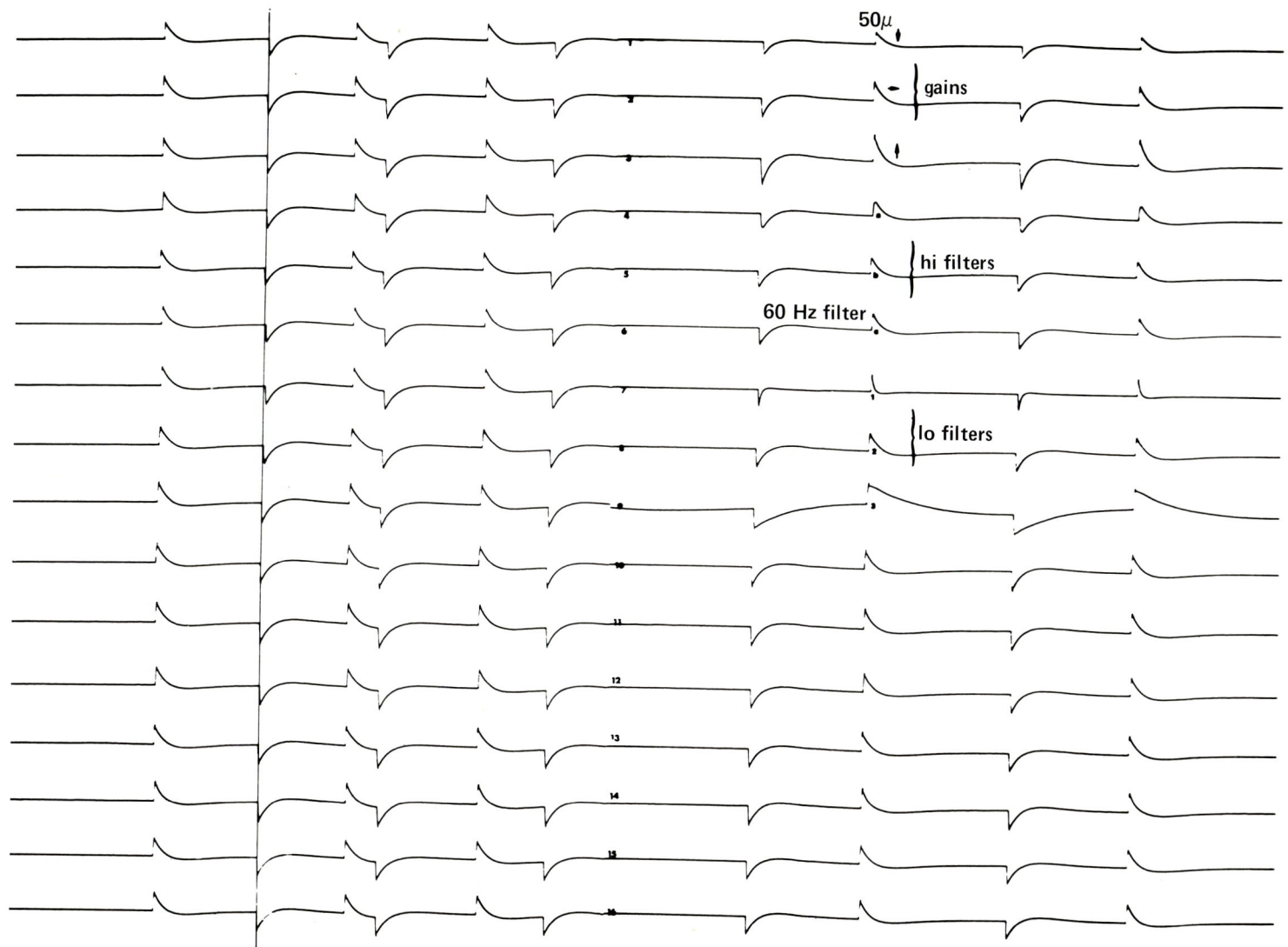

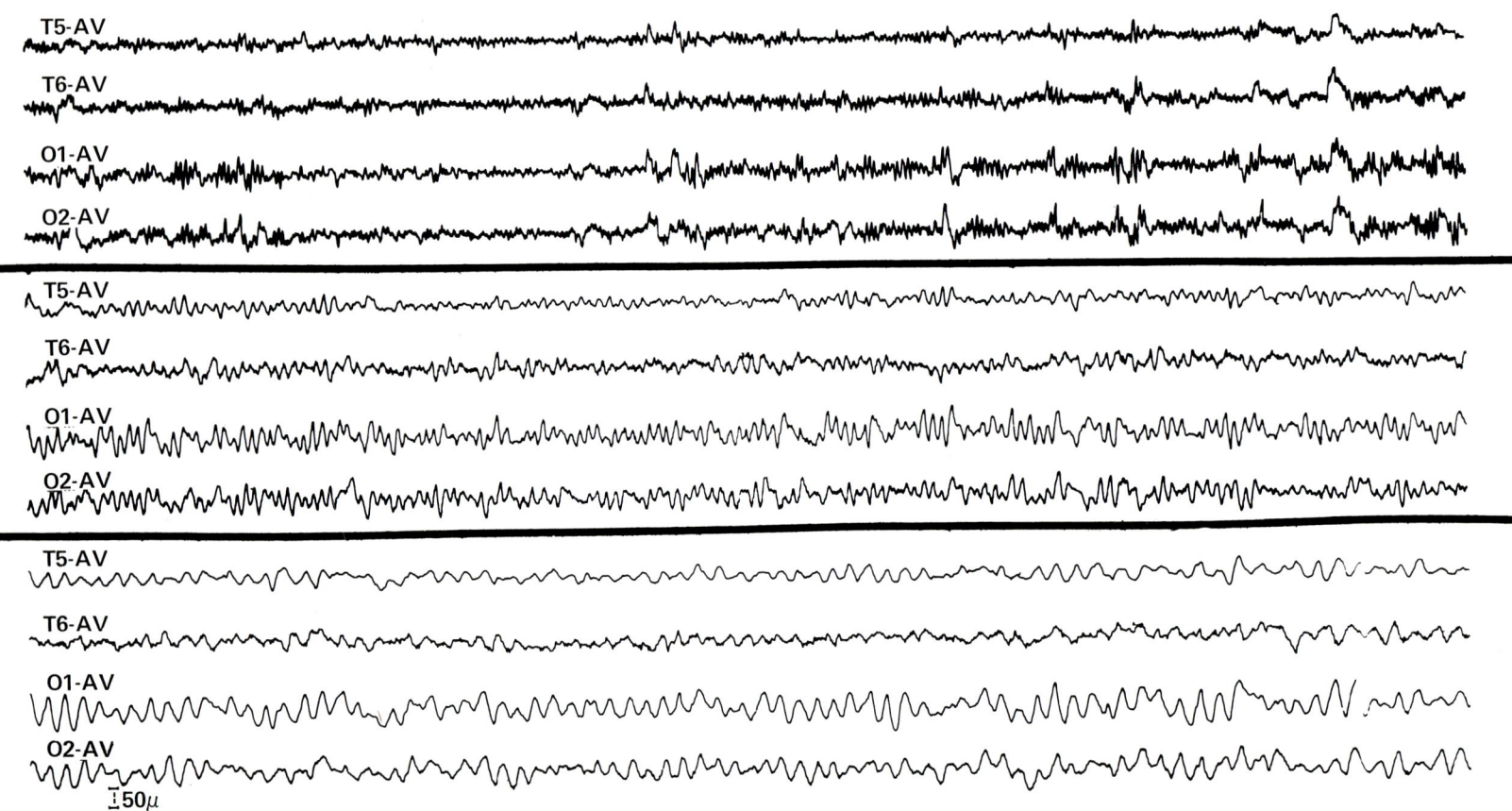

FIG. 11. Three samples of EEG from the same patient. Paper speed has varied.

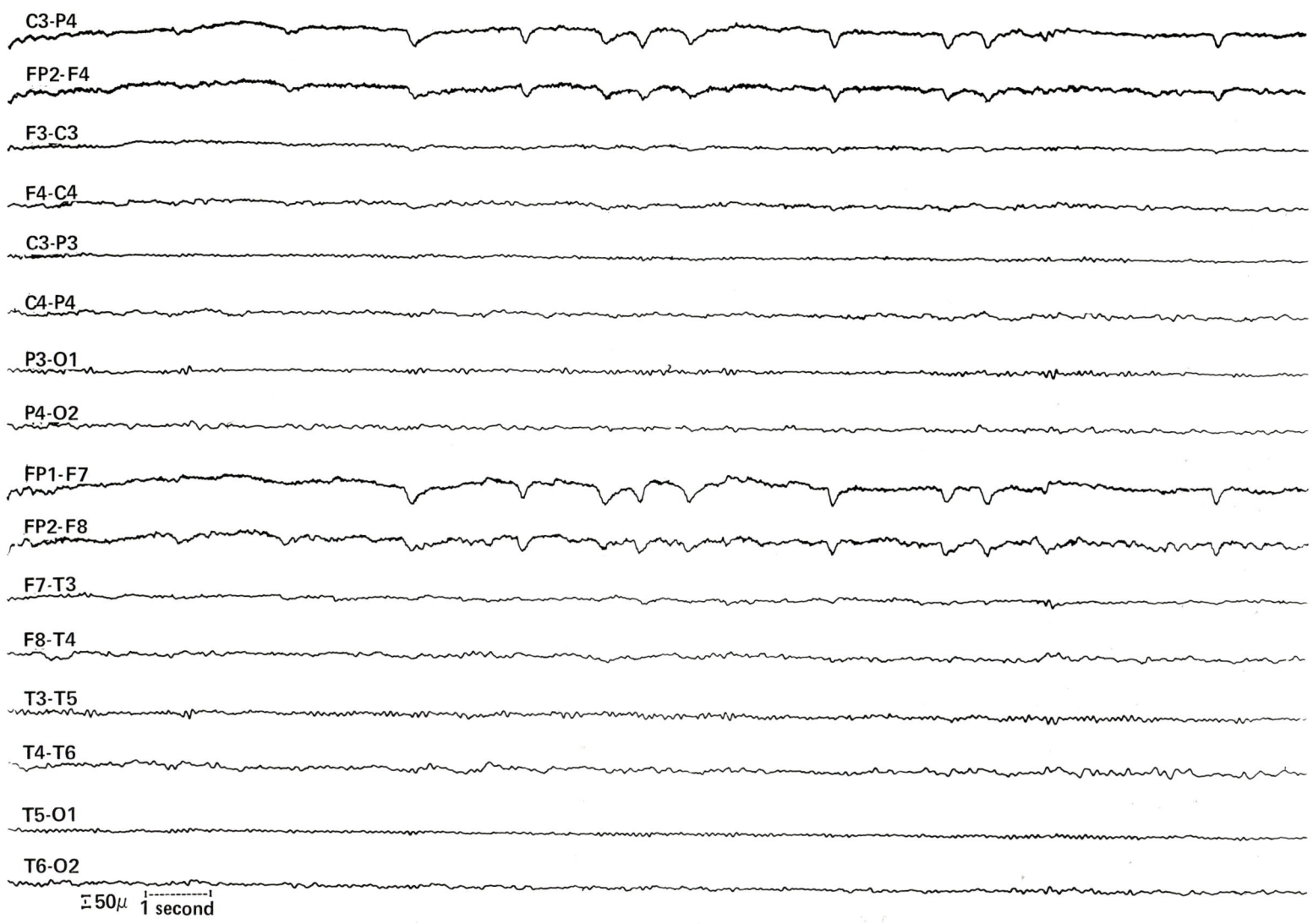

FIG. 12. EEG recorded with sensitivity set at a low value *(see text)*.

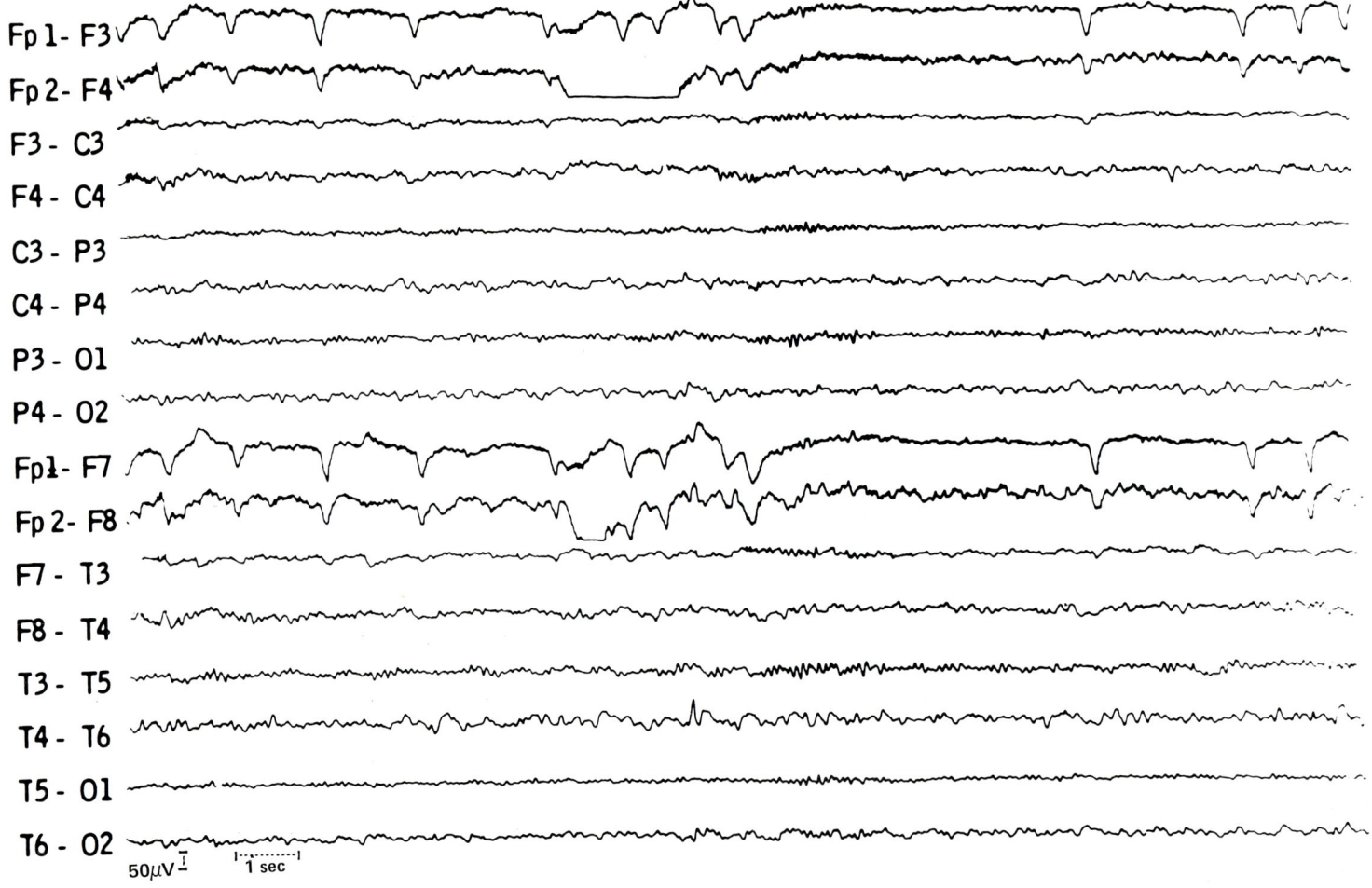

FIG. 13. Increased sensitivity improves perception of abnormality.

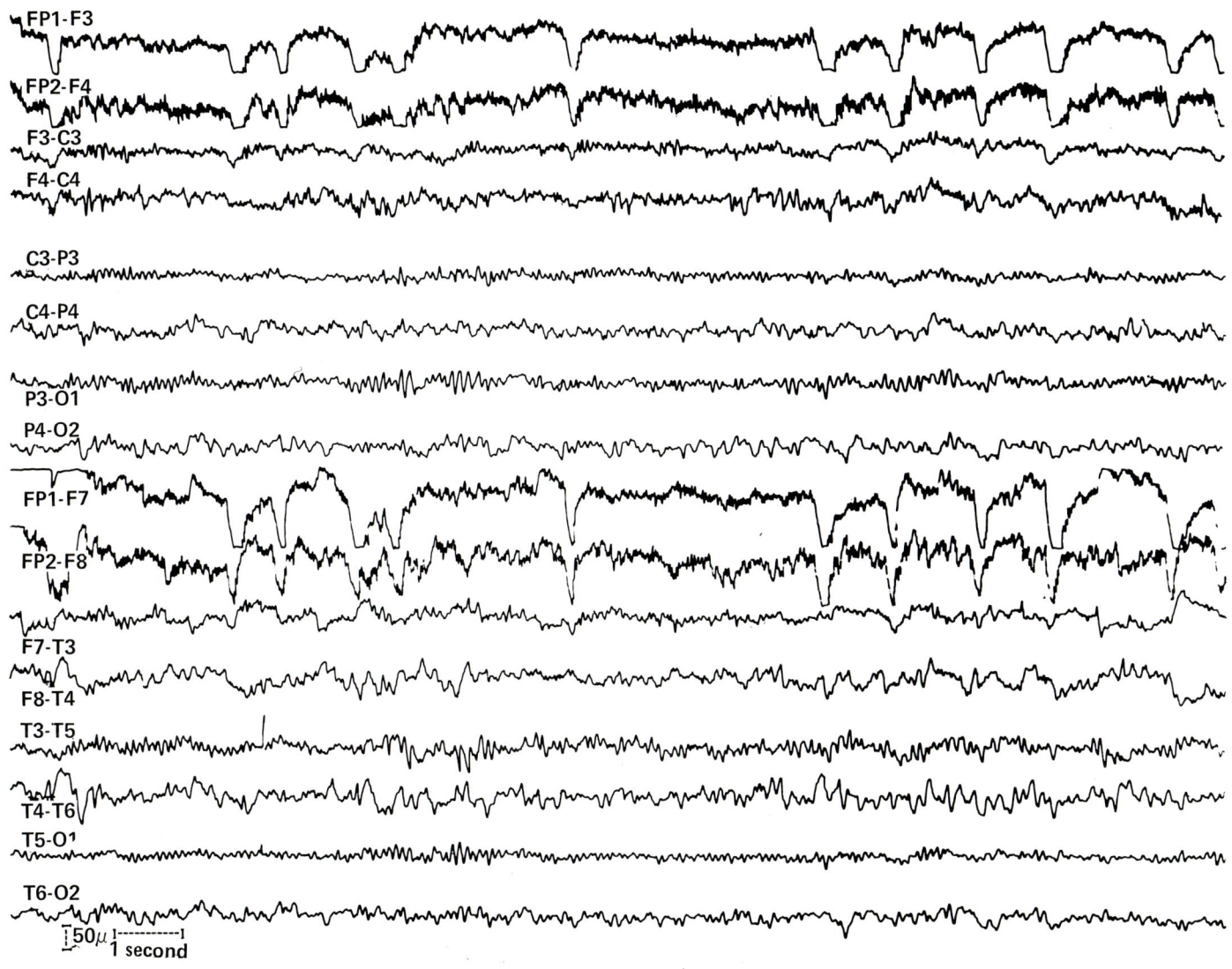

FIG. 14. Further increase of sensitivity in the initially low voltage record of Fig. 12 yields more information *(see text)*.

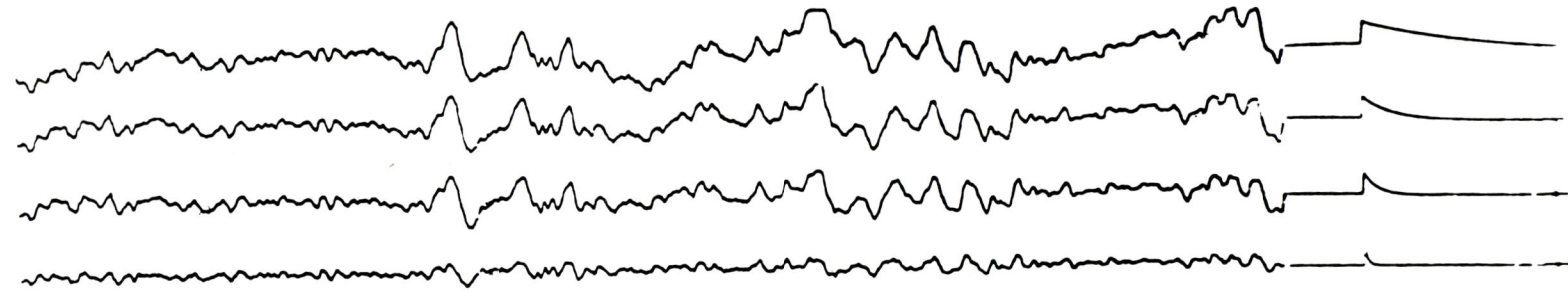

FIG. 15. Effect of different low frequency filters (time constants) on identical inputs.

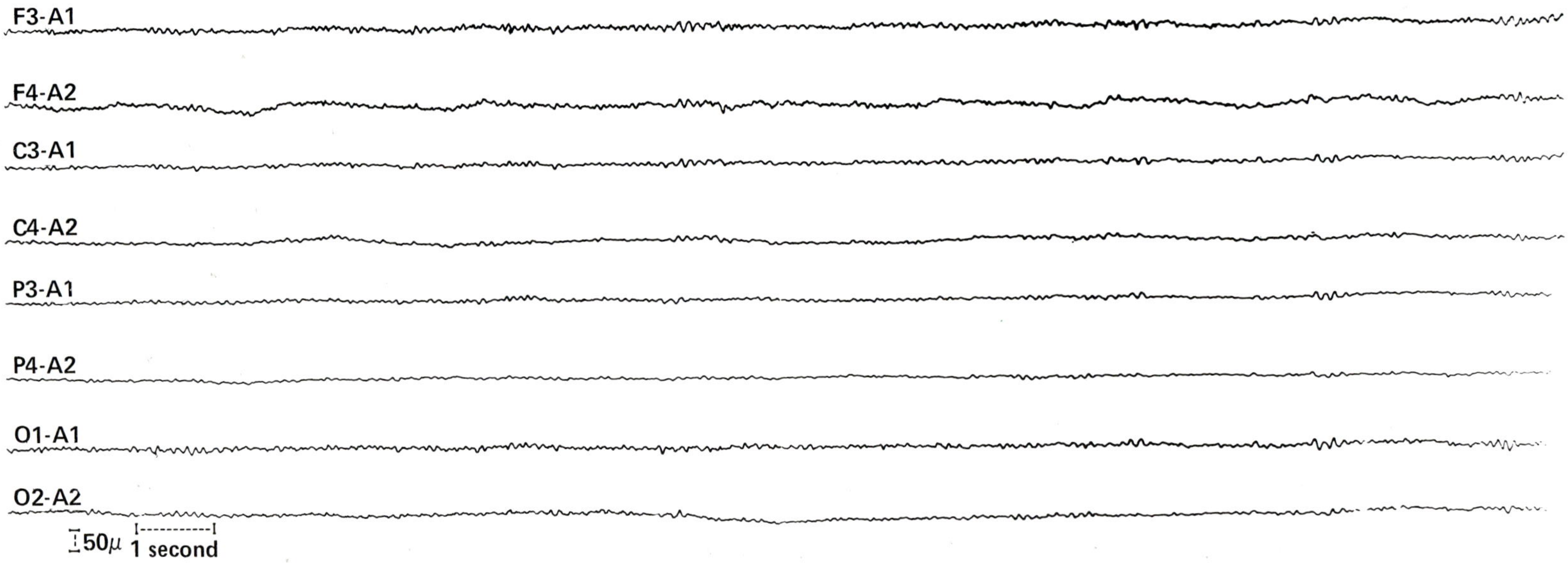

FIG. 16. Failure to note changes in state of the patient can lead to misinterpretation *(see text)*.

Fig. 15 shows a recording from C_3-A_1 during sleep at four different time constants—1.0, 0.3, 0.16, and 0.03 sec from above down. There is very marked attenuation of the delta activity at the shortest time constant. For most clinical work it is justifiable to use a time constant of 0.3 sec.

8.1 The state of the patient—awake, drowsy, sleeping, or comatose—and any change thereof should be noted by the technologist on the EEG recording. Any commands or signals to the patient and any movement or clinical seizure activity or absence thereof should also be listed on the record.

The record in Fig. 16 is from a patient in a complete unrousable coma shortly before death. It is *not* from a normal patient with eyes closed. Observations on patient status by the technologist are of the greatest importance.

9.1 Needle electrodes are not recommended for use under ordinary laboratory conditions. They should only be used when completely sterilized and when the technologist who employs them has been taught the exact techniques as well as the disadvantages and hazards of their use. Anteroposterior alignment of the needles is important, and misalignment may cause amplitude asymmetries or distortions.

When using needle electrodes the following points must be remembered:

1. Needles carry infection—certainly of hepatitis and possibly of syphilis. It is essential to fully sterilize the needles to kill hepatitis virus.
2. Inserting needle electrodes can be very painful. All interpreters should have the most incompetent technologist in the department insert 17 or more needles in them and then have an EEG recorded.
3. Needle electrodes may be thought easy to put in, but they fall out easily, too. It is easy to miss an artifactual asymmetry that may occur. Such asymmetry has recently been shown to occur if pairs of needles are not parallel with the points in the same direction.
4. Because needle electrodes are thought to be so easy to use, they are the most likely to lead to poor recordings.

ACKNOWLEDGMENT

The editors are grateful to Shirley Oliver, R. EEG T., Supervisory Technologist, Electroencephalograph Department, Health Sciences Center, Winnipeg, Canada, for providing the prints for the illustrations used in this chapter.

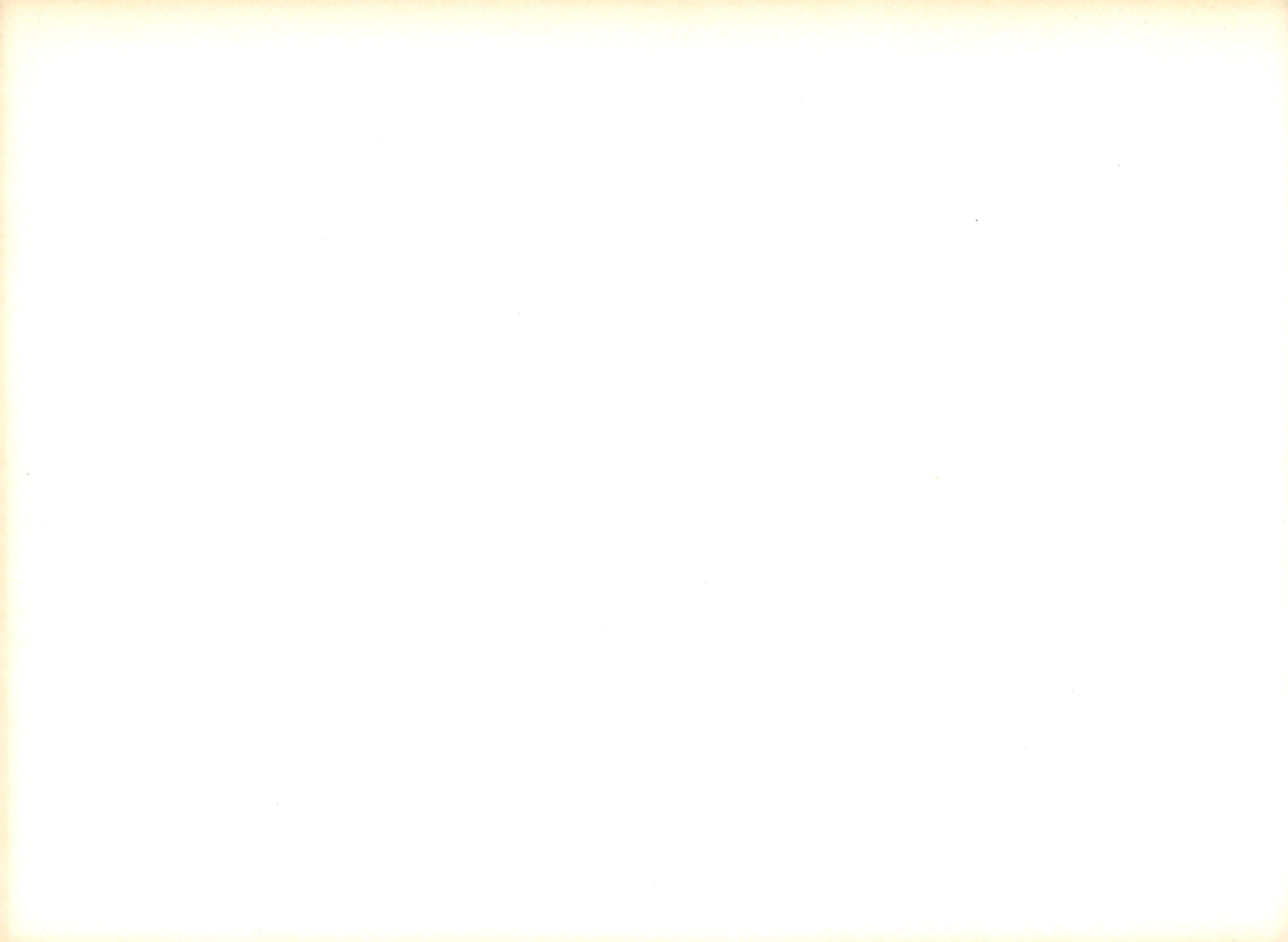

Chapter 3

Basis for Visual Analysis: Polarity Convention, Principles of Localization, and Electrical Fields

Robert L. Maulsby

Department of Neurology, Wayne State University School of Medicine, and Harper Hospital EEG Laboratory, Detroit, Michigan 48201

Polarity Convention 28
Electrical Fields 28
    Methods of Recording Electrical Fields 29
        Referential Method 29
        Differential Method 30
    Constructing Electrical Fields 31
    Localization of Electrical Fields 32
Summary and Practical Problem 35
References 36

EEG interpretation involves recognition of voltage, frequency, wave form, temporal pattern, polarity, and localization of the electrical events recorded from the scalp. Of these, polarity and localization present the most difficult challenge to the student. In spite of the difficulties, it is very important to appreciate these parameters since the distinction between an abnormal and a normal event often rests upon them. For example, a sharp, pointed wave in the occipital region during sleep may be normal or abnormal, depending upon polarity (positive sharp waves here are normal). Or a sharp negative transient recurring in the rolandic region on one side during sleep would be abnormal, but if located near the vertex, may be normal.

POLARITY CONVENTION

The process of determining polarity and localization proceeds as a single mental operation during visual analysis since some idea or inference of location is necessary in order to determine polarity and vice versa, but it is convenient to begin with a discussion of polarity per se, considering first how the EEG instrument responds to polarity of input. For a more detailed discussion of polarity, the reader is referred to articles by Knott (1) and MacGillivray (2).

Figure 1 illustrates the convention by which differential amplifiers used in EEG instruments respond to input signals. The two input leads of the EEG amplifier are termed lead 1 and lead 2 or grid 1 and grid 2. By convention, when lead 1 is more negative than lead 2, the EEG pen will deflect upward as illustrated in the top center of Fig. 1. From this convention, the other logical possibilities follow: when lead 1 becomes positive with respect to lead 2, the pen goes down; negativity in lead 2 drives the pen down; positivity in lead 2 causes an upward deflection; identical polarity in both leads produces no deflection. Using chain-linked amplifiers, as illustrated in the right side of Fig. 1, is a common practice in EEG. Polarity of the common lead between two amplifiers is then quickly appreciated by pen deflections: when the pens move towards each other, the common lead is negative with respect to the other two inputs; and, similarly, diverging pens signal positivity at the common input.

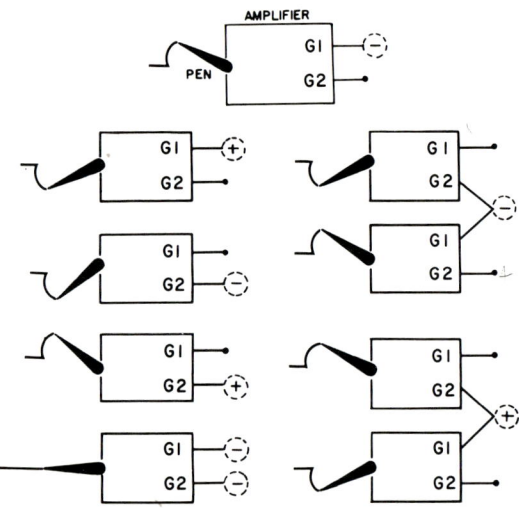

FIG. 1. EEG amplifier polarity convention. Amplifiers are represented by boxes with recording pens on the left and inputs on the right labeled G1 (grid 1) and G2 (grid 2). See text for explanation.

ELECTRICAL FIELDS

Unfortunately, the electrical events on the scalp do not usually resemble little spots of positivity or negativity as illustrated above. Instead, most EEG waves (normal or abnormal) occupy wide areas on the scalp which may affect the input leads of several amplifiers simultaneously. A priori knowledge of the typical spread or field of the electrical event helps the interpreter determine its source. Indeed, any EEG wave that does not produce a typical electrical field on the scalp suggests artifact.

Localized EEG waves may be thought of as arising from electrical

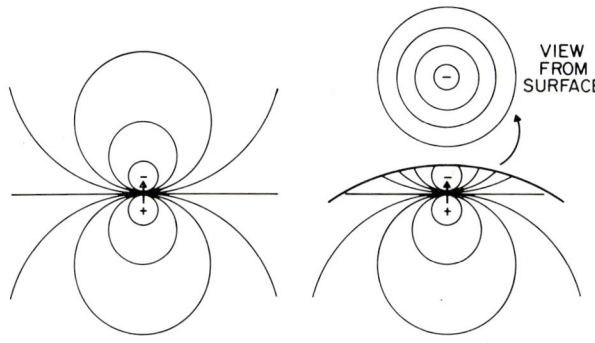

FIG. 2. Potential distribution around hypothetical dipoles located in an infinite conductor or near the surface of a spherical conductor. The circular lines surrounding positive and negative ends of the dipole represent isopotential lines.

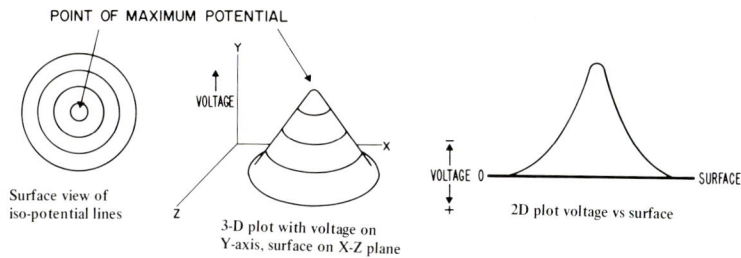

FIG. 3. Several ways of graphically representing electrical fields on a surface. Isopotential contour lines *(left)*, three-dimensional plot with voltage on Y-axis, surface on X-Z plane *(center)*, or a two-dimensional plot of voltage along a line on the surface *(right)* are more commonly used in EEG literature.

dipoles (or sheets of dipoles) within the cortex (3–5). Although this is a gross oversimplification of the underlying neurophysiological events (see chapter 15 by Goldensohn), it is a useful concept for analyzing the EEG on the scalp.

Figure 2 illustrates a hypothetical dipole (simultaneous negative and positive discharges occupying two separate points in space) within an infinite conductor and near the surface of a sphere. The lines or circles around the positive and negative ends of the dipole represent isopotential contours. Groups of vertically oriented cortical neurons and their dendritic processes would be analogous to a dipole near the surface of a sphere *(shown on the right)*. In this model, the isopotential lines intersect the surface and appear as a target-shaped field when viewed from above, with maximum potential near the center, and decreasing voltage levels in concentric circles around this. Most abnormal EEG events (spikes and sharp waves) appear to arise from this type of dipole with the negative end toward the surface and the positive pole deep inside (undetectable). The actual shape of the field is usually not circular, as illustrated here, but may be bean- or cigar-shaped or any other irregular contour. See the article by Gloor (4) for a more complete discussion of dipoles on the surface of the scalp.

Graphic representation of electrical fields on the surface may take several forms, as illustrated in Fig. 3. For the remainder of this chapter, most illustrations are in the form of a two-dimensional plot of voltage-versus-surface, as seen in the right in Fig. 3.

Methods of Recording Electrical Fields

Referential Method

Figure 4 illustrates the referential method of recording (the so-called monopolar technique). A two-dimensional graph of a hypothetical electrical field is depicted on the left, with electrode positions on the surface labeled *A* through *G* and a reference electrode, *R*,

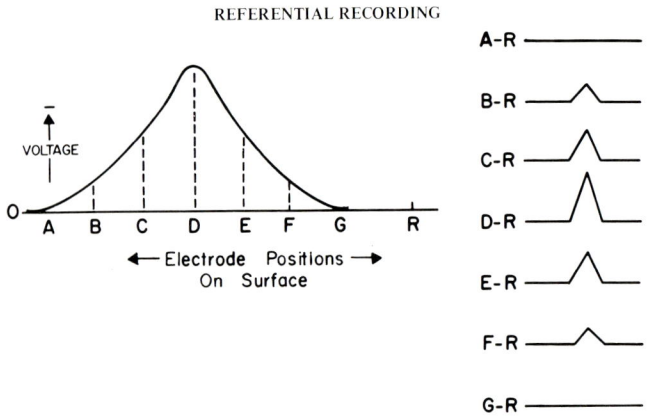

FIG. 4. Referential method of recording. Hypothetical electrical field *(left)* and simulated recording from this field *(right)*. The field represents the potential spread at the peak of the sharp wave in the recording.

at a point remote from the field. This slice through the electrical field represents an instant in time with potential maximum above electrode *D*. On the right in Fig. 4 are simulated recordings at the various electrode sites using the inactive reference electrode as a common indifferent reference. The simulated recording gives a straight forward representation of this surface negative field: no deflections at electrodes *A* and *G*, which are at zero potential; maximum deflection at electrode *D*; and intermediate height of deflections at the other electrodes.

Referential recording gives the most accurate representation of an electrical field in terms of voltage and wave shape and is particularly good for displaying widespread fields (6). The major disadvantage of referential recording is difficulty in locating a good reference site, free from artifacts (cardiac or myogenic) and outside the electrical fields generated by the brain. A rule-of-thumb for quickly assessing the adequacy of a reference site is to scan all channels for events that are represented equally in all channels ("contaminated" reference) or events that have apparent phase reversals in different channels ("active" reference). If such are noted, the reference site is bad and another should be chosen.

Differential Method

Figure 5 illustrates the "bipolar" or differential method of recording an identical electrical field. Only active sites *A* through *G* are used; these are subtracted from each other sequentially in the simulated recording on the right. Here, deflections are in the direction of the slope of the potential field, and their amplitude is determined by the difference in potential between the two electrodes rather than

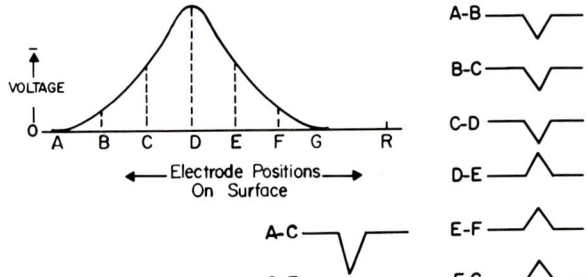

FIG. 5. The differential or "bipolar" method of recording. Electrical field *(left)*, closely spaced bipolar chain recording *(right)*, widely spaced bipolar derivations *(bottom center)*.

the absolute potential at any one electrode site. For instance, the first channel (*A* minus *B*) shows a downward deflection since grid 2 (connected to electrode *B*) is more negative than grid 1 (electrode *A*). *B* minus *C* and *C* minus *D* show similar downward deflections for the same reason, but *D* minus *E* yields an upward deflection because grid 1 is now more negative than grid 2. At this point in the tracing, where deflections of the pens are in opposite directions, there is an apparent "phase reversal." The phase reversal refers only to the deflections of the pen and not to the electrical field; a better term would be inflection of potential gradient. In interpreting differential recordings, this inflection point represents the location of the maximum voltage of the electrical field. The electrode that is common between the two channels involved in the inflection (or phase reversal) is the electrode overlying this maximum point (electrode *D*).

In the lower portion of Fig. 5, a three-channel tracing with wider electrode spacing is illustrated (electrodes *B*, *D*, and *F* are omitted). Here, an inflection of potential gradient is also noted with respect to the first and third channels, and an isopotential channel intervenes. The isopotential channel (*C* minus *E*) results from equal voltages entering the input of both leads of this amplifier. The interpreter, noting such an inflection with an isopotential channel in between, simply infers that the potential maximum is halfway between the two electrodes connected to the equipotential channel: halfway between *C* and *E* is position *D*, the area of maximum potential.

Bipolar or differential recording has an advantage of showing minor differences between electrode sites, and it is also a quick way to localize the maxima of fields since phase reversals or inflection points seem to attract the human eye. The disadvantages are many: it is difficult to directly infer the voltage of any event; the wave shapes may be quite distorted; and false localizations sometimes occur. Rules-of-thumb for reading differential recordings include: (a) pay no attention to amplitude of deflection, only direction, and (b) if there is no inflection point or phase reversal in a straight line sequential chain of electrodes, form no opinion about the distribution of the electrical field along that chain.

Constructing Electrical Fields

The experienced EEG interpreter "senses" the electrical field of significant events in the recording by scanning the channels from top to bottom at one instant in time. He can then construct a graph of the electrical field mentally or on paper, as illustrated in Fig. 6, from either the referential or differential recording. After practicing this on paper for many different events, it becomes easier to construct them in the mind. Referential recording *(on the left)* is easily trans-

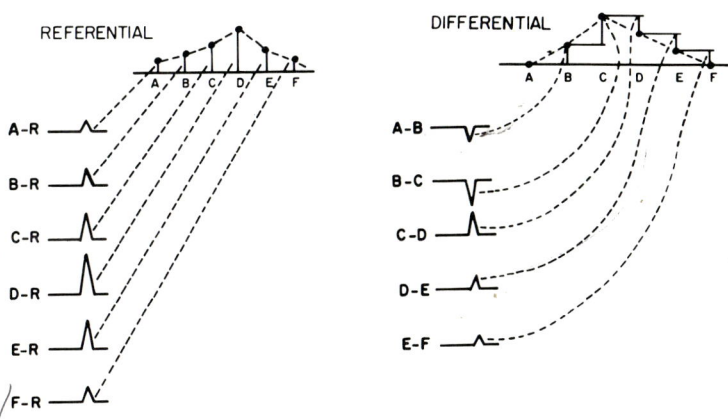

FIG. 6. Graphic construction of electrical fields from EEG recordings. See text for details.

ferred into a two-dimensional graph of voltage versus electrode position by simply placing the amplitude of the deflection on top of a line representing electrode positions. Constructing graphs from a differential recording is more difficult. First, the interpreter has to assume that one end of the electrode chain is at zero potential (not always true). In the sample on the right, one assumes that the potential of electrode *A* is zero and places a dot above this electrode on the horizontal axis of the graph. The deflection in channel *A* minus *B* is then graphed above electrode *B* in the appropriate direction (*B* more negative than *A*), and a construction line is then drawn horizontally from this level to the next electrode position. The deflection in *B* minus *C* is then added to the horizontal construction line, yielding the potential at position *C,* and another construction line is drawn horizontally from there to the next position. The deflection of *C* minus *D,* being of opposite direction, is then drawn below the previous construction line to yield the potential at electrode *D,* etc.

Localization of Electrical Fields

Figure 7 illustrates the most precise way to localize the maximum of an electrical field with the minimum number of electrodes. At the top, a hypothetical field is graphed over electrodes *A* through *E* with maximum at electrode *C*. In the middle of the figure, electrodes *A* through *C* are depicted on the surface with three different possible locations of an electrical field represented by concentric circles of isopotential lines ("targets"). Any of these three locations are possible: on the left, *C* is exactly in the center of the field; in the middle, the field lies slightly below electrode *C,* and on the far right, the maximum voltage is above electrode *C*. Fields in either of these three different locations would yield the same potential dis-

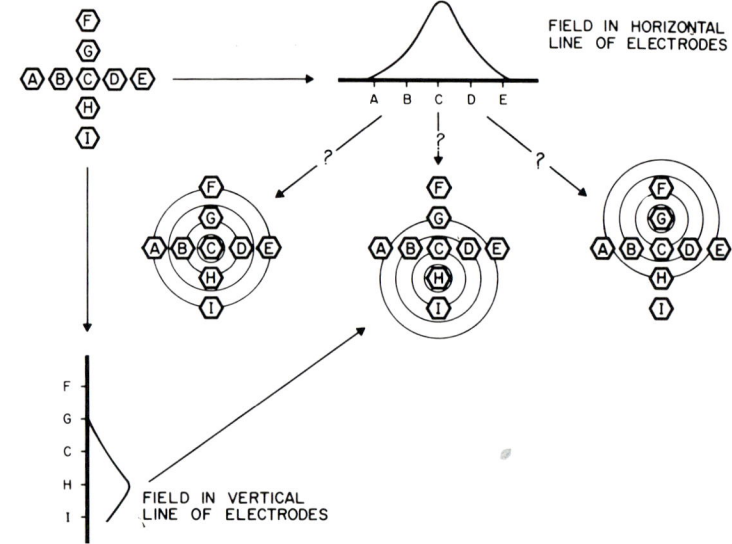

FIG. 7. Localization of field maximum point by electrodes arranged in X and Y axes.

tribution graph drawn at the top of the figure. In order to determine which of these three possibilities is most accurate, one must add additional electrodes (*F* through *I*) on an axis that is perpendicular to the original chain (*A* through *E*). Recordings from electrodes in the chain *F* through *I* might yield a field graph as illustrated in the lower left portion of this figure, showing a maximum at electrode *H*. Now from the information obtained from both chains of electrodes, one can infer that the representation in the center is the most accurate in this case—the field maximum was below electrode *C* and close to electrode *H*.

This format of arranging electrodes in fairly straight chains over the scalp crossing at right angles to each other is the best way to localize a focus with accuracy. The standard positions may be connected in chains to amplifiers in this manner or additional electrodes may be added if the chains do not completely cross the apparent field. For example, a spike focus in the left occipital region can be adequately graphed in the horizontal direction by connecting electrodes around the back of the head (T3–T5–O1–OZ–O2–T6–T4). The perpendicular chain (C3–P3–O1), however, does not completely cross the field, and an additional electrode is needed below electrode O1 towards the neck to adequately demonstrate the field in X and Y directions.

Not all electrical fields are unipolar. If the sheet of cortical elements generating an event lies at right angles to the surface of the head (as in the side of a sulcus), a horizontal or oblique dipole field may appear on the scalp. In these fields there is a simultaneous surface negative and surface positive area at different locations on the scalp as depicted in Fig. 8. In the case of a horizontal dipole, the positive and negative areas will be approximately equal in amplitude, but if one end is closer to the surface as in an oblique dipole, that portion of the field will be higher in voltage.

Figure 9 illustrates one of these complex fields. On the left, bipolar or differential recording reveals a surface negative spike near T3 and a simultaneous positive maximum near C3. Average reference (AR) recording on the right shows the referential representation of this spike.

Figure 10 is the construction of the potential field shown in the previous figure. On the left, the AR tracing was made at double speed to facilitate measurement. On the right the deflections of the pens at various electrode sites were plotted on a graph representing surface of the scalp in the transverse direction from the left ear

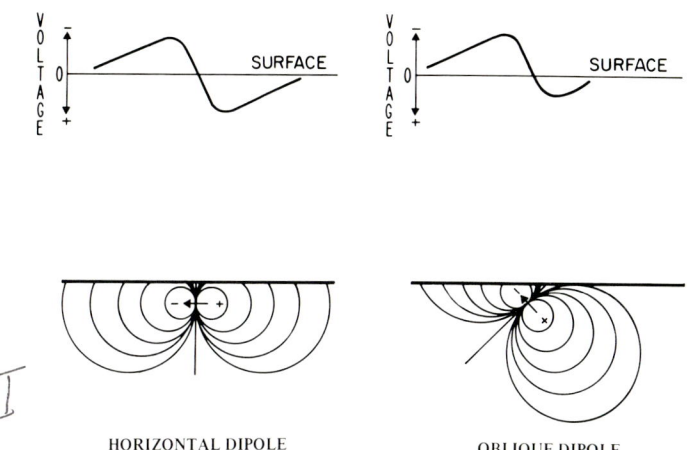

FIG. 8. Theoretical fields produced by horizontal *(left)* or oblique *(right)* dipoles near the surface. Note that the point on the surface directly over the center of the dipole is usually near zero potential and lies about halfway between the simultaneous positive and negative maxima.

across the top of the vertex. Note the similarity of this field to those that would be produced by horizontal or oblique dipoles.

Localization of the electrically active region is assumed to be halfway between the maximum negative and maximum positive poles of this graph or at the point where zero potential exists between these two maxima, i.e., near electrode C5. In this case one might postulate the event on the cortex is predominantly surface negative and that in order to produce such an oblique field with the negative end towards the temporal region and the positive end above, it would most likely be located above the sylvian fissure as the cortex invaginates in to blend with the insular area.

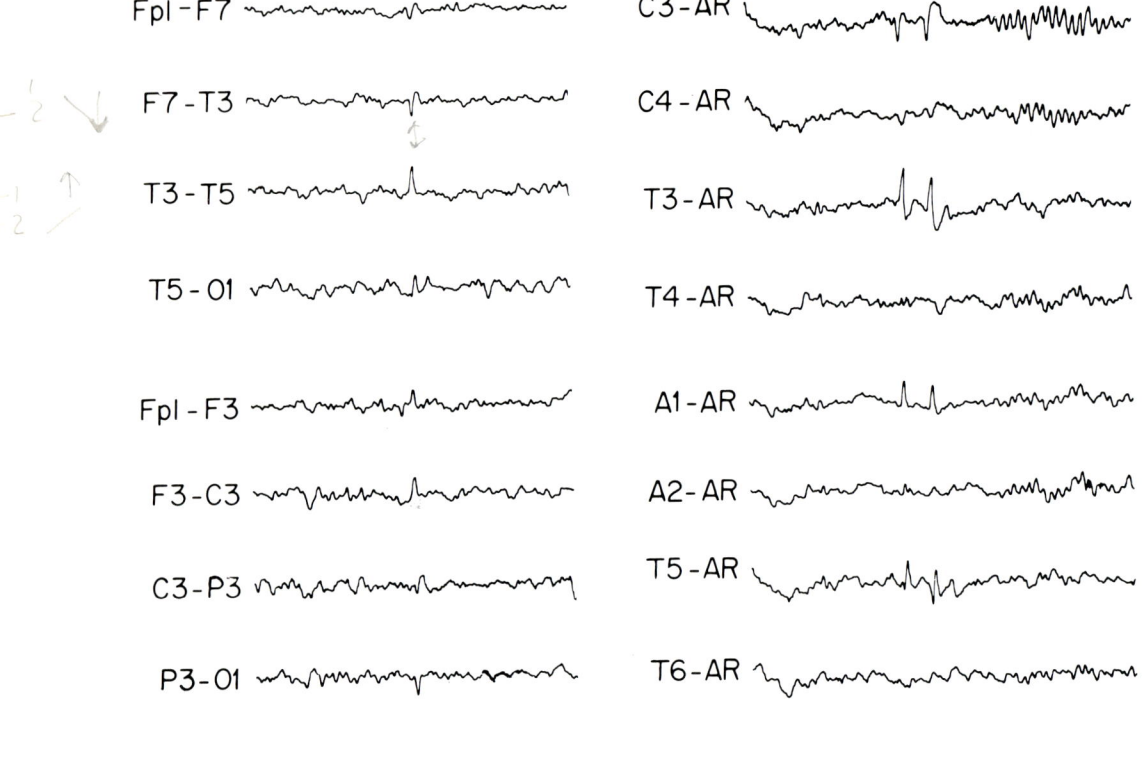

FIG. 9. Sample of an EEG recording from a child showing simultaneous positive and negative spikes. Differential recording on the left and referential recording on the right utilizing a common AR.

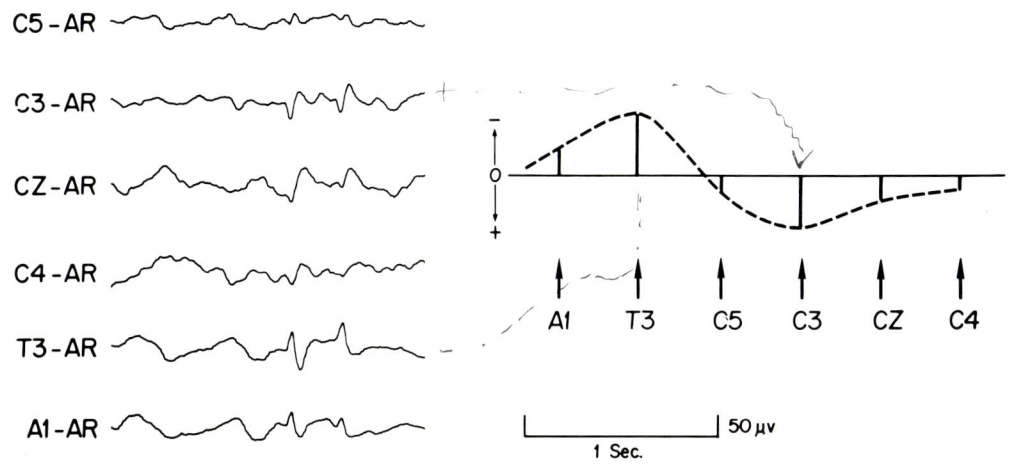

FIG. 10. Graphic construction of the field from the same EEG illustrated in Fig 9. On the left a double-speed tracing was used for easier measurement of pen deflections at the peak of the spike potential. Vertical lines in the field plot on the right are proportional to the maximum pen deflection of the spike (measured from assumed base line to the peak).

SUMMARY AND PRACTICAL PROBLEM

Competent visual analysis of EEG tracings demands attention to polarity, knowledge of typical electrical fields, and ability to localize fields accurately. The student should practice construction of electrical fields from EEGs at every opportunity with the goal of incorporating this in his mental processes as he views an EEG tracing. Both referential and differential recording techniques should be used in every case.

Figure 11 is a hypothetical problem to begin this practice. On the left, electrodes A through I are arranged on a surface in an X–Y format with a remote electrode, R, assumed to be outside of the field of interest. On the right, simulated recordings using both referential and differential techniques are depicted for a single electrical event, i.e., the same field recorded in two different ways. On the lower left hand side of the figure, vertical and horizontal axes are suggested, on which the potential fields may be plotted for practice in localization. When this is done, it will be noticed that in the chain, A through E, a maximum is indicated halfway between electrodes C and D; and in the chain, F through I, a maximum occurs at electrode H. These observations mean that the maximum of the potential field lies on a line halfway between electrodes C and D, perpendicular to chain A-E, and on another line through electrode H, perpendicular to the chain F-I. Where these two lines intersect (*just to the right of electrode* H) the field is assumed to be maximum.

POLARITY, LOCALIZATION, AND FIELD THEORY

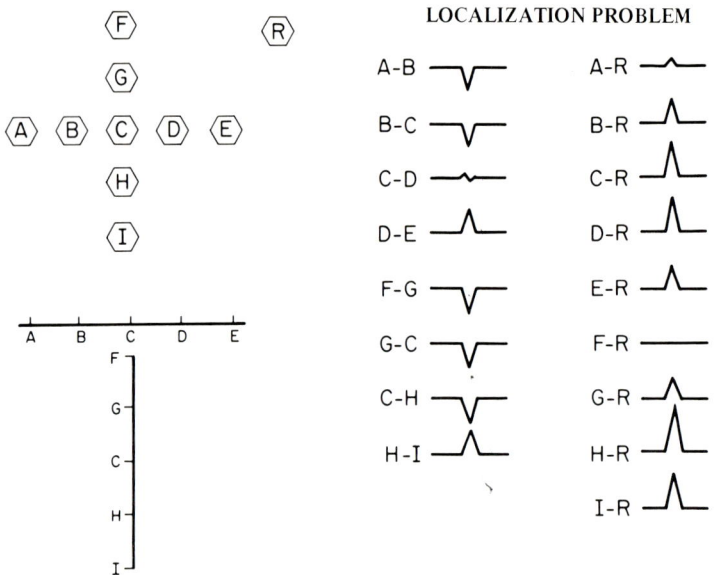

FIG. 11. Localization problem assuming electrode positions diagrammed in the upper left hand corner and recordings obtained by differential and referential methods on the right. Coordinates for plotting the field in horizontal and vertical directions are suggested in the lower left.

REFERENCES

1. Knott, J. R. (1969): Electrode montages revisited: How to tell up from down. *Am. J. EEG Technol.*, 9:33–45.
2. MacGillivray, B. (1974): Traditional methods of examination in clinical EEG. In: *Handbook of Electroencephalography and Clinical Neurophysiology*, Vol. 3, Part C, edited by A. Remond, pp. 22–57. Elsevier, Amsterdam.
3. Brazier, M. A. B. (1949): A study of electrical fields at the surface of the head. *Electroencephalogr. Clin. Neurophysiol. (Suppl.)*, 2:38–52.
4. Gloor, P. (1971): Volume conduction theory and recording principles. *Spike and Wave*, Special Issue No. 2:1–48.
5. Magnus, O. (1961): On the technique of localization by electroencephalography. *Electroencephalogr. Clin. Neurophysiol. (Suppl.)*, 10:1–35.
6. Osselton, J. W. (1969): Bipolar, unipolar and average reference recording methods II: Mainly practical considerations. *Am. J. EEG Technol.*, 9:117–133.

Chapter 4

Artifacts: Activity of Noncerebral Origin in the EEG

Michael G. Saunders[*]

Formerly, Section of Electroencephalography; Department of Physiology, and Computer Department, Faculty of Medicine, University of Manitoba, Winnipeg, Manitoba, Canada

Causes and Forms of Artifact	38
External	38
Instrumental	39
Electrodes	43
EEG Machine	43
Physiological	46
Skin	46
Muscle Artifact	51
Eye Artifacts	56
Tongue and Mouth	61

[*] This chapter was posthumously edited by John R. Knott, Professor-Emeritus, Departments of Neurology and Psychiatry, University of Iowa, Iowa City, Iowa 52242; Presently Department of Neurology, Tufts University School of Medicine, Boston, Massachusetts 02111.

EKG Artifact 63
　　Mixed Causes 63
　　　Pulse Artifact 63
　　　Ballistrocardiograph Effect 66
　　　Respiratory Pump Artifact 66
　　　Artifacts of Spontaneous Movement 66
Conclusion 66
Acknowledgment 67
References 67

Artifact can so obscure an electroencephalogram (EEG) record that it is unreadable and unuseable. It may be a nuisance, making reading more difficult and interpretation less certain, or in some instances it can mimic abnormal brain activity so exactly that misinterpretation results.

Knowledge of the multiplicity of different causes and patterns of artifact is essential for the technologist and the interpreter, and both have the responsibility for recognition of artifact appearing in the EEG. Whereas the technologist must be able to identify artifact and take steps to remove the cause, something that requires much competence, the interpreter should be alert to the simulation of cerebral activity by extracerebral generators and should work with the technologist for ever improving EEG quality.

CAUSES AND FORMS OF ARTIFACT

The difficult components of EEG analysis are the conversion of the EEG patterns into meaningful clinical information and the separation of true EEG activity from artifact, which is recorded activity appearing at the output of the EEG but not generated by the brain. What we deal with here is the illustration of principles, since it is not possible to demonstrate all possible examples. Some artifacts and their occurrence can relate to individual technologists, to specific types of electrodes and equipment, or even to a specific laboratory environment. It is profitable for every EEG laboratory to make its own *Atlas of Artifacts*.

There are three basic causes of artifact (1–3):

1. external,
2. instrumental, and
3. physiological.

These may, to compound the confusion, sometimes be combined.

External

The most obvious externally introduced artifact is 60-Hz interference (4). With modern EEG equipment—usually having 60-Hz notch filters—this artifact should rarely appear in routine work. It is no longer necessary to screen recording rooms unless, for example, unshielded electric cables are in the walls of the room or a very high energy radio-frequency (RF) generator is nearby. Electromagnetic fields produce 60- or 120-Hz artifact and are difficult to shield. They can be induced by nearby fan or air conditioning motors. Another common cause is from the ballasts of fluorescent lights. When these lights are in the ceiling of the room below the recording room, the cabling, the ballast, and the discharge light are unseen but may be within a few inches of the patient. It is better to have suspended incandescents in rooms below recording rooms.

Sixty-hertz interference in only one or two channels is frequently due to unequal electrode resistances (Fig. 1). A check of resistance (impedance) values by either built-in test devices or external meters is necessary. It is more important to have all electrode resistances equal than necessarily to have them all of low value. When using the "common average reference" (so-called Goldman-Offner or average potential reference), inherent inequalities in input resistance of the reference lead cause this system to be more susceptible to 60-Hz interference. This type of interference also occurs if lamps or photic stimulators are placed on the EEG console or near the patient's head.

In the Intensive Care Unit (ICU) or Coronary Care Unit, the problems may be far more difficult to control (5,6). This is particularly true when sensitivities of 1 or 2 $\mu V/mm$ are used. Respiratory pumps, pump infusers, heating or cooling blankets, electrocardiogram (EKG) monitors, and so on, all induce 60-Hz interference. When 60-Hz interference occurs it must be eliminated if possible—especially when looking for electrocerebral silence (ECS). This involves first keeping the EEG input cable far away from power cables. Sometimes it may be necessary to progressively unplug one piece of equipment after another, until the problem is resolved. None except the respirator is vital for support for several minutes. Even the respirator can be turned off and hand bagging of oxygen substituted. The technologist must, in collaboration with the ICU staff, intelligently control the environment during the EEG recording. It is for the benefit of the patient and the physicians to produce good ICU records, and all must work to this end.

Other external artifacts can arise from electrostatic potentials developed by clothing. This is particularly true when humidity is low and when clothing made from artificial fabric is worn. The potentials may come from the clothing of the patient but more usually from another person nearby—a nurse, parent, or technologist. The rule must be, No movements of persons in the recording room. Any necessary movements must be observed and noted on the EEG.

The types and forms of artifacts from voltages built up by electrostatic effects of movement are of every conceivable type. Even one simulating a spike-and-slow-wave complex has been seen. The need for continual careful observation of the patient and notation on the record by the technologist is essential. Recording in darkened rooms with awkward viewing windows between the patient and the technologist does not enhance this process. It is advantageous to have the patient and technologist (and equipment) in the same room.

Numerous other causes, such as "spike" discharges from intravenous drips (5,7,8) (Fig. 2), potentials developed in electrode wires swaying in the breeze from a fan, from nearby TV stations or radar transmitters (RF overload), radio paging, even from the voltages developed in telephone lines as the bell rings (5) (Fig. 3), must be known about and recognized by the interpreter and the technologist.

Instrumental

The artifacts from instrumental causes can be generated in any part of the recording system—electrodes, electrode cables, switches,

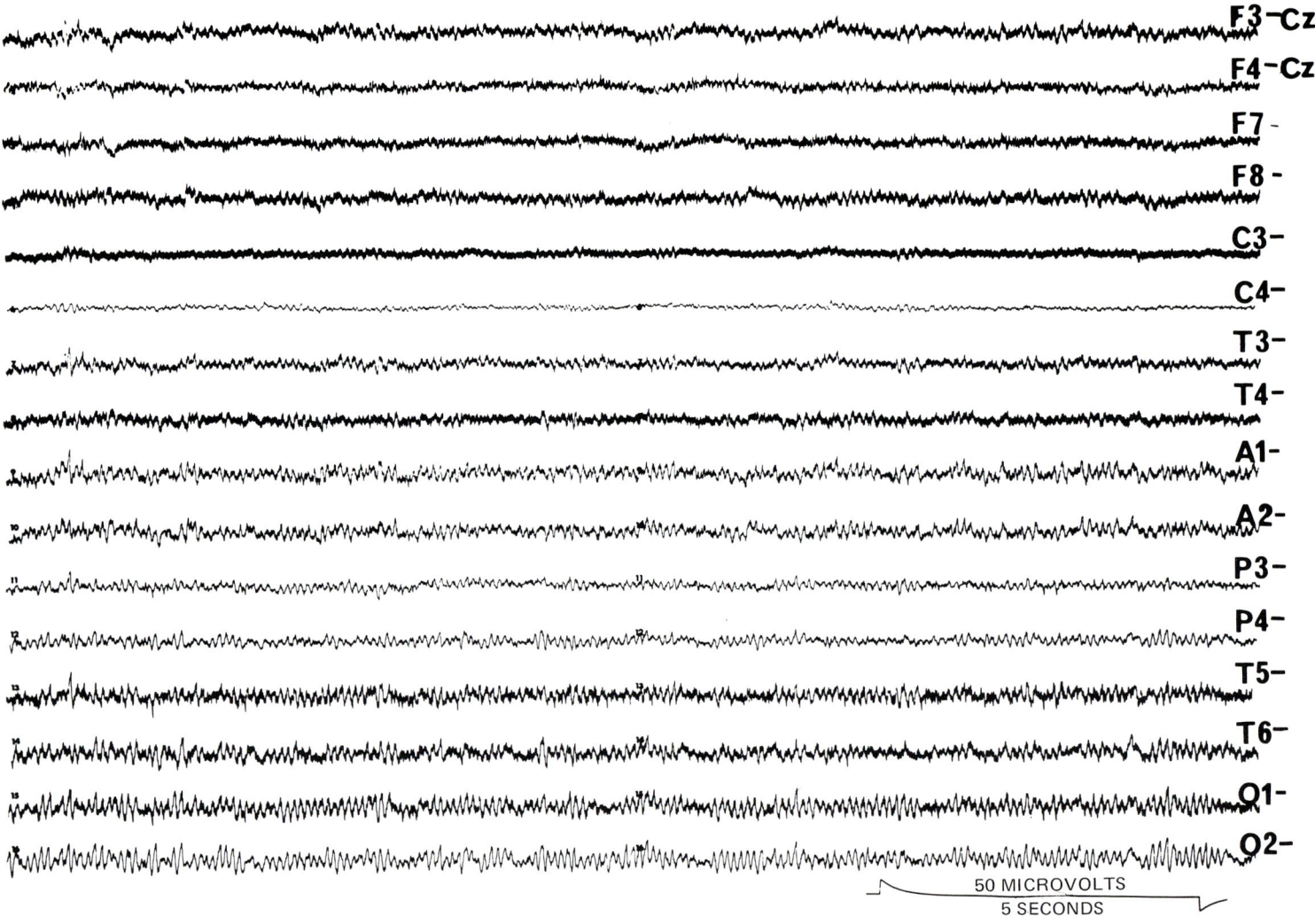

FIG. 1. Sixty Hz artifact in several channels is introduced by unequal electrode resistances. This record was taken without use of 60-Hz notch filters. With careful application of the electrodes this level of artifact usually can be avoided. Cz is a reference lead connected to input terminal 2 of each channel in this recording.

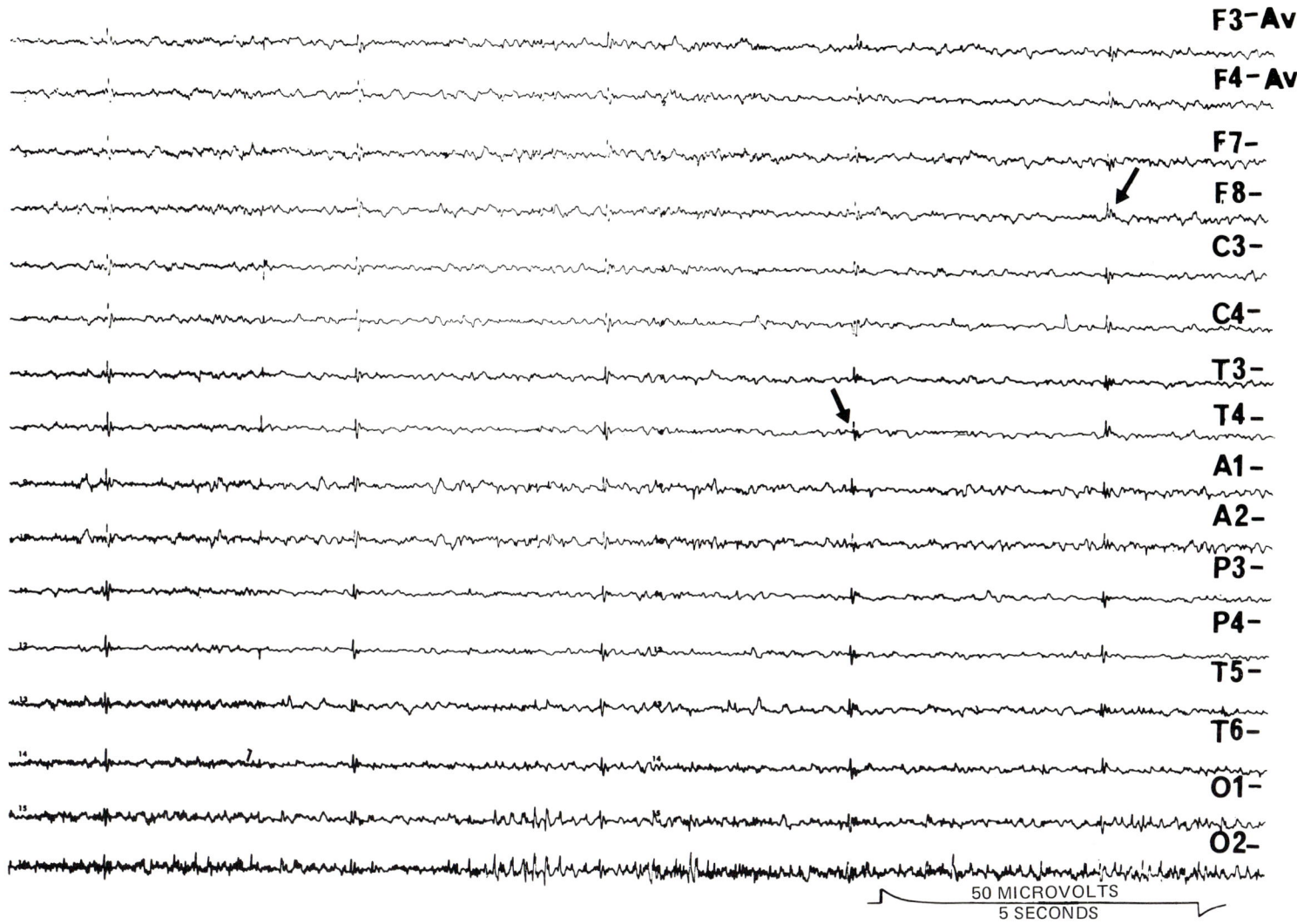

FIG. 2. Periodic spike-like artifacts, two of which are indicated by the arrows, are produced by the drip of intravenous saline. An average potential reference lead is connected to input terminal 2 of each channel in this recording.

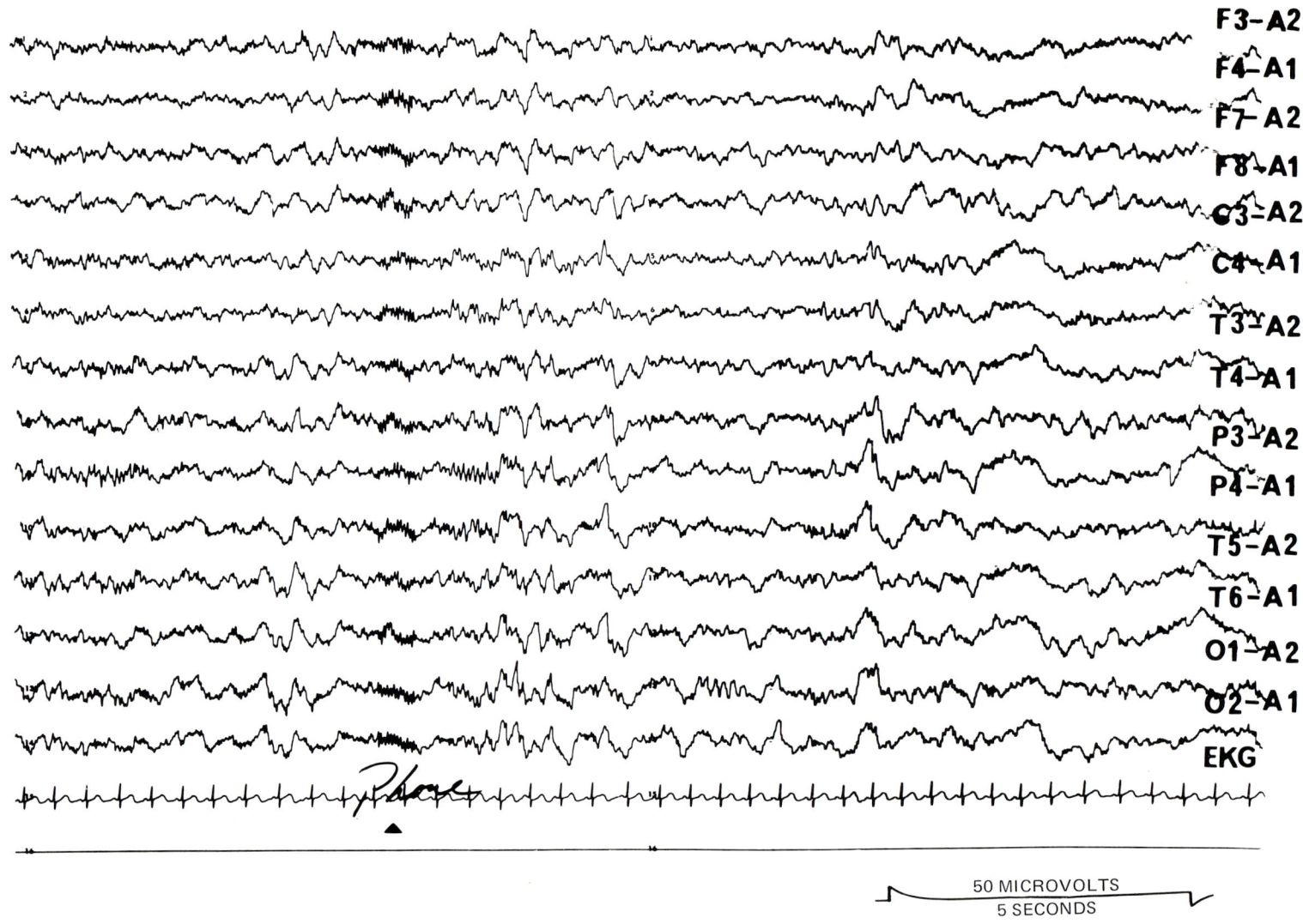

FIG. 3. Artifact produced by the ringing signal of a telephone. This may not be noticed by the technologist if the bell is muted. It may or may not repeat regularly, depending on the switchboard system.

amplifiers, oscillographs, and pens. It is not possible to describe all causes since there are so many. All types and forms of artifact patterns result. Some of the wave forms simulate brain activity so exactly that there can be interpretative error. Some are easily recognizable and of passing annoyance. Others, although of recognizable form and origin, obscure the EEG patterns to make the record uninterpretable.

There are two major subgroups of instrumental artifacts—those related to the electrodes and those from the EEG instrument.

Electrodes

The artifacts from electrodes depend on the type of electrode. Most electrodes can produce "popping" (Fig. 4) and may even cause repetitive spike-like discharges. Monopod or pad electrodes are susceptible to movement artifact and sliding potentials when they are not well applied with their rubber headbands. Silver-silver chloride electrodes may occasionally produce rhythmic delta/theta patterns, presumably when an area of chloride is chipped or dissolved off to leave bare silver. Needle electrodes have a tendency to fall out and produce spurious asymmetries. Sweat in contact with stainless steel needles can cause most bizarre patterns, and an example is shown in the section on sweat artifact (Fig. 7). The significant features are almost always caused by instability of electrode-scalp interface. Dirty electrodes are a common cause, as is evaporating electrolyte.

Electrode wires produce artifact from the static and capacitive potentials generated when the conductors move against the insulating sheath. It is possible to obtain wires in which the effect is negligible, but most leads produce movement potentials. These artifacts can mimic brain activity very exactly. Unless the technologist is observant confusion may occur about the cause. If only one lead is moving, the pattern may appear only in one channel, depending on the montage. This fact should lead to suspicion of artifact. Several wires may sway to produce effects in several channels. Recognition of the cause may then be difficult. Usually the artifact of delta and/or theta activity appears with a distribution in the different channels that is unlike the distribution produced by any disease process. Wire movement may also induce movement of electrode-scalp interface.

Another electrode-generated artifact occurs if the electrolyte (usually NaCl) contacts two metals, e.g., silver or gold (the electrode) and copper (the wire). This must be particularly watched for, especially in "home-brewed" electrodes.

EEG Machine

Artifact from the EEG machine can occur in any component from the electrode box to the pen system. Each machine may have individual idiosyncracies and be prone to certain types of artifact, although this is rare. There are several causes of artifact—poor switch contacts, vacuum tube or transistor changes, breakdown of capacitors, or development of incorrect feedback loops.

Usually the artifacts are recognizable by their unphysiological form (Fig. 5). They can obscure the EEG activity and make interpretation difficult or impossible. One or more channels may be affected. Occasionally the artifact can mimic brain activity, and its presence can only be recognized by its persistence in a sequence of records from different patients.

The effect of changes at interfaces is usually from wearing away of silver plating in switches to leave bimetallic surfaces. Alternatively, oxidation or sulfiding of the silver may occur. Even the gold plating of plug board connectors may deteriorate and cause intermittent contact. The modern techniques of soldering connections reduce the problem of cold soldering or crystallization causing intermittent contact. Frequently, judicious application of antioxidant oils to the con-

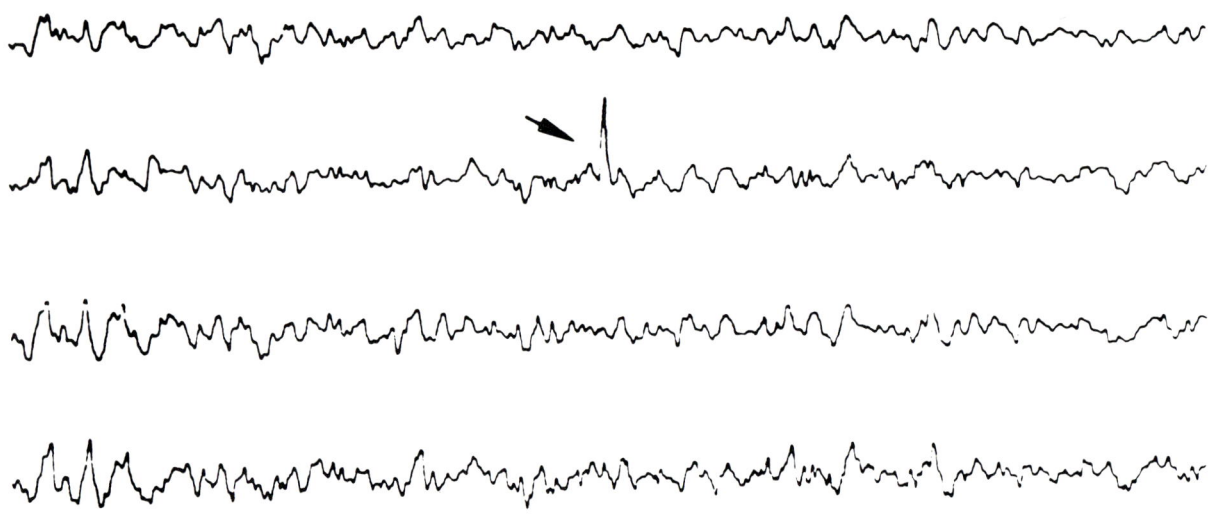

FIG. 4. An isolated "pop" of an electrode indicated by the arrow. It is usually easy to recognize due to its almost right angle upshoot from an imaginary baseline plus its superimposition on (not modification of) the EEG patterns.

tacts will cure the fault. The best modern switches minimize these problems.

Vacuum tubes are not used in the newest machines; however, many older instruments still in service use input stage tubes that may generate noise or produce asymmetries attributable to impedance variations. These are usually seen during calibration. The cause can be traced by substituting appropriate modules of different channels. It is desirable to have spare tubes and/or modules for replacement. Transistors can become noisy although reliability is now very high. As channels are now modularized, fault finding by substitution is simple and does not require a knowledge of electronics. Capacitors can develop faults similar to those of transistors. Again, this is increasingly uncommon. The continually improving quality of components is increasing machine reliability and reducing artifact from this source. Such improvements are in part an offshoot of the space program and of computer technology.

Some EEG machines are designed to require a feedback stabilizing loop through a ground electrode. The Offner Type T was the first to use this system. If a ground electrode was not used or if its resistance was too high, oscillation could occur in the theta and alpha frequency ranges. One, several, or all channels could be affected, and the spurious pattern could simulate atypical brain activity. When evaluating ECS such oscillatory effects could be most confusing. Machines not using ground feedback loops can produce oscillatory effects when a reference electrode is of high resistance.

Three other machine-oriented problems can cause misinterpreta-

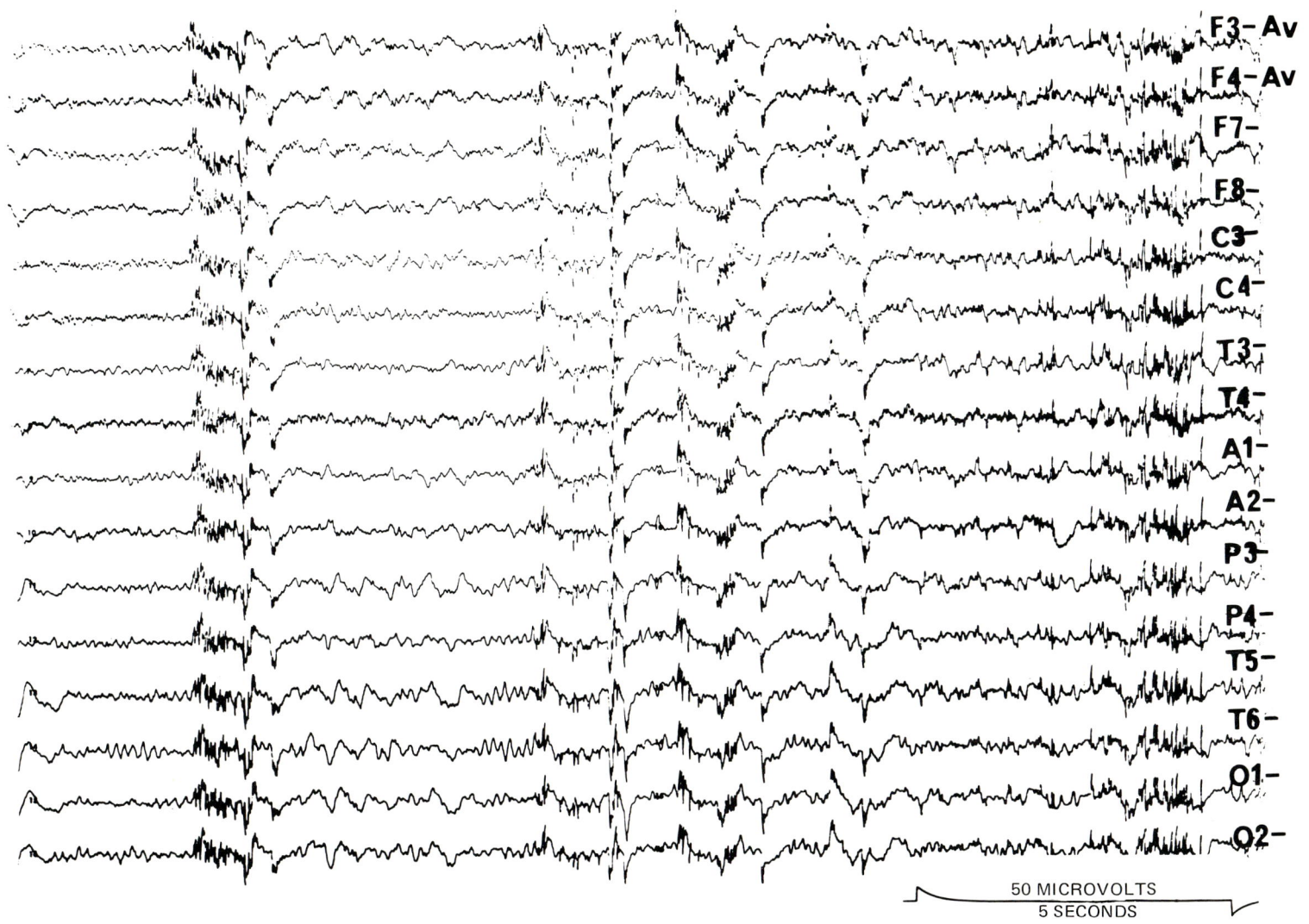

FIG. 5. High voltage repetitive discharges produced by poor contact in a master switch plug and socket and affecting all channels. With such artifacts, although they are obvious, there may be great difficulty in finding the cause and curing it. An average potential reference is connected to the input terminal 2 of all channels in this recording.

tion of EEG activity. One is incorrect adjustment of the gain control on one or more channels. This should be noted by the interpreter since he/she should always start reviewing the record by looking at the calibration signals. If the gains are changed during recording this must be noted on the EEG at the time. The return to the previous level must also be noted. Calibration at the end of the record should be regarded as mandatory.

A malfunctioning galvanometer with a loose pen holder or cracked bearing may give correct calibration for large signals and inadequate movement for small signals. This causes the affected channel to lose low amplitude fast patterns and give a false impression of asymmetry. Calibration at 5 or 10 as well as 50 μV shows the presence of this defect, and such calibration pulses at beginning and end of the record should routinely be included.

Misalignment of the pens can also produce misinterpretation, particularly of the origin and spread of fast transients. Here sharp waves or spike discharges falsely appear to start earlier in one channel. A false assumption of a primary area of discharge may result. Examples of this effect are difficult to find in EEG departments with well-trained technologists who take care of their EEG equipment and with well-trained interpreters who examine calibrations carefully.

An effect causing misjudgment can occur if ink in one pen flows too freely. The impression that the channel shows more activity is an illusion, but it can be disconcerting and requires careful examination of the record to demonstrate that this is indeed an illusion.

Physiological

All living cells have electrogenic properties. Only when relatively rapid changes in cellular metabolism or status occur are the potentials recordable on standard EEG equipment. Due to the frequency response of the EEG equipment the changes must last longer than 10 msec and less than 2 to 3 sec. As a result many physiological phenomena, from peripheral nerve action potentials to changes in areal blood flow, are not recorded by the EEG equipment. A number of other noncerebral electrogenic activities do occur and can cause appearance of artifact in the EEG (9,10).

As with other artifacts they may be of passing annoyance, they may be such that EEG activity is partly or wholly obscured, or they may be so similar to EEG activity that misinterpretation can result.

Skin

The skin can produce artifact in two ways.

1. Movement of muscles, such as the frontalis and temporalis, can cause the electrodes to move on the skin. These movements set up variations in the electrode contact potentials. The effects are generally obvious since muscle activity usually appears concomitantly. The voltages may be so large and irregular that the pens reach full excursion (Fig. 6). The recording becomes virtually uninterpretable in this case.

2. Sweating can produce several effects. The sweat with its high NaCl and lactic acid content can react with exposed metal of the electrodes and produce not only huge base-line sways but even rhythmic potentials (Fig. 7). Unchlorided silver and stainless steel electrodes are prone to this type of interaction. Sweat on an exposed electrode wire made of copper produces the effect even more markedly and can also set up oscillatory effects.

The common artifact produced by sweating is from the electric potentials developed by active sweat glands as well as skin potentials. There also is change in skin–electrode interface and electrolyte. The

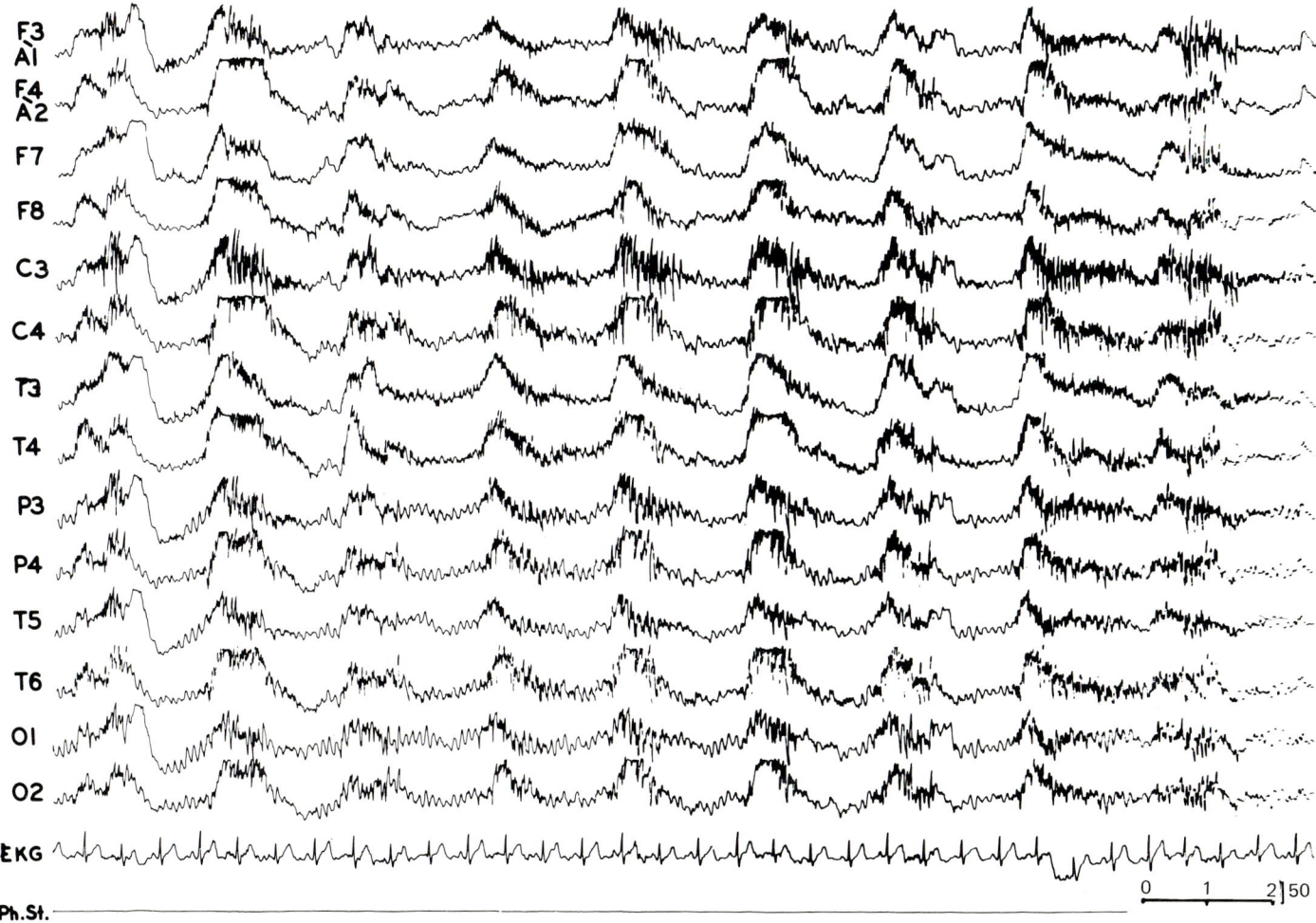

FIG. 6. Excessive movement and muscle artifact make the record uninterpretable. Only the most obvious abnormalities or gross delta asymmetries might be seen. In the lower right-hand corner, the horizontal line indicates time in seconds and the vertical line indicates the amplitude produced by a 50 μV input. The reference lead connected to input terminal 2 in the upper 14 channels is attached to the ear lobe ipsilateral to the designated scalp lead.

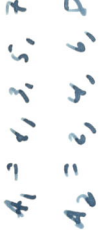
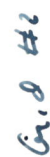
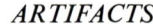

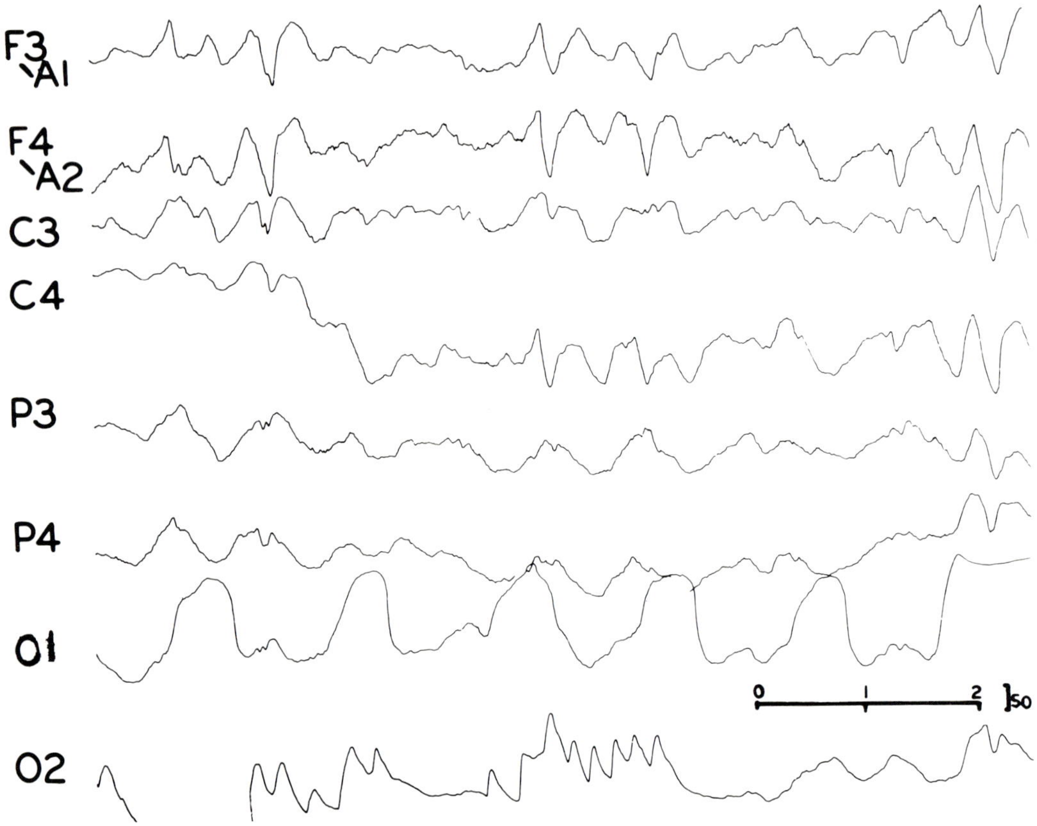

FIG. 7. EEG from a patient on dialysis after a suicidal dose of phenobarbital. During continuous EEG monitoring, there was a phase of profuse sweating. This very acid sweat attacked the stainless steel electrodes to produce bizarre patterns affecting particularly channels 4, 7, and 8. The same effect at lower amplitude could simulate EEG abnormality. Time and amplitude indicators are the same as for Fig. 6. A1 is connected to input terminal 2 of channels 1, 3, 5, and 7. A2 is connected to input terminal 2 of channels 2, 4, 6, and 8.

forehead is the most active region, but all areas of the head are capable of sweating.

The artifact is typically registered as long duration slow activity, smooth in outline, and of high amplitude. Recognition is usually simple because of the very low frequency of the artifact (Fig. 8).

Difficulty can arise when there is unilateral sweating and a delta-producing lesion is suspected (Fig. 9). There can be simulation of the delta activity produced by a cerebral abscess. Differentiation between localized sweat artifact and EEG abnormality is made by looking at activity in adjacent brain areas. Lesions will show some

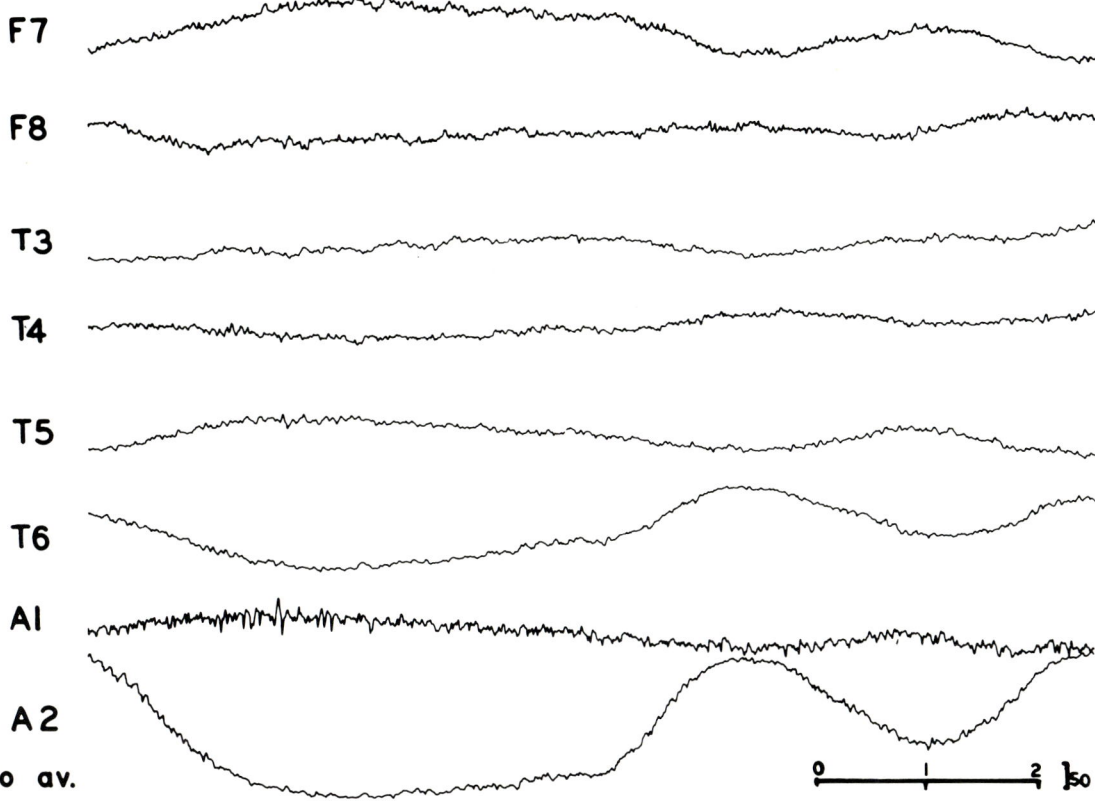

FIG. 8. The typical, very long duration baseline sway produced by sweating. An average potential reference is used for the input terminal 2 of each channel. Time and amplitude indicators are the same as for Figs. 6 and 7.

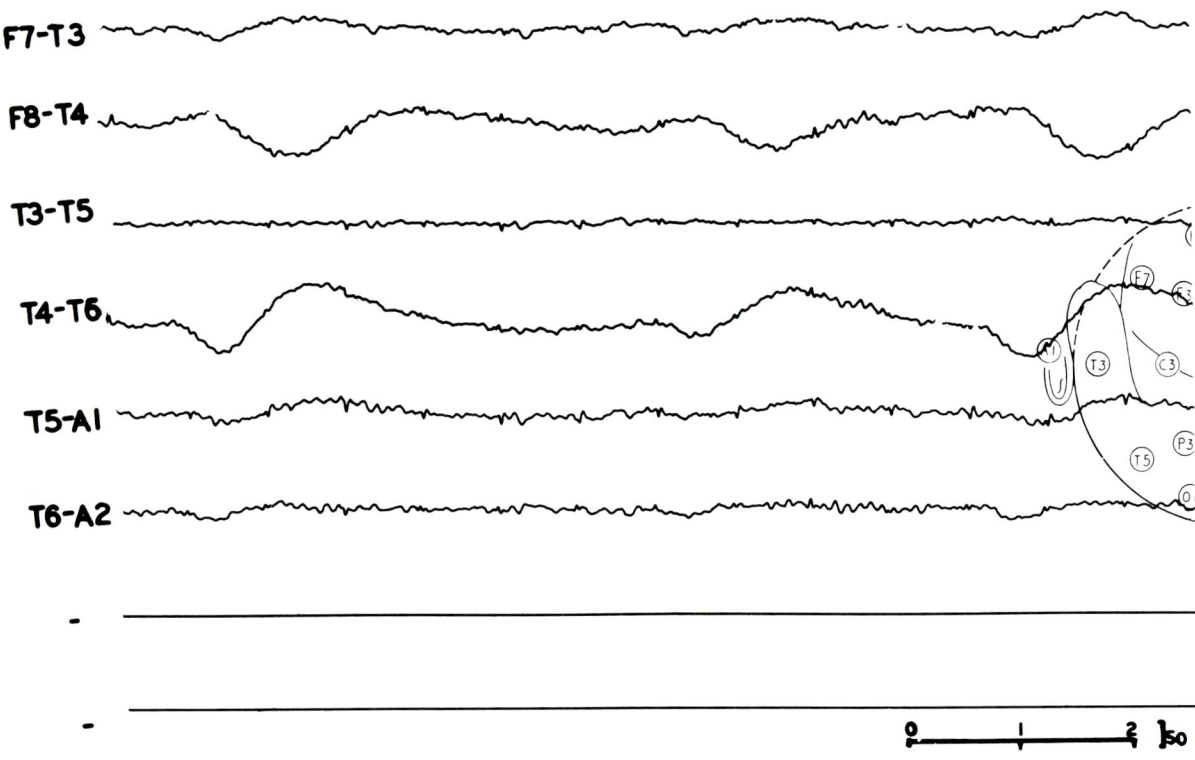

FIG. 9. Asymmetric sweating simulating focal delta activity of cerebral origin (channels 2 and 4). Time and amplitude indicators are the same as for Figs. 6, 7, and 8.

delta activity and abnormal theta patterns in these areas. Theta activity is not produced by active sweat glands. When persistent sweat artifact accompanies diffuse theta and/or delta activity, the possibility of profound hypoglycemia must be considered.

The low resistance of sweat can cause reduction in amplitude of recorded patterns especially with scalp-to-scalp montages. This must be seriously considered when local diminution of activity appears in the record. Subdural hematomata, cephalohematomata, bruising of the scalp, and large prosthetic bone repairs can all cause similar asymmetries.

Reduction of sweat artifact can be produced by cooling the patient, drying the scalp with alcohol, careful use of antiperspirant sprays, and/or overbreathing. Delta activity from cerebral tissue is not reduced by these procedures.

Muscle Artifact

The electrical discharge from muscle is the most common artifact seen in EEG recordings. Its presence may be engendered in the patient by tenseness of the technologist as well as natural or pathological anxiety of the patient or by rigidity or spasticity from neurological disease. It sometimes is worse when needle electrodes cause local "splinting" reactions, as in temporalis muscle. Muscle artifact from tenseness can usually be abolished or adequately diminished if the technologist takes time to explain the procedures and makes an effort to establish rapport with the patient. Unfortunately, this necessary personal involvement is too often forgotten.

The amount of artifact varies from continuous high amplitude deflections that obscure all EEG activity to little bursts that may mimic cortical spiking (4).

Muscle activity in the EEG can be produced by the frontalis, occipitalis, temporalis, nuchal, and auricular muscles. The temporalis muscle has a particularly wide distribution that underlies the temporal, central, and parietal areas of the scalp. In some patients the Cz and Pz positions are the only ones not over muscle. The muscles under the zygoma can produce artifact in sphenoidal leads as can the nasopharyngeal muscles with nasal leads. Artifact in these leads may simulate temporal lobe discharges, and considerable caution must be taken to exclude this artifact before identifying temporal lobe abnormality.

A common muscle artifact is seen in the frontal or anterior temporal leads. These small spikes are reputedly from action of the external ocular muscles. They are not from the cortex. An example is shown in Fig. 10.

Individual sporadic muscle twitches or short bursts of rhythmic myogenic potentials (Fig. 11) can present a more difficult interpretive problem. Probably, not infrequently, true cortical spiking has been thought to be muscle artifact or the artifact to be cortical spiking. The characteristics of short duration, surface negativity or biphasicity, sharp point, and local origin may cause suspicion of local cortical irritation. Differentiation is made by the high degree of localization to one electrode and absence of other local abnormality such as, in the case of the artifact, theta activity, sharp waves, or fast activity. Also when of muscle origin, rather than cortical origin, bursts of more easily recognizable muscle artifact often appear from the same leads in other parts of the EEG record. The technologist helping the patient to relax can cause muscle artifact but not cortical spiking (11) to disappear.

The presence of low amplitude muscle artifact can be of diagnostic value on occasion since the triad of this artifact, low amplitude EEG patterns, and tachycardia are evidence in favor of an anxiety state. The periodic unilateral bursts of muscle activity associated with facial myokymia provide evidence for dysfunction of the brainstem (12).

During photic stimulation, myoclonic jerking (photomyoclonic or photomyogenic response) can produce patterns mimicking those of paroxysmal cortical discharges (13). An electrode movement component is often present to produce large slow waves. The jerking may be from small muscle groups around the eyes and in the frontalis but can involve many muscles elsewhere in the body. When complexes appear during photic stimulation, it is desirable to record from the forehead and from regions around the eyes to check activity close to the source of the artifact. The photic stimulation should also be stopped suddenly since the myoclonic response stops with the light flashes, unlike some cortical discharges induced by photic stimulation.

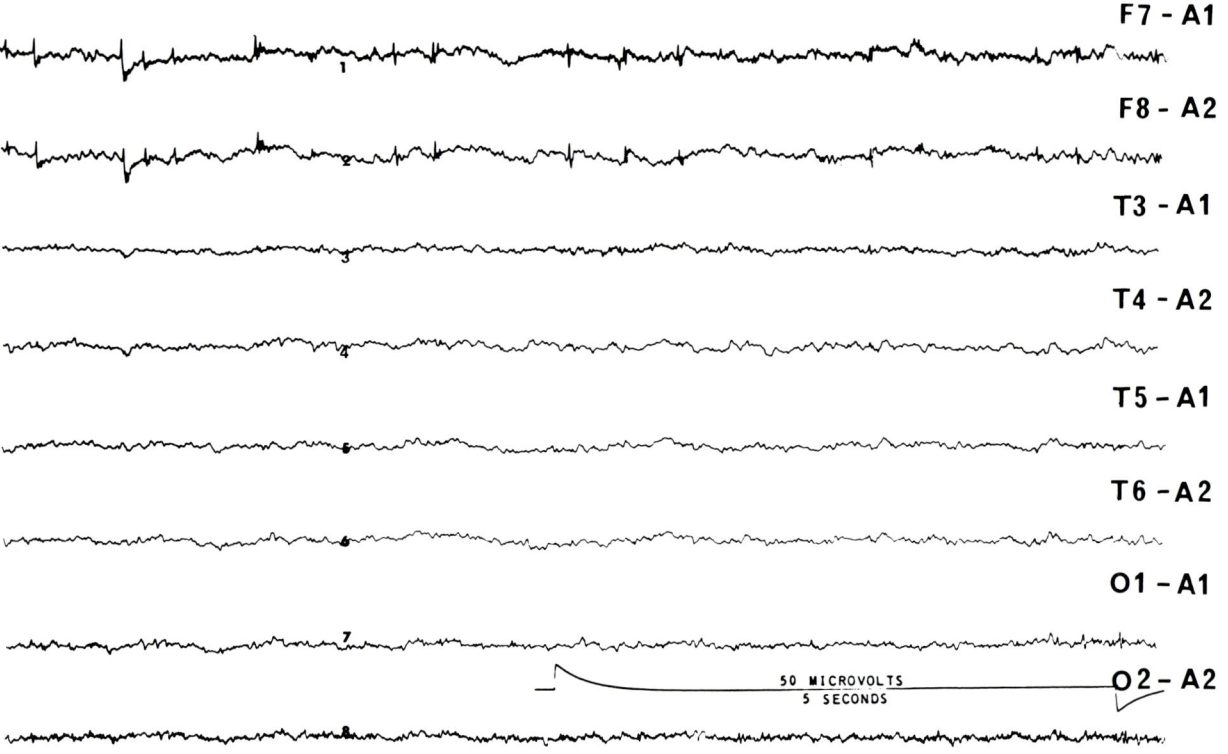

FIG. 10. Small spike-like myogenic discharges recorded from the F7 and F8 leads.

One of the most disconcerting forms of muscle artifact is seen in patients after acute cerebral anoxic episodes when intense shivering or decerebrate rigidity has set in. Since the EEG may be of critical diagnostic or prognostic value, it is essential to completely suppress the artifact. In such cases, succinylcholine or curare administered intravenously with assisted breathing of pure oxygen may be given during the recording (5). The improvement in ability to read the EEG patterns or discern their absence is dramatic (see also Chapter 7). An example of the use of the muscle relaxant is shown in Fig. 12A and B.

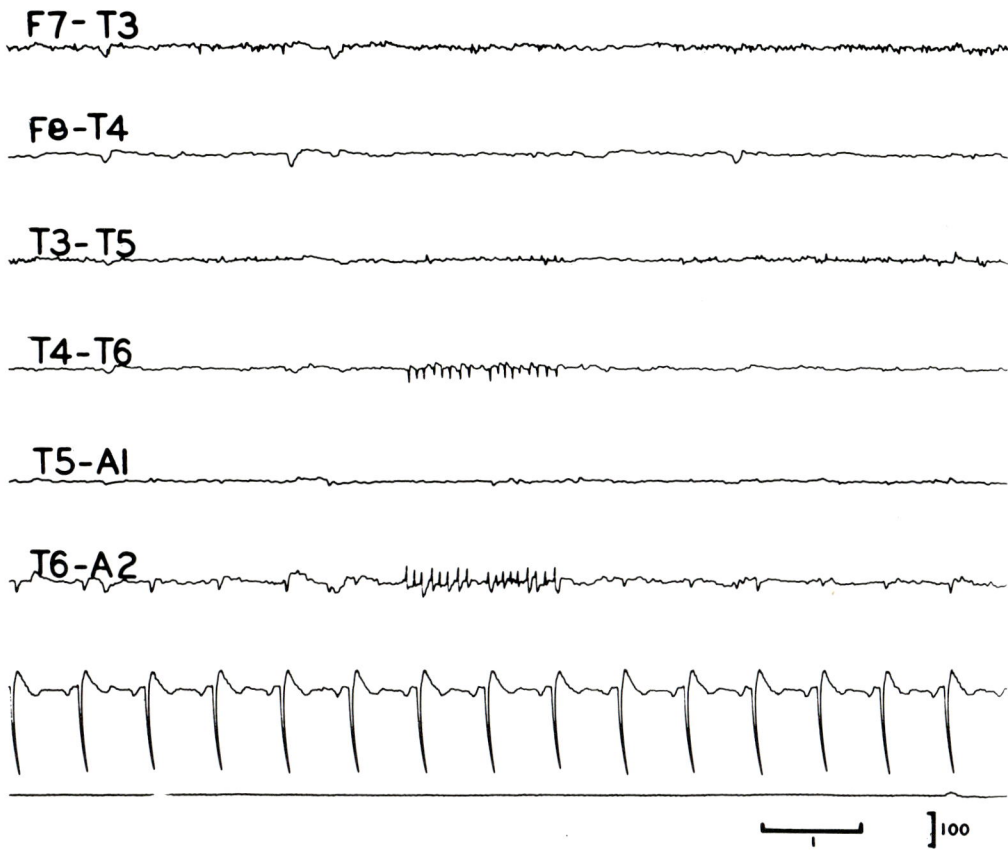

FIG. 11. A burst of myogenic "spikes" localized to a single electrode (T6) position. In the lower right-hand corner the horizontal line indicates 1 sec, and the vertical line indicates 100 μV for the upper six channels. EKG is recorded in channel 7.

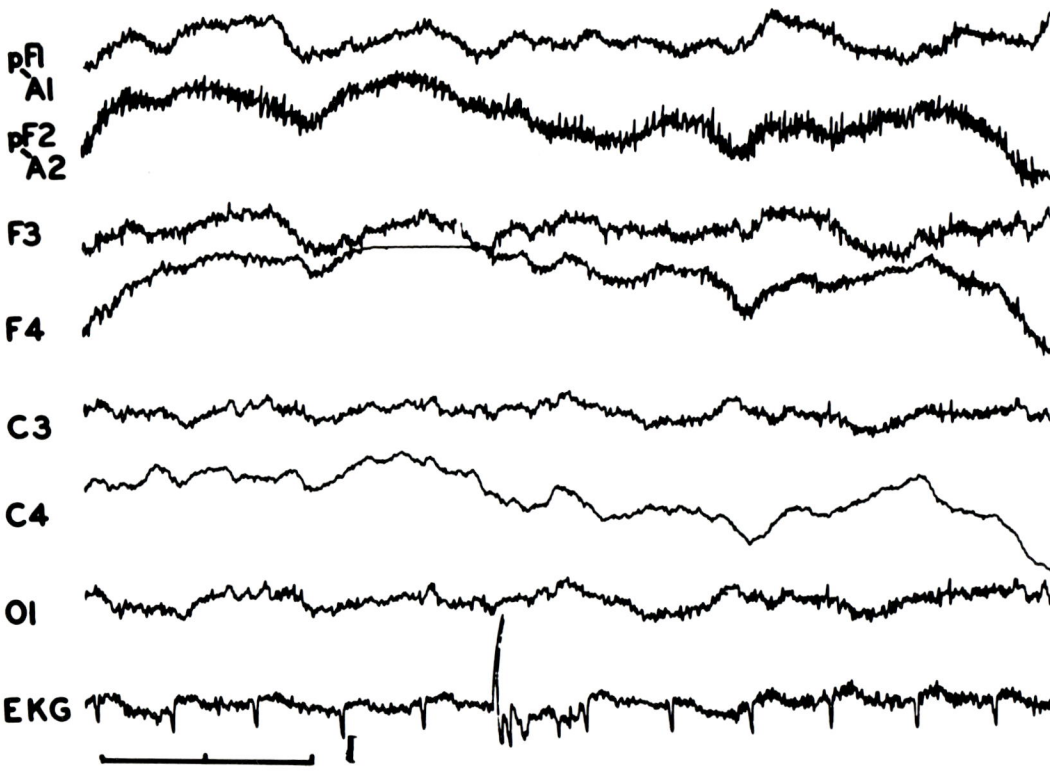

FIG. 12A. A recording from a moribund patient in the ICU. ECS was being questioned. The muscle artifact makes accurate assessment of EEG activity impossible. In this figure as in **B,** A1 is the reference lead in input terminal 2 of channels 1,3,5, and 7, and A2 is the reference for channels 2,4, and 6.

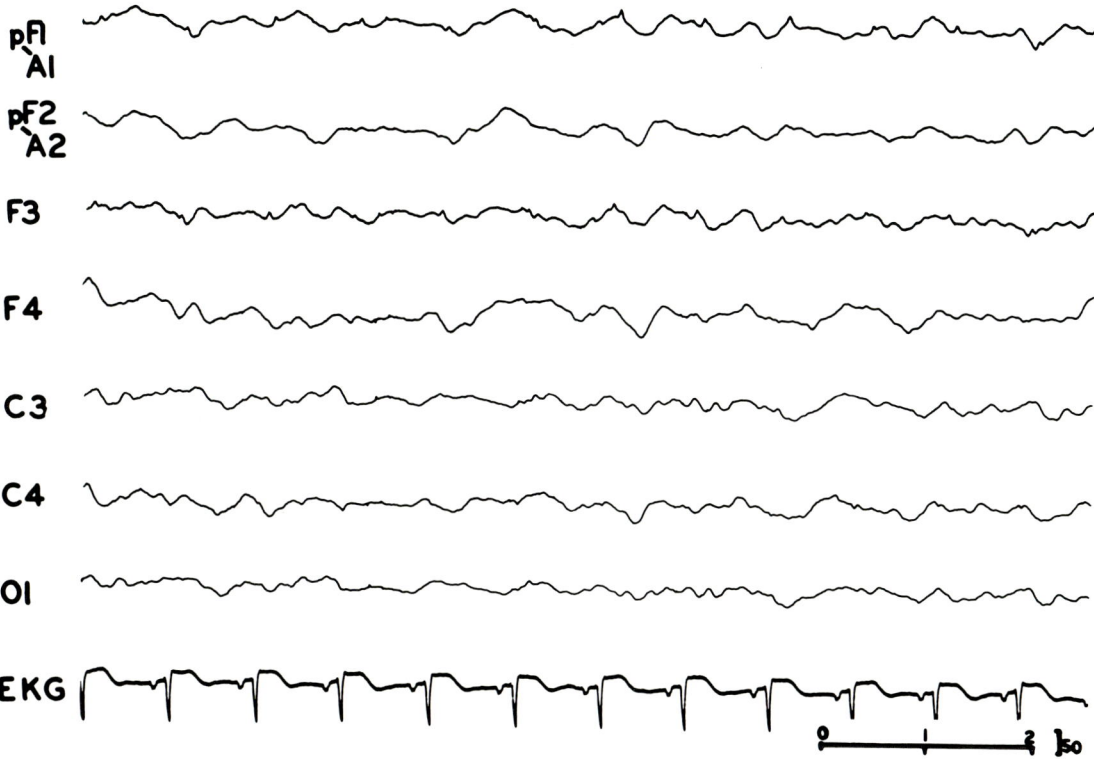

FIG. 12B. A recording from the same patient as in **A** after succinylcholine given intravenously has completely abolished the muscle artifact, thereby permitting demonstration of the brain activity. A mechanical respirator was used throughout the procedure. Time and amplitude indicators are the same for **A** and **B**.

Eye Artifacts

These are from three sources—eyelid movement, eyeball movement, and the electroretinogram. The last is usually of little consequence in routine EEG practice.

Eyelid movement and eyeball movement are difficult to separate functionally, although separate potential processes are related to each. As is well known, closure of the lids reflexly causes upward rotation of the eyeball. However, partial lid closure, which is often associated with a slight tremor, can produce rhythmic theta-like activity in the frontal leads. In blepharospasm this effect can be very marked. Delta and theta range activity (Fig. 13) may appear in the frontal leads sometimes and even in the ear leads. The voltage distribution is the clue to the artifactual nature. It is greatest around the eyes and shows phase reversal across the eye sockets (13). The technologist should recognize the possibility of this artifact simulating frontal slow activity, particularly if it is rhythmic, and should watch the patient's eyes carefully and, if necessary, gently hold the lids closed and feel for eyeball movement (Fig. 14).

The most common and obvious artifact produced by the eyeball occurs with the normal eye blink. The exact cause of this artifact is not known for certain, but it is usually considered caused by rotation of the eyeball, which is electrically polarized between the cornea and retina. The eyeball may be represented as a small battery, electrically positive at the cornea and electrically negative at the retina. As this battery rotates the moving electrical field that extends through the surrounding tissues constitutes the source of the eye blink potential (14). It should not be forgotten that one-eyed patients produce a unilateral artifact (Fig. 15). One-eyed persons also produce unilateral eye tremor patterns (Fig. 16). The triphasic sharp waves of hepatic coma (Fig. 17) can look very much like the eye artifact, but show no phase reversal in leads above and below the eyes. Identification of vertical eye movement and its differentiation from true frontal-polar slow waves can be best achieved by recording Fp1 to A1, a lead below the left eye to A1, and the homologous derivations on the right. True slow activity of cerebral origin is in-phase in leads above and below the eyes. Eye movement artifact shows phase reversal.

Since the eyeball is a voltage source, movement in any direction produces electrical field changes. Lateral eye movement shows up best in the lateral frontal or anterior temporal leads. Since normal lateral eye movements tend to be jerky, their pattern is relatively easy to recognize. The lateral movement produces potentials of opposite phase and of highest amplitude in left and right lateral frontal regions (Fig. 18). With the eye movement deflections, there may also be electromyogram "spikes" at F7 and F8 from the periocular musculature.

Whereas normal small saccadic movements of the eyes may produce no noticeable changes in the EEG, nystagmus can produce rhythmic artifacts. The form of the artifact depends on the pattern of movement of the nystagmus (15). Since some nystagmoid movements increase on lateral gaze and may only be apparent then, bursts of rhythmic slow activity can be produced by the patient squinting sideways. The technologist and interpreter must be aware of this. Nystagmus artifact should be suspected as a possible cause of frontal and anterior temporal theta and/or delta patterns, particularly if the left and right patterns are out of phase. However, bear in mind that intracranial lesions can produce slow wave abnormalities *and* nystagmus. The complexity of patterns produced by nystagmus is further emphasized when it is realized that eye opening and eye closing may cause nystagmus to appear or disappear. The technologist should be taught to recognize nystagmus and to look for it.

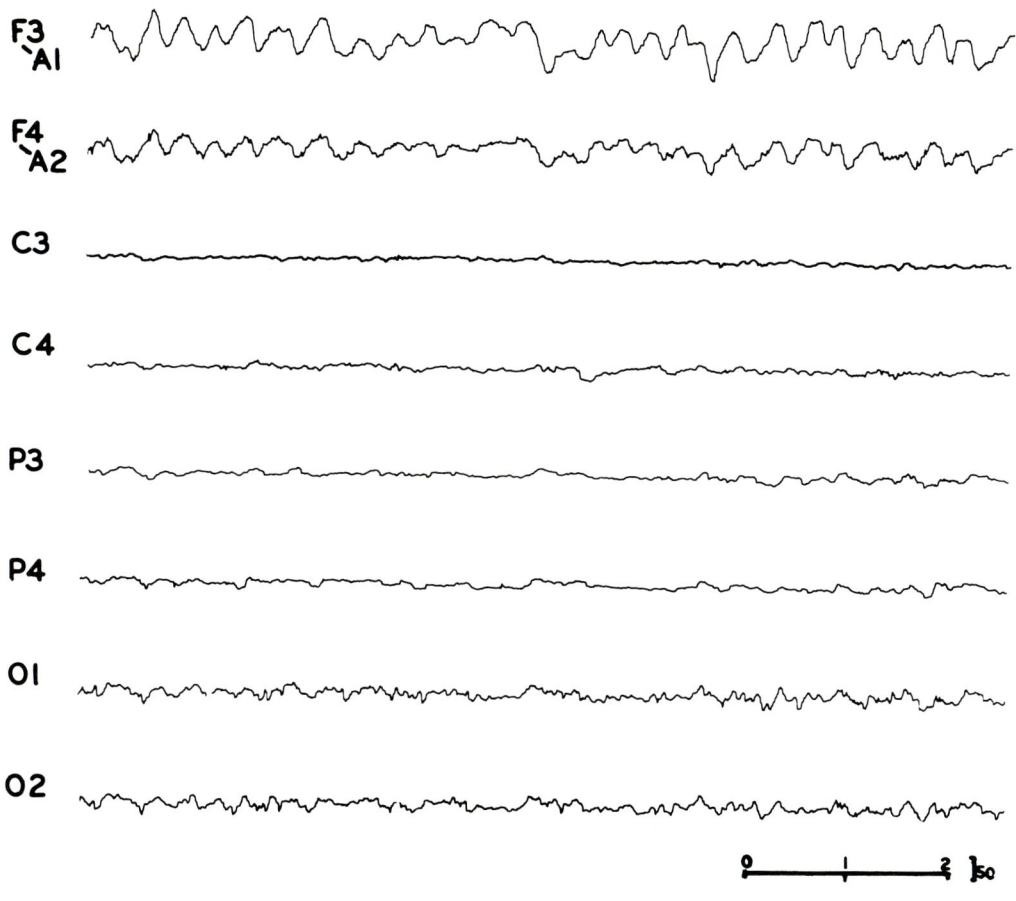

FIG. 13. EEG from a patient with blepharospasm. The artifact in the frontal leads closely simulates abnormal brain activity. A1 is the reference lead in input terminal 2 of channels 1,3,5, and 7, and A2 is the reference lead in channels 2,4,6, and 8. In the lower right corner, the horizontal line indicates time in seconds, and the vertical line indicates an amplitude of 50 µV.

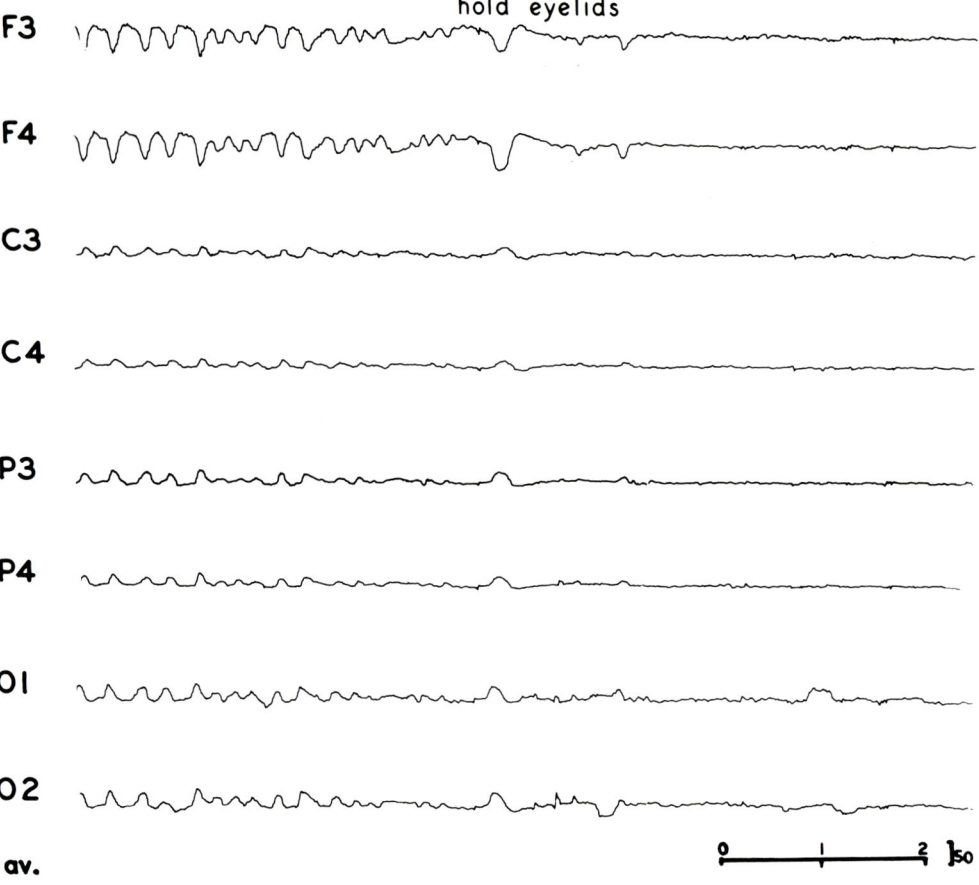

FIG. 14. Artifact due to rhythmic eye movement is abolished after the technologist holds the patient's eyelids closed. An average potential reference is used in input terminal 2 of each channel. Time and amplitude indicators are the same as for Fig. 13.

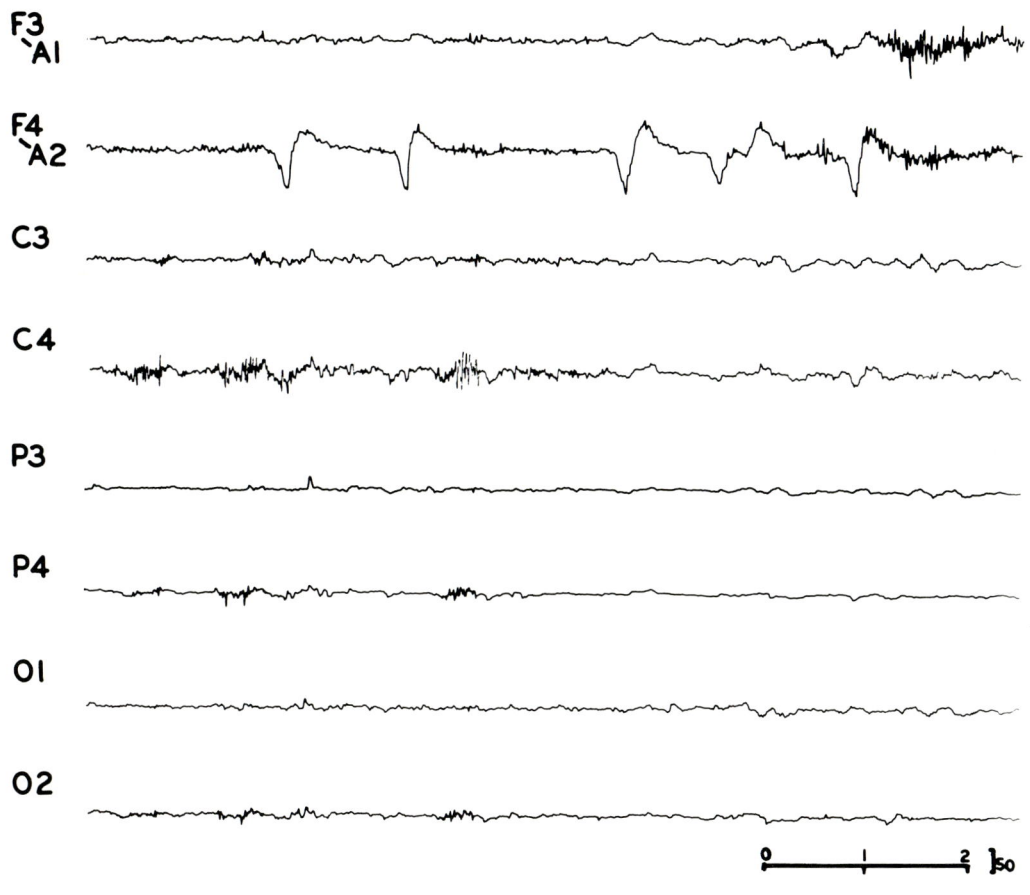

FIG. 15. Eye blink artifacts appear on the right side only (channel 2) in recording from a patient whose left eye had been enucleated. A1 is the reference lead in input terminal 2 of channels 1,3,5, and 7, and A2 is the reference lead for channels 2,4,6, and 8. Time and amplitude indicators are the same as for Figs. 13 and 14.

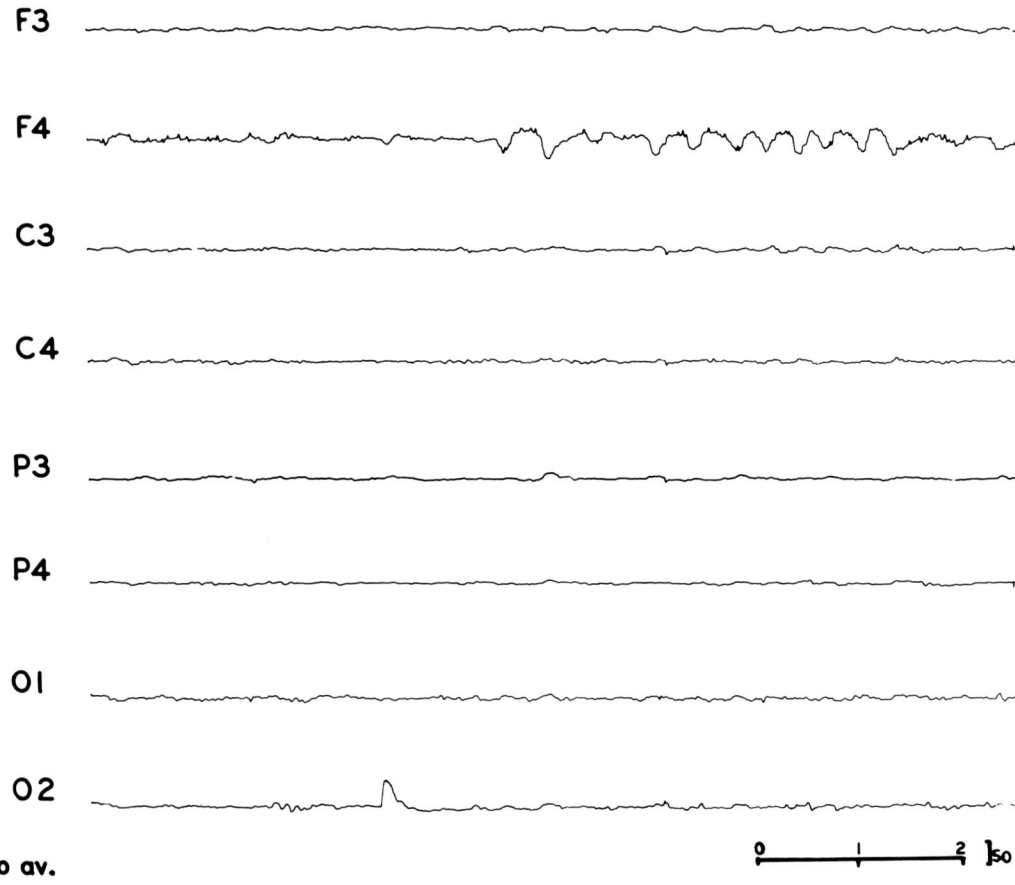

FIG. 16. Eye movement artifact producing unilateral frontal rhythmic slow activity (channel 2) in recording from a patient whose left eye had been enucleated. The single upward deflection in channel 8 is an electrode artifact (O2). An average potential reference lead is connected to input terminal 2 of each channel. Time and amplitude indicators are the same as for Figs. 13, 14, and 15.

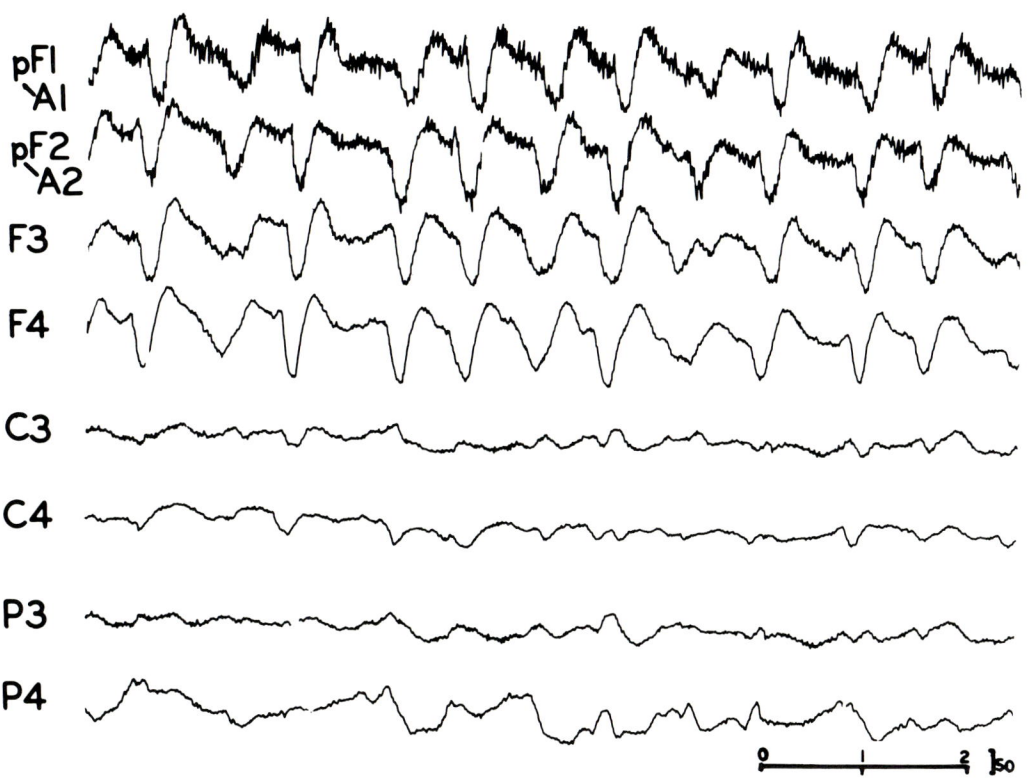

FIG. 17. Recording from a patient with hepatic coma showing frontal waves of cerebral origin that resemble eye blink artifacts. A1 is the reference lead in input terminal 2 of channels 1,3,5, and 7, and A2 is the reference lead for channels 2,4,6, and 8. Time and amplitude indicators are the same as for Figs. 13 to 16.

Tongue and Mouth

In the very young the most common artifact arises from sucking (16), presumably from lip and cheek movements and muscle contractions but also possibly associated with movement in the large potential field that exists in the mouth from the production, flow, and distribution of saliva. The artifact is usually recognized by the technologist, and it can be monitored by placing an electrode near the mouth or by using a "dummy" connected to a strain gauge.

The palatine muscles and pharyngeal muscles in cases of palatal myoclonus can produce spike-like discharges in the ear leads, but their rather typical very short duration should make one suspect artifactual cause (17,18).

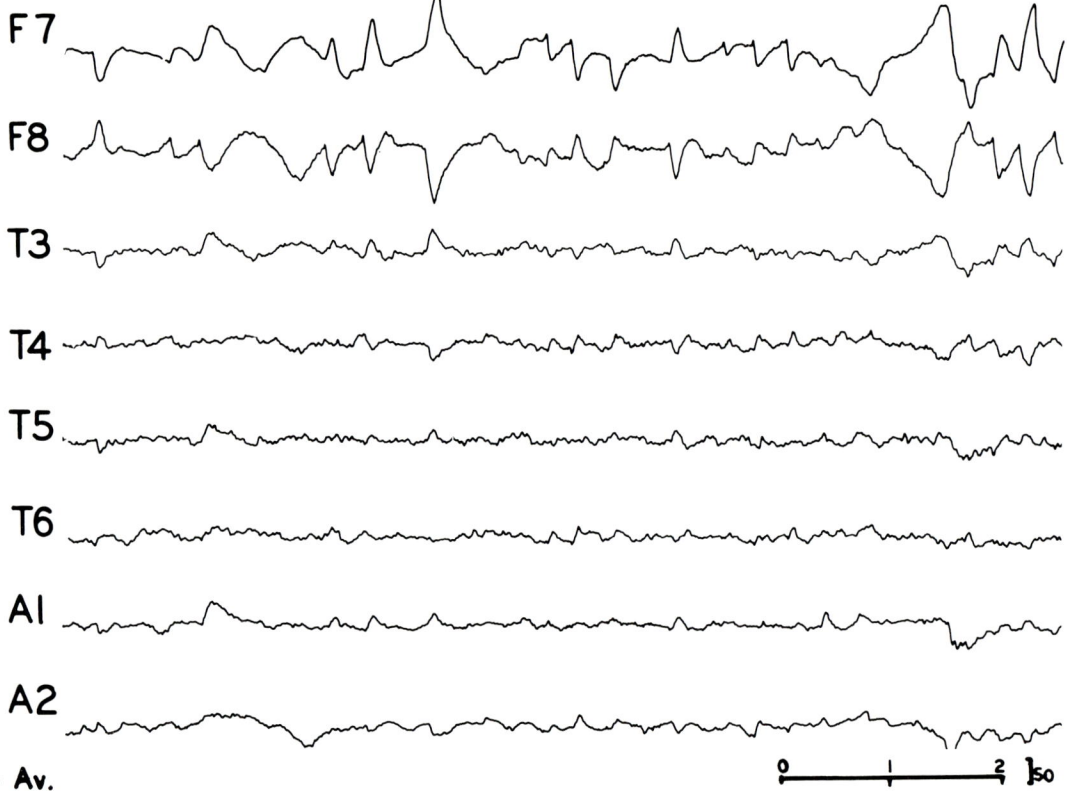

FIG. 18. Artifact from lateral eye movement appears best in F7 and F8 leads, and the deflections are out of phase in these two leads. An average potential reference lead is connected to input terminal 2 of each channel. Time and amplitude indicators are the same as for Figs. 13 to 17.

In the adult, movements of the tongue in the mouth, licking movements, and even movements of artificial dentures produce potential changes that distribute over the head and affect the ear leads predominantly (10,15,18,19). The patterns produced by tongue movements (glossokinetic potentials) are not always easy to recognize although they tend to be of very low frequency and may be associated with muscle artifact. They are usually distributed symmetrically on the two sides of the head, but if the movements take place more to one side of the mouth, lateral dominance of the activity may occur. It is probable that tongue movement artifact is more common and more often interpreted as abnormal EEG activity than realized. The technician should watch for tongue movement and if in doubt ask the patient to say "lilt" to see if the activity in question can be reproduced (15,18,19).

EKG Artifact

In some individuals, particularly those who are fat and have short necks, the EKG field is rather large over the head. An R wave of the QRS complex may appear in the EEG record. It is of highest amplitude in the A1 and A2 leads, and usually it is positive in A1 and negative in A2 (Fig. 19). Frequently, the artifact is of sufficient amplitude to be obvious, and it may inject into all channels with ear reference montages. Joining both ear electrodes may reduce the amplitude of the EKG markedly, but analysis of EEG abnormality can be more difficult. In young persons, sinus arrhythmia may produce great variability of the R-R interval, and the artifact can resemble EEG spike activity. The electrical axis of the R wave may vary with breathing so that the R wave may appear for one or two beats and then disappear for several. Again, intermittent cortical spiking may be simulated in this way.

The presence of the R wave artifact in the ear leads is usually only irritating as a superimposed but recognizable pattern, but sometimes, particularly when ear reference leads are being used, a confusing picture may result. An extrasystole artifact may superimpose on an alpha wave to simulate a sharp wave, or a small R wave may appear fortuitously in front of a delta wave and look like a spike-and-slow-wave complex. R wave artifacts that mimic temporal lobe spikes are uncommon, but misinterpretation of this artifact as temporal lobe abnormality is a serious error. Generalized dysrhythmic EEG activity may be simulated by a very dysrhythmic EKG. Every precaution must be taken to avoid such errors of interpretation, and the simplest and most reliable way is to record a simultaneous EKG in one channel (5,6).

Mixed Causes

A number of artifacts can occur due to interaction between instrumental and physiological processes. Some, such as sweat and electrode artifacts, have been referred to. Three other artifacts are noteworthy.

Pulse Artifact

When an electrode is placed over a pulsating artery or tissue, minute movements occur at the electrode–tissue interface. A sliding potential is set up that appears in the appropriate lead. This artifact has different forms, but that shown in Fig. 20 is typical. There is usually a steep upslope and slower delay, but the reverse may occur or the wave may be symmetrical. Use of very short time constants may convert this pattern to a series of short pulses simulating sharp waves. Usually the frequency and form readily identify the artifact. However, if the heart beat is irregular and/or the cardiac output

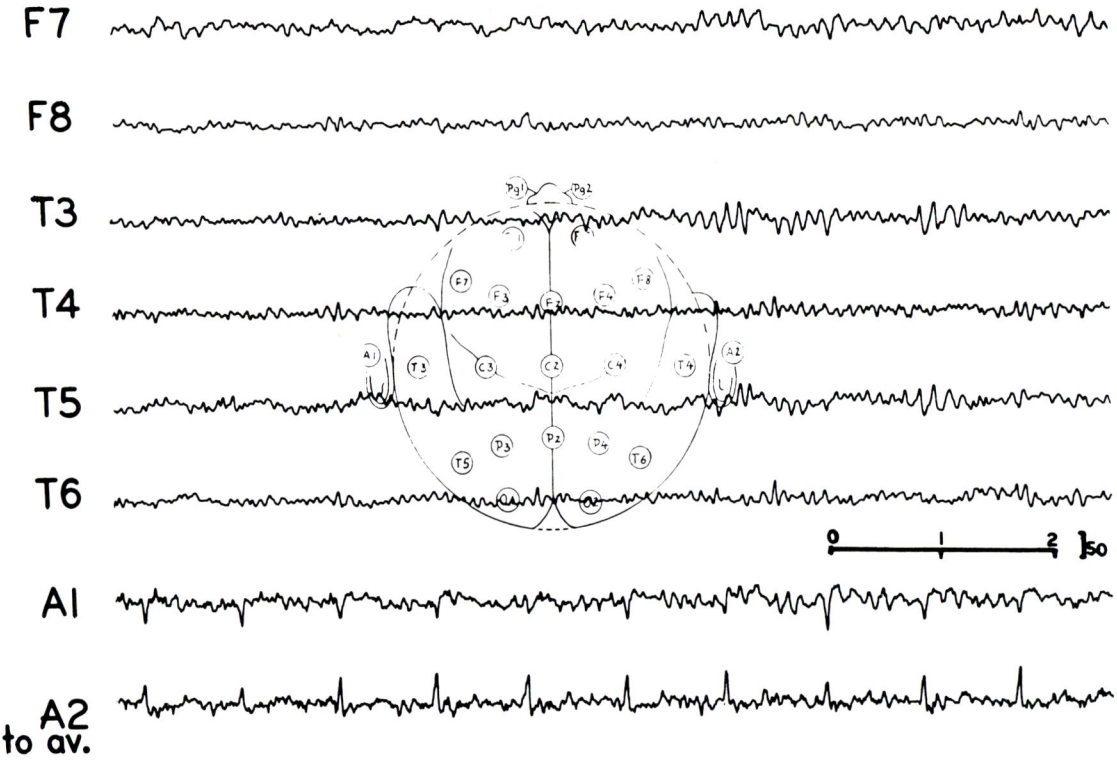

Fig. 19. Rhythmic artifact due to the R wave of the EKG is picked up in A1 and A2. Note the phase reversal due to the zero axis of the generator passing roughly through the middle of the head in most persons. An average potential reference lead is connected to input terminal 2 of each channel. Time and amplitude indicators are the same as for Figs. 13 to 18.

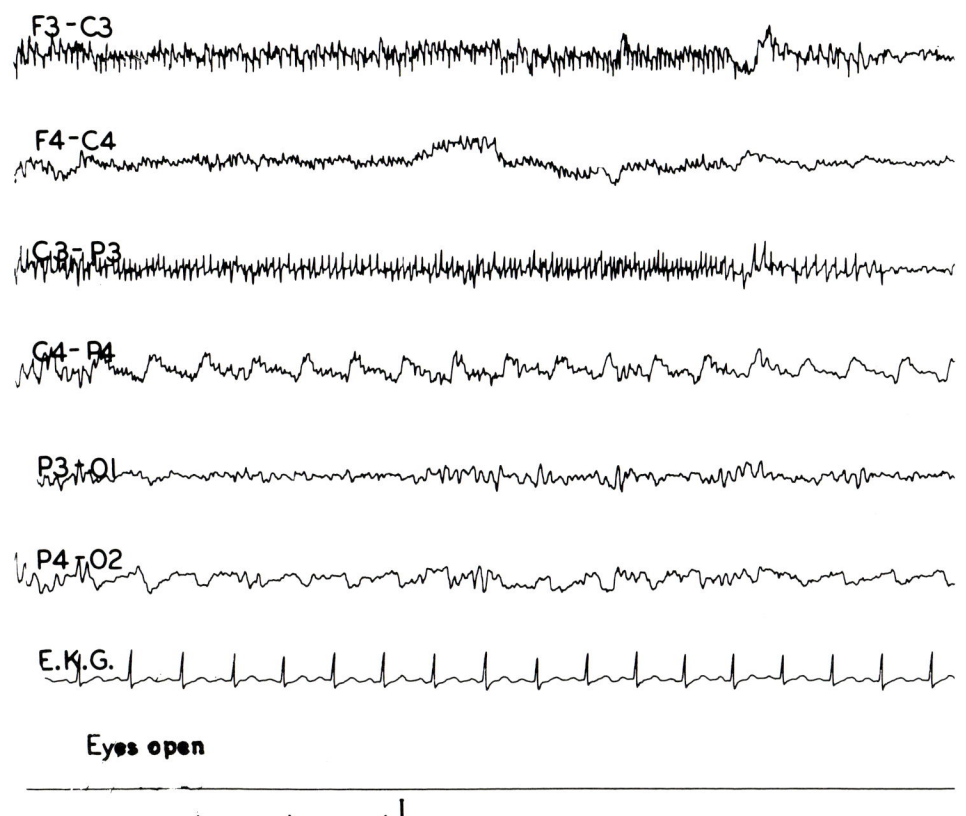

FIG. 20. An example of a pulse artifact (channels 4 and 6). The repetition rate is the same as the EKG monitored in channel 7. Time and amplitude indicators are the same as for Figs. 13 to 19.

causing the arterial pulse wave is irregular, the pulse artifact can simulate closely local delta activity of cerebral origin. The nature of the activity is identified with certainty by recording the EKG simultaneously, bearing in mind that the start of the pulse wave does not coincide with the R wave but is delayed by about 200 to 300 msec.

Ballistocardiograph Effect

This artifact is only seen when recording at the high gains used for detecting ECS (6). It is due to microscopic movements of electrodes or electrode wires from the recoil effect of the beating heart. Rhythmic activity of low amplitude is seen that simulates brain activity. The artifact is detected by simultaneously recording the EKG and noting its repetitive form coincident with each heart beat.

Respiratory Pump Artifact

Artifact generated by the respiratory pump in the ICU can also produce artifact that simulates suppression-burst type of EEG activity (5,20). This artifact takes many different forms varying from one to two rhythmic delta waves to short runs of activity simulating sleep spindles. Noting each respiratory pump action on the EEG can identify the cause in most cases, but stopping the respirator for 20 to 30 sec or hand bagging may be necessary.

Artifacts of Spontaneous Movement

A final group of artifacts to note are those produced by spontaneous and usually repetitive movements of the scalp, head, or body causing electrode and electrode wires to move (8,16). The most common causes are tics and tremors.

The tics usually cause simple muscle twitches, sometimes with superimposed slow waves from electrode movements. Should the electrode wires move, electric potentials can be set up in the wire to produce a further slow wave pattern at the end of the complex. Differentiation is made by noting the coincidence of timing and by the laterality—the side of the twitch is almost always the side producing the major artifact. With irritative cerebral discharges the EEG spike complex is contralateral to the twitch.

Rhythmic artifact due to tremor may be produced by an electrode wire moving in its insulation (a capacitive effect) and also by minute change at skin–electrode interface (a combined battery-resistance-capacitive effect). Frequently one lead tends to show the effect more than others. The lead that is most affected is fortuitous; but occasionally the artifact can appear in a lead that, on clinical grounds, one would expect to show abnormality. High electrode resistances tend to increase the amplitude of the artifact. Identification of the cause depends to a large extent on the technologist observing the movements, but also can be checked by having an electrode on a part of the body that moves but that is remote from the head. Simultaneous activity will be recorded. Parkinsonism is the most common cause of this artifact, and the most common frequency of tremor encountered in this disease is around 6 Hz, but lower frequencies can also occur. Frequencies higher than 7 Hz from tremor are uncommon.

CONCLUSION

There is little doubt that even the most skilled interpreter can be confused by the presence of subtle artifact mistakenly thought to be cerebral in origin or by cerebral abnormality that may be thought to be artifact. Identification is best made at the time of recording and requires technologists of ample skill, training, and experience. The electroencephalographer also should be prepared to go to the laboratory, to the bedside, or to the ICU to assist the technologist in the solution of the more difficult problems. The results of incorrectly calling a normal EEG "abnormal" because of failure of artifact identification are likely to be detrimental to the patient and may lead to further unnecessary tests, administration of inappropriate medication, or prolonged hospitalization. It is equally serious to err on the side of calling a record "normal" when abnormality produced by a lesion is overlooked or "written off" as an artifact. Obviously it is best, with the proper care and concern of the interpreter and the technologist, to attempt to identify artifacts. When uncertainty cannot be avoided, it is best to defer an opinion.

ACKNOWLEDGMENT

The editors are grateful to Shirely Oliver, R. EEG. T., Supervisory Technologist, Electroencephalograph Department, Health Science Center, Winnipeg, Canada for providing the prints for the illustrations used in this chapter.

REFERENCES

1. Cooper, R., Osselton, J. W., and Shaw, J. C. (1974): *EEG Technology,* 2nd ed., pp. 96–105, 148–155. Butterworths, London.
2. Kiloh, L. G., McComas, A. J., and Osselton, J. W. (1972): *Clinical Electroencephalography,* 3rd ed., pp. 47–50. Butterworths, London.
3. MacGillivray, B. B. (1974): "Traditional Methods of Examination in Clinical EEG, Vol. 3, Part C," In: *Handbook of EEG and Clinical Neurophysiology,* edited by A. Remond, pp. 88–109. Elsevier, Amsterdam.
4. Gibbs, F. A., and Gibbs, E. L. (1950): *Atlas of Electroencephalography, Vol. 1, Methodology and Controls,* pp. 324. Addison-Wesley, Reading, Mass.
5. Bennett, D. R., Hughes, J. R., Korein, J., et al. (1976): In: *Atlas of Electroencephalography in Coma and Cerebral Death,* Chapter 4. Raven Press, New York.
6. Oliver, S. (1973): Artefacts in EEG recordings in intensive and coronary care units. *Spike and Wave,* Special Issue, 9:23–45.
7. Redding, F. K., Wandel, V., and Nasser, C. (1969): Intravenous infusion drop artifacts. *Electroencephalogr. Clin. Neurophysiol.,* 26:318–320.
8. Goldensohn, E., and Koehle, R. (1975): *EEG Interpretation: Problems of Overreading and Underreading,* Section I. Futura Publ., Mount Kisco, N.Y.
9. Saunders, M. G. (1971): Physiological artefact. *Spike and Wave,* Special Issue, 4:58–77.
10. Brittenham, D. (1974): Recognition and reduction of physiological artifacts. *Am. J. EEG Technol.,* 14:158–165.
11. Johnson, T. L., Feldman, R. G., and Sax, D. S. (1973): Reduction of muscle artifact in electroencephalographic recording. *Am. J. EEG Technol.,* 13:13–25.
12. Espinosa, R. E., Lambert, E. H., and Klass, D. W. (1967): Facial myokymia affecting the electroencephalogram. *Mayo Clin. Proc.,* 42:258–270.
13. Bickford, R. G., and Klass, D. W. (1964): Eye movement and the electroencephalogram. In: *The Oculomotor System,* edited by M. Bender, pp. 293–302. Harper, (Hoeber) New York.
14. Peters, J. R. (1967): Surface electrical fields generated by eye movements. *Am. J. EEG Technol.,* 7:27–40.
15. Klass, D. W., and Reiher, J. (1968): Extracerebral uses for electroencephalography. *Med. Clin. N. Am.,* 52:941–948.
16. Kagawa, N. (1973): EEG recording in the neonate. *Am. J. EEG Technol.,* 13:163–176.
17. Joynt, R. J. (1959): An EEG artefact in palatal myoclonus. *Electroencephalogr. Clin. Neurophysiol.,* 11:158–160.
18. Westmoreland, B. F., Espinosa, R. E., and Klass, D. W. (1973): Significant prosopo-glossopharyngeal movements affecting the EEG. *Am. J. EEG Technol.,* 13:59–70.
19. Klass, D. W., and Bickford, R. G. (1960): Glossokinetic potentials appearing in the electroencephalogram. *Electroencephalogr. Clin. Neurophysiol.,* 12:239.
20. Sims, J. K., Aung, M. H., Bickford, R. G., Billinger, T. W., and Shattuck, C. M. (1973): Respirator artifact mimicking burst-suppression during electrocerebral silence. *Am. J. EEG Technol.,* 13:81–87.

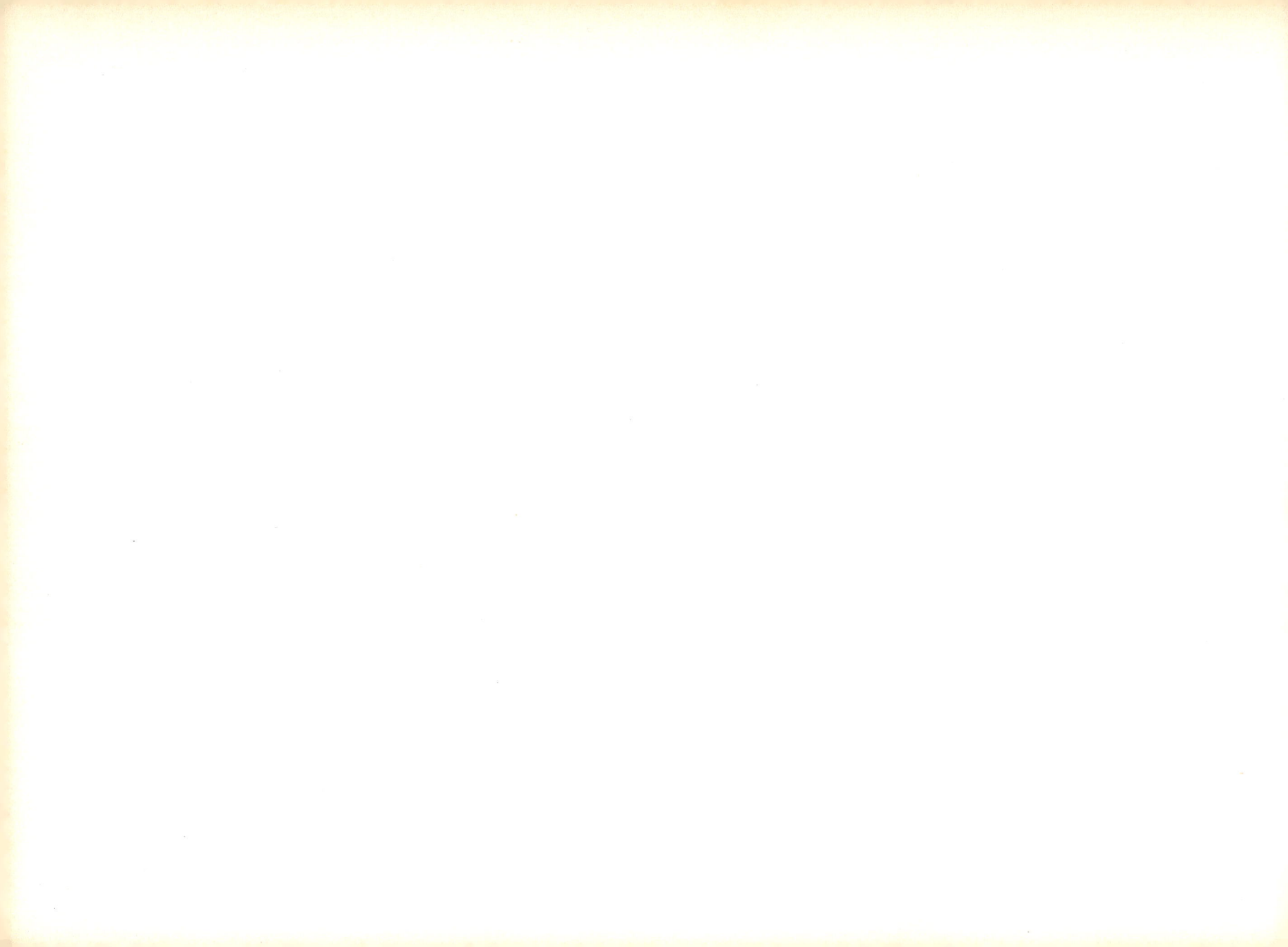

Chapter 5

An Orderly Approach to Visual Analysis: Parameters of the Normal EEG in Adults and Children

Peter Kellaway

Division of Neurophysiology, Department of Neurology, Baylor College of Medicine, Texas Medical Center, Houston, Texas 77030

Features of the Normal EEG.. 73
    Alpha Rhythm.. 73
        Normal Parameters of the Occipital Alpha Rhythm.................... 74
        Frequency of Alpha Rhythm in Children............................. 75
        Frequency of Alpha Rhythm in the Elderly........................... 76
        Alpha Rhythm Voltage... 76
        Regulation 77
        Locus 80
        Mu Rhythm.. 80
        Temporal Alpha Activity 80
        Bilateral Symmetry 81

Beta Activity	82
Beta Activity During Sleep	84
Frontal and Frontocentral Theta Activity	87
Posterior Slow Waves	90
Anterior Slow Activity in Children	100
The Ideal EEG	102
Lambda Waves	103
Temporal Slow Activity: A Normal Finding in the Elderly?	103
Hyperventilation Response	109
Activity of Drowsiness, Arousal, and Sleep	112
Activity of Drowsiness (Stage 1 Sleep)	112
Monorhythmic Slow Activity	112
Paroxysmal Slow Activity	115
Activity of Arousal	119
Postarousal Hypersynchrony	121
Activity of Sleep	124
Vertex Sharp-Wave Transients of Sleep	124
Spindles	127
Fast Activity During Sleep	132
Positive Occipital Sharp Transients of Sleep	135
Occipital Transients of Sleep	138
The Meaning of "Normal" and the Significance of Deviations from the Norm	139
Genetic Factors	140
Sex	140
Ontogenetic Factors	140
Metabolic and Homeostatic Factors	141
Sleep and Wakefulness	141
Psychoaffective State	142
Extrinsic Factors	143
Acknowledgment	143
References	143

Reading an electroencephalogram (EEG) should be a rational and systematic process involving a series of simple analytic steps that serve to characterize the electrical activity in terms of a consistent set of parameters. The data thus obtained are then subjected to a series of comparisons with data expected for the age and "state" of the patient.

Table 1 outlines the essential parameters used to characterize the various elements or activities of the EEG. On the basis of this cumulative analysis, it can be determined if the EEG is within the range of normal variation for age. If it is not, the characteristics of the deviation(s) from normal are specified.[1] The nature of the EEG abnormality is characterized first in general terms: diffuse, focal, lateralized, regional (e.g., bifrontal), or a combination of these. The character of the abnormality is then specified more precisely according to a schema similar to that in Fig. 1. Only at this point is the available clinical information incorporated into the analytic process. The EEG findings are correlated with the clinical information to derive a "clinical impression," i.e., an assessment of the probable significance of the EEG findings in terms of the patient's clinical history and findings.

In practice, the age and state of the patient are noted first, and this should be the only extraneous information required before the EEG is analyzed. The age of the patient is provided by the patient data sheet, which should be part of the EEG record.[2] The younger the patient, the more critical it is that age information be precise. In the newborn, age should be specified in days since delivery; in infants of 1 to 3 months, it should be given in weeks, and in those 3 to 36 months, stated in months. This progressively decreasing degree of precision reflects the fact that the landmarks of ontogenetic development of the EEG in the newborn are clearly differentiated in weekly or biweekly epochs but become progessively less sharply delineated with increasing age; for example, there are clearly defined differences between the EEGs of a premature infant of 35 weeks' and one of 36 weeks' conceptional age, but there are no important or sharply delineated differences between the EEGs of a child of 3 years and one of 4 years.

The "state" of the patient refers to the clinical assessment of the patient's general state of consciousness; this should be specified in terms of "alert," "lethargic," "stuporous," "semicomatose," etc., on the clinical data sheet accompanying the record. The patient's state also refers to the physiological variations of alertness and levels of sleep that occur during the recording, which are noted by the technol-

TABLE 1. *Essential parameters of EEG analysis*

1. Frequency or wavelength
2. Voltage
3. Wave form
4. Regulation
    a. Frequency
    b. Voltage
5. Manner of occurrence (random, serial, continuous)
6. Locus
7. Reactivity (eye opening, mental calculation, acapnia, sensory stimulation, movement, affective state)
8. Interhemispheric coherence (homologous areas)
    a. Symmetry
        1) Voltage
        2) Frequency
    b. Synchrony
        1) Wave
        2) Burst

---

[1] This specification should be incorporated into the EEG report as the "technical impression" (Fig. 1).

[2] Both age and date of birth should be recorded.

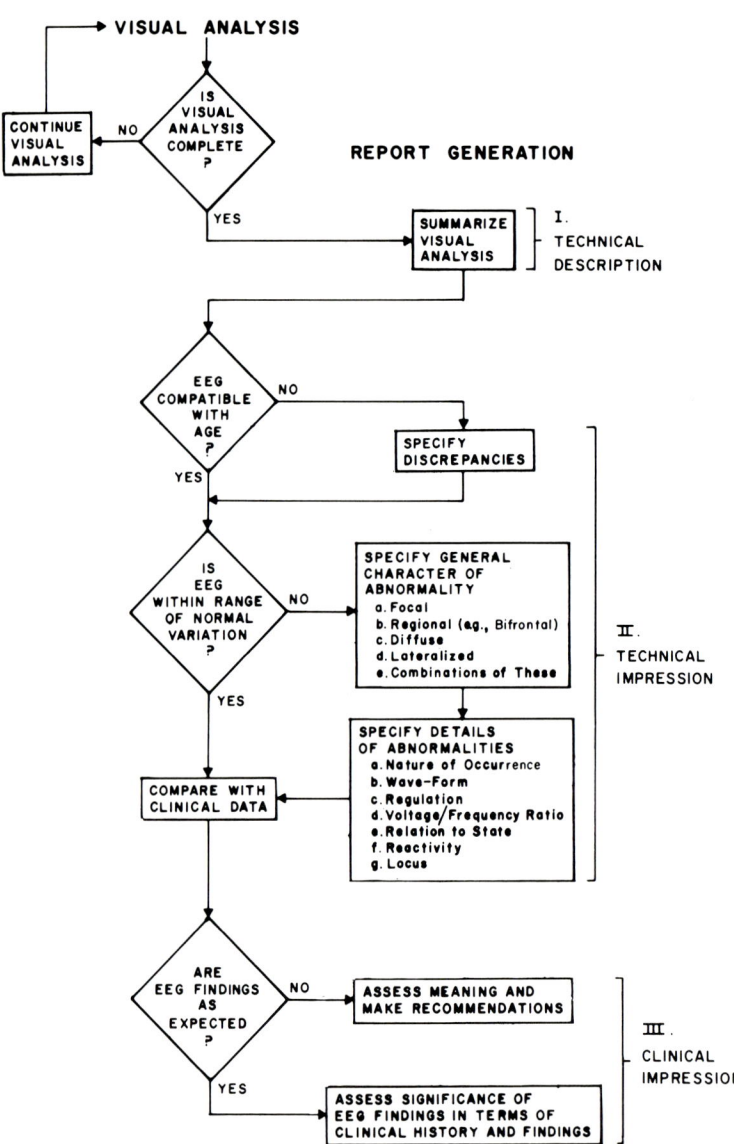

FIG. 1. Flow chart, illustrating the systematic process underlying generation of the clinical EEG report. Four steps are involved: (a) visual analysis of the essential parameters of the EEG (Table 1); (b) summarization of this analysis in the form of a technical description; (c) generation and statement of a technical impression, e.g., "Paroxysmal generalized 3-Hz spike-and-wave dysrhythmia, with no focal or lateralizing features, present only during sleep and photic stimulation"; and (d) assessment of the significance of the EEG findings in terms of clinical history and findings.

ogist. The importance of these data and their proper notation on the record is discussed in detail elsewhere in this volume.

Although these two items of information (the patient's age and state of consciousness) are essential to interpretation of the EEG, it is a good teaching exercise and a test of analytic acumen occasionally to read a record when only one or neither of these two items is known. Attempting to specify the age or, more easily, the physiological state of the patient according to the characteristics of his EEG activity sharpens analytic technique and subjective criteria.

The fact that *age* is an important determinant of the characteristics of the EEG has been known since Berger's early studies in 1932. The electrical activity of the brain, awake, asleep, and in response to stimuli, varies considerably with age; a particular activity or pattern that is normal at one age may be quite abnormal at another.

In the premature infant, the age factor is critical. In reading the records of such infants, the initial step is to pose the question, can the conceptional age (gestational age plus time since delivery) be determined from the characteristics of the EEG? Absence or distortion of features that normally make this possible is evidence of abnormality, as are differences between the maturational characteristics of the various stages of the awake/sleep cycle in the same infant (dyschronism). At the other end of the age spectrum, EEG features such as focal, episodic, temporal slow activity may be within the normal range for an elderly person but are clearly outside the normal range for a young adult.

The *state of alertness* or of altered levels of consciousness, physiological and pathological, is also a critical factor in EEG interpretation. The obvious situations are the well-known alpha-type record and the spindle sleep-like patterns that may be seen in comatose patients and that, in spite of their "normal" appearance, have precise pathological significance in the altered states of consciousness in which they may be found. Less well recognized are the dramatic EEG changes sometimes seen in young children in association with changes in affective state and with subtle physiological alterations of cerebral state that are antecedent to the onset of clinically evident sleep.

FEATURES OF THE NORMAL EEG

Before the various features of the normal EEG of adults and children are described and discussed, it is important to recognize that the identification of a particular activity or phenomenon may depend on its "reactivity" (Table 1). An important element of the recording and its analysis is the testing of the reactions, or responses, of the features of the EEG to various physiological changes or provocations. These include eye opening and closing, repetitive movements of extremities, visual scanning, sensory stimulation, and hypocapnia produced by hyperventilation.

Specification of the reactivity of a given activity, rhythm, or pattern is essential to the identification and subsequent analysis of the activity and may clearly differentiate it from another activity with similar characteristics. For example, occipital slow waves intermixed with the alpha rhythm that block with the alpha rhythm when the eyes are opened may be a normal finding in a child, but similar slow waves that do not block may be pathological. Similarly, a run of rhythmic, high-voltage, monomorphic 3 to 4 Hz waves in the frontal leads occurring in association with arousal may be normal in a young child, but a similar burst occurring spontaneously and not associated with arousal may be abnormal.

Alpha Rhythm

The occipital alpha rhythm should be the starting point of visual analysis. The initial question should be, is there an occipital alpha rhythm present, and are its characteristics appropriate for the age of the patient? If there is little or no occipital alpha rhythm, is it a result of the eyes being open (reactivity) or the patient's being drowsy or asleep (state)? Could it be an idiosyncrasy of a normal adult (genetic?); or finally, is it an abnormal finding?

Some individuals (adults, rarely children) who are apparently normal show no alpha activity, at least under the conditions of routine clinical recording. Other individuals, also apparently healthy, may show brief episodes of occipital alpha activity only during hyperventilation or, transiently, upon arousal from sleep.

In addition to providing clues concerning the patient's affective state (anxiety) or level of arousal, the presence and character of the occipital alpha rhythm are critical determinants in evaluating the significance of other activities present. Thus the presence of some low-voltage 5 to 6 Hz frontocentral activity in an adult may, in the transient absence of an occipital alpha rhythm, merely signify that he is drowsy; however, in the total absence of an occipital alpha rhythm, it may have pathological significance. Similarly, the meaning of the frontocentral theta activity would be more ominous if the occipital alpha rhythm were itself slow, e.g., 7 Hz. It is important to remember that the occipital alpha rhythm may remain unchanged in conditions that produce marked slowing of activity in anterior derivations. Thus slowing of the occipital alpha rhythm usually denotes a more serious change than if its frequency were maintained.[3] Conversely, preservation of the occipital alpha rhythm in the presence of marked slowing elsewhere usually is considered a favorable finding.

Normal Parameters of the Occipital Alpha Rhythm

The normal range for the frequency of the occipital alpha rhythm in adults is usually given as 8 to 13 Hz. The distribution curve for

---

[3] There are exceptions of course. A notable example is the slowing of the occipital alpha rhythm that may be the first sign of intoxication with phenytoin.

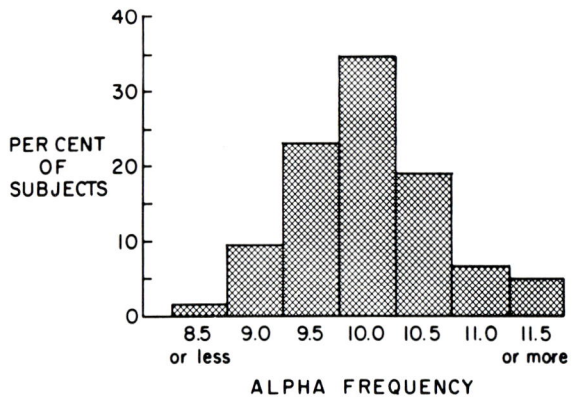

FIG. 2. Distribution of the mean alpha frequency in a series of 200 volunteer flight personnel, ages 24 to 35 years, on active duty in the US Air Force (144 pilots and 56 navigators).

the mean alpha rhythm frequency in a series of 200 selected adult males is shown in Fig. 2. Note that the incidence of an alpha rhythm as slow as 8 Hz is less than 1%. The maturational curve for occipital alpha rhythm frequency (Fig. 3) shows that the lower limit of the adult range is usually reached by age 3 years, and that there is generally a progressively slower increase in frequency with increasing age throughout childhood. The curve has an overall parabolic course, the rate of change diminishing after late adolescence. In late life, the frequency of the occipital alpha rhythm tends to decrease, and this change appears to be related to changes in cerebral metabolic rate (1–7).

Although population studies indicate that an 8-Hz alpha rhythm may be found in normal, asymptomatic young adults, in clinical practice this should always raise the suspicion that the alpha rhythm has slowed which, statistically, is more likely. It has been demon-

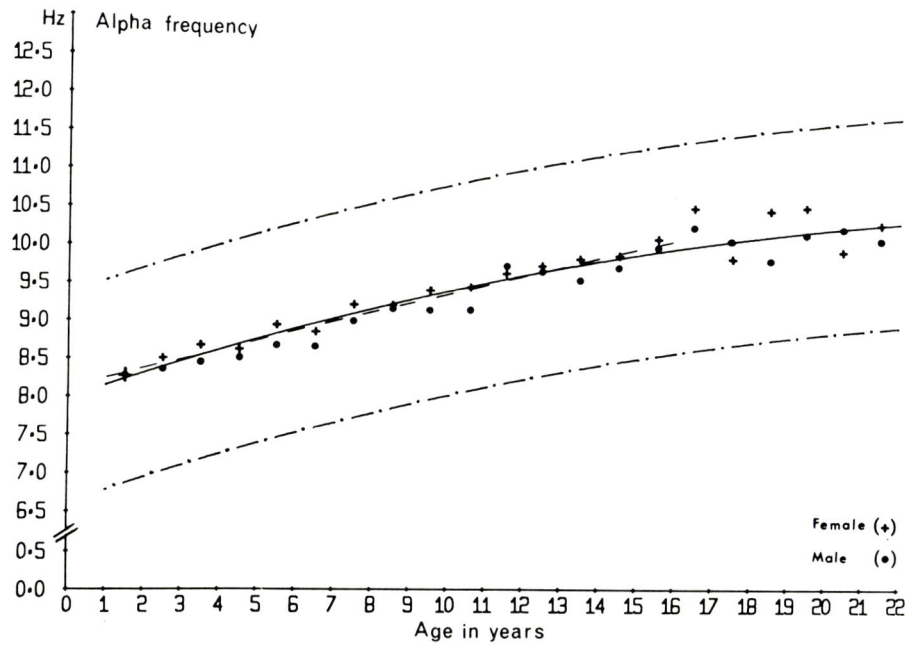

FIG. 3. Alpha frequency in relation to age in highly selected normals (continuous line). The diagram is based on a second-degree polynomial (parabolic function). The dot-dash lines indicate 95% confidence limits.

strated that the frequency of the occipital alpha rhythm is closely related to cerebral blood flow, and that if cerebral perfusion falls below a certain critical level, the occipital alpha rhythm slows. The relationship of alpha rhythm frequency to the adequacy of cerebral perfusion has been demonstrated repeatedly in patients with cardiac failure; pacemaker or cardiac implants often produce an increase in alpha rhythm frequency of as much as 2 Hz (8). As certain drugs (particularly phenytoin) approach toxic levels, the alpha rhythm slows without other changes occurring in the EEG. Thus if alpha rhythm frequencies are at the low end of the normal spectrum for age in patients on such drugs, the possibility of toxic effects should be considered.

Frequency of Alpha Rhythm in Children

The relationship of the occipital alpha rhythm frequency to age in normal control subjects is shown in Fig. 3. The curve fits a second-degree polynomial (parabolic function); the graph shows the range of frequencies encountered and the mean values for each age. Occipital rhythmic activity responsive to eye opening appears in approximately 75% of normal infants between the third and fourth months after (term) birth. Initially this activity is not well sustained and has a frequency of approximately 3.5 to 4.5 Hz. The alpha rhythm frequency increases rapidly, reaching 5 to 6 Hz in approximately 70% of children by 12 months of age. At age 36 months, 82% of normal term infants show a mean occipital alpha rhythm frequency of 8 Hz (range, 7.5 to 9.5 Hz). In infants and young children, the occipital alpha rhythm may totally block with the eyes open, and slower activity may be mistaken for the occipital alpha rhythm. For this reason, a portion of the awake record should be run during passive eye closure. An infant or very young child usually does not close his eyes until he becomes drowsy and is ready to fall asleep, and at this time, the occipital rhythm may slow considerably before disappearing. By age 9 years in 65% of controls, the mean alpha rhythm frequency is 9 Hz. In approximately 65% of controls by age 15 years, the mean is 10 Hz (9,10).

Frequency of Alpha Rhythm in the Elderly

Extrapolation from the parabolic curve describing the age/alpha rhythm frequency relation (Fig. 3) to determine the age at which the frequency of the occipital alpha rhythm might begin a decline suggests that the critical age is approximately 58 years (9,10). However, in healthy elderly individuals (70 to 85 years of age) the predominant occipital alpha rhythm still has a mean frequency of approximately 9 Hz (1–7). On the other hand, in this same age group, subjects with known organic brain syndromes consistently show a slower alpha rhythm, with a mean of approximately 8 Hz (1–7).

Alpha Rhythm Voltage

Absence of an alpha rhythm, or even a very low voltage alpha rhythm, is not encountered when recordings are made directly from appropriate regions of the brain in unanesthetized persons. Indeed, a striking number of alpha rhythm generators exist in the cortex and the depths of the brain, and they produce remarkably high voltage rhythms (11). On the other hand, the voltage of the alpha rhythm as recorded at the scalp occasionally barely exceeds the noise level of the amplifiers in apparently healthy individuals (12).

Recent normative studies showed that 6 to 7% of healthy adults have alpha rhythm voltages of less than 15 μV at the scalp (13). It must be kept in mind, however, when considering voltage characteristics of a given activity, that interelectrode distance is a factor that influences the actual voltage measured, depending on the size of the potential field and the position of the electrodes in relation to that field (Fig. 4). In discussing voltage, the electrode placements used in measuring the voltage should be specified. Using the P4–O2 derivation, 75% of a normal adult series were found to have alpha rhythm voltages of 15 to 45 μV (13).

Children rarely show low-voltage alpha rhythms (less than 30 μV). In their control group, Petersén and Eeg-Olofsson (10), using the T5–O1 derivation, found no children with voltages less than 20 μV; only 1.3% of the children had voltages of 20 to 30 μV, and each was more than 12 years of age.

In this same series, the average alpha rhythm voltage in children ages 3 to 15 years was 50 to 60 μV. Approximately 9% of the children of this age (predominantly ages 6 to 9 years) showed alpha rhythm voltages of 100 μV or more. High voltage should not, in itself, ever be considered an abnormal finding. However, paroxysmal bursts of 9 to 12 Hz activity having a wider areal distribution than the occipital alpha rhythm (Fig. 5) are abnormal (14). This pattern, associated with epilepsy, can be clearly differentiated from a normal alpha rhythm on the basis of its distribution, paroxysmal features, and lack of reactivity to eye opening.

The voltage of the occipital alpha rhythm diminishes with increasing age, probably in large part reflecting changes in the density of

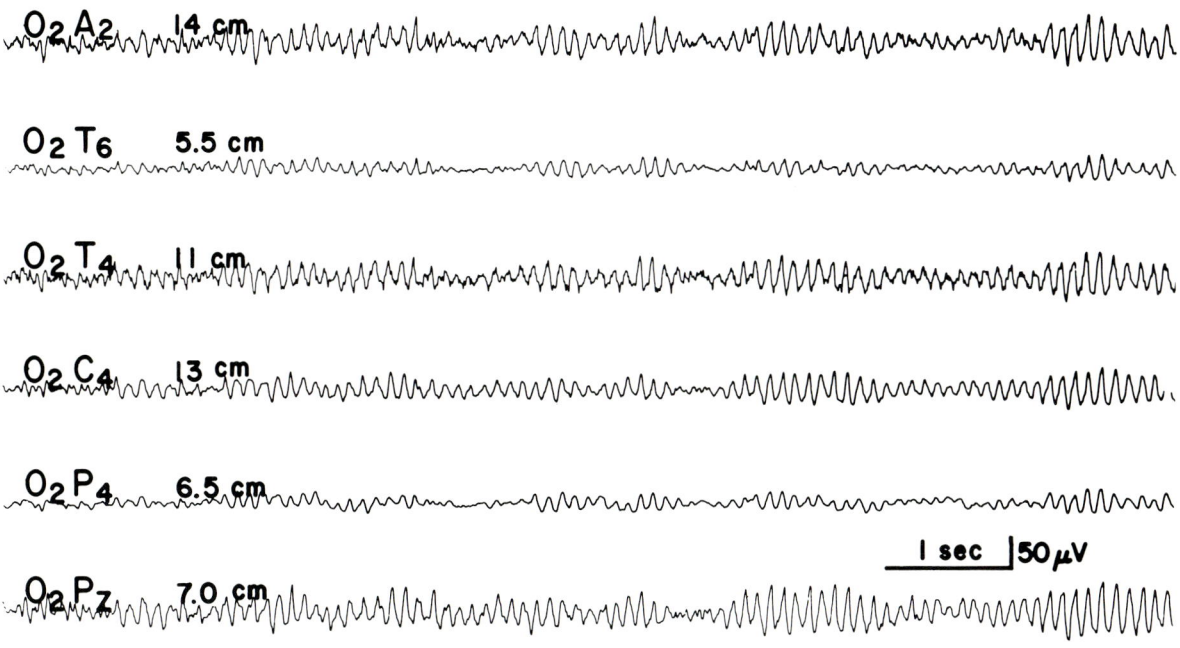

FIG. 4. Effect of interelectrode distance on recorded amplitude of alpha rhythm. Note that this is not the only factor determining amplitude; the geometry of the potential field is also a factor. This is illustrated by the fact that although the interelectrode distance between O2 and PZ is half that between O2 and A2, the recorded amplitude is actually somewhat greater.

the bone and increased electrical impedance of the intervening tissue rather than a decrease in the electrical activity of the brain. This impression rests on the observation that during electrocorticography, the voltage is not appreciably reduced in older patients who have shown low-voltage alpha rhythms at the scalp. The relation between EEG voltage and the impedance of the intervening tissues is discussed in more detail in the section that deals with bilateral voltage asymmetry (see below).

Regulation

Good regulation of frequency[4] and voltage[5] of the occipital alpha rhythm is characteristic of EEGs of approximately 80% of young

---

[4] "Good" regulation is defined in terms of frequency as follows: a sustained rhythm in which the mean frequency does not vary more than ± 0.5 Hz (as measured during any 2-sec epoch in which the activity is sustained).

[5] Regulation in terms of voltage refers to the smoothness of the envelope of the waxing and waning of voltage that the alpha rhythm typically shows.

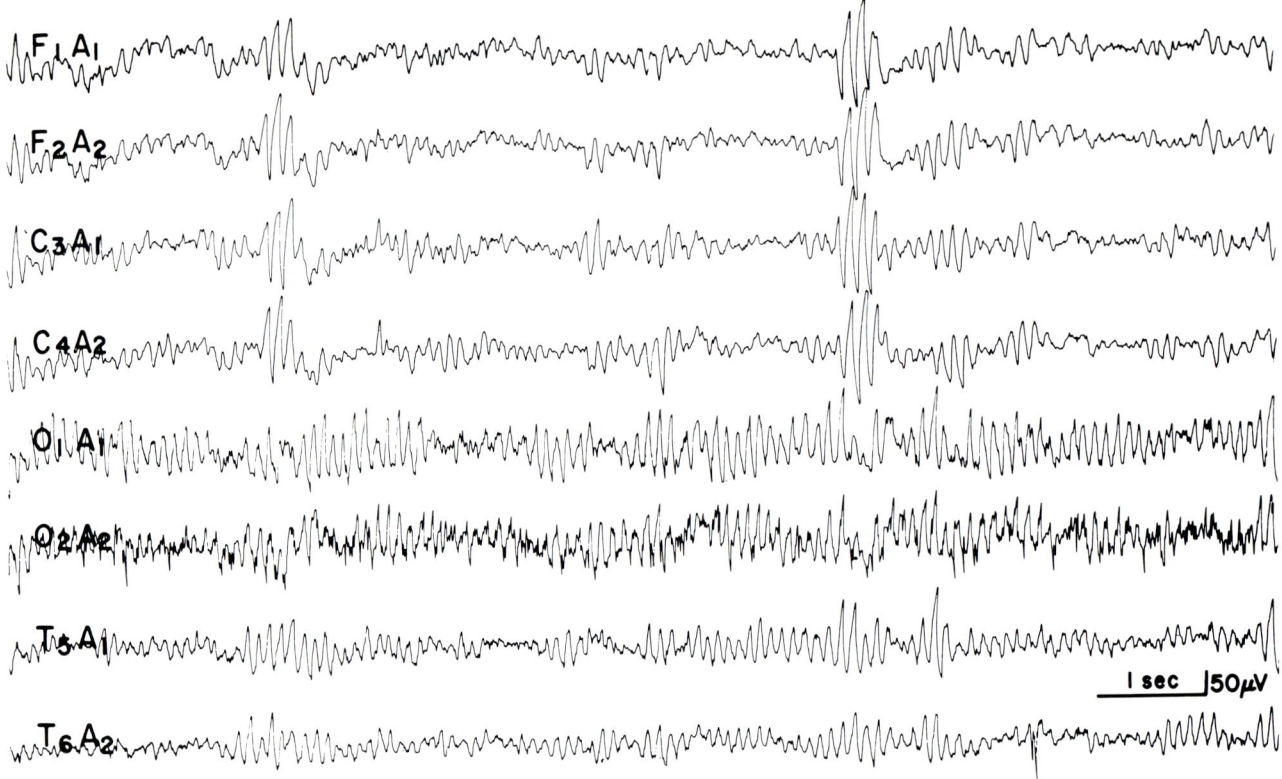

FIG. 5. Paroxysmal generalized 8-Hz rhythmic activity in 21-year-old male with generalized seizures. Clinical attacks were associated with an initial buildup of rhythmic, frontal-dominant but generalized, high-voltage, 8–10 Hz activity.

adults (9,10). With increasing age, there is a tendency for alpha activity to become less well regulated.

As mentioned above, the peak frequency of the occipital alpha rhythm is remarkably constant and, in healthy individuals, shows virtually no variation throughout the day or over long periods (15–18). Precise computer analytic techniques have indeed illustrated that the peak alpha rhythm frequency may increase in women during the initial phase of the menstrual cycle, but the change is so small

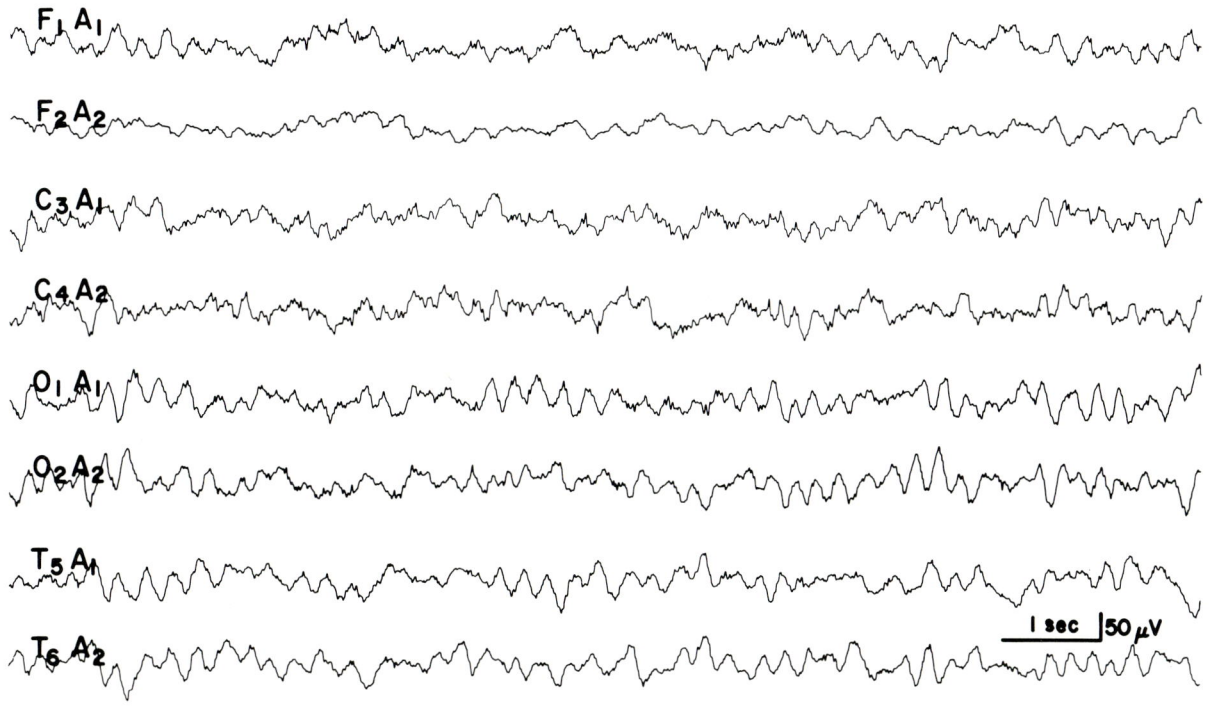

FIG. 6. Normal EEG of an awake asymptomatic 9-month-old infant, eyes closed. The almost monorhythmic occipital activity with little or smoothly contoured amplitude modulation is typical of the age group 4 to 24 months.

(+ 0.3 Hz) it escapes notice with routine visual analysis (15–18). The *stability* of frequency regulation of the alpha rhythm does fluctuate somewhat throughout the day and in relation to certain physiological changes (e.g., the menstrual cycle). Regulation is also affected in some individuals by mental activity and anxiety. Thus the general comments concerning "regulation" of the alpha rhythm refer to conditions of recording that approach the optimal conditions for "good" regulation: a quiet, nonstressful environment, eyes closed, the subject at rest but still alert.

Both voltage and frequency regulation of the occipital alpha rhythm are good from the ages of approximately 6 months through 3 years. During this age period, the occipital activity may be almost monorhythmic, and the voltage variation is usually smoothly contoured (Fig. 6). From ages 3 to 14 years, poor regulation (particularly of voltage) is common in normal subjects, and the regulation in approximately 33% of individuals in this age group is poorer on the low-voltage side (9,10).

Locus

The occipital region is the site of maximal alpha rhythm voltage in 70% of adults and 95% of children. During late life, the maximal voltage may be temporal in asymptomatic individuals; and in some elderly subjects, the maximal voltage may be in the central region. Some evidence suggests that central alpha activity, with little or no occipital alpha rhythm, may be an abnormal finding during late middle age and old age.

There are at least three independent rhythms of alpha activity frequency that may be recorded from the scalp in normal individuals. In addition to the generally predominant occipital rhythm, there are often clearly differentiable temporal and central rhythms. These independent rhythms may, and usually do, have mean frequencies close to that of the occipital alpha rhythm, but there are sometimes differences of up to 2 Hz in normal individuals.

Mu Rhythm

The mu rhythm,[6] a central rhythm of alpha activity frequency (usually 8 to 10 Hz) (Fig. 7), is present in approximately 19% of young adults (13). It is less common in the elderly and in children. A well-defined mu rhythm occurs in only 5% of normal children less than 4 years of age, and the incidence increases little up to the age of 8 years. Between 8 and 16 years, the incidence increases from 7% to the adult figure of 18%. It is more common in females than males throughout childhood and adolescence (the incidence is approximately twice as great in females at age 14) (9,10).

The voltage characteristics of the mu rhythm resemble those of the occipital alpha rhythm. The mu rhythm does not block with eye opening but blocks unilaterally with movement of the opposite extremity. Its presence relates to the level of attention and is enhanced by immobility (19).

In infants in whom the occipital "alpha" rhythm is still only 4 to 7 Hz, a low-voltage, fairly well organized and sustained activity of 8 to 9 Hz may be present in central regions. However, it lacks the characteristic wave form of mu rhythms and may or may not be ontogenetically related to them. This activity can best be seen with the derivation C3–C4.

Temporal Alpha Activity

Independent, low-voltage rhythms of alpha activity frequency also occur in the scalp EEG recorded from the temporal region. In the elderly, these rhythms may have a higher voltage than the occipital alpha rhythm, and the activity may tend to occur in runs or bursts that are sometimes quite asynchronous on the two sides. This temporal alpha activity often persists during drowsiness, after the occipital alpha rhythm has disappeared.

Enhancement of temporal alpha activity in the elderly may be associated with the normal aging process, or it might be a sign of altered function of some subtle brain processes not evident on routine clinical evaluation. We consider this activity within the range of

---

[6] Synonymous with wicket, comb, and arcade rhythms and *rythme en arceaux,* these names were derived from the distinctive wave form of this activity. The Greek letter mu (μ) now designates this rhythm because the symbol resembles the wave form and conforms with the practice of using Greek letters to name specific EEG activities.

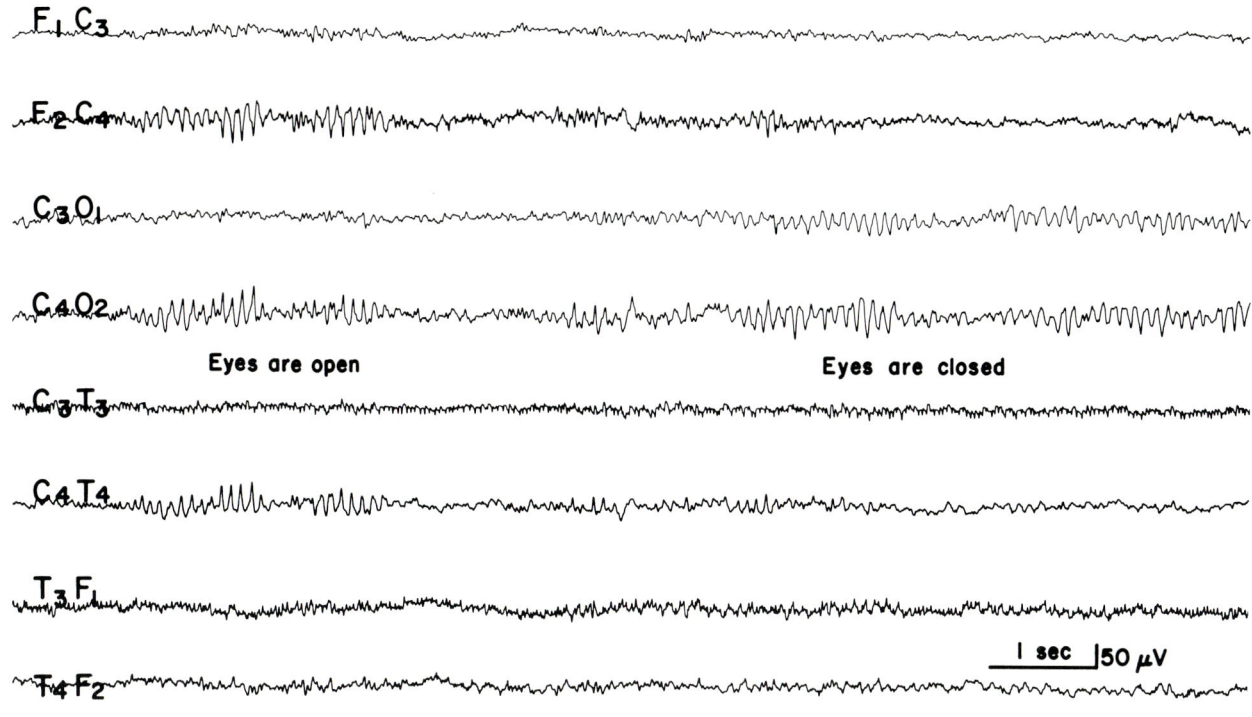

FIG. 7. Episode of mu rhythm occurring during a period when eyes are open and occipital alpha rhythm is blocked. EEG of asymptomatic 25-year-old female. Mu-rhythm asymmetries of this degree are not uncommon in normal subjects.

normal variation (see discussion of temporal slow activity in the elderly).

Bilateral Symmetry

Asymmetry of occipital alpha rhythm voltage on the two sides occurs in 60% of adults; in 50%, the right side shows the higher voltage (without consistent correlation with handedness). The asymmetry between sides is generally less than 20%,[7] and only 17% of normal adults show differences greater than this. In only 1.5% is the asymmetry more than 50% (13).

---

[7] The difference between the two sides, expressed as the percent of the high side.

In practice, asymmetry of 50% or more should be regarded as clinically significant until proved otherwise. An additional consideration is the side of the low voltage. As there is a statistical probability that the alpha has a higher voltage on the right side in a given individual, asymmetries of 35 to 50% should be considered suspicious if the right side has the low voltage.

In 95% of normal children, the alpha rhythm voltage has an asymmetry between sides of up to 20%. In 98% of these children, the lower voltage is on the left side, and there is no relationship to handedness. In the 5% of children with asymmetries of more than 20%, none showed a difference of more than 50%. The same rule mentioned above for adults should be used in the assessment of asymmetries in children when the low voltage appears on the right side, for the likelihood that the right side should be the high side is 98:2 (9,10).

A difference in the thickness of the skull on the two sides may be a major factor in determining the presence of voltage asymmetry. Using an ultrasonic-pulse technique, it was shown that differences in skull thickness of more than 33% in homologous regions of the two sides may occur in normal individuals; the left is more commonly the thicker side (in approximately 72% of cases). Differences of skull thickness of this degree can account for voltage asymmetries of 20 to 70% (20). Thus difference of bone thickness on the two sides not only accounts for asymmetries encountered in normal subjects but may mask or simulate abnormality. In the absence of actual measurements of bone thickness, asymmetries of less than 50% must be regarded as being of doubtful diagnostic significance. Special vigilance should be kept for the presence of subgaleal swelling due to hematoma, leakage during an infusion into a scalp vein, etc., as these also greatly reduce the apparent voltage of the EEG activity recorded by overlying electrodes.

Asymmetry of the mu and temporal alpha activity is the rule rather than the exception, and predominance of the activity on one side is not uncommon in asymptomatic individuals. For these reasons, asymmetry of the mu and temporal alpha activity should be interpreted with caution, especially in children. In prolonged (36-hr) and serial studies in children, the mu rhythm sometimes showed higher voltage on one side (even to the point that it appeared unilateral) for prolonged periods and then showed predominance on the opposite side (21,22). Such findings may well be significant in terms of subtle brain functions, but the clinical electroencephalographer should not conjecture about the presence of focal cortical lesions. Admittedly, there appear to be cases such as Gastaut et al. (22) originally described in which the mu rhythm appears to be enhanced at or near the site of a craniocerebral injury, but by far the greatest percentage of unilaterally predominant mu rhythms are not associated with evident cortical lesions. It must also be remembered that high voltage of the mu rhythm on one side may result from an underlying or subjacent skull defect (e.g., burr hole) that provides a low-resistance pathway for activity in cortex underlying the region of absent bone. Mu rhythms are often enhanced during and following hyperventilation, and this may further mislead the inexperienced electroencephalographer into an assumption of abnormality.

Temporal alpha activity in young adults is usually fairly symmetrical on the two sides. However, elderly persons, in whom the voltage of this temporal activity may be greater than that of the occipital alpha rhythm, may show alternating voltage lateralization; in 80%, the left side shows higher voltage. (This is discussed further in relation to temporal slow activity in the elderly.)

Beta Activity

Activities with frequencies higher than 13 Hz are commonly present in the EEGs of normal adults and children. Three distinct frequency bands in the beta activity range may be distinguished: a common 18 to 25 Hz band, a less common 14 to 16 Hz band, and a rare 35 to 40 Hz band. High-voltage activity in the first two frequency bands is present at the cortex in unanesthetized man, particularly in the pre- and postrolandic cortex. This fast activity is greatly attenuated in the scalp EEG, and in 97 to 98% of normal adults and children, the voltage in the awake EEG is less than 20 μV; in 70% it is 10 μV or less (recorded between closely spaced scalp electrodes) (9,10,13).

Beta activity with a voltage of 25 μV or more is usually regarded as abnormal in the clinical EEG. Although statistically such findings are outside the range of normal variation, little is known about the significance of high-voltage beta activity. The early literature documents a significantly higher percentage of "fast" EEGs in epileptic individuals than in normal controls and implies that a fast EEG (a record having much beta activity with a voltage of 25 μV or more) may be considered supportive evidence for a diagnosis of epilepsy. The fact is, however, that "fast" EEGs also occur with a greater incidence than in normal controls in a number of other, nonepileptic conditions (23–25), and fast EEGs have no correlation with epilepsy in children (26–30).

The presence of beta activity at amplitudes of 25 μV or more is currently of little or no diagnostic utility (except when drug ingestion is suspected). Thus if a patient with a differential diagnosis of syncope versus epilepsy is referred for EEG studies, the finding of excessive voltage and a prevalence of beta activity in no way clarifies the diagnosis. Similarly, the impression that high-voltage beta activity may have some specific significance for the diagnosis of "minimal brain dysfunction," dyslexia, behavior disorder, or hyperactivity has no established basis; the finding neither proves nor illuminates the diagnosis.

There is evidence that beta activity is a multifactorial genetic effect, with an age factor responsible for its penetrance (31), but the relationship to age is complicated. For example, whereas beta activity is a predominant feature of the EEG of the premature and term infant, it is barely evident in the EEGs of young children. It may be increased in voltage and persistence in the precentral region in middle-aged and elderly females, but it tends to have a low voltage during old age, especially in males (1–7).

It should be kept in mind when evaluating beta activity that many commonly used drugs (e.g., barbiturates, benzodiazepines, chloral hydrate) increase the amplitude and thus apparently the "amount" of beta activity (32). Because the incidence of beta rhythms with amplitudes much above 20 μV is statistically low in normal individuals, the presence of such activity suggests the possibility of drug ingestion. Although the 18 to 25 Hz band is the one most generally affected, some drugs also increase the 14 to 16 Hz activity.

In the presence of skull defects, beta activity in the area of the defect or adjacent to it may be enhanced as a consequence of the low-impedance pathway. Defects of dura, bone, and scalp enhance beta activity more than other, lower frequency activity (33), which has led to erroneous identification of so-called "foci of fast activity" in patients with surgical or traumatic skull defects.

Beta activity of 18 to 25 Hz usually increases in amplitude during drowsiness, light sleep, and rapid eye movement (REM) sleep, and decreases during deep sleep. When a barbiturate or other beta-enhancing drug is administered to promote sleep during the EEG examination, the resultant fast activity increases with the onset of light sleep, markedly decreases during deep sleep, and then remains prominent after the patient is aroused. In sleep studies, this effect of sedation has been particularly pronounced in children.

Beta activity should have the same frequency on both sides; however, even in normal individuals, the voltage may display asymmetry: it may be as much as 35% lower on one side. Such asymmetries probably are largely explainable on the basis of differences in skull thickness, as described above for the alpha rhythm. On the other hand, a consistently low voltage on one side (with the difference between sides being greater than 35%) that is focal, regional, or hemispheric is often a useful diagnostic feature; it indicates cortical injury (e.g., acute contusion or ischemia, or the presence of a subdural or epidural fluid collection). Focal, regional, or hemispheric depression of beta activity may also occur transiently following a focal epileptic seizure. Beta activity is generally the first to show diminished voltage in the presence of a cortical injury or subdural or epidural fluid collection; its presence on the low-voltage side can therefore be helpful in assessing the significance of a voltage asymmetry of other background activity in the same region (if the latter is borderline in degree). In this regard it must be remembered that beta activity amplitude is particularly susceptible to the presence of subgaleal fluid, and special care should be taken by the technologist to note the presence of scalp swelling—its location, extent, and degree.

Beta activity, especially when frontocentral in origin, is predominantly out of phase in the two hemispheres; as a consequence, its amplitude is greater in the paired interhemispheric frontal derivation than in either frontal electrode paired with an "indifferent" electrode or with another adjacent scalp electrode (Fig. 8).

Beta activity in the 14 to 16 Hz band is usually most marked in the frontocentral region but may show maximum voltage elsewhere—even in the occipital region. The location of the maximum potential field does not appear to have particular physiological or pathophysiological significance. Beta activity in this band, when present, is usually enhanced by hyperventilation and indeed may become clearly evident only during this procedure. It may be present during sleep but should be distinguished from sigma activity, which by definition occurs only in bursts.

Activity in the 35 to 40 Hz band is rarely seen in clinical EEGs. When it is, it is observed only in adults and is reported to be associated with organic psychosis or "dull psychopathy" (34). It has not been reported in any series of normal adults or children.

Beta Activity During Sleep

The 18 to 25 Hz activity in the awake EEG usually is enhanced during stages 1 and 2 sleep, and tends to decrease during the deeper sleep stages.[8] In infants older than 6 months, the onset of sleep is marked by increased beta activity in the central and postcentral regions (35). The frequency of this activity is usually 20 to 25 Hz; in infants of 12 to 18 months (the age at which beta activity is usually maximally expressed), it may have a maximum amplitude of 60 μV (Fig. 9). This activity diminishes in both incidence and voltage with increasing age, and beta activity amplitudes exceeding 5 to 10 μV are rare after age 6 years. Again, the diagnostic utility of beta activity during sleep is limited. Focal, regional, or hemispheric depression (defined as being at least 50% lower on one side) of beta activity is a reliable indicator of abnormality, and it is usually accompanied by "depression" of other background activity on the same side. It is a sign either of cortical depression (contusion, ischemia, atrophy, or cystic defect) or of the presence of an intervening fluid collection somewhere between the cortex and the electrode sites. Conversely, high-voltage, generalized but anterior dominant, fast activity may be a sign of "brain damage." In children, a mixture of 18 to 25 and 14 to 16 Hz beta activity with sigma activity of 10 and 14 Hz may occur during sleep in a pattern that has been called "continuous

---

[8] REM sleep is rarely seen in routine clinical EEG recordings of adults and children because time and other factors usually do not permit this stage to be reached. However, when REM is recorded, beta activity equal to or greater than that seen in the awake record is usually present.

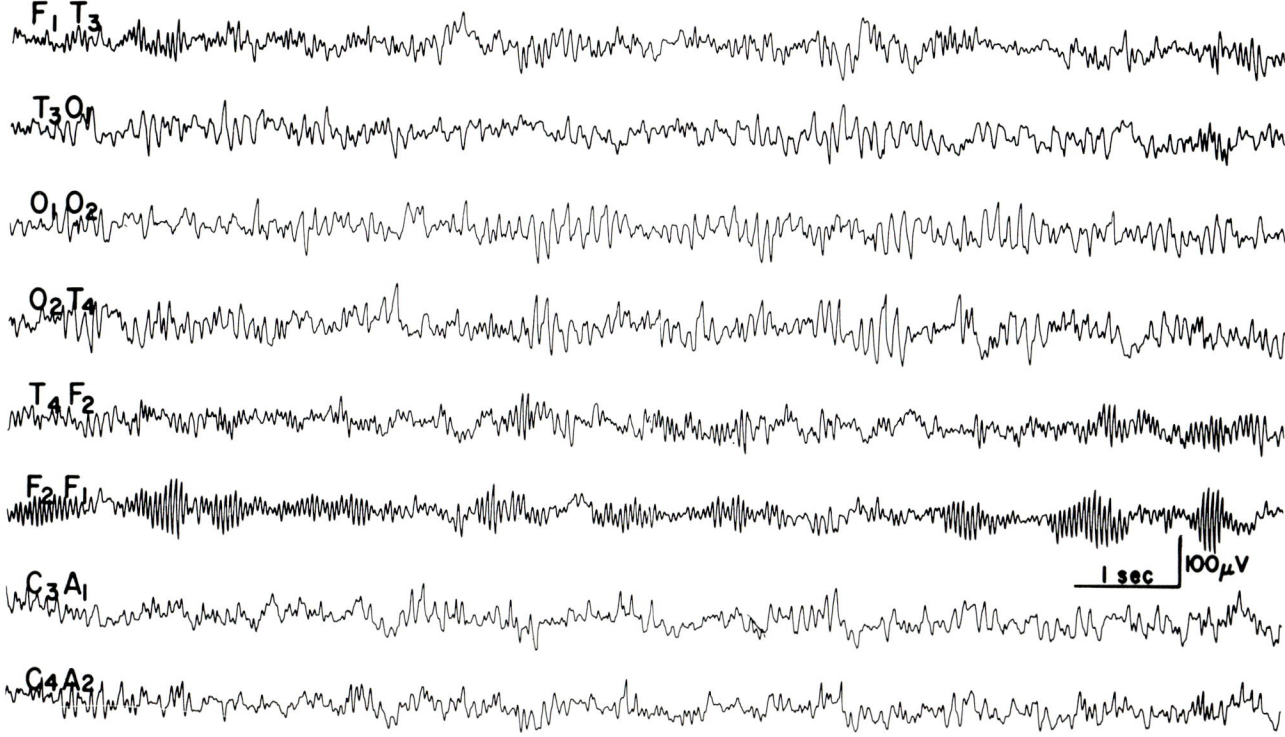

FIG. 8. Frontal beta activity in 12-year-old male, referred for abdominal pain and receiving diphenoxylate and atropine (Lomotil®). Note high amplitude of the beta activity in paired frontal derivations as compared with ipsilateral derivations.

spindling and fast activity" (36). This abnormal finding is seen in certain cases of cerebral palsy and mental retardation. The continuous sigma activity may be the predominant feature of the pattern and has led to the name "extreme spindles," which has been applied to essentially the same phenomenon (37). The interpretation of pronounced fast rhythms—but not so pronounced as to qualify as "continuous fast activity and spindling"—in children during sleep is an unresolved problem. Whatever the voltage and duration of the beta activity, the effects of any drugs the patient may have been taking, as well as any used to promote sleep for the purpose of the EEG

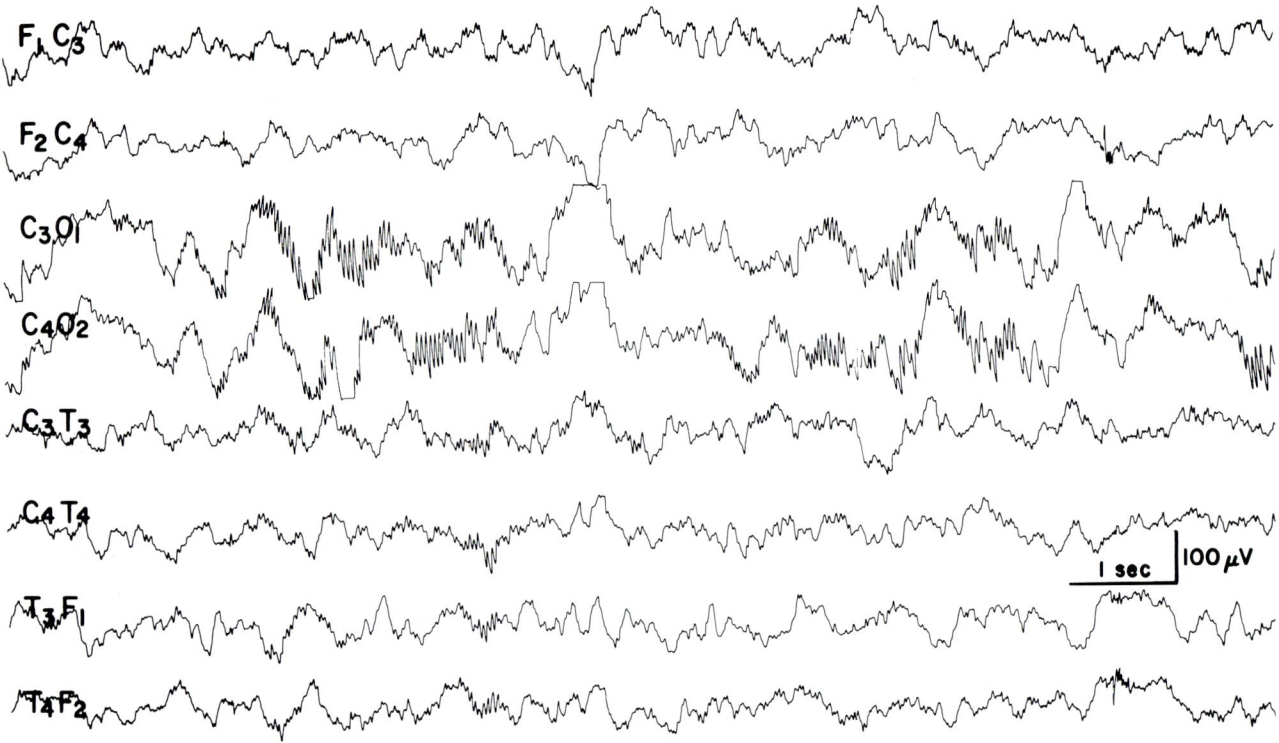

FIG. 9. Posterior 20–22 Hz activity present almost continuously but tending to show bursts of high voltage. Asymptomatic 18-month-old female.

study, should be taken into account. The electrographic effects of a given drug dose are different in different individuals, even if dose–weight schedules are used. There have been no definitive studies to determine if these differences relate to drug level in the blood or to differences in the response of the brain to equivalent levels. In children given sedation for sleep in the EEG laboratory, beta activity may become very pronounced if sleep does not ensue after a reasonable period (approximately 35 min). Similarly, beta activity may become greatly enhanced in the postsleep record when the child is awakened.

Frontal and Frontocentral Theta Activity

Most normal young adults show traces of 6 to 7 Hz random activity but no activity slower than this. In approximately 35%, some low-voltage (less than 15 μV) 6 to 7 Hz waves may be present in the frontal or frontocentral region with the eyes closed and in the presence of a well-sustained occipital alpha rhythm (13,38). The 6 to 7 Hz activity in the frontocentral region tends to become sustained and higher in voltage with the onset of drowsiness, but this effect can usually be recognized because the occipital alpha rhythm concomitantly becomes intermittent or disappears. In patients in whom the alpha rhythm is low in voltage or poorly sustained, the onset of drowsiness can be determined objectively by using eye electrodes to detect the slow, pendular eye movements which accompany the onset of the drowsy state.

In young adults and particularly in children, heightened emotional states enhance frontal theta activity in the 6 to 7 Hz range (39–47). Moreover, some normal individuals show marked frontocentral rhythmic theta activity (with the eyes open) while carrying out certain tasks. It has not been established whether this latter effect results from a change in affective state related to the task or is a concomitant of some other aspect of brain function.

Since the routine clinical EEG examination generally does not encompass evaluation of "affective state" or even of "vigilance" during the recording, the presence of some 6 to 7 Hz random or rhythmic activity in the routine EEG cannot be regarded as having pathological significance. As mentioned above, approximately 35% of young, non-drowsy, asymptomatic adults show some very low voltage (less than 15 μV) 6 to 7 Hz activity in the frontal or frontocentral region in the environment of a quiet, smoothly operating, clinical EEG laboratory. In 10%, the voltage is 15 to 25 μV, and the activity tends to occur in rhythmic serials. The extent to which more-sustained, higher-voltage (greater than 15 μV), 6 to 7 Hz rhythms reflect the patient's emotional state (39–47) or some other physiological condition cannot be assessed properly unless specific procedures are carried out. Hence there is no clear-cut endpoint at which frontal theta activity can be specified as abnormal. This problem is particularly important in children, who are especially prone to increased theta activity in highly emotional states and in whom frontal theta activity was once identified as an abnormality having a specific association with behavior disorders. Indeed the presence of this "abnormality" in the EEG was originally thought to be "evidence of the organic nature of the behavior disorder present" (48). Clearly, enhanced theta activity in such children might result from emotional upsets engendered by the behavior problem and its consequences rather than from pathologically altered brain function. The clinical interpretation of anterior theta rhythms in the EEGs of children was overly influenced by a series of early reports, beginning with that of Jasper et al. in 1938 (48), which reported that such activity was more pronounced and more prevalent in children with behavior problems than in normal, age-matched controls. It is clear that Jasper et al. and subsequent investigators regarded this theta activity as evidence of "fundamental brain pathology." Lindsley and Cutts, for example, reported that although occasional brief runs of 5 to 8 Hz waves in frontal and central regions are not unusual in normal subjects, they should be considered abnormal "if they are present as much as 10% of the time in well-organized 'runs' or 'bursts' " (49). This concept has been reiterated ever since (usually without critical reappraisal) as a criterion of abnormality in children. However, the runs of 6 Hz activity shown in Fig. 10 are comparable to those Lindsley and Cutts described as abnormal. The tracing in this figure is from the EEG of an asymptomatic 19-year-old male. Such rhythmic activity appears in approximately 15 to 20% of asymptomatic children and adolescents between age 8 and 16 years; serial studies indicate that

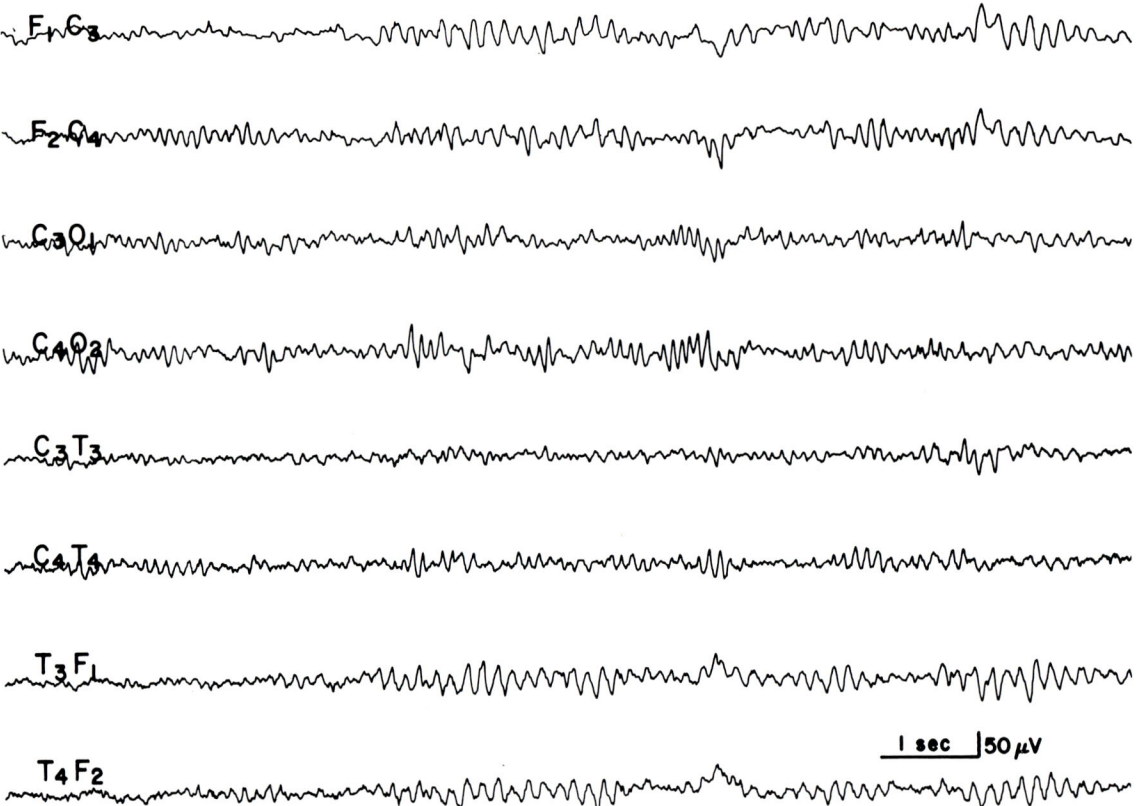

FIG. 10. Monomorphic, rhythmic 6–7 Hz moderate-voltage activity, occurring in fairly prolonged runs in the frontal leads in asymptomatic 19-year-old male pilot. Theta activity of this degree occurs in young adult asymptomatic individuals but usually is not so continuous nor pronounced at this age as in this subject.

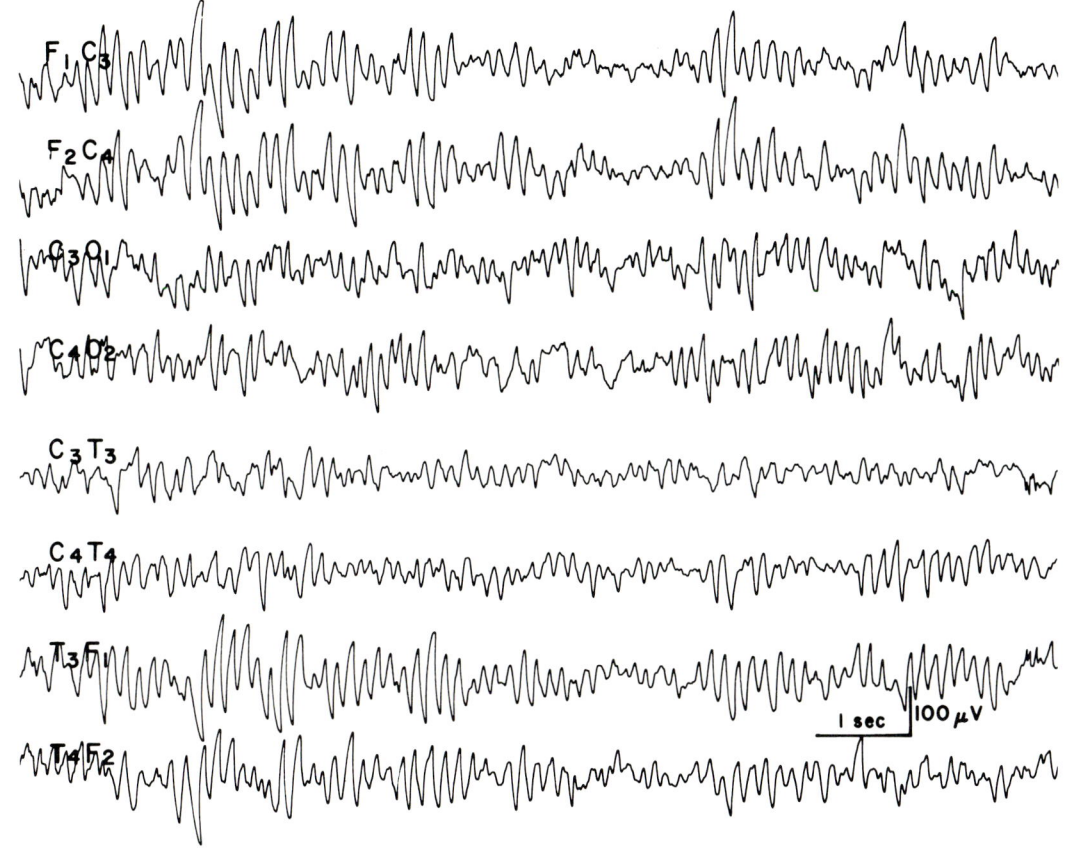

FIG. 11. Monomorphic, rhythmic, high-voltage 6–7 Hz activity in 9-year-old male. Rhythmic 6–7 Hz activity, similar to that seen in Fig. 10, occurs commonly in this age group but usually not so continuously as in this subject. This high-voltage, frontal theta activity is outside the range of normal variation for any age.

the occurrence of such rhythms is age-related, appearing in a given child at a certain age, increasing to a peak voltage at approximately age 8 years, and tending to diminish and finally disappear thereafter (9,10).

Thus age and ontogenetic processes are factors in the appearance of this type of anterior theta rhythm. Evidence also indicates that genetic factors may be an influence (50). The problem is: at what point do frontal 6 to 7 Hz rhythms—because of high voltage, unusual persistence, or paroxysmal regulation—qualify as evidence of abnormal function?

Monomorphic, rhythmic 6 to 7 Hz activity occurring in high-voltage (greater than 100 μV) paroxysmal bursts in the frontal or frontocentral region (Fig. 11) is not typically seen in normal children (zero incidence in controls). The two extremes of rhythmic theta activity occurrence are shown in Figs. 10 and 11; however, all degrees of theta activity may be encountered in pediatric practice. At what rate of amplitude change, maximum voltage attained, degree of persistence, or combination of these does such activity have diagnostic significance? The problem is compounded by the fact that such rhythms are potentiated during drowsiness and by hyperventilation, and what may be a "baseline" rhythm awake and at rest may become paroxysmal during stage 1 sleep or when overbreathing. Clearly, the true meaning of such rhythms must await development of a more sophisticated knowledge of neuropsychiatry. In clinical practice, the electroencephalographer should not be misled by poorly controlled studies that purport to show that monomorphic frontocentral activity of 4 to 6 Hz (which interrupts and exceeds in peak amplitude the background activity) is correlated with clinical epilepsy. Activity of this description is seen as often in children referred for problems other than epilepsy. Nor should the electroencephalographer be led into false syllogistic thinking—i.e., that since a significant incidence of such theta rhythms has been reported in epileptic patients, other disorders that display such rhythms must be epileptic in character.

Posterior Slow Waves

Perhaps no EEG finding has been more misunderstood and misevaluated to the detriment of the patient than slow activity in the parietooccipital and occipitotemporal regions. The interpretation of such activity in children, adolescents, and young adults continues to be fraught with difficulties. Perhaps the problem can be clarified by reviewing how some of the difficulties arose.

In 1938, Jasper and associates (48), beginning with the premise that "the important electrical signs of brain dysfunction given by the electroencephalogram might contribute to our understanding" of certain primary behavior disorders, studied 71 children between the ages of 2 and 16 years who had been admitted to the Bradley Home with a primary diagnosis of behavior problem. For controls, a comparison was made with the EEGs of "40 normal children of comparable age, 70 normal adults, and 219 patients with other nervous or mental disorders." As a pioneer effort, this study was important chiefly in terms of its heuristic value. The authors' conclusion that "abnormal brain function as revealed by the electroencephalogram is an important component in the majority of a group of problem children whose disorder had been considered as primarily psychogenic previous to using this method of diagnosis" was to have a far-reaching influence on future studies, and for a long time no systematic attempt was made to examine this concept or its implications. A long series of papers reported similar findings and reached similar conclusions, each tending to repeat the errors in the research design of the original study without, however, the extenuating circumstance of being the first to deal with the subject.

The errors of experimental design in the original study of Jasper et al. (48) were largely a reflection of the lack of knowledge at this very early point in the history of clinical electroencephalography. Thus although the authors were concerned about the intelligence of the subjects, they did not control for state (e.g., drowsiness, alertness) and did not appear to make significant adjustments of EEG criteria in terms of age. Consequently, although the study included children as young as 2 years, the authors considered, for the purpose of their study, that the EEG was abnormal if the waves below 7 Hz occurred in more than 10% of at least 100 sec of record.

The fundamental limitations of this original study and many since were the small size of the control group and the basis of the criteria of abnormality. Further, in all the studies, there is the pervading concept that the "abnormalities" are signs of damage. The evidence for this concept was not conclusive, only circumstantial, and included some statistical conceptualizations of questionable validity.

The occipital slow activity seen by Jasper et al. (48), Lindsley and Cutts (49), and other early workers studying children who had behavior problems was not well characterized and, in fact, consisted of several types, ranging from continuous delta activity with no alpha rhythm to episodic delta activity with a continuous superimposed alpha rhythm of normal frequency. Clearly, several varieties of occipital or posterior slow activity may be present in children; furthermore, there are numerous permutations of amplitude, wave form, incidence, and posterior areal distribution that cannot be combined into a single category of abnormality without regard for age and state.

The weight of the statistical evidence (48,49,51–53) appears to confirm a greater incidence of posterior slow activity in children with behavior disorders than in selected controls of the same age. The character of the deviation and its degree vary considerably, however, and probably do not reflect a unitary pathophysiological mechanism, even in terms of "brain damage" or lack of it. The evidence of Aird and Gastaut (54), Wiener et al. (38), and Sutter and Harrelson (55) suggests that asymptomatic children with no antecedent history of brain insult may show posterior slow activity, and this slow activity appears to be age-related. It is likely that some of the types of posterior slow activity described in problem children reflect *simply that the subjects are children of a certain age.*

The interpretation of posterior slow activity can be made coherent only if its characteristics are clearly defined in terms of the analysis schema outlined in the introduction to this chapter. As a starting point: some posterior slow activity, intermixed with the alpha rhythm, is present in the EEGs of 7 to 10% of highly selected normal young adults (18 to 30 years of age). The type of activity present in 90% of these individuals consists of moderate-voltage (defined as no more than 120% of the alpha rhythm voltage) fused waves intermixed with the alpha rhythm (which is often superimposed on them). These waves have been called "polyphasic waves" (9,10), or "posterior slow of youth" (54). An example of this type of activity in a normal young adult is shown in Fig. 12. This type of posterior slow activity is rare in normal adults after age 21 years but has a 15% incidence in individuals 16 to 20 years old (9,10).

Such waves are uncommon in children below age 2 years, but they are maximally expressed (in amplitude and incidence) between 8 and 14 years (see Fig. 16B); they occur more often in females than in males. It is common for the amplitude and incidence of posterior polyphasic waves in a child to diminish as the recording proceeds. The basis for this change is not clear; it may reflect a change in the anxiety or stress level of the child (56; see also refs. 39–47).

A practical point to remember is that the potential field of posterior polyphasic waves is such that they appear to be much more pronounced when recorded from C3–O1 or C4–O2 than from scalp-to-ear derivations (e.g., O2–A2). These waves block with eye opening and disappear with the alpha rhythm during drowsiness and light sleep. They are not always symmetrical or synchronous on the two sides, but the asymmetry should not be consistently more than 50%. They are accentuated by overventilation and possibly by stress (56; see also refs. 39–47).

If polyphasic or fused waves were the only type of occipital slow activity encountered in children, the difficulty of interpreting children's EEGs would be considerably lessened. However, occipital slow

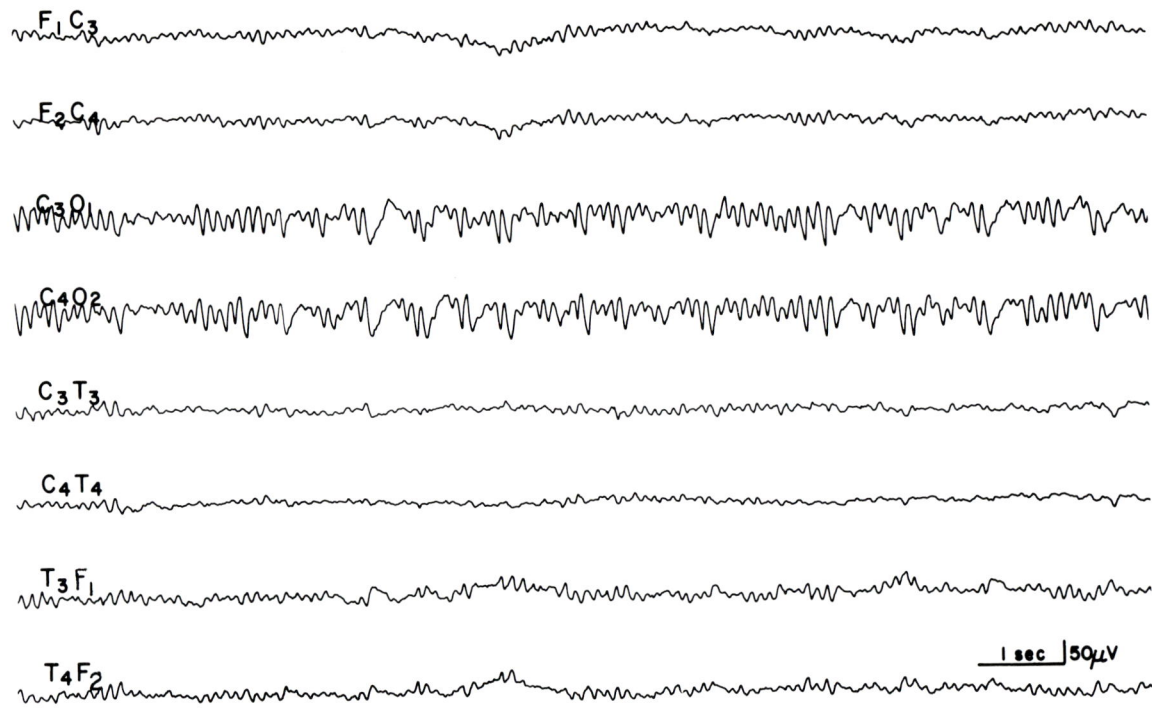

FIG. 12. "Posterior slow waves of youth" in 18-year-old asymptomatic female. Long interelectrode distances and the central-occipital derivations emphasize this type of slow activity.

activity may be present in numerous permutations of amplitude, wave form, occurrence, and topography, rendering it difficult to distinguish between normal and abnormal findings.

In terms of manner of occurrence, there is an occipital slow activity that is semirhythmic in character and is a normal finding between the ages of 1 and 15 years (9,10); this is discussed in detail later. Except for this age-related finding, in the awake state there should be no *rhythmic* component in the occipital regions which has a frequency slower than that of the normal range (for age) of the occipital alpha rhythm.

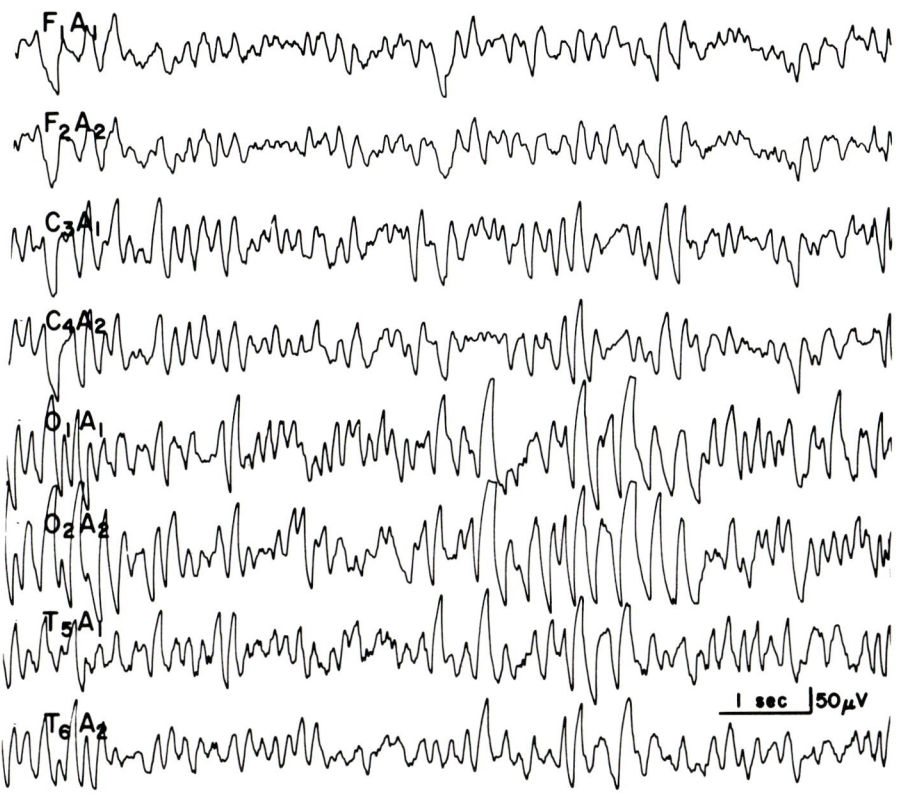

FIG. 13. A: This EEG is outside the range of normal variation for age (8 years 1 month) because of high-voltage (three times the alpha-rhythm amplitude) rhythmic 4-Hz waves, which are not seen in normal children.

Random, occipital slow activity may be present in normal children in a wide range of wave forms, voltages, and wavelengths, and the problem of interpreting the meaning of such activity is complicated by the fact that in children, the occipital region appears to be a common site for the EEG expression of disordered function. Thus, following closed head injury or hypoxia or in the various encephalitides, occipital slow activity may be the initial and the last persisting EEG sign of dysfunction resulting from the brain insult. However, because of the wide range of normal variation in the amount and character of occipital slow activity in normal children of various

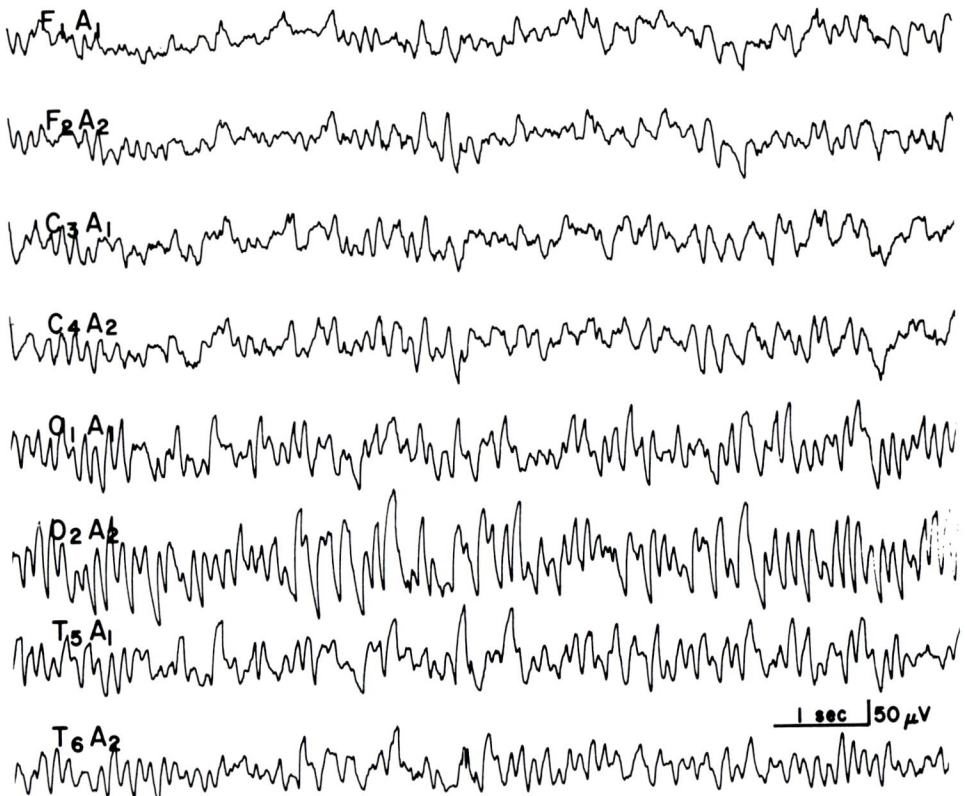

FIG. 13. B: The occipital slow activity occurs chiefly at 5–6 Hz; although it sometimes exceeds voltage of the occipital alpha rhythm, it is within the range of normal variation for age (8.5 years). Occipital slow activity is usually of higher voltage on the right side; this degree of asymmetry causes no concern. Based on amount, frequency, and voltage of the occipital activity, this EEG is slightly slow.

ages and under various conditions, it is often difficult to assess the significance of random occipital slow waves. Nevertheless, it is possible to provide some guidelines for interpretation on the basis of studies of normal children and the experience gained from prospective serial studies of children with various types of brain insult.

Serial observations dating from the time a brain insult is incurred permit us to define certain features of occipital slow activity that are more characteristic of abnormal than normal function. Thus when the slow activity deviates from that commonly seen in normal children, it can be expressed in terms of: (a) complexity and variability

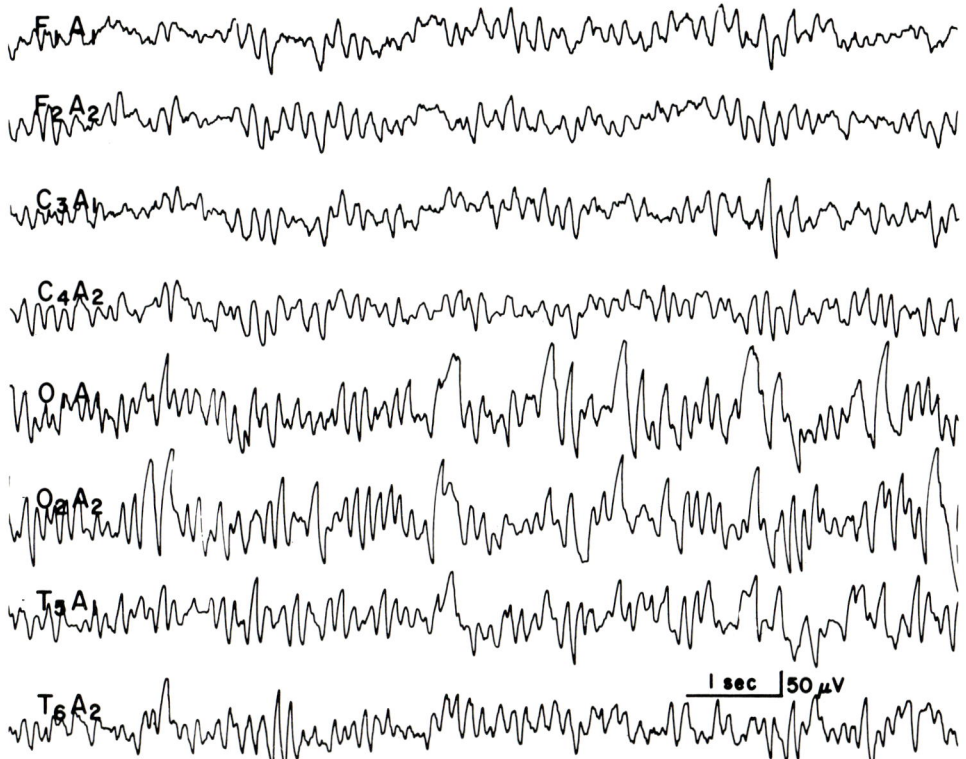

FIG. 13. C: The occipital slow activity (3–4 Hz) is polymorphic, asynchronous, and over 300 μV. These features are outside the range of normal variation for age (8 years); however, the slow activity in anterior derivations is well within the range of normal.

of wave form; (b) incidence (How often do slow waves occur within a given time epoch, e.g., 10 sec?);[9] (c) voltage ratio (Is the voltage of the slow activity greater than 1.5 times the voltage of the occipital alpha rhythm?); (d) persistence (Does the occipital slow activity persist with the eyes open?); (e) synchrony (Is the occipital slow activity synchronous on the two sides?); and (f) symmetry (Is the occipital slow activity predominant on one side?) (Figs. 13 and 14).

Any or all of these factors and their degree of expression may be utilized to formulate an index of abnormality. When this index

---

[9] In the age group 6 to 24 months, awake, occipital activity is monorhythmic, and with the eyes closed, there should be no random slow waves with a duration of >0.25 sec and an amplitude >1.5 times that of the alpha rhythm. This is not true of light sleep, in which random delta waves characterize the occipital derivations (35).

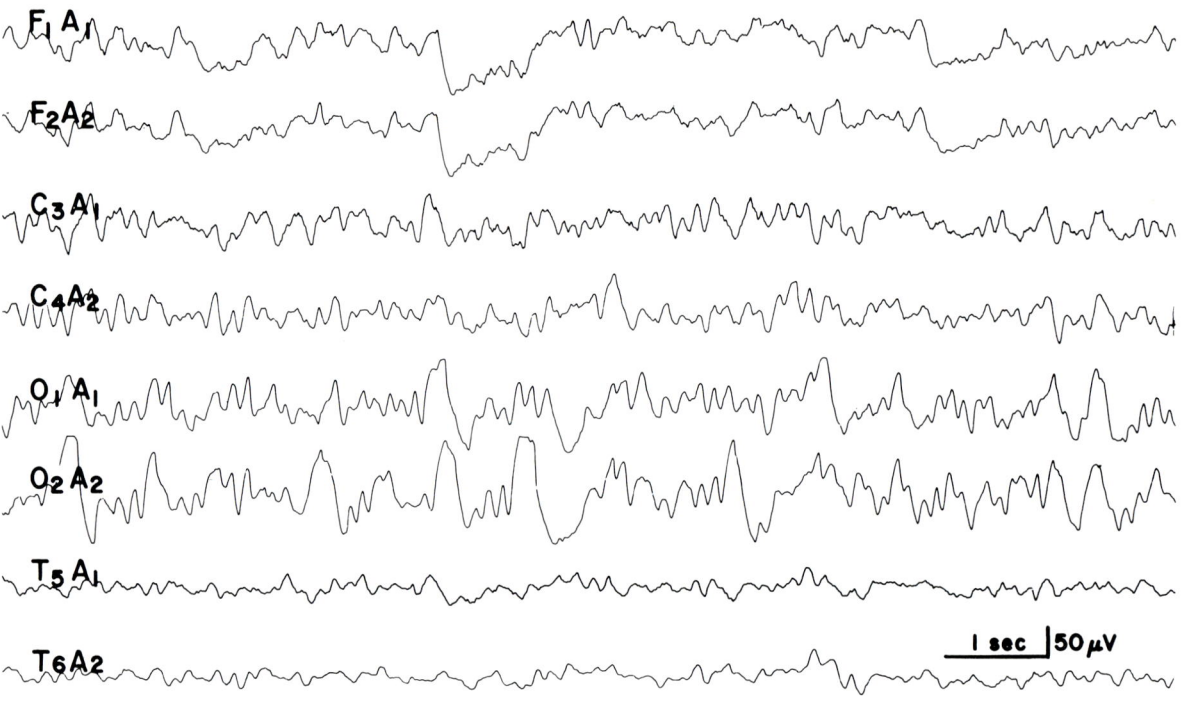

FIG. 13. D: In this 8-year-old child, high-voltage, random, 2.5–3.0 Hz asynchronous waves in the occipital derivations are abnormal, even though the slow activity in anterior derivations is within the range of normal variation. Diagnosis: meningitis.

is high, there should be no difficulty with evaluation. A definitive statement of normal or abnormal cannot be made, however, about many electrograms encountered in clinical practice. The term "borderline" is sometimes applied in this situation, but the clinical utility of this designation is doubtful.

When serial EEGs are made following a brain injury, after brain surgery, or in various disease states (e.g., encephalitis), this index of abnormality can be employed effectively. *It is much less useful if the EEG is an isolated diagnostic study.* In the latter circumstance, even if the electroencephalographer can conclude with confidence that an EEG is outside the range of normal variation in terms of the occipital slow activity present, the diagnostic significance (or clinical meaning) of such a finding is not *ipso facto* clearly evident. If, for example, the patient was referred to the EEG laboratory be-

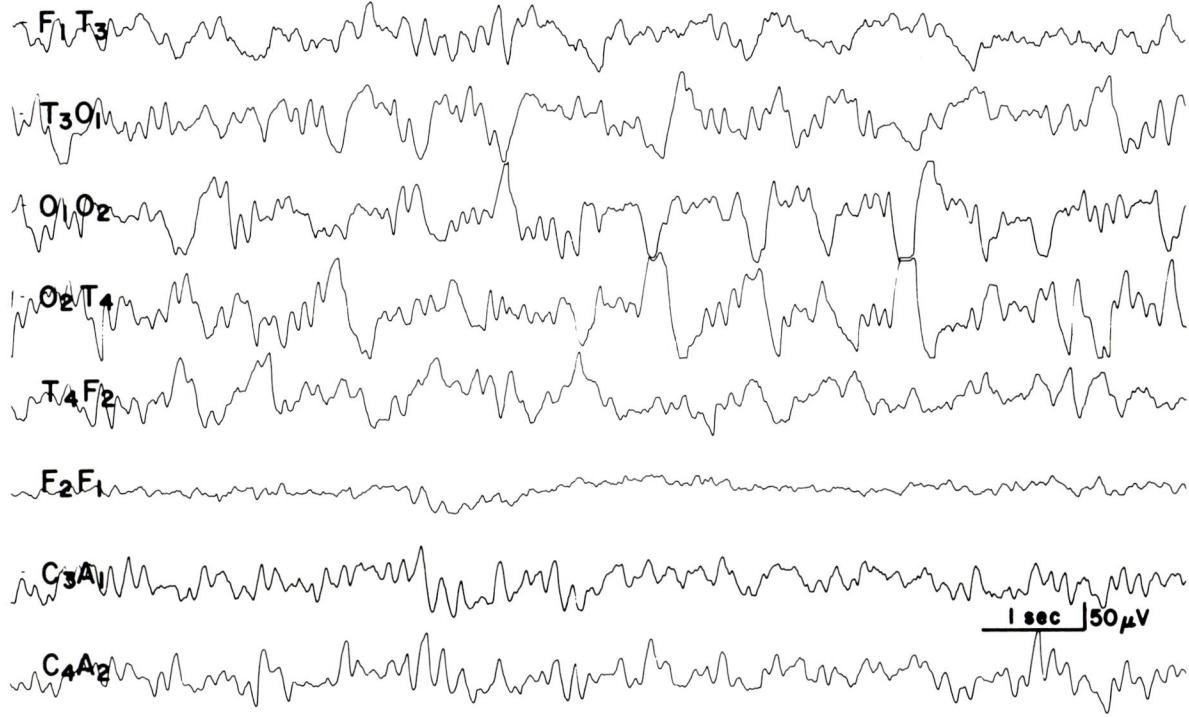

FIG. 13. E: Same patient as in D. In scalp-to-scalp derivations, amount and degree of occipital slow activity are obvious. Note that duration of some waves exceeds 0.75 sec.

cause of "possible seizures," does the presence of an occipital dysrhythmia—or for that matter any nonspecific dysrhythmia—help establish a diagnosis of epilepsy? Occipital slow dysrhythmia, as an isolated finding, occurs as often in children who are referred for behavior disorder or learning disability and who do not have seizures as it does in epileptic children (Table 2). Even in instances of known epilepsy, the finding of an occipital slow dysrhythmia does little to illuminate the diagnosis. The occipital dysrhythmia may be bilateral, but even this does not establish that the patient has a "generalized" epilepsy. The patient may also have an occult focus not revealed

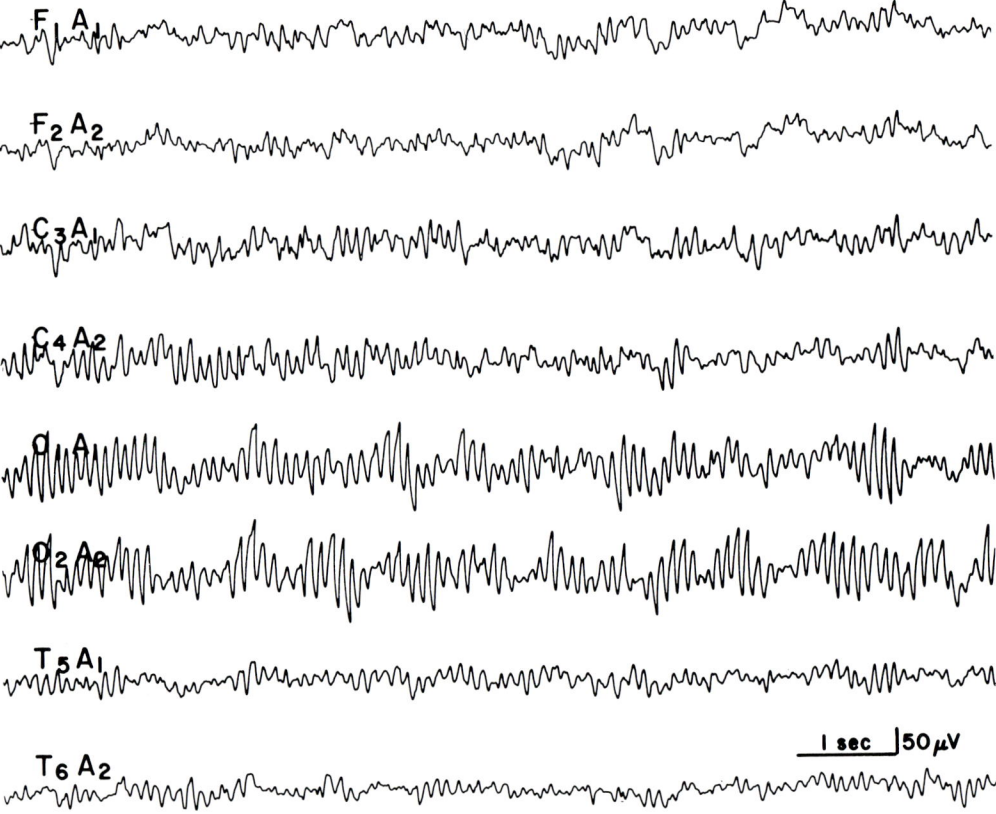

FIG. 13. F: For comparison, a "supernormal" EEG in boy aged 7 years 9 months. Occipital slow activity is minimal and masked by continuous alpha rhythms. The amount of slow activity seen in anterior derivations is within range of normal variation up to age 16 years.

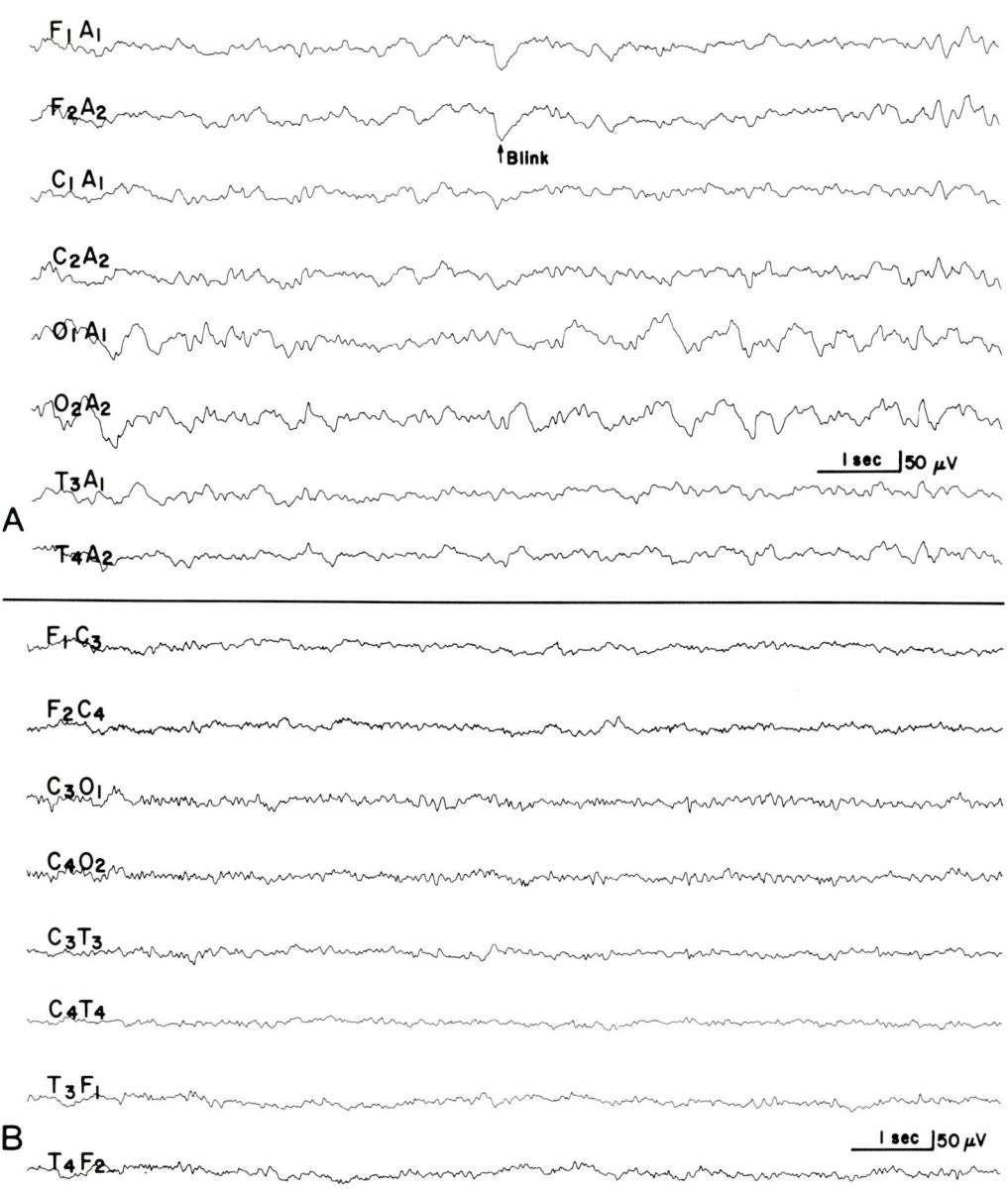

FIG. 14. A: Polymorphic slow activity in occipital leads is often difficult to evaluate if low in voltage and random in occurrence, as in this 14-year-old male. The slow activity is different from that shown in Fig. 12 (normal for age 18 years) and from that in Fig. 16B (normal for age 10 years). The occipital slow activity in this tracing, made 6 hr after injury, typifies that seen soon after closed head injury (concussion) occurring in late childhood or adolescence. This slow activity usually resolves within 10 days. **B:** Same patient as in **A**. Note that 7 days after injury, occipital slow waves have disappeared. The alpha rhythm is somewhat slow, poorly sustained, and poorly organized, but "normal" for age.

TABLE 2. *EEG findings in children with known seizures compared with other children commonly referred for EEG studies (Age group: 3 to 16 years)*

EEG findings	Epilepsy (%) (N = 3,046)	Primary behavior disorders (%) (N = 2,626)	Learning and communication disorders (%) (N = 3,148)	Questionable seizures (%) (N = 1,163)
Normal	39.6	66.9	65.8	64.0
Nonspecific dysrhythmias	19.0	19.9	21.0	24.0
Foci	29.8	7.5	8.0	8.7
Spike-wave	4.8	1.8	1.9	3.0
Other	7.8	0	0	0.3

Note that the incidence of nonspecific dysrhythmias is approximately the same for all groups and is similar to the incidence (16%) given by Wiener et al. (38) for normal children.

in the EEG study. In such a case, it is possible that the occipital dysrhythmia does not relate directly to the patient's epilepsy but results from some other intercurrent factor, e.g., phenytoin intoxication.

The foregoing is prelude to a plea: we must raise the criteria for what is rated as abnormal in children and indicative of disease or disorder. We should also use more caution in assigning significance to such findings. Examples of various degrees and types of slow activity encountered in children of a given age are shown in Fig. 13. The samples illustrate the range from "supernormal" to clearly abnormal. It would be more useful if the various types of occipital slow activity could be illustrated for each age. In addition to *random* slow waves, occipital or "posterior" *rhythmic* slow waves are seen in normal children (9,10). Episodic rhythmic 2.5 to 4.5 Hz mono- and polymorphic low-to-moderate voltage waves (< 100 μV) occur in the parietooccipitotemporal region (usually maximal at O1–O2) in approximately 25% of normal awake children ages 1 to 15 years. Such activity is most prominent in those 5 to 7 years old. Runs of this activity rarely last more than 3 sec and are present only 2% of the time (9,10). Hyperventilation generally causes this activity to become more continuous and higher in voltage.

Anterior Slow Activity in Children

It has long been known that the amount of slow activity in the EEGs of children decreases with increasing age, and that the persistence and frequency of the slow activity vary in different areas. Both of these facts are clearly illustrated in Fig. 15, a graphic representation of the findings of an early frequency–analysis study by Gibbs and Knott (57). This figure may be regarded as a fairly good approximation of the frequencies present and their degree of expression in various regions at different ages. It does not, however, provide information concerning the wave form of the activity, its voltage, or the manner of its occurrence (random, continuous runs, etc.), all of which are critical elements of visual analysis and essential to clinical evaluation of the EEG.

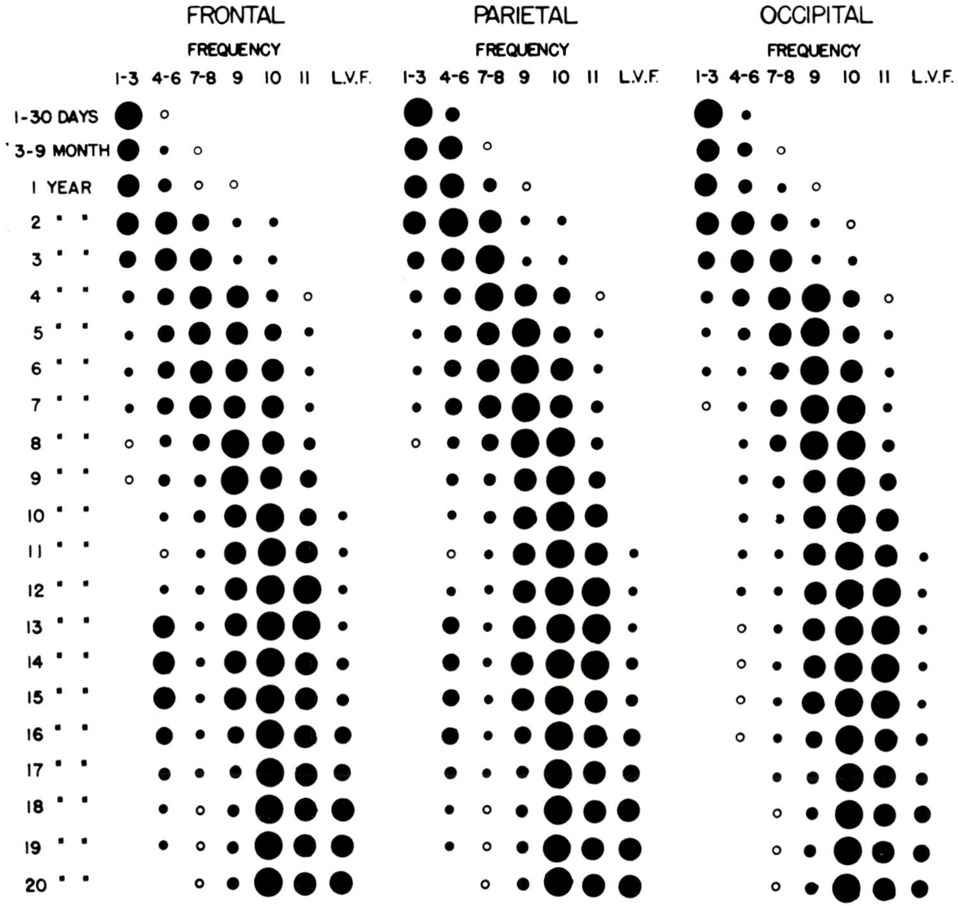

FIG. 15. Graphic summary of early frequency-analysis study of Gibbs and Knott (57). The designation PARIETAL refers to parietal bone of the skull. Actual electrode locations are approximately those of the C3 and C4 positions. At the time this study was made, temporal derivations were not used routinely by this group.

Another important aspect of assessing the amount of slow activity in the EEG is the frequency/voltage ratio. It has become the practice for clinical electroencephalographers to rate an activity as having high or low voltage in relation to its frequency. Thus at the two ends of the EEG frequency spectrum, a 25 Hz activity is regarded as being high in voltage if it is 30 μV in amplitude, but a 1 to 2 Hz wave of similar amplitude is considered low in voltage. This convention grew out of the everyday experience of recording the EEGs of human subjects: beta activity is generally much less than 25 μV in amplitude; hence anything more is "high voltage." On the other hand, 1 to 2 Hz waves of over 800 μV are common during physiological (sleep) and abnormal conditions in man. The convention has significance in terms of the power–spectral characteristics of the EEG. The clinical electroencephalographer assesses the significance of slow activity in relation to its voltage; this frequency/voltage ratio is an important component of the set of mental templates (one for each age range) which he must develop in order to have a consistent basis for evaluation. The age range to which each such template can be applied varies with age, owing to the fact that the *range* of normal variation is different at different age levels.

The Ideal EEG

When evaluating the amount and duration of slow activity present relative to the age of the patient, it is helpful to use the concept of the "ideal" EEG for each age as a standard of comparison. "Ideal" is not used to convey "perfection" (particularly in a clinical sense) but is employed in the platonic sense of "prototype." The "ideal" is based on what 75% of asymptomatic children of a given age show in terms of the slow activity present in the various derivations. Approximately 5% of normal children (same age) show less slow activity than the "ideal" and have EEGs that more closely approximate the adult pattern (these are sometimes called "supernormal" EEGs) (9,10). Another 15% of normal children show slightly more slow activity than the "ideal," and 5% show moderately increased amounts of slow activity. These general concepts have been adopted, modified, and expanded by our colleagues and collaborators in Sweden and underlie their categorizations of "slightly increased slow" and "moderately increased slow" (9,10). The bench-mark papers of Petersén and his collaborators provide the essential data on which the kind of mental template required for the evaluation of children's EEGs can be developed.

Petersén and Eeg-Olofsson (9,10) rated the amount of nonrhythmic (random) slow activity in the EEGs of children in their normal series as "minute," "normal," "slightly increased (SIL)," and "moderately increased (MIL)" for age. Of their highly selected healthy children, approximately 87% had random slow activity in an amount rated as normal for age. Approximately 8% had less slow activity than this, and 4.3% had slightly more nonrhythmic slow activity; in 0.5% of the series, the random slow activity was MIL. This compares with our own concept of the "ideal" EEG and the range of normal variation that was developed from studies of asymptomatic but not highly selected children. Petersén and Eeg-Olofsson found that the incidence of SIL and MIL is greatest in children between 6 and 11 years of age and is significantly higher in females than males.[10]

Comparison of Petersén's prototype EEG samples of "normal," "slightly increased," and "moderately increased" slow activity with our own prototypes indicates that the highly selected healthy children in the Gothenburg series (9,10) showed less random slow activity than did our unselected asymptomatic children. If the criteria offered by the Gothenburg study of highly selected children are used as a

---

[10] This finding is in accord with our concept that the *range* of normal variation itself varies with age.

basis of interpretation in routine clinical practice, considerable caution must be exercised when categorizing an EEG of a given child as "outside" the range of normal variation; care should be taken here because the "pathological" significance of an abnormal EEG, which is too readily equated with brain "damage" or at best "dysfunction," is often based on simplistic reasoning. The talent of the clinical electroencephalographer is measured not so much by an ability to make a visual analysis of the tracing but by an ability to determine what the findings mean in a particular patient under particular circumstances in relation to a particular clinical history. The characteristics of the EEG are determined by numerous influences, not the least of which may be the uniqueness of the laboratory environment. Factors that determine the characteristics of an individual's EEG at any point in time are discussed in the final section of this chapter.

It is beyond the scope of this chapter to attempt to convey the "ideal" and the "range of normal variation" for each age. Figure 16 illustrates the concept for a single age level.

Lambda Waves

When a person's eyes are open, especially if the room is well illuminated, sharp waves with a duration of 160 to 250 msec may be recorded in the occipital regions bilaterally. These sharp transients, designated lambda waves, are particularly likely to be present if the patient is looking at a patterned design, e.g., a perforated acoustic-tile ceiling. The necessary condition for generation of these waves is saccadic movements of the eyes. In her initial description of lambda waves, Gastaut described them as "biphasic or triphasic potential variations with a small initial positive phase and a prominent subsequent negative phase" (58). More recently, using computer techniques it was shown that the lambda waves are multiphasic, with the most prominent phase being surface-negative in the occipital region (59,60). However, most of the numerous studies concerning lambda waves recorded from the scalp in human subjects (61–67) describe them as predominantly surface-positive at the occipital electrodes (Fig. 17). Routine experience indicates that the duration and wave form of lambda waves vary considerably among individuals and that, in children particularly, the highest amplitude and sharpest component is generally surface-negative in the occipital derivations. Lambda waves are much more commonly seen in children aged 2 to 15 years than they are in adults; they are rarely seen in routine EEGs of elderly people. With long interelectrode distances (e.g., C3–O1), lambda waves with voltages as great as $65\mu V$ may be seen in children (Fig. 18).

In a routine clinical EEG, lambda waves may be quite asymmetrical on the two sides and indeed may be present only on one side. This asymmetry may lead to the misinterpretation of lambda waves as a focus of abnormal activity. This is especially likely to occur if the technologist or the electroencephalographer fails to note that this activity occurs only during the eyes-open condition. If there is any doubt concerning the nature of the activity, then eye closure, diminution of illumination, or having the patient stare at a blank white card should eliminate lambda waves but have no effect on the incidence or amplitude of abnormal occipital spikes.

Temporal Slow Activity: A Normal Finding in the Elderly?

With increasing age, a significant number of individuals show episodic, irregular slow activity in the temporal regions, usually with maximum voltage in the midsylvian region. A 50-year-old subject typically shows a series of EEG changes in the temporal regions during the next 15 years of life. The sequence of changes may be

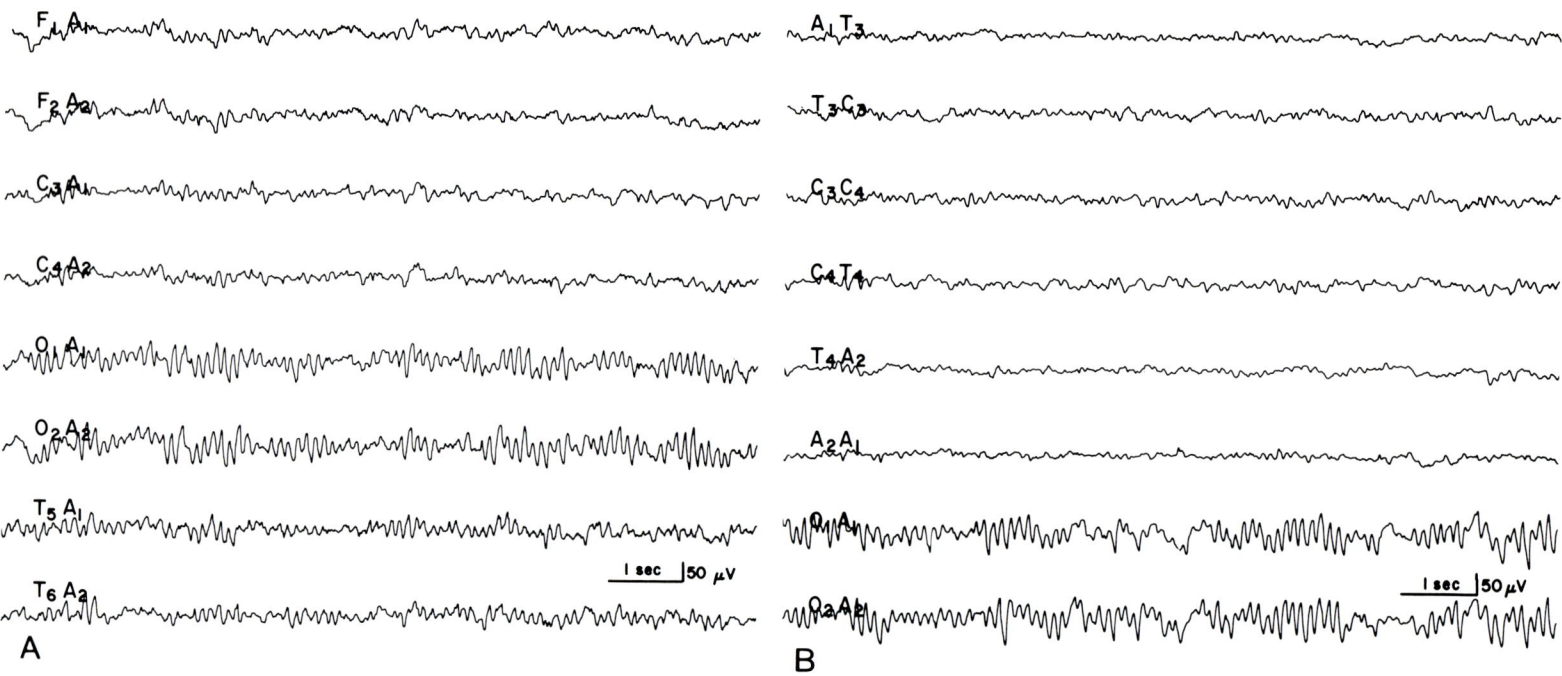

FIG. 16. A: "Supernormal" EEG for age (10-year-old female). More slow fused (polyphasic) activity could appear in the occipital leads, as in **B**, or more random 4–6 Hz moderate-voltage activity in the anterior leads and yet remain within the range of normal for age. **B:** This EEG shows more "posterior slow waves of youth" than in **A** but has slightly less anterior slow activity. Asymptomatic male, aged 10 years 2 months. **C:** *(Facing page.)* Moderately increased slow activity, random moderate-voltage 4–6 Hz activity, and some slower low-voltage fused forms in anterior derivations. Occipital derivations show moderate amounts of polyphasic slow activity. Age: 9 years 8 months.

as follows: first to appear might be episodic, temporal 8 to 10 Hz waves of higher voltage than the occipital alpha rhythm. With time, some episodic activity that is usually a subharmonic frequency (4 to 5 Hz) of the alpha rhythm may then appear. This mixed alpha/theta activity is usually more marked on the left side, is enhanced by overventilation, and may persist when the occipital alpha rhythm disappears during drowsiness. The episodes are usually quite brief, ranging from two to three waves to rarely more than six or seven. Overventilation increases their voltage and persistence. Enhanced temporal alpha activity is not a constant feature. Episodic temporal

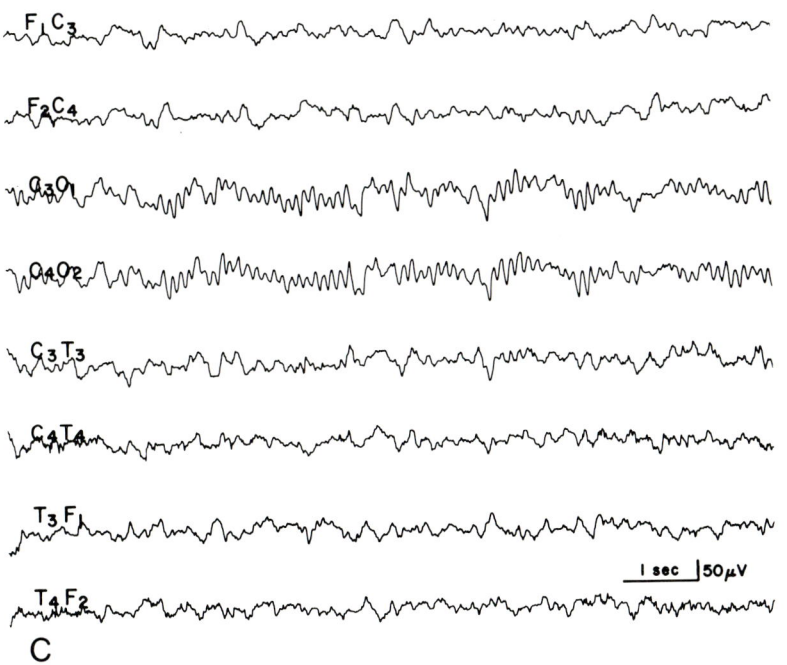

FIG. 16. C: *(See legend facing page.)*

theta activity of this type, called sylvian theta activity by Gastaut et al. (68), may remain unchanged for many years (up to 20 years in our experience), or it may become higher in voltage, more polymorphic, and more persistent.

Because independent temporal focal slow activity may be seen in aged but asymptomatic individuals, Obrist (3–5) and others (69) suggested that it is a normal accompaniment of the aging process. Others (68,70–73), beginning with Gastaut et al. (68), suggested that temporal EEG changes are associated with cerebrovascular insufficiency. If indeed a group of individuals with carotid insufficiency are compared with an age-matched group who have no evidence of cerebrovascular disease, we find that the age incidence of temporal slow activity is shifted to the left in the carotid insufficiency group, and there is a greater overall incidence of this type of activity (Crawley and Kellaway, *unpublished observations*). Furthermore, if, in a series of subjects 50 to 70 years old the individuals who show temporal slow activity are compared with those who do not, there is a 35% higher incidence of hypertension, coronary insufficiency, peripheral artery occlusion, and other evidence of systemic vascular disease in those with the temporal slow activity (Crawley and Kellaway,

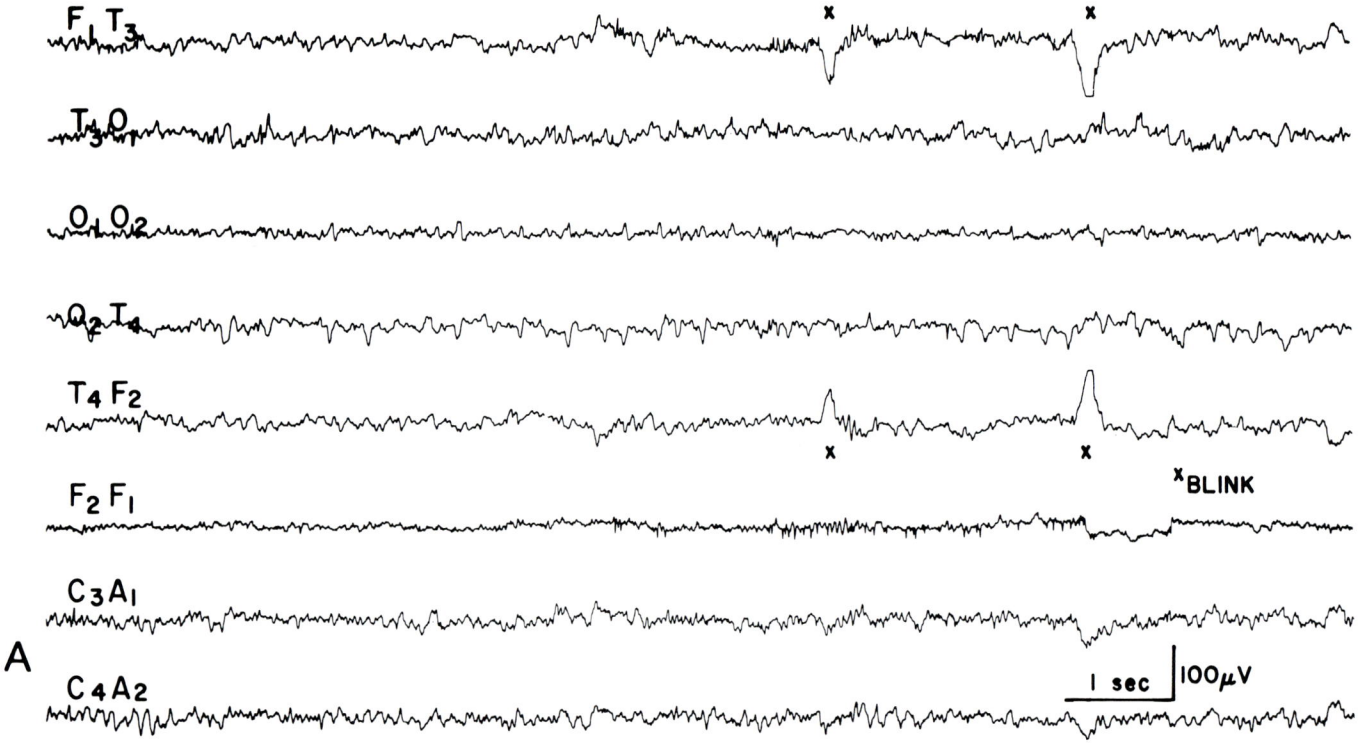

FIG. 17. A: Lambda waves in a patient looking at a pattern (e.g., ceiling tile). Asymptomatic 25-year-old female. B: *(Facing page.)* Recording designed to provide greater definition of lambda waves. Asymptomatic female, aged 12 years. Note that lambda waves are often polyphasic, and in this child the predominant phase is positive at the occipital electrode.

unpublished observations). However, the predominantly left lateralization of the temporal slow activity appears to have no relationship to the side on which the first or any subsequent transient ischemic attack or completed stroke might occur. These observations, made during the last 16 years, are based on pre- and postsurgical EEG studies in more than 1,500 patients with carotid insufficiency and on serial EEG studies in a group of 200 executives aged 45 to 75 years. However, there has never been a well-designed prospective

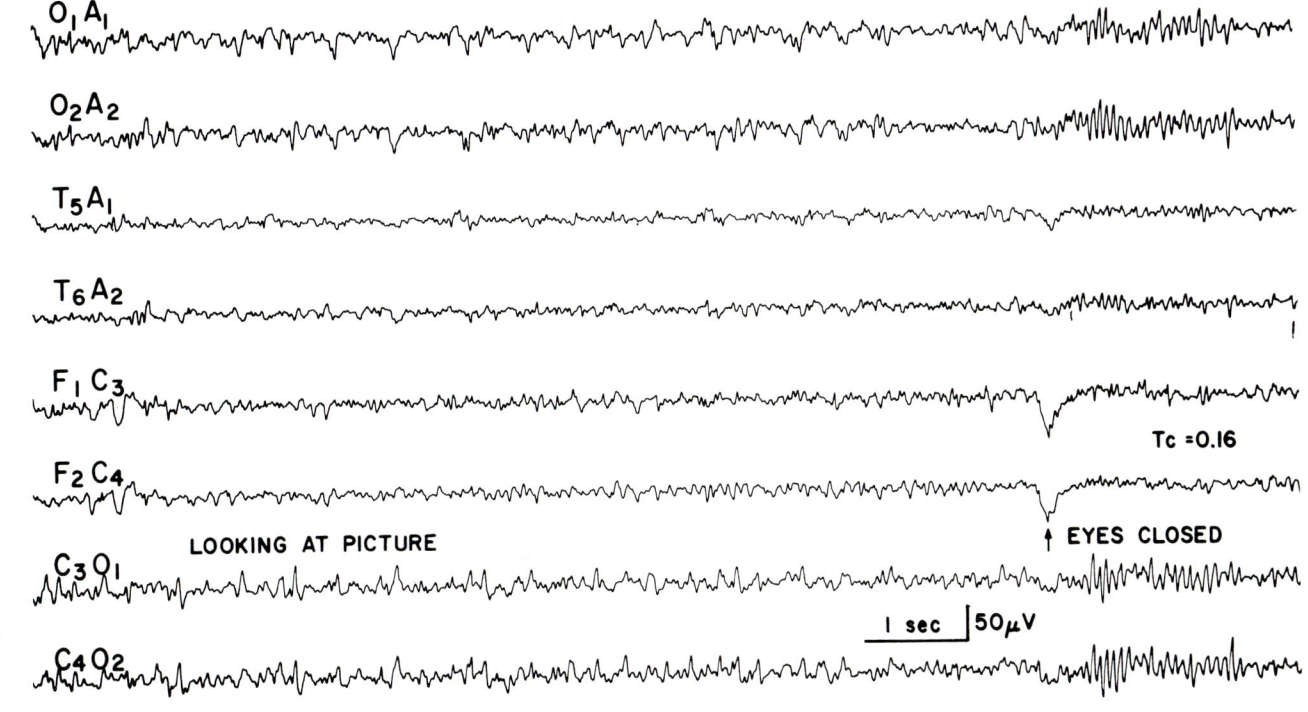

FIG. 17. B: *(See legend facing page.)*

and longitudinal study, and so the descriptive data mentioned above have not been published. To be useful, such a study would have to include measurements of regional blood flow, quantitative EEGs, and neuropsychological evaluations. In the absence of such data, the clinical electroencephalographer faces the problem of interpreting the significance, if any, of various degrees of temporal slow activity in a high percentage of middle-aged and elderly patients. It is common practice to report some temporal theta waves and possibly a few temporal delta waves as normal findings in elderly patients. The problems of how much slow activity is allowed and how old the patient must be for the findings to be considered normal are currently being neglected; as a consequence, there is an enormous variability

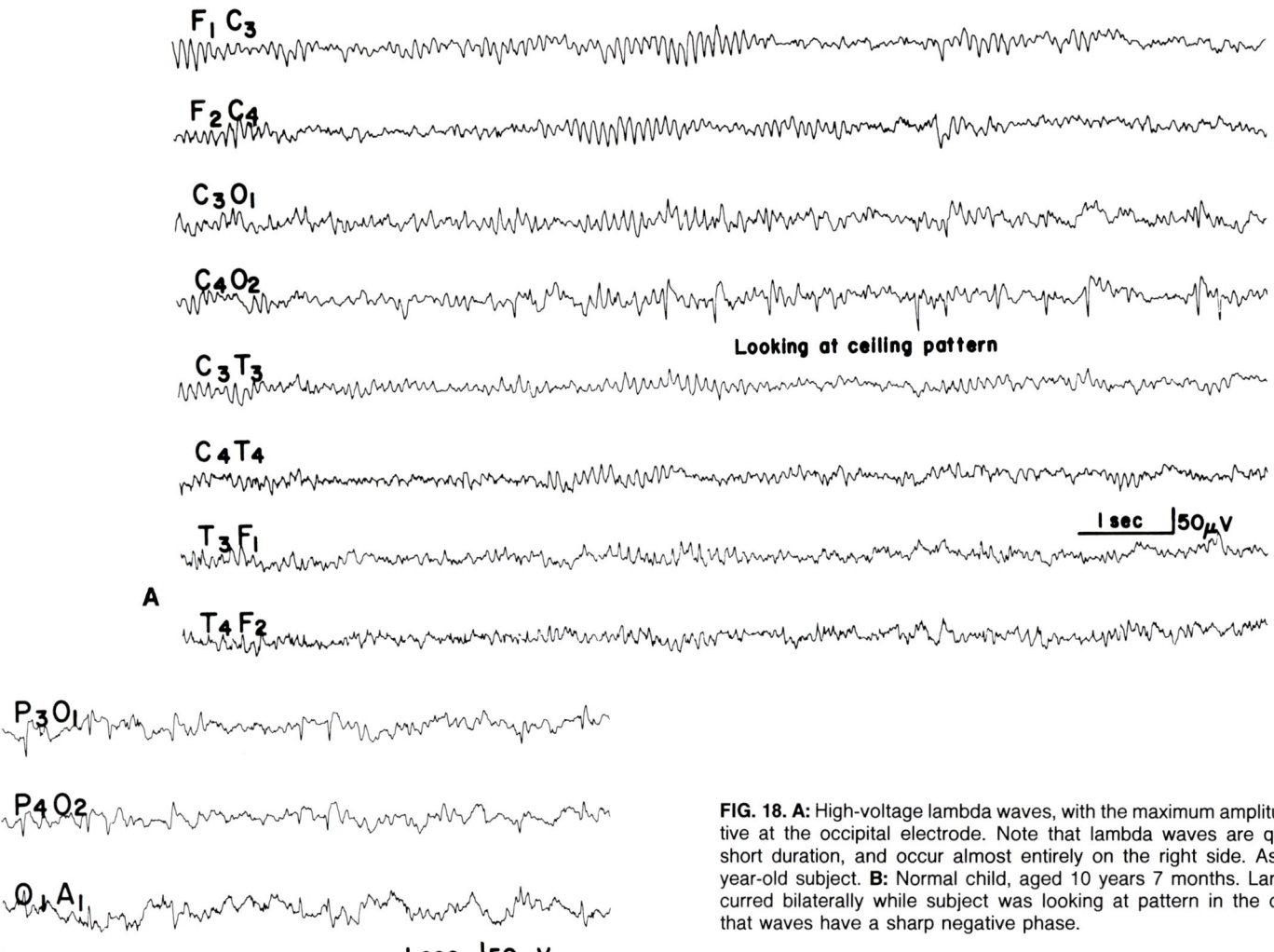

FIG. 18. A: High-voltage lambda waves, with the maximum amplitude phase negative at the occipital electrode. Note that lambda waves are quite "sharp," of short duration, and occur almost entirely on the right side. Asymptomatic 15-year-old subject. **B:** Normal child, aged 10 years 7 months. Lambda waves occurred bilaterally while subject was looking at pattern in the ceiling tile. Note that waves have a sharp negative phase.

in the way individual electroencephalographers evaluate this type of finding.

When episodic 4 to 5 Hz low- to moderate-voltage waves are seen in the temporal leads bilaterally or with a marked predominance on one side (usually the left) in individuals 50 years old or more, it is reasonable to report their presence and to note that "such activity may occur in asymptomatic individuals in this age group." When the activity is present in younger adults, or if there is episodic temporal delta activity, the suspicion of "clinically significant" abnormality is increased. It is important also to recognize that, because temporal slow activity occurs in middle-aged and elderly individuals, such findings in patients of this age group who are referred because of head injury or possible cerebral metastases are *unlikely* to be related to these etiologies and therefore carry the same meaning here as would a normal EEG.

A case in point is a 65-year-old male patient who was in the hospital for gallbladder surgery. He fell out of bed one morning and bruised his forehead; he was not unconscious but seemed confused for several minutes after getting back into bed. The EEG (made on the afternoon of the same day) showed a well-regulated 9 Hz occipital alpha rhythm, with some episodic, low-voltage 3 to 5 Hz waves in the left temporal region and some rare activity of similar frequency that occurred independently in the right temporal region. Statistically, there is a high likelihood that such EEG findings in a man of this age predated the injury; also, focal episodic left-lateralized temporal theta activity is an unlikely consequence of an acute closed head injury. Follow-up EEGs 5 and 10 days later showed no change.

Another case is a 72-year-old woman with a history of breast cancer and bilateral mastectomy, referred for EEG studies because of attacks of dizziness and headaches. Tentative diagnosis was possible cerebral metastasis. The EEG showed an 8 Hz alpha rhythm, with some moderate-voltage (85 μV maximum) 4 to 5 Hz waves that appeared episodically in the left and right temporal regions independently but were much more marked on the left side where there were also occasional low-voltage 3 to 4 Hz waves. The EEG report indicated that these findings were probably not related to the presence of cerebral metastasis but that a follow-up study at 4 weeks might be helpful in this regard. Over a period of 18 months, the patient continued to complain of headache and dizziness, but several EEGs failed to show any change. Over the next 3 years, the patient's symptoms showed some fluctuation but no progression. The EEG remained essentially unchanged.

In this sense, then, it is appropriate to treat as "normal" much of the temporal slow activity seen in middle-aged and elderly patients. However, the more that temporal slow activity differs from the simple prototype shown in Fig. 19, the more it should be considered with suspicion. The slower the activity, the greater the voltage, the more complex the wave form, and particularly the more continuous it is, the less reasonable it becomes to regard the finding as being within the range of normal variation for age.

Hyperventilation Response

Throughout the literature of pediatric electroencephalography, the response to hyperventilation is cited repeatedly as partial or complete supporting evidence of brain abnormality in children. Historically, this concept had its origin in the early report of Lindsley and Cutts (49):

> Overbreathing in some cases produced what we have called a "hyperventilation effect." This is defined as a distinct change (usually abrupt) in the electroencephalogram, consisting of a sequence of slow waves, ranging in frequency from 2 to 8 per second and usually of a magnitude considerably above anything of similar frequency occurring in the records before hyperventilation. The "hyperventilation effect" may persist as a continuous series of rhythmic slow waves or may consist of repeated

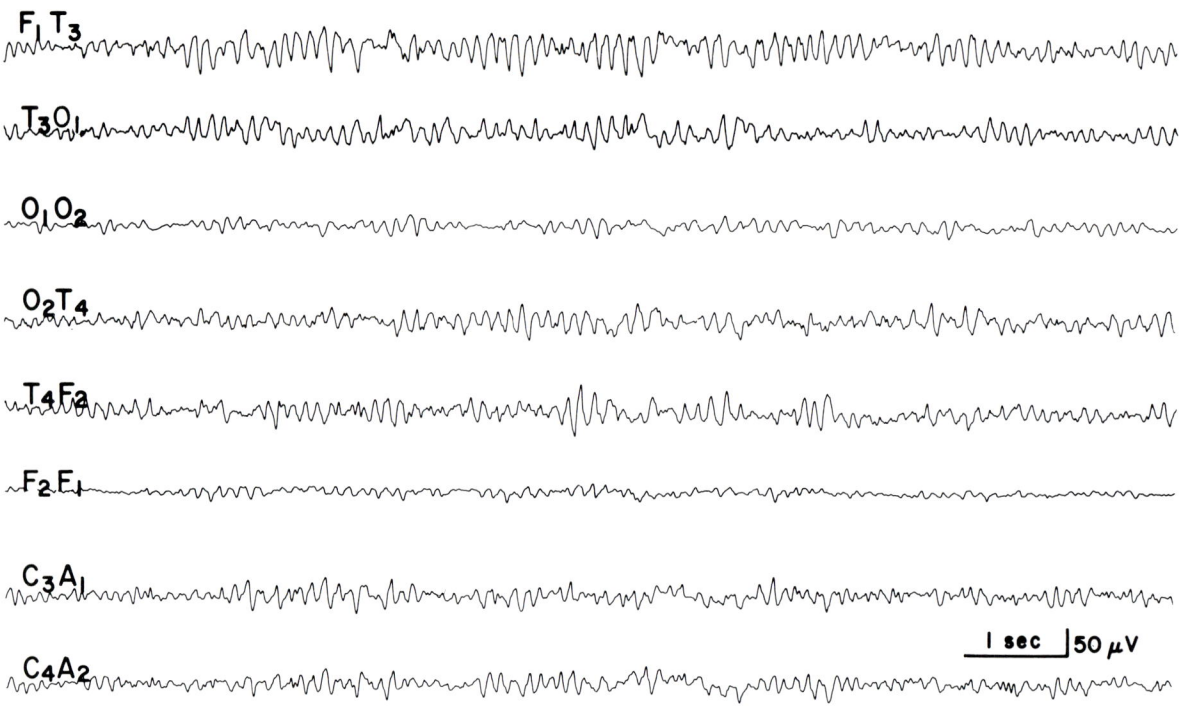

FIG. 19. Temporal alpha and fused slow activity on left and occasionally independently on right side in a 60-year-old male with occlusive carotid disease, more marked on right.

bursts of slow waves at irregular intervals. Two measurements were made, one of the duration from the beginning of hyperventilation to the onset of the "effect," the other of the duration from the cessation of hyperventilation to the disappearance of the "effect."

Lindsley and Cutts employed 1.5 min hyperventilation unless a marked effect appeared before that time, in which case the subject was told to stop overbreathing and to remain quiet until the record returned to the original state. They found that behavior-problem children showed a more abrupt and greater buildup of slow activity and demonstrated more prolonged effects after cessation of hyperventilation than normal control children.

The subjects were instructed "how to hyperventilate or overbreathe

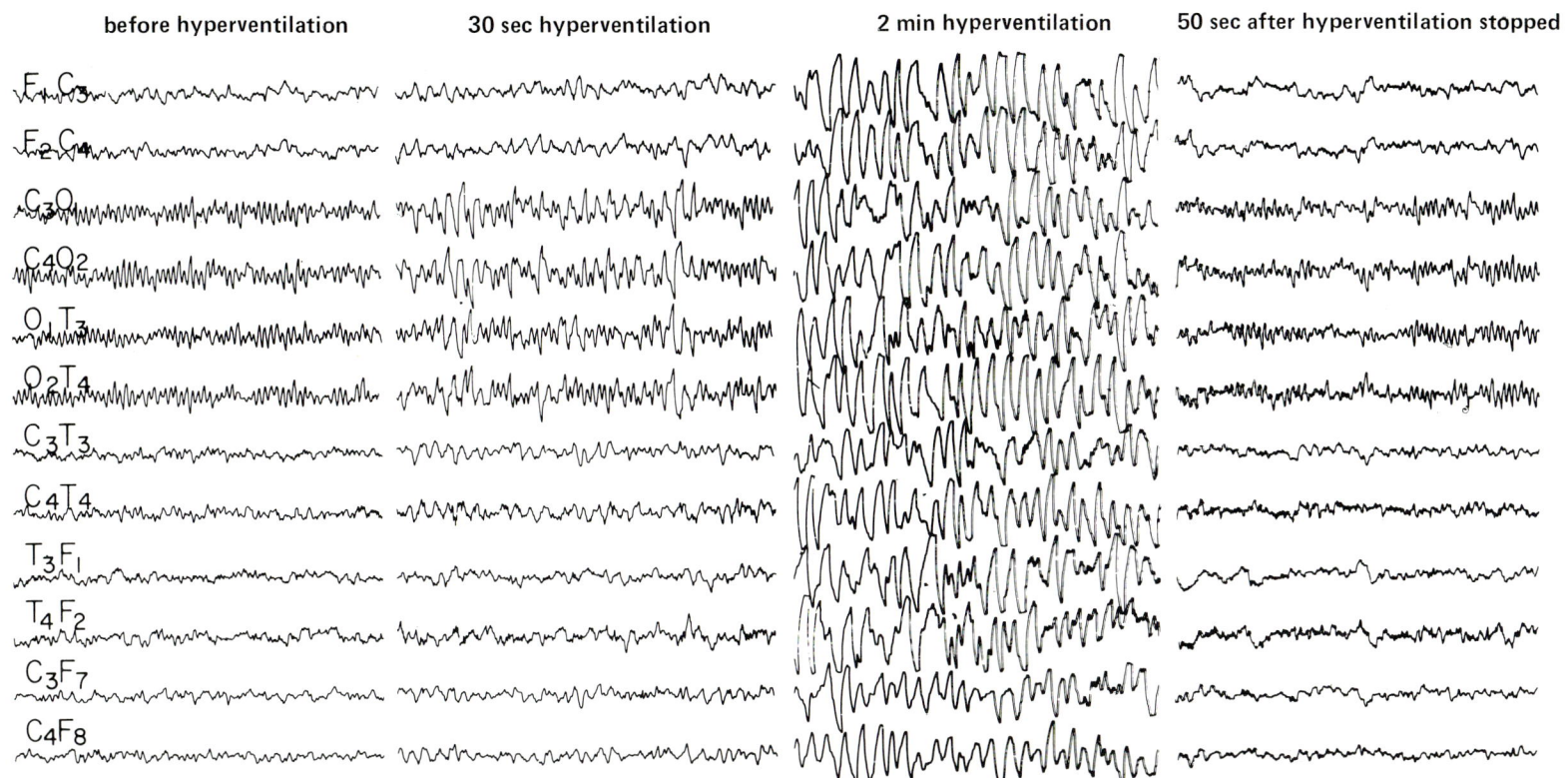

FIG. 20. Example of pronounced overventilation response that may occur in children 8 to 12 years of age. Female, aged 9 years 6 months at time of EEG with serum glucose of 110 mg %, now 25 years old. No history of seizures nor evidence of CNS disease. Note initial posterior slowing, typically seen in children, is quite marked after only 30 sec overventilation. Some frontal delta activity continues 50 sec after overventilation stopped.

at a relatively uniform depth and constant rate," but no measurements were made to determine the blood CO_2 or pH changes, nor were the blood–glucose levels measured at the time of the test. It is now known that all of the measures of "hyperventilation effect" used by Lindsley and Cutts (i.e., abruptness of the change, amplitude and slowness of the waves produced, and degree of persistence of the effect after overbreathing stopped) are determined by the effectiveness of the overbreathing in producing a change in blood CO_2 as well as by the level of blood glucose at the time of the test. It is difficult to judge the degree of hypocapnia (blood CO_2 reduction) produced by a given hyperventilation effort (74), particularly in children; the rate, depth, and consistency of the respiratory effort are extremely difficult to gauge and compare without measuring the respiratory exchange or blood pCO_2 changes. Even if attempts are made (which is rare in most clinical laboratories) to standardize the performance of overbreathing, the effect on blood chemistry is unpredictable (75), and an uncertain relation exists between the levels of peripheral and cerebral blood gases owing to cerebral vasoconstriction, indeed the main basis of the effect (76).

The blood-glucose level is also important in determining the degree of response to hyperventilation (77–79). Most routine EEG studies of children do not control for this factor, but even in adults a low blood-glucose level (< 80 mg/100 ml) favors the appearance of slow waves, and a high level (> 120 mg/100 ml) tends to inhibit or prevent such an effect (77).

If effective overventilation is obtained in children, slow waves appear much more abruptly and are more pronounced than in adults, and the slowing outlasts overbreathing for a longer time than the slowing produced by a similar degree of overbreathing in adults (80). The degree and abruptness of the response seem to relate directly to age (80–83). Indeed, when the blood pCO_2 change produced by overbreathing is measured, there is a linear relationship between age and the effect produced (84,85). Practically speaking, under routine laboratory conditions, where respiratory effort and effect are not measured, the most pronounced responses to overventilation usually occur in children 8 to 12 years of age (10,81,86) (Fig. 20).

Practical experience has shown that in routine diagnostic electroencephalography, interpretation must allow wide latitude for the degree of slowing and the abruptness and duration of the hyperventilation effect. *Only the elicitation of abnormal wave complexes (spike-and-slow-wave, sharp-and-slow-wave) or clear focal or lateralizing changes can be considered unequivocal evidence of abnormality.* Even paroxysmal slow bursts are not acceptable evidence of abnormality, as these may be elicited in normal children under certain circumstances (9,10). Yet "susceptibility to hyperventilation" (87) and other characterizations of pronounced overventilation responses continue to be used as diagnostic EEG parameters in the evaluation of children (88).

Although prominent slow activity occurs less commonly in adults than in children, it too should be regarded with the same degree of caution. An abrupt, pronounced or prolonged buildup of slow waves should never in itself be considered a basis for classifying as abnormal an EEG in an adult, and certainly should *never* be considered a criterion for the diagnosis of epilepsy. If the blood glucose is near normal and the pronounced or prolonged slowing persists, there may be some reason to suspect abnormal brain function. In the absence of direct measurement of the blood pCO_2 level, however, only elicitation of a focal abnormality or production of an abnormal wave pattern can reliably indicate disordered brain function.

Activity of Drowsiness, Arousal, and Sleep

Activity of Drowsiness (Stage 1 Sleep)

Monorhythmic slow activity. The state termed "drowsiness" in adults and children—with slow, pendular eye movements—is associated with the disappearance of the occipital alpha rhythm and the appearance of some rhythmic and semirhythmic theta activity in the central or frontocentral regions. "Drowsiness" is usually defined as a "presleep" state, or a prodromal or twilight condition between being awake and asleep. In infants and young children, overt signs of "drowsiness" may not be evident even though the EEG shows changes indicating that the child is falling asleep. Because "drowsiness" commonly conjures up a certain "heavy-lidded" appearance and because, on the contrary, infants may have their eyes wide open and be irritable and restless during a variable period before onset of clinical and electrographic sleep, we use the less common term "hypnagogic" to refer to this state (35). A smooth transition from the hypnagogic state to sleep may not occur, especially in the strange environment of the EEG laboratory; instead, the child may fluctuate between sleep, arousal, and transitional states. A steady state of slow-wave sleep (stages 2, 3, and 4) may not appear under ordinary conditions in the EEG laboratory for intervals ranging from a few minutes to an hour or longer.

In order not to be misled by the sometimes dramatic changes in the EEG that occur during transition between wakefulness and sleep, the clinical electroencephalographer must know the EEG patterns and their variations that are possible during this state in children of various ages. The electroencephalographer can better understand and interpret what transpires if the entire process of falling asleep is recorded. The irrational, if economical, practice of turning off the instrument while waiting for the child to fall asleep may also result in loss of critical data: an important electrographic event may occur only once or only during one stage of the sleep cycle. Furthermore, the child sometimes drops precipitously into deep sleep with a consequent omission of the more productive stages 2 and 3 of sleep.

The changes that take place in the transient stage between wakeful-

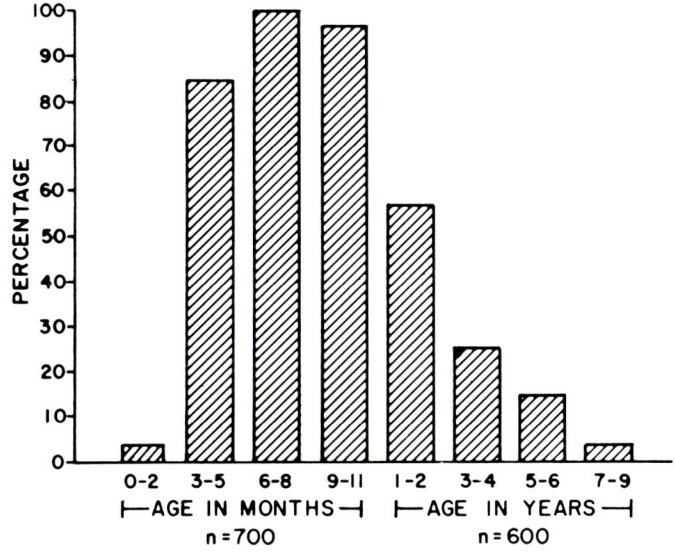

FIG. 21. Age distribution and incidence of sustained monorhythmic slow activity of drowsiness in asymptomatic children.

ness and sleep are best understood in the light of changes with increasing age from birth onward. Once a sustained, reasonably rhythmic, occipital activity appears at approximately 3 months of age, the onset of the hypnagogic state is marked by sustained, monorhythmic, 4-Hz generalized activity. When this activity first appears, the frequency is 3 to 4 Hz, and it increases in older children to 4 to 5 Hz. Approximately 30% of 3-month-old infants show this hypnagogic hypersynchrony, the degree of its expression and duration varying in a single infant at different times and on different days. It may be seen in normal children up to age 12 to 13 years but is increasingly rare after 11 years, when it appears in only 10% of

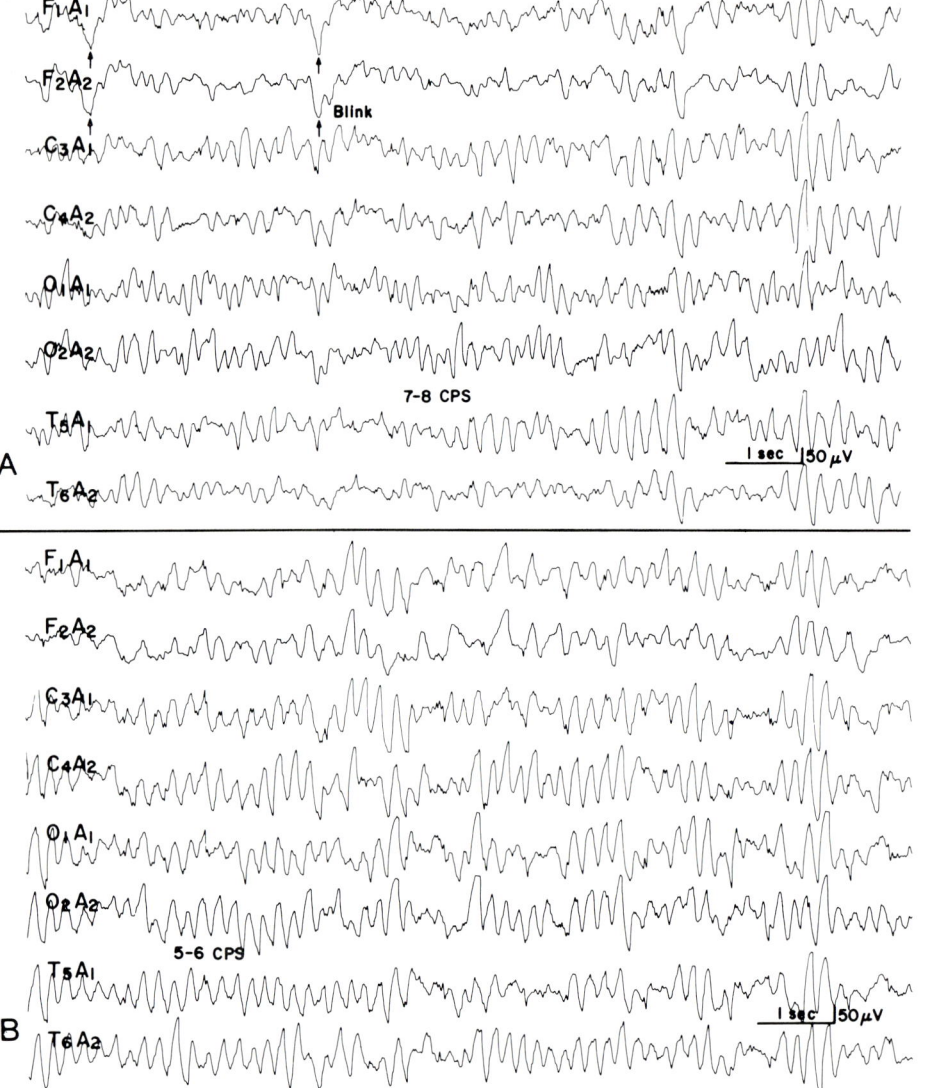

FIG. 22. A and **B:** Slowing of the occipital alpha rhythm as record shifts from awake state (first two-thirds of **A**) to drowsy state (last part of **A** and all of **B**). Asymptomatic female, aged 28 months.

healthy children. Figure 21 shows the incidence of this drowsy pattern in our own series of 1,000 healthy children. The relation to age resembles that reported by Gibbs and Gibbs in asymptomatic children (89) and by Eeg-Olofsson et al. in highly selected normals (90).

In some children, the occipital alpha rhythm may slow as "drowsiness" ensues (Fig. 22), and at a time when anterior derivations show the more usual 4 to 5 Hz hypnagogic hypersynchrony, the occipital derivations may show some high-voltage, less well regulated, slower (3 to 4 Hz) activity. In healthy children, the latter effect occurs in not more than 3% prior to the onset of sleep, but occurs in approximately 6% following arousal. It commonly occurs during a transient episode of arousal. In our own series of healthy children, each one with this pattern was less than 4 years of age.

More commonly, as a shift toward sleep takes place, the occipital alpha rhythm becomes less persistent, and a central or frontocentral rhythm of 4 to 6 Hz develops; this rhythm may have a high voltage (200 μV) and persist. Examples of monorhythmic drowsy patterns in children of various ages are shown in Figs. 22 and 23.

Paroxysmal slow activity. Gibbs and Gibbs (89) and Kellaway and Fox (35) were first to describe paroxysmal slow bursts during drowsiness in normal children. The latter authors described it as follows:

> The onset of the hypnagogic phase is signaled by a general reduction in the amplitude and rhythmicity of the activity of all areas. This relative "quiet" may then be broken by paroxysmal bursts of high voltage sinusoidal waves which involve all leads but which are greater in amplitude in the precentral or central regions and generally more strongly expressed in the frontal than in the occipital regions.
>
> These paroxysmal bursts may reach extremely high voltages when maximally expressed (in excess of 350 microvolts) and therefore constitute a possible source of error both for the interpretation of sleep where this is sought and for the interpretation of waking records where the oscitant state may intervene without true sleep ensuing.
>
> . . . The appearance of such bursts in the period just preceding true sleep, or at its onset, or at a time when the electrogram shows other evidence of the hypnagogic state, is never considered an epileptiform manifestation unless accompanied by spike discharges in some form. Long experience has shown that if a patient with established petit mal epilepsy shows abnormal paroxysmal activity during sleep the spike component is always strongly in evidence and the epileptiform serials persist into fairly deep levels of sleep. A distinguishing characteristic then of the pre-oscitant paroxysmal episodes is that they make a brief appearance at the onset of sleep and do not persist into deeper stages.

The example of paroxysmal drowsy waves illustrated in the report of Kellaway and Fox (35) is shown in Fig. 24. The paroxysmal activity in this sample, which we considered representative for age (35 months), has a frequency of 4.0 to 4.5 Hz and shows maximum voltage in the central regions and a spindle-like waxing and waning of amplitude typical of the drowsy pattern seen in this series of asymptomatic children.

More complex wave forms, slower wave bursts, and a more frontal dominant distribution of the activity may also be seen in normal children. The example of paroxysmal slow activity illustrated by Gibbs and Gibbs (89) shows some waves at the end of the bursts as slow as 2.5 to 3.0 Hz and some complex wave forms with faster components superimposed on, or intermixed with, the slow waves. Figures 25 and 26 show examples of activity of this type in drowsy asymptomatic children. It is difficult to distinguish between such bursts and a pattern described by Gibbs and Gibbs (91) which they designated "pseudo petit mal." They characterized the pattern as "paroxysmal diffuse 3–4 per second slow waves, with a poorly developed spike in the positive trough between the slow waves, occurring in drowsiness only . . . and most prominent in the parietal [central—C3–C4] areas." Gibbs and Gibbs saw this pattern only in children between age 3 months and 9 years, and in only 0.1% of normal children aged 0 to 14 years. Eeg-Olofsson et al. (90), however, found similar activity during drowsiness in 7.9% of 599 highly selected normal children aged 1 to 16 years. The highest incidence (12%)

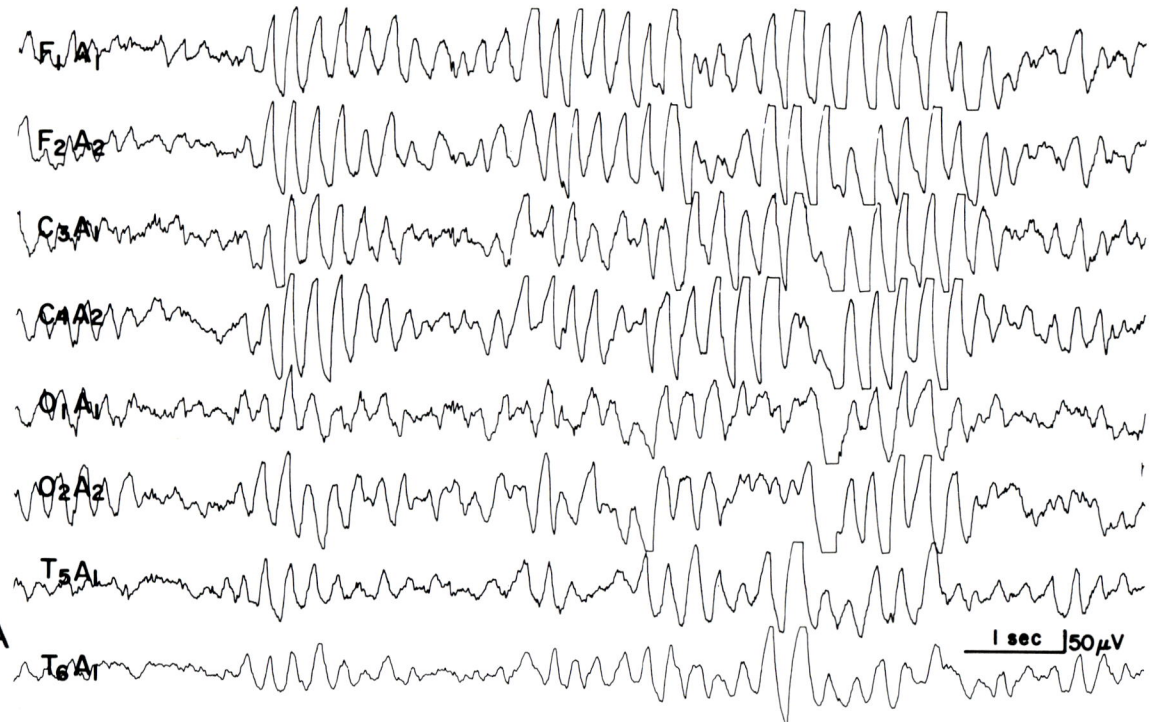

FIG. 23. A: Almost continuous "hypnagogic hypersynchrony" in asymptomatic 6-month-old infant.

was in children aged 4 to 5 years. These authors describe this "drowsy" pattern as consisting of bursts of 2 to 4 Hz waves of 100 to 300 μV, with a spike or spike-like component appearing briefly, early or late, in the burst. The pattern disappears as soon as drowsiness is replaced by deeper sleep. A wide diversity of patterns of paroxysmal drowsy bursts may occur in normal children, ranging from a common type with occasional notching of the slow waves to bursts with polyspike-like components (Fig. 26).

Figure 27 illustrates the incidence of "paroxysmal hypnagogic hypersynchrony" in asymptomatic children of different ages. The heavily shaded bars show the incidence of what Brandt and Brandt (92) called the "severe" type, i.e., slow bursts with sharp or "spike-

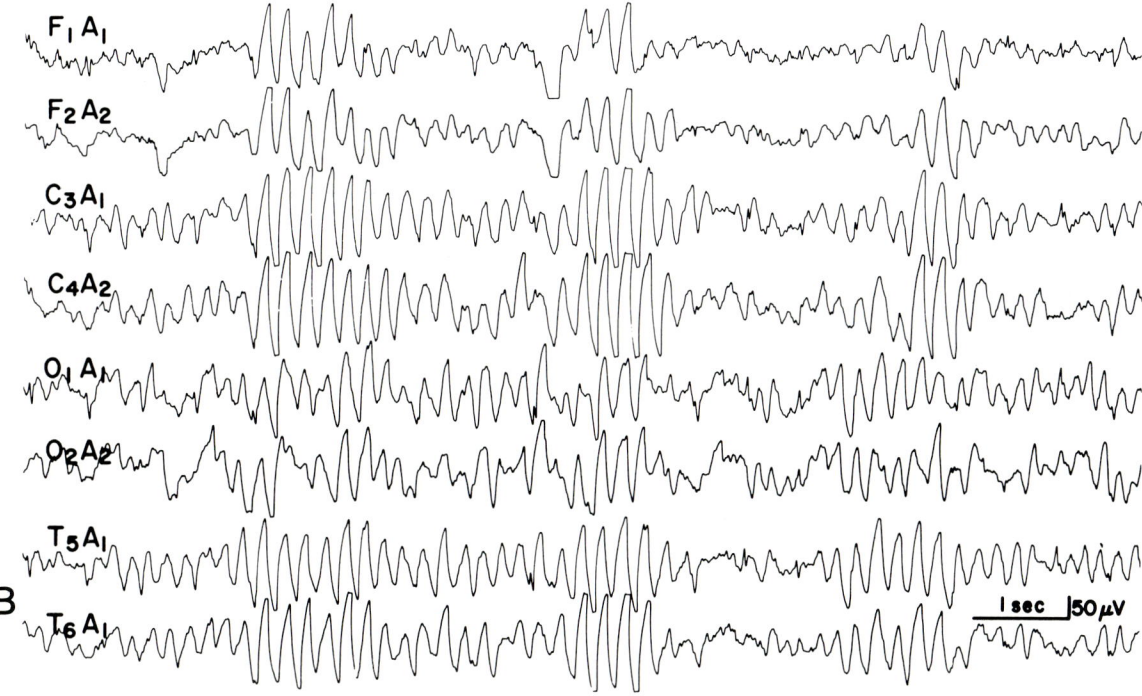

FIG. 23. B: Continuous "drowsy" pattern in asymptomatic 12-month-old infant.

like" components. The percentage approximates that found by Eeg-Olofsson et al. in their highly selected normal children (90).

In routine clinical practice, if such bursts occur only during drowsiness or at the onset of sleep, they cannot be considered evidence of abnormal function and certainly cannot support a clinical diagnosis of epilepsy. Even bursts with a clearly defined spike component fitting Gibbs and Gibbs' definition of "pseudo petit mal" have only a tenuous association (10%) with febrile convulsions. According to Gibbs and Gibbs (91), the incidence of epileptic (other than febrile) convulsions is only 7% greater in children with "pseudo petit mal" bursts than in children with normal EEGs, a difference that is not statistically significant.

From age 3 months to 6 years, patterns of drowsiness may vary from time to time in the same child. If sleep begins abruptly, little

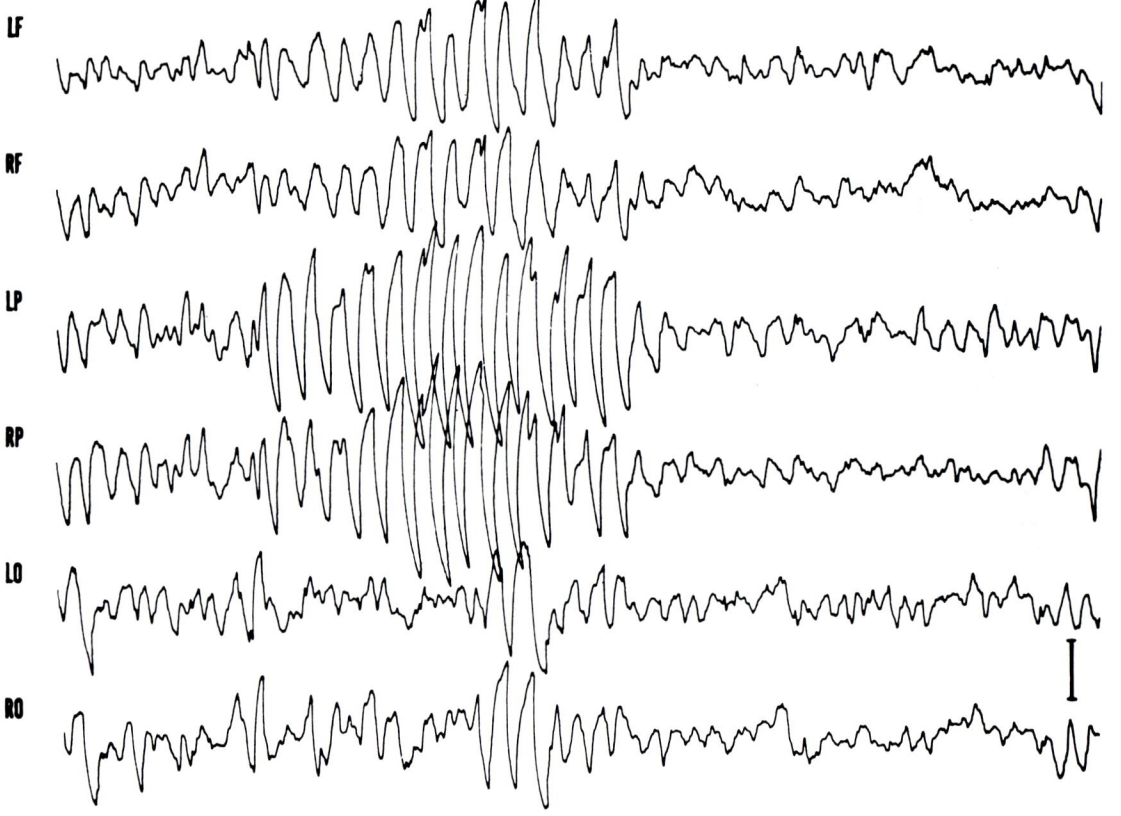

FIG. 24. Paroxysmal "hypnagogic hypersynchrony" in an asymptomatic female, aged 35 months. From Kellaway and Fox (35).

hypersynchrony of any type may be seen. If the onset of true sleep is delayed, continuous, rhythmic, high-voltage, slow or paroxysmal slow activity may persist for prolonged periods. Transient arousals (Fig. 28) frequently elicit a paroxysmal type of slow pattern; thus it is important for the technologist to make note of such arousals and for the electroencephalographer to watch for artifacts associated with such a change of state.

Arousal from any level of sleep in infants and children is always associated with a paroxysmal change. This may be a single, high-voltage sharp-wave transient similar to that in adults, or it may be

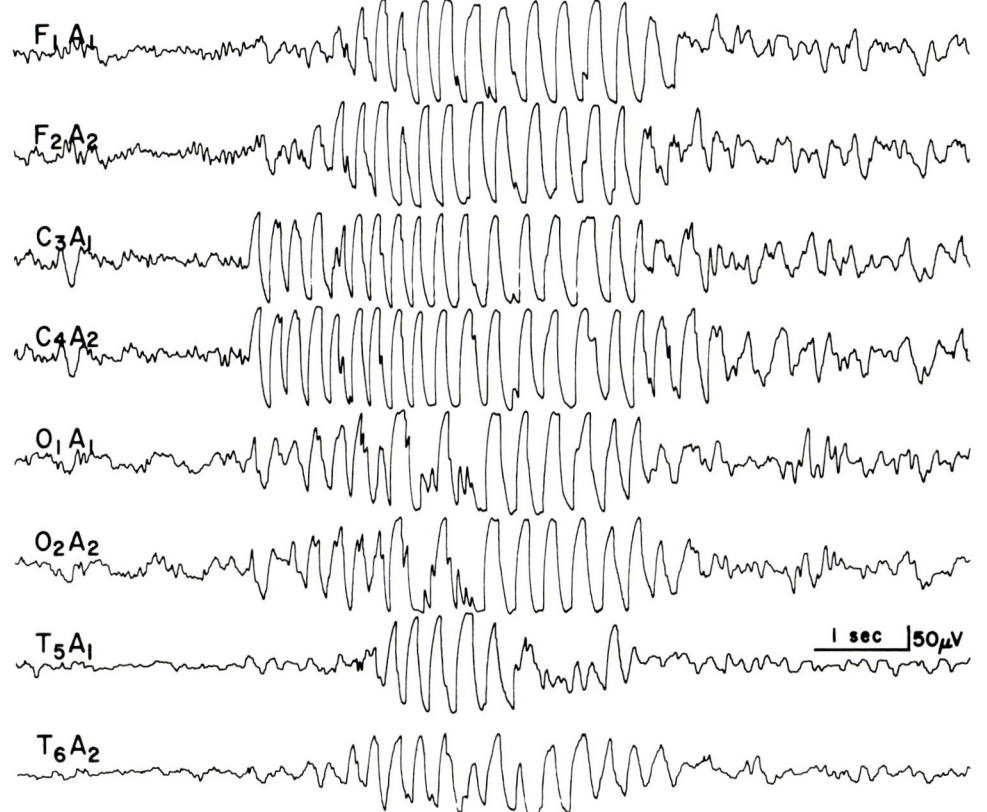

FIG. 25. Paroxysmal "hypnagogic hypersynchrony" in 14-year-old female, asymptomatic at the time of the EEG and in 10 years since tracing was made. No family history of seizures. Complex, paroxysmal slow bursts of this type, occurring only in drowsiness, are rare at this age (see Fig. 27).

a complex three-phase change, which, if unexpected or unrecognized as an arousal event, may be misinterpreted as abnormal (Fig. 29A and B).

In general, the ages with pronounced arousal patterns coincide with those for hypersynchronous slow drowsy patterns.

Activity of Arousal

Loomis and co-workers (93) were the first to show that reactive arousal involved a more or less complex electrographic pattern, rather than a simple and immediate transition from "sleep" to "waking"

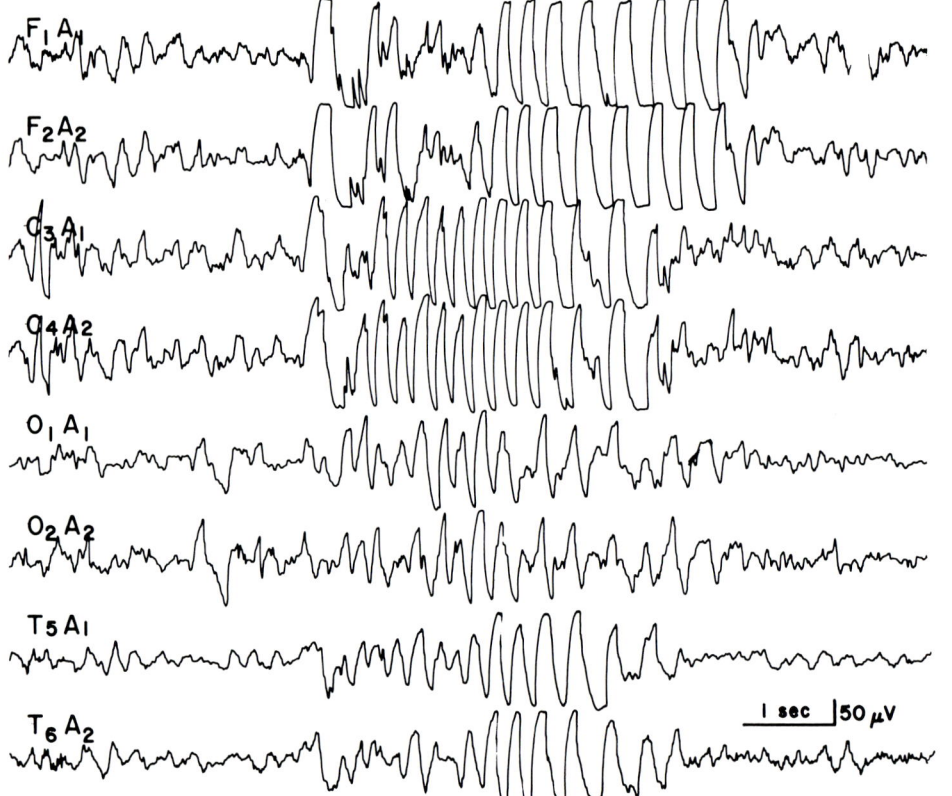

FIG. 26. Complex wave configurations such as in O1 and O2 and low-voltage spike-like components seen in other derivations are most common in drowsy, asymptomatic children between the ages of 4 and 9 years. Asymptomatic 7-year-old male.

activity. In adults they observed an initial diphasic slow wave followed by a series of rapid oscillations of "about 8 to 14 per second," the total pattern occurring maximally in the central regions "but appearing at lower amplitude in the frontal, occipital, and temporal areas also."

This phenomenon appears prominently in children but varies somewhat in character and degree with age. The initial "slow" component, sometimes erroneously referred to as the K complex, is discussed later in relation to the spontaneous, bicentral sharp-wave transients of early sleep. The "fast" component represents, as the original work-

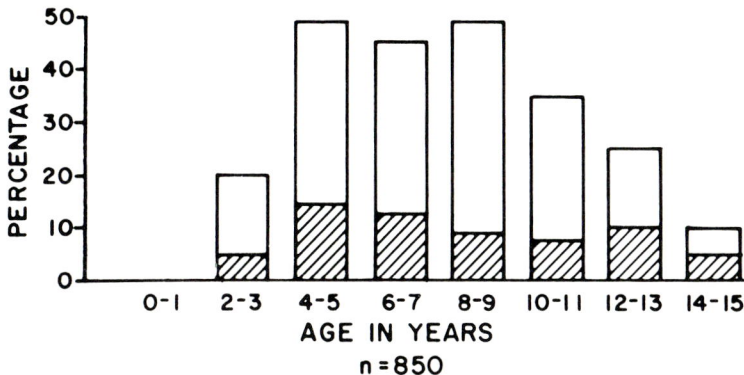

FIG. 27. Percentage of asymptomatic children of various ages who show paroxysmal slow bursts in drowsiness. Shaded areas show percentage having sharp or spike-like components intermixed with slow waves, as in Figs. 25 and 26.

ers hinted, a process associated with a greater degree of arousal. Thus the slow-transient component may represent the only response to a stimulus (e.g., a loud sound), with no clinical signs of arousal and indeed no transition to a lighter stage of electrographic sleep (Fig. 30A). The fast component, on the other hand, is always accompanied by clinical or electrographic evidence of partial or full arousal.

Neither component of the electrographic arousal reaction is clearly defined before age 2 months. During the first 8 weeks of life, and especially during the first 6 weeks, the transition from sleep to waking is characterized only by a degree of desynchronization. Sometime between the 8th and 12th week rudimentary diphasic slow-wave responses to applied stimuli may occur; moreover, at about this time, the first signs of a definite rhythmic hypersynchrony similar to that of the drowsy state make their appearance in the immediate postarousal state. However, the slow component of the arousal reaction is rarely well defined before age 3 months.

The faster component of the arousal reaction usually does not appear before age 7 months. Initially rudimentary, it consists of a few moderately high voltage sinusoidal waves of 4.0 to 4.5 Hz in the frontocentral region, superimposed on a slower irregular background activity (Fig. 30B).

With increasing age, this "fast" component of arousal increases in frequency until it reaches the adult rate of 8 to 10 Hz. In children, it is maximal in the central region (C3–C4), and its field is such that its voltage is higher at F4–F3 than at P4–P3. Its appearance is transitory, and its duration is usually no more than 4 to 5 sec. Occasionally the duration of the runs of this activity may be as long as 30 sec (35).[11]

Postarousal hypersynchrony. In children, the "fast" component of the arousal pattern is quickly followed by what would be called a "paradoxical arousal response" in adults. Thus as the child awakens, a high-voltage, monomorphic, quite slow rhythm (2.5 to 3.5 Hz) appears in the frontal regions (Fig. 29A), and as further arousal ensues, the rhythmic slow activity becomes less slow and moves posteriorly, the voltage and persistence of the rhythm progressively diminishing in anterior derivations. In infants and children in whom continuous "monorhythmic slow" or "paroxysmal slow" activity occurs during drowsiness, there may be similar episodes of postarousal hypersynchronous slow activity of similar frequency (35).[12]

A graphic depiction of the various components of arousal and awakening patterns in children is shown in Fig. 30. These components may be aborted at any point in the process. If an external stimulus triggers the arousal (if there is a sudden sound, if the child's name is called, or if he is touched), a diphasic sharp-wave transient appears

---

[11] This is probably the same arousal rhythm that White and Tharp (94) reported in a series of children with "minimal brain dysfunction"; they did not study its incidence in a matched control group.

[12] In infants when this phase of postarousal slow activity is over, passive eye closure should be done in order to determine the frequency of the occipital alpha rhythm.

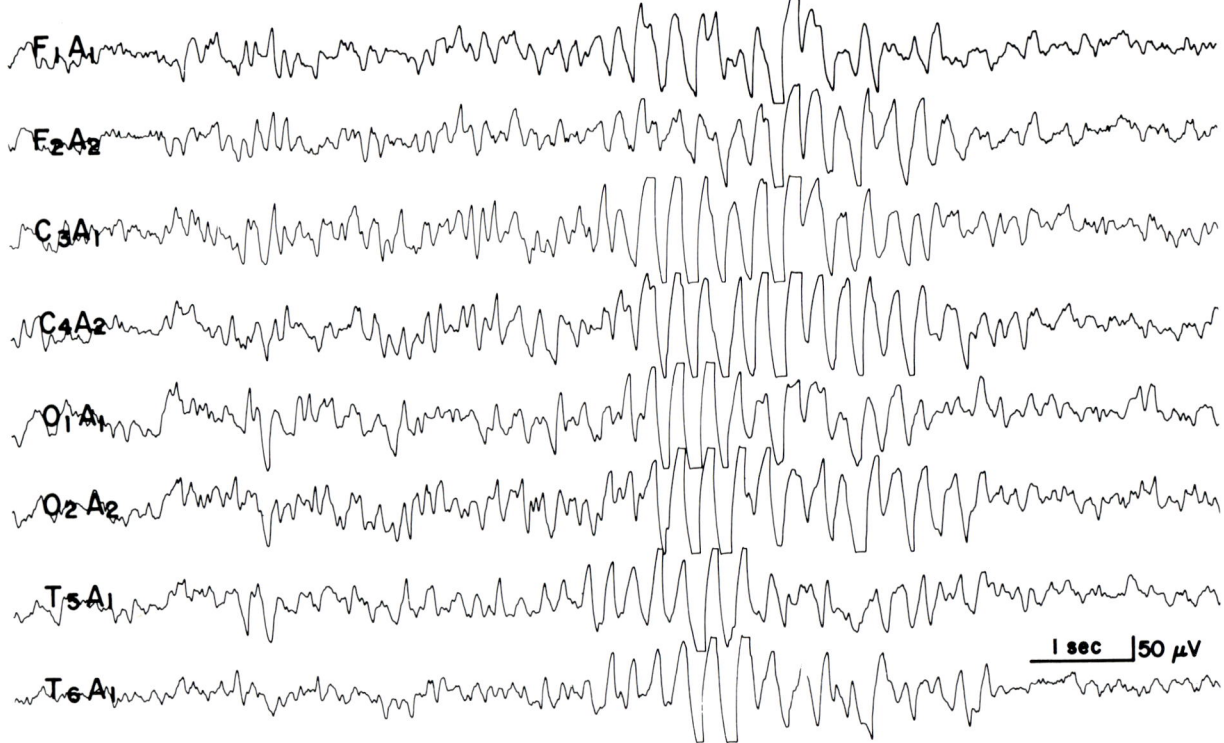

FIG. 28. Transient arousal in asymptomatic male, aged 7 years. Just prior to beginning of sample, child had been asleep (stage 2). A brief period of desynchronization is followed by some central and occipital alpha activity lasting 2–2.5 sec and, in turn, by a high-voltage, central-dominant, "drowsy" burst lasting about 3 sec; then sleep resumes.

in the region of the vertex; if no arousal effect is produced, the background EEG activity reverts immediately to its prestimulation character (as in Fig. 30A). Presumably a further degree of arousal is signaled by the appearance of the "fast" central component (as in Fig. 30B), and overt signs of arousal (e.g., movement or eye opening) do not occur until the hypersynchronous slow activity appears (Fig. 30C). *Spontaneous* arousal may occur without the appearance of the diphasic central (vertex) sharp-wave transient.

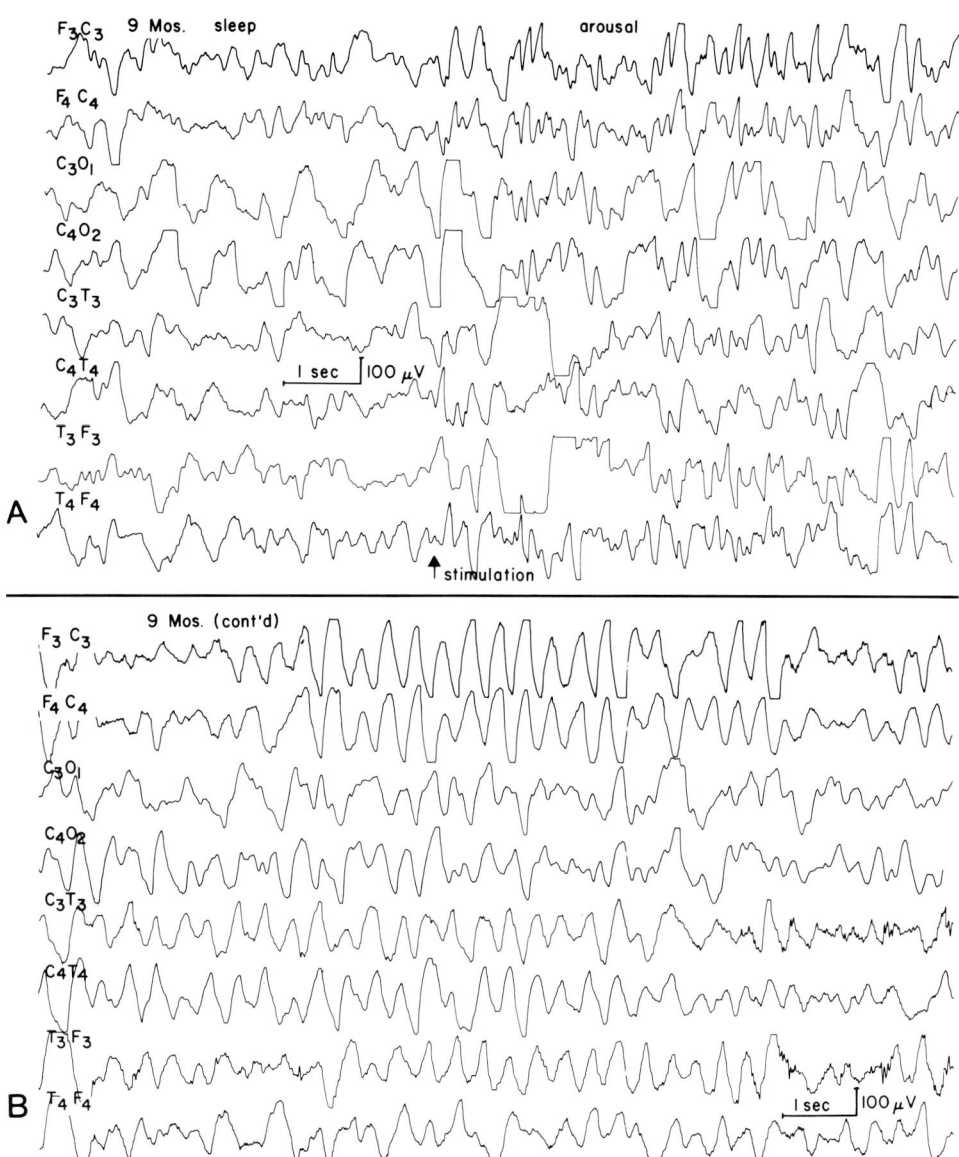

FIG. 29. **A** and **B**: Arousal from stage 4 sleep in response to a loud handclap (↑ stimulation). Asymptomatic 9-month-old male. Note initial train of central rhythmic 6.5–7 Hz activity after stimulation, followed by generalized, but frontal dominant, rhythmic, 3–4 Hz activity lasting about 11 sec. Full sequence of arousal changes is diagramed in Fig. 30.

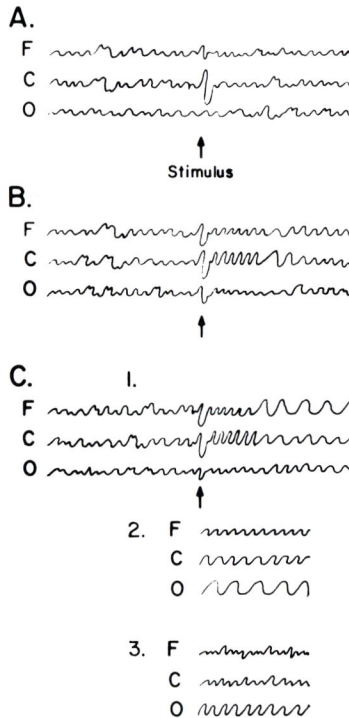

FIG. 30. Diagrammatic representation of degrees of EEG arousal in children. **A:** Vertex transient elicited by stimulus (e.g., handclap), with no change in sleep pattern. **B:** Central, rhythmic "fast" 6–8 Hz activity follows vertex transient, then quick reversion to sleep pattern of prestimulus level. **C:** Vertex transient and "fast" component are followed by high-voltage, rhythmic, frontal-dominant delta activity [1], which shifts posteriorly as anterior rhythms increase in frequency [2]; finally, the characteristic awake pattern is reached [3]. Child may appear to be clinically awake soon after rhythmic frontal-dominant delta activity appears.

In adults, the arousal pattern depends on the level of sleep that preceded the arousal. Arousal from stage 1 (drowsiness) is not associated with any change other than a reversion to the awake alpha rhythm pattern (Fig. 31). Once the spindle stage has been reached, an attenuated form of the arousal patterns seen in children may occur: there may be an initial diphasic central sharp-wave transient, followed by a brief train of waves of alpha activity frequency that occur *in the frontocentral region,* and there may be one or two high-voltage, frontal slow waves (1.5–3.0 Hz). Examples of adult "arousal" patterns are illustrated in Figs. 31 and 32.

A postarousal, frontocentral burst of 4 to 5 Hz waves of brief duration may occur in young adults and is fairly common in adolescents. The only figures on the incidence of this type of postarousal burst in asymptomatic subjects are those of Gibbs and Gibbs (89), who found the bursts to be present in at least 40% of subjects 10 to 14 years of age.

Activity of Sleep

Vertex sharp-wave transients of sleep. The onset of stage 2 sleep is signaled by the appearance of bilaterally synchronous sharp-wave transients in the central region (Fig. 33). They are maximal in voltage in the C3 and C4 electrode positions, but when they are of high voltage, as they sometimes are in young children, they may be evident over a wide area of the frontocentral region. These sharp waves are usually diphasic, with an initial surface-negative deflection followed by a low-voltage, surface-positive phase. The sharp wave may be followed by a slow, surface-negative wave and/or a sleep spindle.

From the time these waves first appear (at approximately 8 weeks postterm), they are bilaterally synchronous and essentially symmetrical on the two sides. With persistent asymmetry of more than 20%, a lesion on the low side should be suspected. Some variable voltage

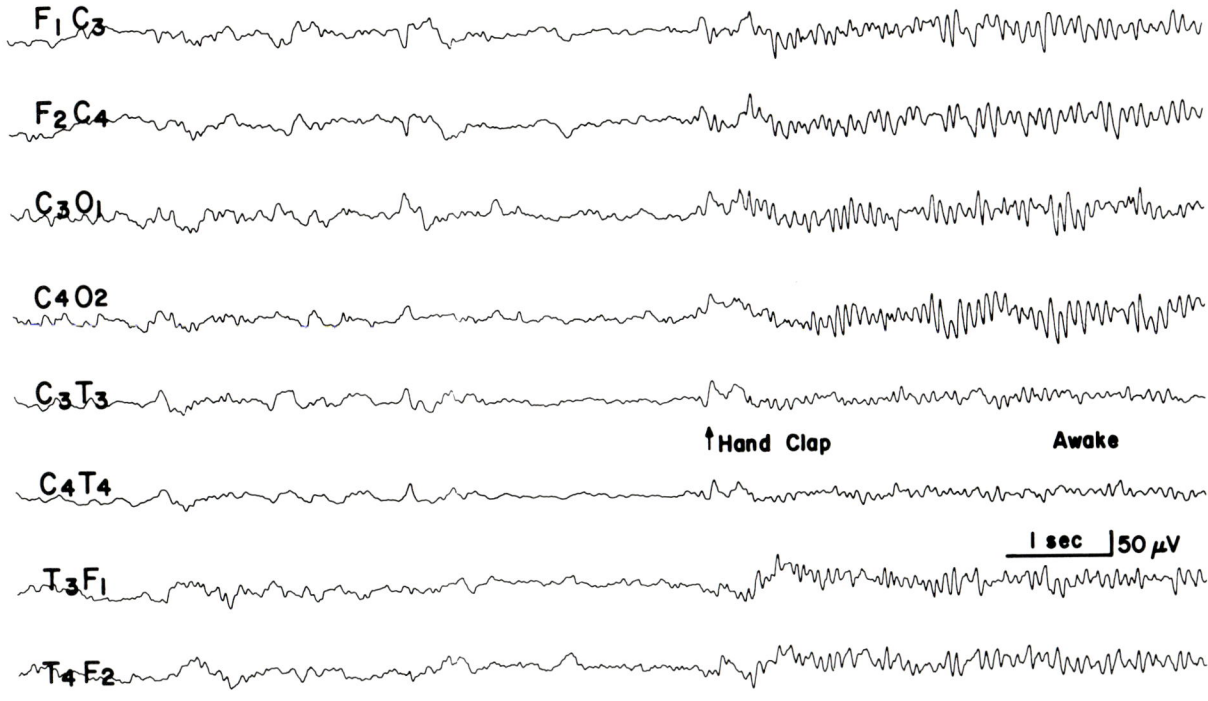

FIG. 31. In stage 1 sleep, arousal is associated with an immediate return of waking pattern without initial high-voltage slow-wave transient.

difference between the two sides is not uncommon in young children, but if the low voltage always appears on the same side, it should be regarded as significant. Unlike other sleep activity (e.g., spindles), vertex transients are always bilaterally synchronous in normal individuals. A breakdown of this synchrony is usually a sign of increased intraventricular pressure (obstructive hydrocephalus). Asynchrony should be distinguished from the situation not uncommonly seen in children in which the vertex transients do not occur on both sides each time. In this situation one or the other side may show more vertex transients (and spindles), but whenever they occur bilaterally they are symmetrical on the two sides. Although this phenomenon—in which an occasional vertex transient (and spindle) may be

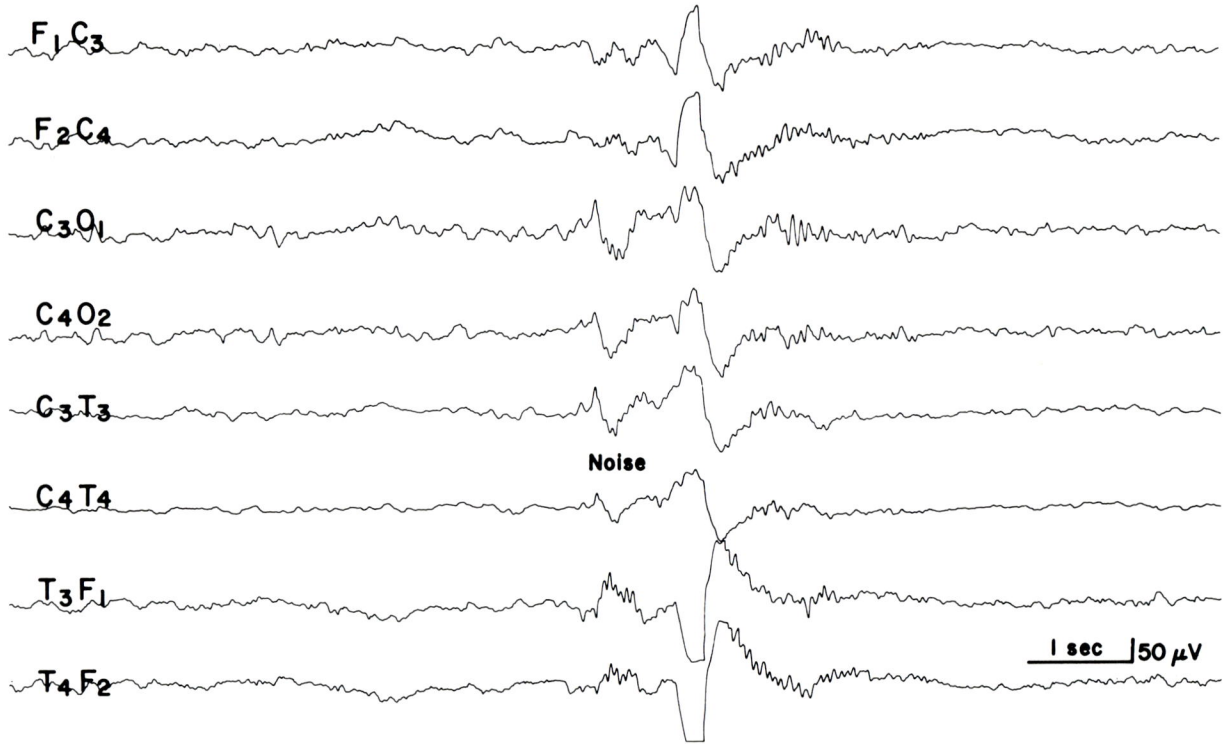

FIG. 32. Abortive-arousal response consisting of a slow-wave transient, maximum in voltage in the frontal leads, followed by a train of 9–14 Hz waves; normal adult. Vertex transient and low-voltage spindle (sigma) activity occur prior to the abortive-arousal response. Such arousal patterns may occur spontaneously.

missing on one side—occurs in apparently healthy children, it is comparatively rare (< 3%) and may indeed be pathophysiologically significant.

The very high voltage that vertex transients may attain in children aged 2 to 4 years may come as a surprise to the electroencephalographer not accustomed to children's records. Caution must be exercised that the high voltage and a sharply peaked wave form not lead to an incorrect interpretation of abnormality. Similarly, these vertex transients in children, unlike the situation in adults, may occur in quick succession (every 1 to 2 sec), and an "interference pattern"

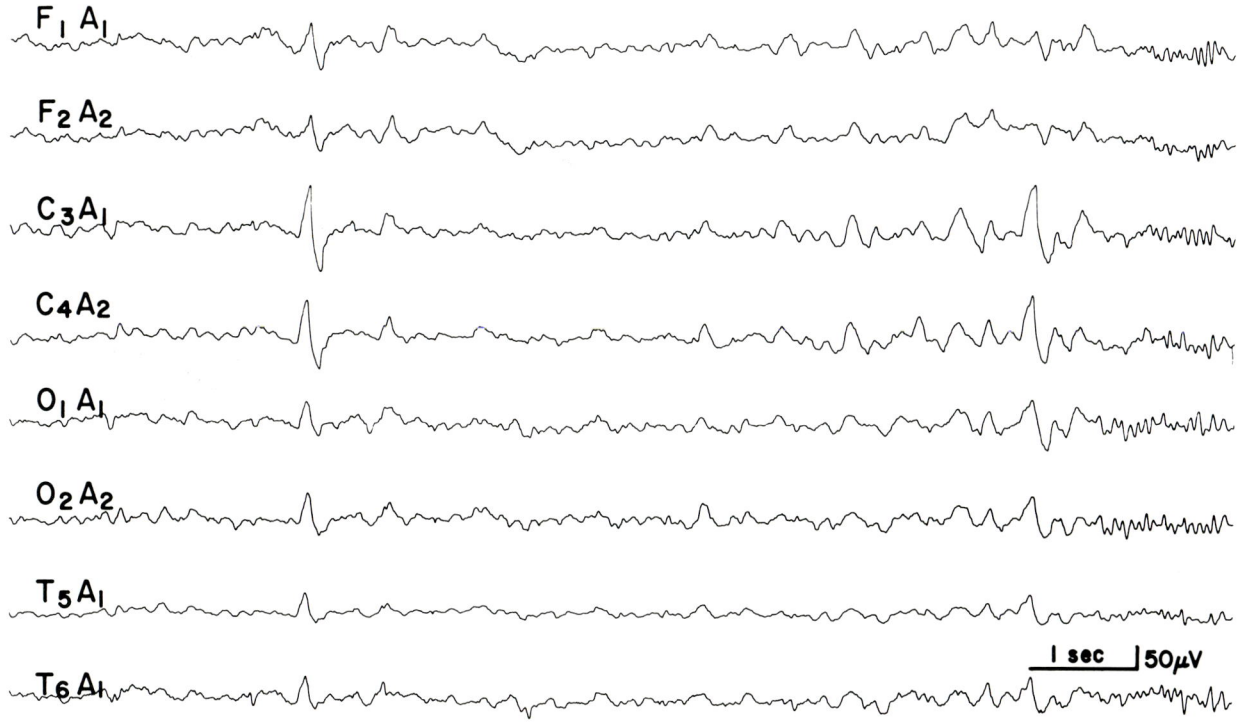

FIG. 33. Example of bilateral vertex transients in asymptomatic 12-year-old female. Note diphasic wave form in central derivations.

may result, giving these waves a complex configuration that seems abnormal (Fig. 34).

The voltage, and to some degree the configuration, of successive vertex transients in any series may fluctuate considerably, and in a given montage it may be difficult to distinguish the vertex transients (Fig. 35) from abnormal sharp-wave discharges arising uni- or bilater- ally from foci in this region (rolandic "spikes"). The problem often can be solved only by mapping the fields of the various sharp waves present.

Spindles. Sleep spindles, at the time of their first appearance at 6 to 8 weeks postterm, are bilaterally asynchronous (35) (Fig. 36); they become increasingly more synchronous during the first year

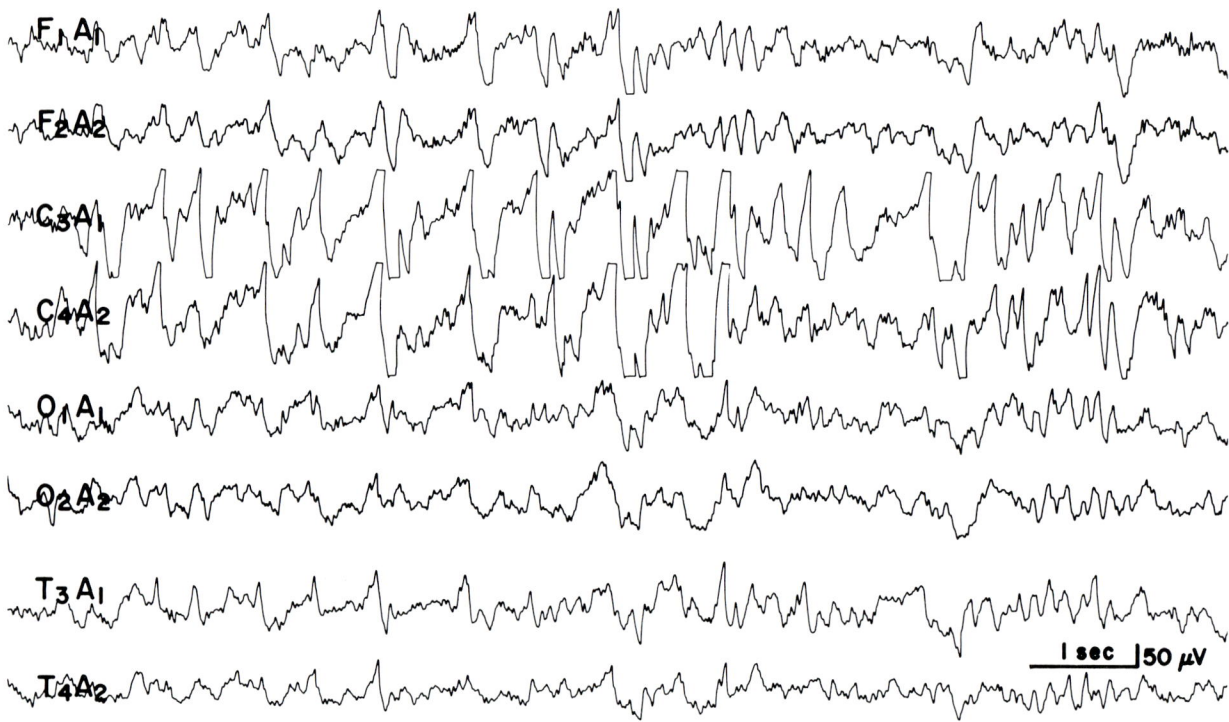

FIG. 34. Vertex transients occurring in repetitive sequence in asymptomatic 11-year-old male. Note variable and often sharp wave form. The higher voltage transients cause blocking at normal gain.

of life, so that by the 18th month, most of the spindles are bilaterally synchronous. Before age 2 years, asynchrony of sleep spindles cannot be considered evidence of abnormality. The wave form and duration of sleep spindles in infants differ from those of adults: the spindles may be 2 to 4 sec in duration and lack the typical fusiform amplitude modulation that gives the adult type of sleep spindle its name. The individual waves of the spindle may be sharply peaked (reminiscent of the mu rhythm) in the surface-negative phase (35) (Fig. 36).

Three types of spindles may be distinguished by their frequency characteristics and potential field. The most common, and usually

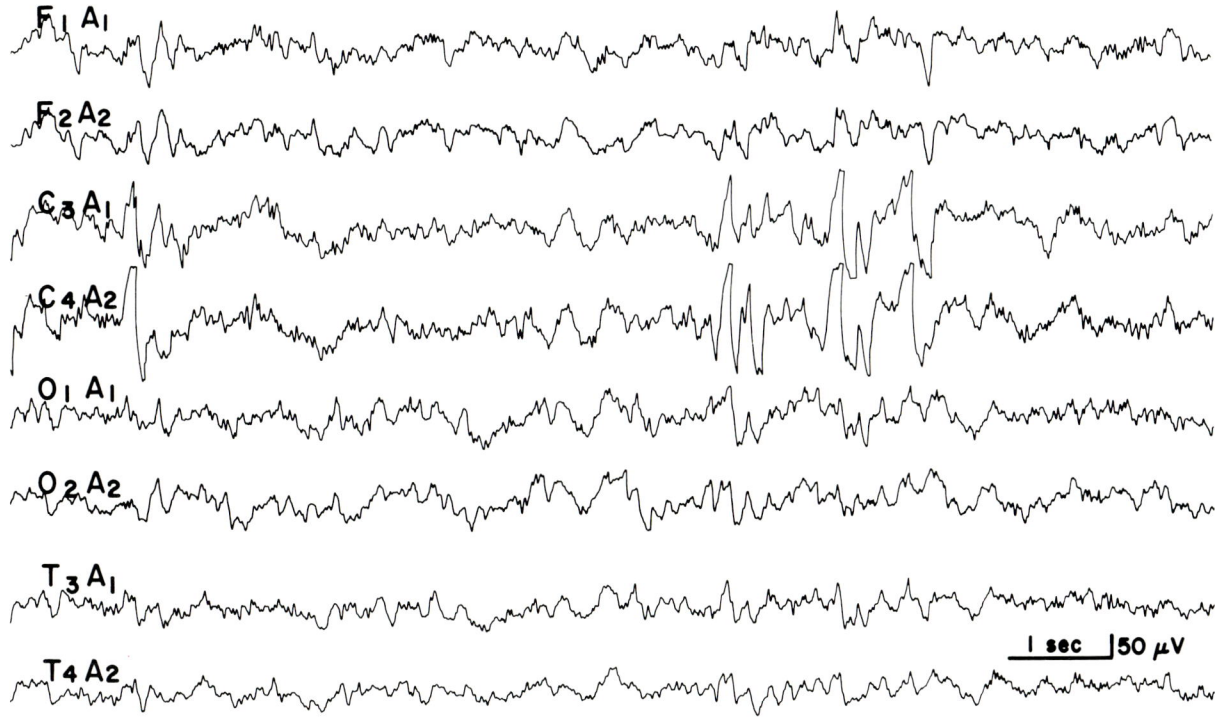

FIG. 35. Characteristically "sharp" appearance of some vertex transients in children is increased in this montage by the admixture of EKG artifact and fast activity. Sample is from asymptomatic female, aged 9 years 6 months (now 25 years old). No evidence of CNS disease.

the only type seen in adults, has a frequency of approximately 14 Hz, and the center of the field coincides closely with the C3 and C4 electrode placements. The presence of the spindle distinguishes stages 2 and 3 sleep, but it is also the distinguishing characteristic of "spindle coma" or "coma sleep" (95).

Spindles that have a fundamental frequency of approximately 10 to 12 Hz and a more anterior locus of origin occur in 5% of normal individuals in the age group 3 to 12 years (Fig. 37). These "frontal" spindles, which are seldom more than 3 sec in duration, should be clearly differentiated from "continuous spindling" or "exaggerated"

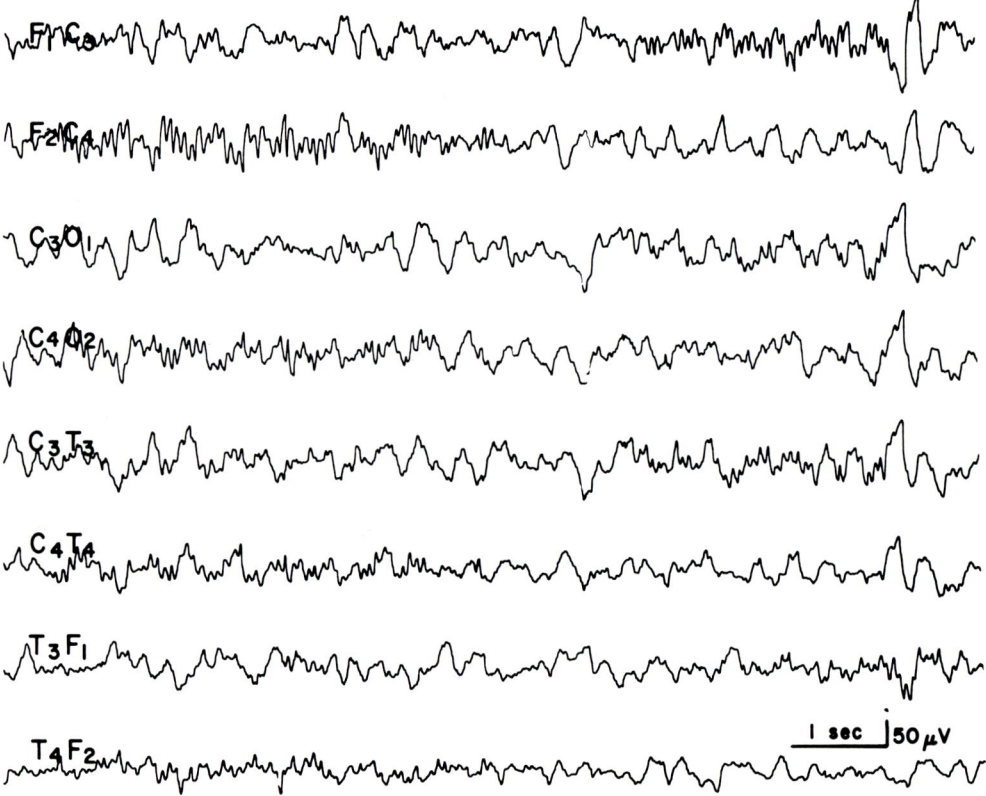

FIG. 36. Typical infant sleep spindles. Note asynchrony (attenuation) between two sides, prolonged duration (> 4 sec), lack of fusiform amplitude modulation, and mu-like wave form.

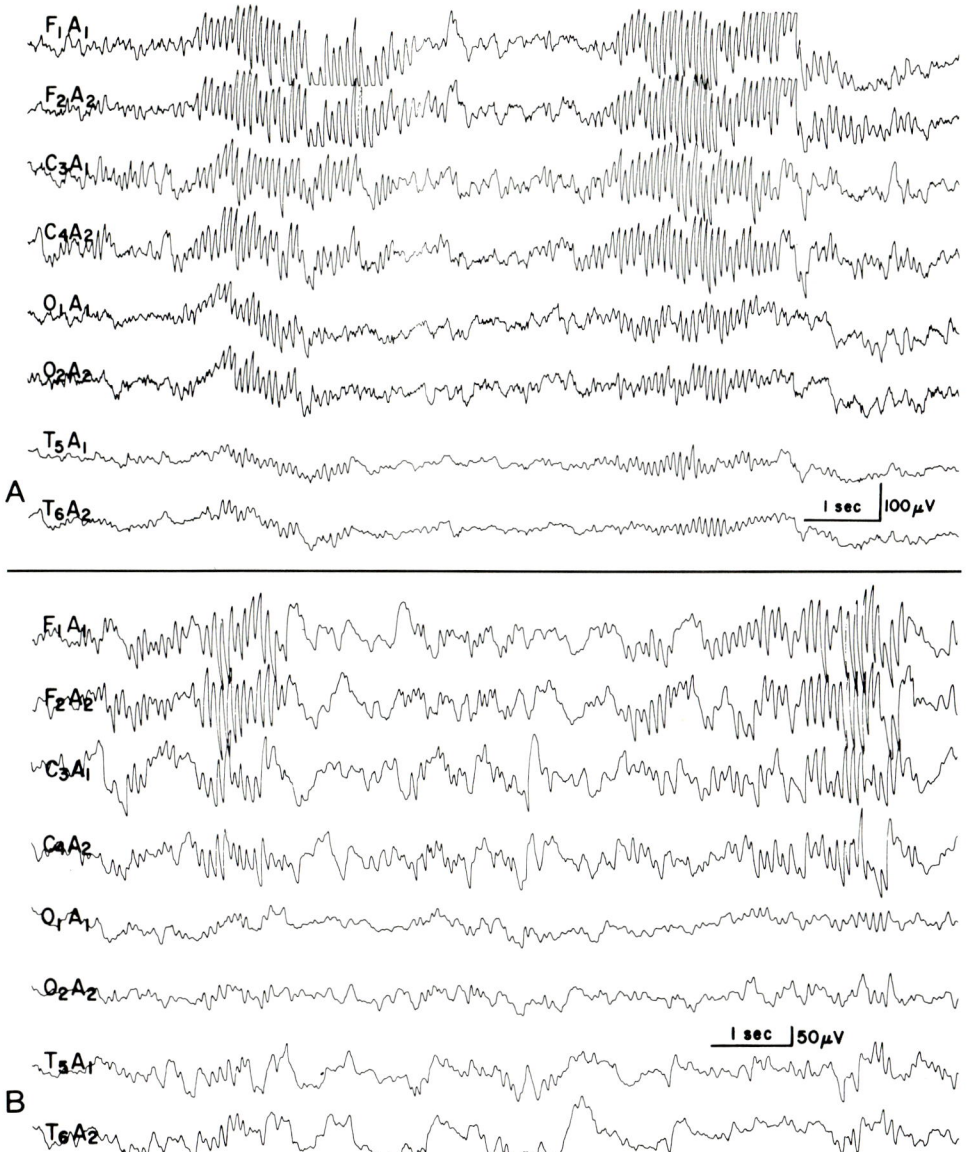

FIG. 37. A: Example of 12-Hz spindles in stage 2 sleep in asymptomatic male, aged 10 years 10 months. These spindles are often high in voltage as compared to 14-Hz central spindles and have larger potential field. **B:** Example of 10-Hz frontal-dominant spindles in asymptomatic 6-year-old male.

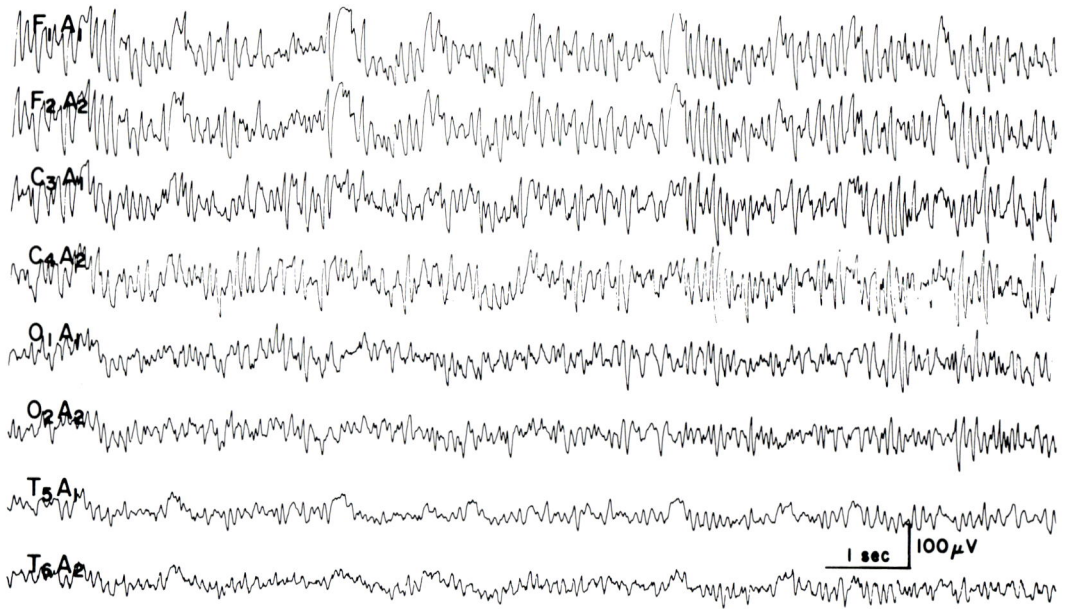

FIG. 38. Almost continuous 10–12 Hz, moderately high voltage, frontal-dominant activity showing a spindle-like amplitude modulation in female, aged 52 years, stuporous from diazepam overdose.

spindles, which are an abnormal finding seen in children with certain types of cerebral palsy and mental retardation. Frontal 10 Hz "spindling" that is almost continuous can result from drug action (e.g., morphine and halothane anesthesia), but the unremitting character of the activity and lack of reactivity to intense stimuli clearly distinguish it from the frontal dominant 10 Hz spindles of sleep (Fig. 38).

Fusiform bursts of 18 to 22 Hz activity in sleep should not be confused with sleep spindles (sigma activity). These are most commonly effects of medication, particularly the phenothiazines and barbiturates (Fig. 39), but they (continuous fast and spindling) are also associated with certain pathological conditions in the absence of drugs.

Fast activity during sleep. Sometime between the 5th and 6th month, many infants begin to show a low-voltage fast activity during the early stages of sleep. This activity occurs in all derivations but is most pronounced in the central or postcentral region (Fig. 9). The frequency averages approximately 28 Hz, but varies as much as ± 6 Hz in different subjects. When the fast activity first occurs, its amplitude is very low (5 μV or less), but relatively high amplitudes (30 μV maximum) may be seen by the 12th to 18th month, when it seems to reach its maximum expression. After age 30 to 36 months,

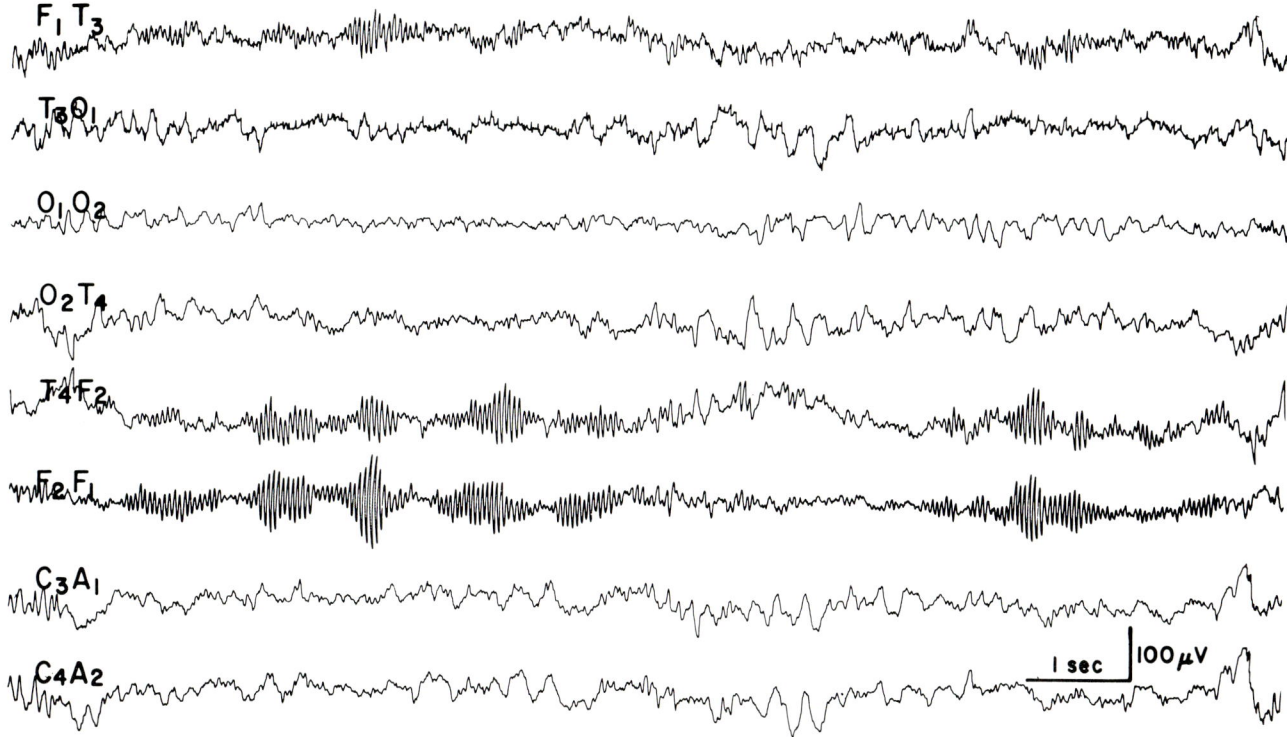

FIG. 39. Barbiturate "spindles" such as those in this figure are sometimes confused with physiological sleep spindles. Note greater amplitude of paired frontal derivations as compared to homolateral frontal derivations—a common finding with barbiturate spindles but not characteristic of sleep spindles. Male, aged 13 years 4 months, with generalized seizures and taking phenobarbital 150 mg/day. Fast activity not present prior to treatment. Sample is from stage 1 sleep.

pronounced fast activity during early sleep is less common, and generally the amplitudes seen are not as great as in the 12 to 18 month age group. Older children are much less likely to show fast activity during early sleep, and after age 7 it is relatively uncommon (35).

When sedation with a barbiturate or other fast activity-inducing drug is used to promote sleep, fast activity is increased in the awake and the sleeping EEG. This fast activity has a frequency chiefly in the 18 to 22 Hz range and a predominantly anterior distribution.

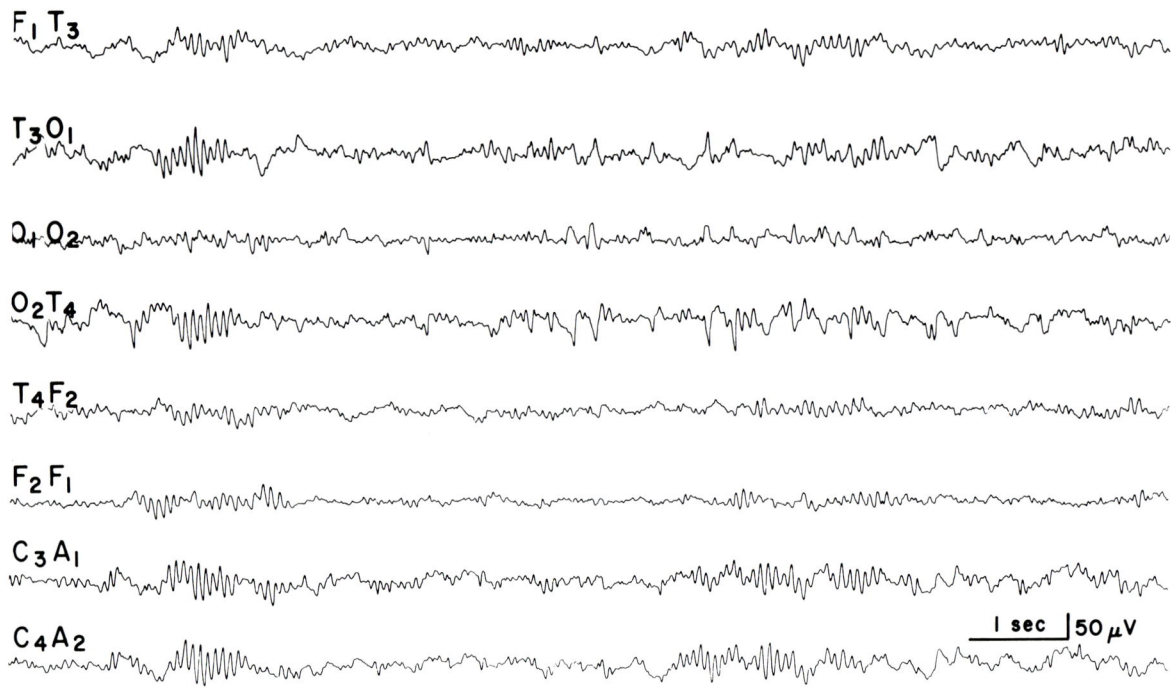

FIG. 40. POSTS during stage 2 sleep (note presence of 14-Hz spindles) in asymptomatic 14-year-old male.

When sedation is administered at some point just prior to or during the recording, the fast activity induced displays maximum voltage during light sleep (stages 2 and 3) and is greatly diminished during deeper sleep. Upon arousal, the fast activity increases again and becomes much more pronounced than in the presleep record—unless there was an inordinate delay in the onset of sleep. Fast activity induced by chronic medication or a drug administered a long time before the recording shows the same diminution during the deep sleep stages but is *equal* during the pre- and postsleep *awake* tracings.

The voltage of both natural and induced fast activity should be essentially the same bilaterally. With a consistent difference of more than 30%, an abnormality on the low side should be suspected, except when the fast activity is confined to a circumscribed focal area, in which case it may be associated with a focal lesion in that

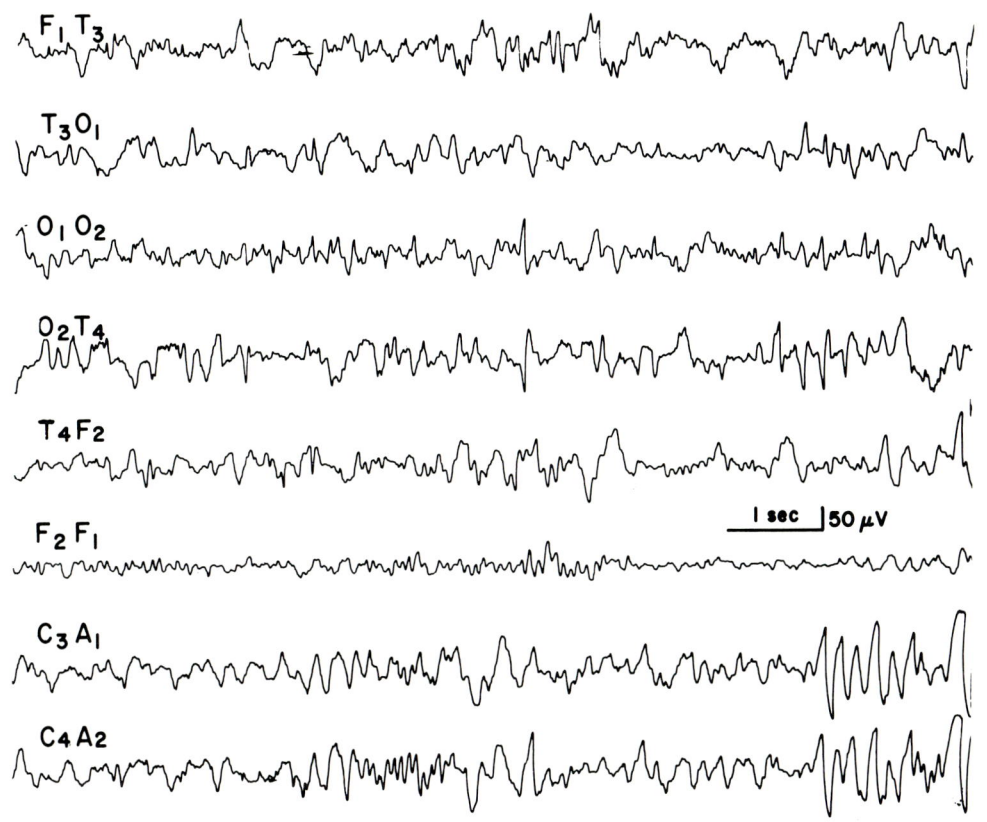

FIG. 41. Asymmetrical POSTS in healthy female, aged 11 years. Note considerable voltage difference between sides, especially of the isolated sharp wave (POST) near center of sample. The fact that the series shows a repetition rate of about 5 Hz at right side of sample and that the sharp waves are positive at O2 provide clues to their identity. However, although positive sharp waves or spikes rarely signify abnormal activity, electrodes near the midline (e.g., O1 or O2) may reveal only the positive end of a dipole, presumably because the negative end lies on the mesial surface of the hemisphere.

region (96). (Beware, however, of the pitfall mentioned elsewhere: the low-resistance pathway provided by a bony skull defect.)

Fast activity of cortical origin is particularly susceptible to the effects of ischemia, hypoxia, contusion, and the presence of subdural fluid. Thus its depression or absence focally or unilaterally may be a useful EEG sign, particularly when interpreted in relation to other findings (e.g., the presence of a slow-wave focus).

Positive occipital sharp transients of sleep. Surface-positive sharp transients, occurring singly or more commonly in runs of 4 to 5 Hz, are often seen in routine EEG sleep recordings (Fig. 40). These

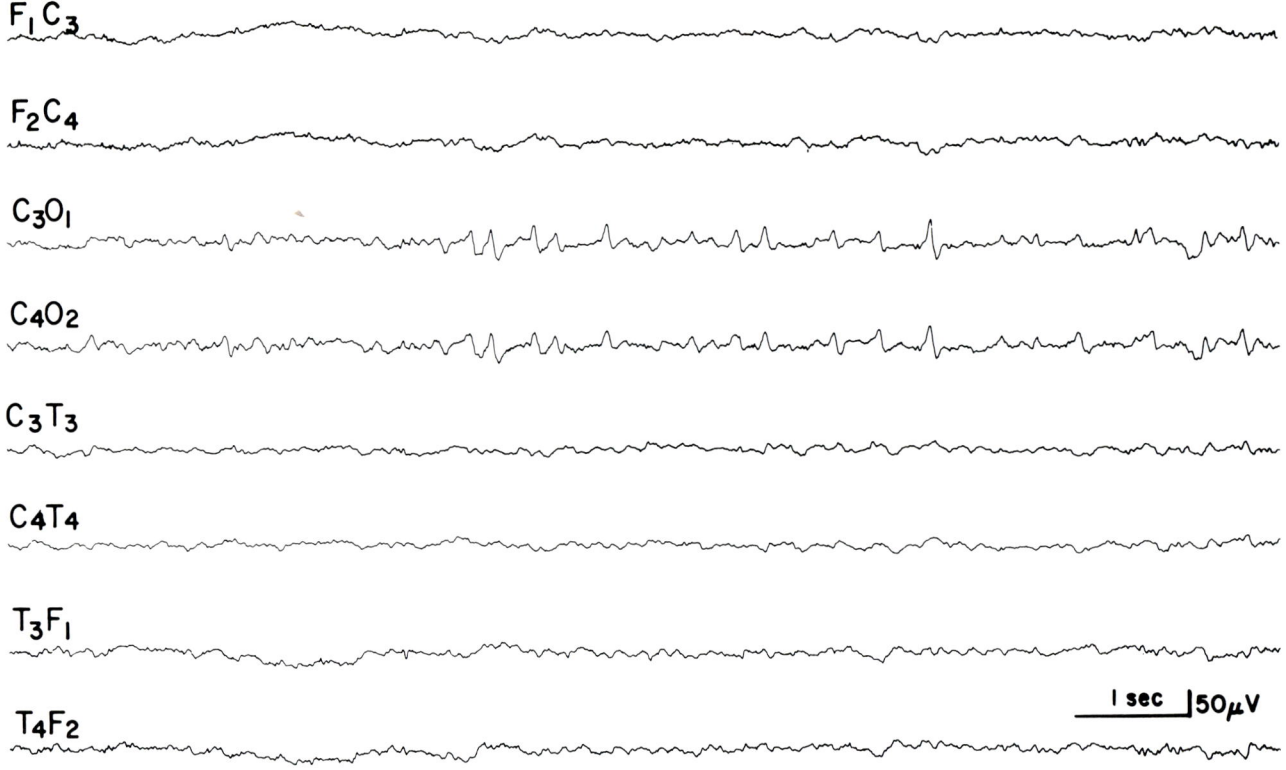

FIG. 42. POSTS, occurring after drowsiness but before spindle sleep had been reached, in asymptomatic 17-year-old female. Note the low-voltage, slightly slow or "drowsy" appearance of the record. Commonly, POSTS appear this way during daytime naps that may occur during routine studies in the typical EEG laboratory.

interesting waves are commonly seen in the EEG laboratory because they are prone to occur during daytime naps and particularly if the patient has been partially aroused and quickly returns to sleep. The pattern occurs in the age group 4 to 50 years and is most common and best expressed in young adults (15 to 35 years). The individual waves show a sharp, surface-positive peak, followed in some instances by a low-voltage, surface-negative peak. The ascending deflection has a somewhat slower time course than the descending phase, so

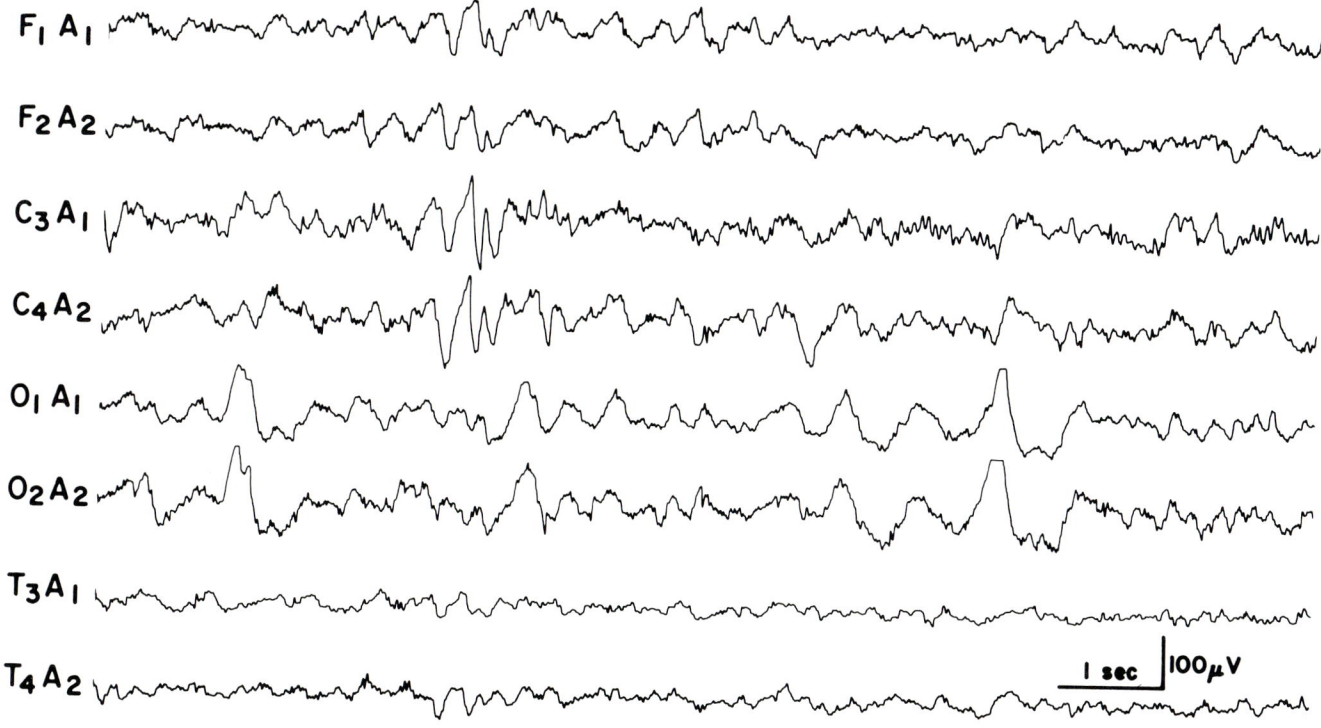

FIG. 43. Cone-shaped, posterior slow transients during light sleep in asymptomatic 35-month-old male.

the resultant wave form may have a checkmark-like shape; some authors refer to them as occipital V-waves of sleep.

Positive occipital sharp transients of sleep (POSTS) (97) are always bilaterally synchronous but are commonly asymmetrical on the two sides (Fig. 41); voltage differences as great as 60% are seen in normal individuals. This may lead to misinterpretation of POSTS as abnormal sharp-wave activity in one or the other occipital region. In this regard, it is important to remember that POSTS may occur at a time when the background activity has an amorphous character that might be thought to be "drowsiness" or a slightly slow awake pattern (Fig. 42).

The helpful distinguishing characteristics of POSTS are: (a) their

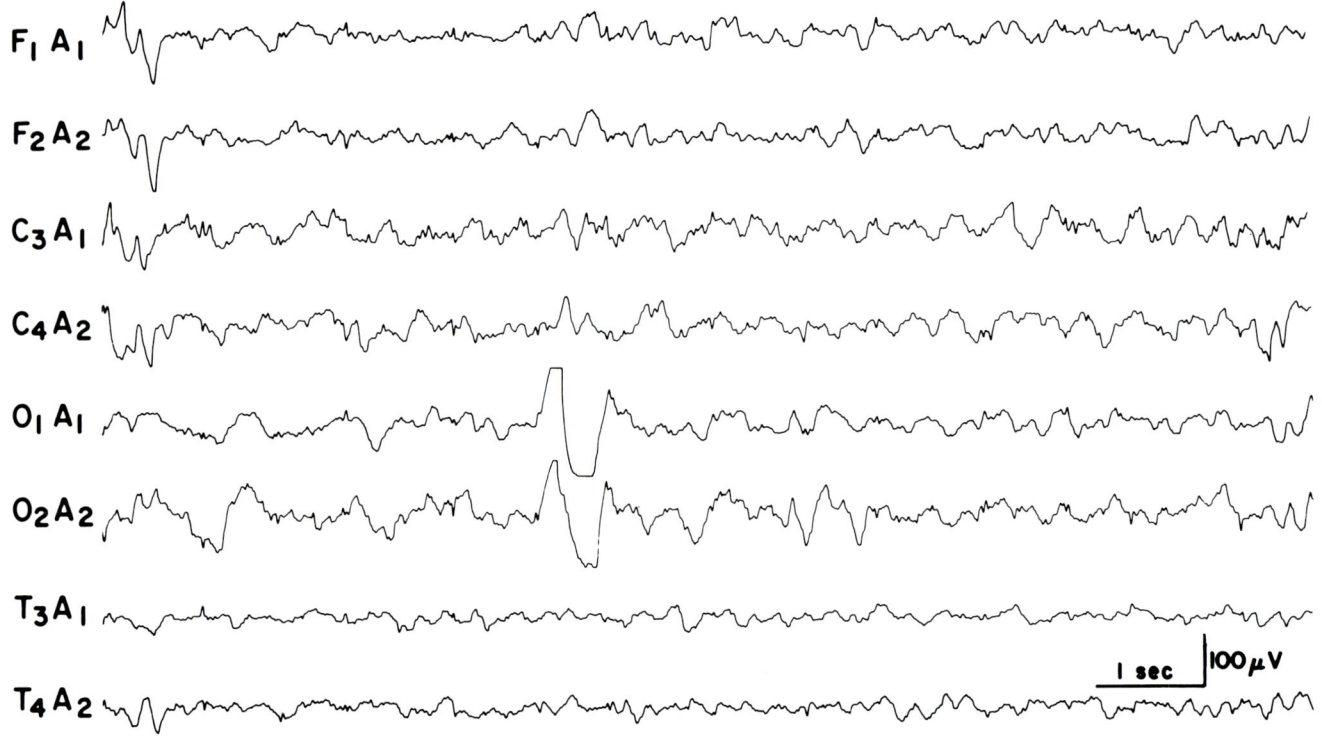

FIG. 44. Diphasic slow-wave transients in occipital derivations in light sleep in same subject as in Fig. 43.

surface positivity (abnormal surface-positive cerebral spikes are rare), (b) the fact that they tend to occur in trains with a repetition rate of 4 to 5 Hz, and (c) their predominantly monophasic checkmark-like wave form.

Occipital transients of sleep. In children, the transition from light to deep sleep may be associated with the bilateral appearance of high-voltage slow transients in the occipital regions (35). These waves vary from a cone-shaped configuration (Fig. 43) to a diphasic slow transient (Fig. 44) reminiscent of a prolonged vertex transient. At first, during light sleep, these transients occur every 3 to 6 sec, but with deepening sleep, they appear more frequently and seem to meld into the continuous, occipital-dominant, random, very slow delta waves of stage 4 sleep.

THE MEANING OF "NORMAL" AND THE SIGNIFICANCE OF DEVIATIONS FROM THE NORM

The purpose of this chapter is to delineate the processes involved in an orderly approach to visual analysis and to provide information concerning the parameters of the "normal" EEG in adults and children. The latter endeavor, if it is to be anything more than a pedagogical exercise, requires some discussion of the meaning of "normal." Perhaps more importantly, some thought should be directed to the meaning of deviations from normative data. Do such deviations always imply *abnormality?* Do they imply that the brain has suffered some sort of insult? Does their presence necessarily mean that they have a causative relationship with the symptoms or signs for which the patient was referred? Certainly the history of clinical electroencephalography has not been distinguished by thoughtful analysis of these problems or even by a critical sense of their significance. Perhaps this has been the natural outcome of the quest for laboratory techniques that can provide "penny in the slot" diagnoses—the kind of explicit certainty that computerized axial tomography apparently is now providing, at a somewhat higher price, for diseases with a morphological signature. From its inception, there has been a tendency in electroencephalography to view minor deviations from the norm as objective evidence of disordered brain function[13]—the result of some past or ongoing pathological process. To some electroencephalographers many EEG findings automatically mean "epilepsy," and to others certain findings (e.g., a spike focus) always imply the presence of a palpable brain lesion. Such concepts are now undergoing thoughtful reappraisal. It is gradually becoming recognized that the EEG characteristics of a given individual are the product of diverse

---

[13] Minor dysrhythmias have been used to "prove" the already tenuous clinical diagnosis of "minimal brain damage."

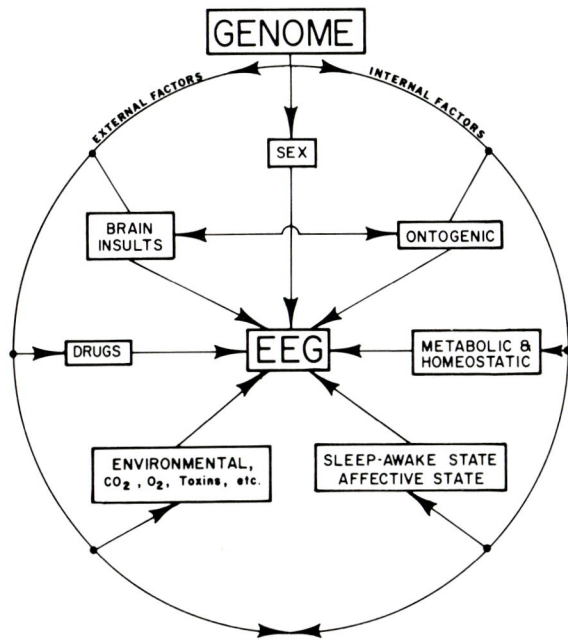

FIG. 45. Factors and their interplay that are known to influence the characteristics of the EEG.

internal and external influences, acting on a genetically determined substrate. These influences may be conceptualized diagrammatically in terms of their interactions. Figure 45 represents an attempt to specify the factors that determine the characteristics of the EEG and to illustrate their interplay.

Many years ago Kennard (98,99) suggested that the "total EEG pattern" may ultimately result from all the "stabilizing" and "disruptive" influences brought to bear on cerebral function. The validity of this concept is being clarified only now.

Genetic Factors

Kennard was also the first to stress the possibility that familial or inherited tendencies may be important in the genesis of some of the deviations from normal (e.g., nonspecific dysrhythmias) seen in children. Her hypothesis was based on the early studies of Davis and Davis (100) and Lennox et al. (101,102), which suggested that the characteristics of the EEG in normal as well as in some epileptic children may be a hereditary trait. Knott and associates (103) also noted a high incidence of EEG "abnormalities" of similar types in the "normal" relatives of children with behavior problems.

Several recent studies indicate that important genetic influences may be operant in determining both normal and some abnormal characteristics of the child's EEG. Various twin studies have demonstrated, in a reasonably convincing way, that the EEGs of monozygotic twins are similar (24,104–106). A significant familial factor has been established for certain abnormal or specific patterns of the child's EEG: 3-Hz spike-and-wave (107–111), midtemporal spikes (112–115), and 14- and 6-Hz positive-spikes (116–118). The most provocative and surprising finding is the genetic or familial factor associated with focal EEG abnormality (113,119). In epilepsy with midtemporal spikes (113), the familial distribution is apparently compatible with incomplete dominance or multifactorial inheritance of an age-dependent abnormality. Clearly, it appears that deviations from "normal" may be the "neurophysiological consequence of a genetically controlled biosynthetic pathway" (111).

Sex

The normative studies of Petersén and Eeg-Olofsson (9,10) showed statistically significant sex differences in the incidence of certain EEG patterns or in their characteristics (e.g., a much higher incidence of mu rhythms and a significantly higher frequency of the occipital alpha rhythms in females). Some of these are mentioned elsewhere in this chapter.

Ontogenetic Factors

Age is a primary factor in determining the characteristics of the EEG: the younger the individual, the more critical the age. In premature infants an age difference of a week may be associated with markedly different EEG characteristics, but there is little difference between the EEG characteristics of an infant at term and one 4 to 5 weeks old. The EEG of an 8-year-old child may be indistinguishable from that of an 11-year-old. The ontogenetic evolution of the EEG throughout infancy, childhood, and adolescence has been well documented (9,10,120).

Less clearly understood is the role that age—degree of cerebral development—plays in determining the characteristics of the EEG in response to a brain insult or injury at various ages, particularly during very early life. For example, when a significant injury is sustained during the perinatal period, it has been demonstrated repeatedly that the EEG initially may manifest abnormality, become normal and remain so throughout early childhood, and then become abnormal again during middle or late childhood. Thus brain damage may not be revealed in the EEG recorded at a given age even though it is in fact present.

The effect of a given insult or injury on the immature brain may be determined in part by the stage of development at the time of the injury. For example, hypsarrhythmia and the characteristic infantile spasms that accompany it may be a manifestation of a wide variety of diffuse cerebral insults operant during the perinatal period and early infancy (121,122). If the same degrees and types of insult are sustained later in the course of cerebral maturation, they do not produce the same types of EEG change or the same types of clinical seizure. Hypsarrhythmia and infantile spasms constitute the reaction of the brain to a nonspecific insult at a certain critical stage of development.

Additionally, the insult may retard or arrest cerebral development, which may be expressed by the persistence of immature EEG characteristics. Walter (123,124) suggested that many of the lesser dysrhythmias of childhood may simply reflect delayed cerebral maturation. He hypothesized that such a delay might occur, even in the absence of a causative brain insult, as a result of "less than optimal trophic influences or systemic growth promoting endocrine and chemical influences." Certainly, deprivation or distortion of sensory input at a certain critical stage of ontogenetic development may engender dramatic electrographic changes (125).

The suggestion has been made, and evidence adduced to support it, that differences in the EEGs of control and, for example, behavior–problem children of a similar age may reflect maturational differences rather than "damage" or dysfunction (126–128). Common experience also suggests that maturational factors are significantly related to minor dysrhythmias, but the nature of this relationship remains obscure. Thus the slow rhythms (e.g., frontal theta activity and posterior slow waves) tend to disappear with increasing age; this was documented in serial studies (Kellaway, *unpublished observations*) and can be inferred from samplings of different age groups (9,10). In practical terms, if minor dysrhythmias are important to the diagnosis and evaluation of behavior disorders, learning disabilities, etc. (as has been suggested), they must then be progressively less so with increasing age.

Epidemiological studies (129–132) of behavior disorders in children yielded some interesting findings that have a bearing on this point. In a study of 482 children selected randomly from households systematically sampled in Buffalo, New York, Lapouse found "a strikingly high prevalence of so-called symptomatic behavior" and pointed out that its "excessive presence in younger as contrasted with older children, and the weak association between these behaviors and adjustment, give rise to the question *whether behavior deviations are truly indicative of psychiatric or organic brain disorder or whether they occur as transient developmental phenomena* in essentially normal children" (132) [italics added]. It seems likely that parallel deviations may occur in the behavior and EEG patterns at a certain time in the life of a young child as coincident manifestations of a transient, ontogenetically determined influence.

Metabolic and Homeostatic Factors

The influences of homeostatic and metabolic factors on the EEG have been well documented and do not require review here. These influences were detailed and discussed in a recent extensive review (133). They become more important in the presence of disease, and it is essential that the electroencephalographer recognize that disease states may affect the EEG secondarily through these factors rather than directly (see Chapter 11).

Sleep and Wakefulness

The characteristics of the EEG, awake and asleep, are considered briefly in this chapter in terms of their interpretation in clinical EEG practice. More extensive treatment of the transformations of the EEG that occur during normal sleep is available in several monographs (134,135).

Psychoaffective State

Kennard (98,99) suggested that anxiety or tension states might importantly influence the EEG characteristics of a child. This possibility has been espoused most persistently by Lairy and Igert (39–41). They drew attention to the fact that occipital slow activity (or "posterior slow activity of youth") appears responsive to psychological factors, and Cohn and Nardini speculated that posterior slow waves constitute "a conditioned response of a disordered brain to the exigencies of interpersonal experiences" (42). Werre (43) reported evidence that, even in adults, posterior slow waves are sensitive to "frustrations"; and Garcia-Badaracco (44) adduced circumstantial evidence to support his view that posterior slow waves are the consequence of frustration as well as evidence of what he calls a "quasi-constitutional sensitivity to frustrations." Speculations aside, it is a common observation that the amount and amplitude of this slow activity may vary throughout a recording, generally being more pronounced at the beginning of the recording period and diminishing with the passage of time. Many factors could account for this phenomenon; there are no controlled studies in this area, but the obvious suggestion is that the slow activity diminishes as the child becomes more accustomed to the unique and unfamiliar circumstances of the laboratory procedure. Carels (45) reported an increase in posterior slow waves in a young adult neurotic patient with each "social encounter," the electrogram becoming more normal in a hospital (protective) environment.

Lairy (40) maintains that posterior slow activity in children with behavior disorders and learning disturbances may reflect the individual's adaptation to stress, and that certain EEG abnormalities may be interpreted as a sign of "impaired adaptation." The prognostic significance of the findings "depends upon the degree of impaired control and the possibilities of recovering equilibrium." In her view, the presence of posterior slow activity implies a more favorable prognosis for therapy than does a "normal" EEG, as she believes these are evidence of "hyperadaptation, which leaves little hope for functional secondary readaptation." Lairy's hypothesis appears to be based largely on intuitional or circumstantial evidence and inferences drawn from her own and others' clinical observations. In spite of the fact that these concepts have yet to be proved by systematic research, they are of heuristic importance and should not be dismissed lightly.

Of all areas of the brain sampled during scalp electroencephalography, the occipitotemporal regions in the child are the most sensitive to hyperventilation (84,85; Kellaway, *unpublished data*); following hypoxia, head injury, or encephalitis in children, the slowing effect persists longest in the occipital region (Kubala and Kellaway, *unpublished data*). Similarly, in leukemia, posterior or occipital slowing of undetermined origin occurs during the acute phase and with exacerbation (Fernbach and Kellaway, *unpublished data*). Each of these organic factors indicates a sensitivity or high reactivity of this part of the brain in children. A similar high reactivity to emotional factors may be present also, as suggested by the findings of Werre (43) in a single subject.

Theta activity has been associated with emotional state by several investigators. Walter (123), for example, reported that he induced bursts of this activity by depriving young children of pleasurable stimuli. Similarly, frustration, annoyance, and embarrassment are reported to cause enhancement of theta activity (46), even in adult subjects (47). Adey et al. (136) and Burch et al. (137) reported increased theta activity in the EEG of an astronaut during launch and the initial hours of space flight, and similar findings have been reported during space flights conducted by the Russians (138). The

78. Brazier, M. A. B., Finesinger, J. E., and Schwab, R. S. (1944): Characteristics of the normal electroencephalogram. II. The effect of varying blood sugar levels on the occipital cortical potentials in adults during quiet breathing. *J. Clin. Invest.*, 23:313–317.
79. Brazier, M. A. B., Finesinger, J. E., and Schwab, R. S. (1944): Characteristics of the normal electroencephalogram. III. The effect of varying blood sugar levels on the occipital cortical potentials in adults during hyperventilation. *J. Clin. Invest.*, 23:319–323.
80. Gibbs, F. A., Gibbs, E. L., and Lennox, W. G. (1943): Electroencephalographic response to overventilation and its relation to age. *J. Pediatr.*, 23:497–505.
81. Brill, N. Q., and Seidemann, H. (1941): The electroencephalogram of normal children: effect of hyperventilation. *Am. J. Psychiatry*, 98:250–256.
82. Von Šimkova, D. (1965): Das EEG bei gesunden Kindern im Alter von 7 bis 10 Jahren. *Psychiatr. Neurol. Med. Psychol. (Leipzig)*, 17:66–71.
83. Götze, W. (1942): Änderung des Hirnstrombildes bei Hyperventilation von hirngesunden Kindern. *Zbl. Neurochir.*, 7:202–207.
84. Daute, K-H., Frenzel, J., and Klust, E. (1968): Über den unspezifischen Hyperventilationseffekt im EEG des gesunden Kindes. I. Stärkegrad. *Z. Kinderheilkd.*, 104:197–207.
85. Daute, K-H., Klust, E., and Frenzel, J. (1968): Über den unspezifischen Hyperventilationseffekt im EEG des gesunden Kindes. II. Strukturbesonderheiten, Schlussfolgerungen. *Z. Kinderheilkd.*, 104:208–217.
86. Fiedlerová, D. (1967): Der Einfluss der Hyperventilation von 3 Minuten auf das EEG-Bild bei gesunden Kindern im Alter von 7 bis 11 Jahren. *Sborn. Lek.*, 4:417–422.
87. Berges, J., Netchine, S., and Lairy, G. C. (1963): Quelques aspects particuliers du tracé E.E.G. chez l'enfant présentant des troubles de la psychomotricité. *Rev. Neurol. (Paris)*, 109:238–246.
88. Hughes, J. R., and Park, G. E. (1968): The EEG in dyslexia. In: *Clinical Electroencephalography of Children*, edited by P. Kellaway and I. Petersén, pp. 307–327. Almqvist & Wiksell, Stockholm.
89. Gibbs, F. A., and Gibbs, E. L. (1950): *Atlas of Electroencephalography, Vol. 1: Normal Controls.* Addison-Wesley, Cambridge, Massachusetts.
90. Eeg-Olofsson, O., Petersén, I., and Selldén, U. (1971): The development of the EEG in normal children from the age of 1 to 15 years: Paroxysmal activity. *Neuropaediatrie*, 4:375–404.
91. Gibbs, F. A., and Gibbs, E. L. (1952): *Atlas of Electroencephalography, Vol. 2: Epilepsy.* Addison-Wesley, Cambridge, Massachusetts.
92. Brandt, S., and Brandt, H. (1955): The electroencephalographic patterns in young healthy children from 0 to five years of age. *Acta Psychiatr. Scand.*, 30:77–89.
93. Loomis, A. L., Harvey, E. N., and Hobart, G. (1938): Distribution of disturbance patterns in the human electroencephalogram with special reference to sleep. *J. Neurophysiol.*, 1:413–430.
94. White, J. C., and Tharp, B. (1974): An arousal pattern in children with organic cerebral brain dysfunction. *Electroencephalogr. Clin. Neurophysiol.*, 37:265–268.
95. Chatrian, G. E., White, L. E., Jr., and Daly, D. (1963): Electroencephalographic patterns resembling those of sleep in certain comatose states after injuries to the head. *Electroencephalogr. Clin. Neurophysiol.*, 15:272–280.
96. Jaffe, R., and Jacobs, L. (1972): The beta focus: its nature and significance. *Acta Neurol. Scand.*, 48:191–203.
97. Vignaendra, V., Matthews, R. L., and Chatrian, G. E. (1974): Positive occipital sharp transients of sleep: Relationships to nocturnal sleep cycle in man. *Electroencephalogr. Clin. Neurophysiol.*, 37:239–246.
98. Kennard, M. A. (1949): Significance of abnormal EEGs in disorders of behavior. *Electroencephalogr. Clin. Neurophysiol.*, 1:118–119.
99. Kennard, M. A. (1949): Inheritance of electroencephalogram patterns in children with behavior disorders. *Psychosom. Med.*, 11:151–157.
100. Davis, H., and Davis, P. A. (1936): Action potentials of the brain in normal persons and in normal states of cerebral activity. *Arch. Neurol. Psychiatry*, 36:1214–1224.
101. Lennox, W. G., Gibbs, E. L., and Gibbs, F. A. (1945): The brain-wave pattern, an hereditary trait: Evidence from 74 "normal" pairs of twins. *J. Hered.*, 36:233–243.
102. Lennox, W. G., Gibbs, F. A., and Gibbs, E. L. (1942): Twins, brain waves, and epilepsy. *Arch. Neurol. Psychiatry*, 47:702–704.
103. Knott, J. R., Platt, E. B., Ashby, M. C., and Gottlieb, J. S. (1953): A familial evaluation of the electroencephalogram of patients with primary behavior disorder and psychopathic personality. *Electroencephalogr. Clin. Neurophysiol.*, 5:363–370.
104. Juel-Nielsen, N., and Harvald, B. (1958): The electroencephalogram in uniovular twins brought up apart. *Acta Genet. (Basel)*, 8:57–64.
105. Heuschert, D. (1963): EEG-Untersuchungen an eineiigen Zwillingen im höheren Lebensalter. *Z. Menschl. Vererb. Konstitutionsl.*, 37:128–172.
106. Dumermuth, G. (1968): Variance spectra of electroencephalograms in twins. In: *Clinical Electroencephalography of Children*, edited by P. Kellaway and I. Petersén, pp. 119–154. Almqvist & Wiksell, Stockholm.
107. Harvald, B. (1954): *Heredity in Epilepsy.* Munksgaard, Copenhagen.
108. Metrakos, J. D., and Metrakos, K. (1960): Genetics of convulsive disorders. I. Introduction, problems, methods, and base lines. *Neurology (Minneap.)*, 10:228–240.
109. Metrakos, K., and Metrakos, J. D. (1961): Genetics of convulsive disorders. II. Genetic and electroencephalographic studies in centrencephalic epilepsy. *Neurology (Minneap.)*, 11:474–483.
110. Metrakos, J. D., and Metrakos, K. (1966): Childhood epilepsy of subcortical ("centrencephalic") origin. *Clin. Pediatr. (Phila.)*, 5:536–542.
111. Metrakos, J. D., and Metrakos, K. (1969): Discussion: genetic studies in clinical

d'un jeune adulte et leur variation quantitative dans le temps. *Acta Neurol. Belg.,* 59:409–413.
46. Faure, J., and Guérin, A. (1958): Au sujet de l'électroencéphalogramme des enfants caractériels. *Rev. Neurol. (Paris),* 99:209–219.
47. Mundy-Castle, A. C. (1951): Theta and beta rhythm in the electroencephalograms of normal adults. *Electroencephalogr. Clin. Neurophysiol.,* 3:477–486.
48. Jasper, H. H., Solomon, P., and Bradley, C. (1938): Electroencephalographic analyses of behavior problem children. *Am. J. Psychiatry,* 95:641–658.
49. Lindsley, D. B., and Cutts, K. K. (1940): Electroencephalograms of "constitutionally inferior" and behavior problem children: comparison with those of normal children and adults. *Arch. Neurol. Psychiatry,* 44:1199–1212.
50. Doose, H., Gerken, H., and Völzke, E. (1972): On the genetics of EEG-anomalies in childhood. I. Abnormal theta rhythms. *Neuropaediatrie,* 3:386–401.
51. Cohn, R., and Nardini, J. E. (1958): The correlation of bilateral occipital slow activity in the human EEG with certain disorders of behavior. *Am. J. Psychiatry,* 115:44–54.
52. Hill, D. (1944): Cerebral dysrhythmia: its significance in aggressive behavior. *Proc. R. Soc. Med.,* 37:317–330.
53. Pavy, R., and Metcalfe, J. (1965): The abnormal EEG in childhood communication and behavior abnormalities. *Electroencephalogr. Clin. Neurophysiol.,* 19:414.
54. Aird, R. B., and Gastaut, Y. (1959): Occipital and posterior electroencephalographic rhythms. *Electroencephalogr. Clin. Neurophysiol.,* 11:637–656.
55. Sutter, C., and Harrelson, A. B. (1966): Occipital slowing in the EEG of 5–15 year olds (teenage slow): a report on this finding in 237 child psychiatric patients. *Electroencephalogr. Clin. Neurophysiol.,* 20:624–625.
56. Netchine, S., and Lairy, G. C. (1975): The EEG and psychology of the child. In: *Handbook of Electroencephalography and Clinical Neurophysiology, Vol. 6: The Normal EEG Throughout Life. Part B: The Evolution of the EEG from Birth to Adulthood,* edited by G. C. Lairy, pp. 69–104. Elsevier Scientific, Amsterdam.
57. Gibbs, F. A., and Knott, J. R. (1949): Growth of the electrical activity of the cortex. *Electroencephalogr. Clin. Neurophysiol.,* 1:223–229.
58. Gastaut, Y. (1951): Un signe électroencéphalographique peu connu: Les pointes occipitales survenant pendant l'ouverture des yeux. *Rev. Neurol. (Paris),* 84:640–643.
59. Lesêvre, N. (1967): Étude de réponses moyennes recueillies sur la région postérieure du scalp chez l'homme au cours de l'exploration visuelle ("complexe lambda"). *Psychol. Franc.,* 12:26–36.
60. Rémond, A., Lesêvre, N., and Torres, F. (1965): Étude chrono-topographique de l'activité occipitale moyenne recueilli sur le scalp chez l'homme en relation avec le déplacement du regard (complexe lambda). *Rev. Neurol. (Paris),* 113:193–226.
61. Barlow, J. S., and Cigánek, L. (1969): Lambda responses in relation to visual evoked responses in man. *Electroencephalogr. Clin. Neurophysiol.,* 26:183–192.
62. Evans, C. C. (1953): Spontaneous excitation of the visual cortex and association areas—lambda waves. *Electroencephalogr. Clin. Neurophysiol.,* 4:111.
63. Green, J. (1957): Some observations on lambda waves and peripheral stimulation. *Electroencephalogr. Clin. Neurophysiol.,* 9:691–704.
64. Rémond, A., and Lesêvre, N. (1956): Remarques sur les conditions d'apparition et l'importance statistique des ondes lambda chez les individus normaux. *Rev. Neurol. (Paris),* 94:160–161.
65. Roth, M., and Green, J. (1953): The lambda wave as a normal physiological phenomenon in the human electroencephalogram. *Nature,* 172:864–866.
66. Scott, D. F., Groetheysen, U. C., and Bickford, R. G. (1967): Lambda responses in the human electroencephalogram. *Neurology (Minneap.),* 17:770–778.
67. Tsai, H-J., and Liu, S-Y. (1965): [Lambda waves of human subjects of different age levels.] *Acta Psychol. Sin.,* 4:343–352. Translated from Chinese by Barlow, J. S. (1971): *Contemporary Brain Research in China,* pp. 50–61. Consultants Bureau, New York.
68. Gastaut, H., Bruens, J. H., Rogers, J., and Giove, G. (1959): Étude électroencéphalographique des signes d'insuffisance circulatoire sylvienne chronique. *Rev. Neurol. (Paris),* 100:59–65.
69. Kooi, K. A., Guvener, A. M., Tupper, C. J., and Bagchi, B. K. (1964): Electroencephalographic patterns of the temporal region in normal adults. *Neurology (Minneap.),* 14:1029–1035.
70. Gastaut, H., and Poirier, F. (1960): The electroencephalogram in cerebrovascular diseases. *Neurology (Minneap.),* 11:110–111.
71. Van der Drift, J. H. A. (1961): Ischemic cerebral lesions. *Angiology,* 12:401–418.
72. Bruens, J. H., Gastaut, H., and Giove, G. (1960): Electroencephalographic study of the signs of chronic vascular insufficiency of the sylvian region in aged people. *Electroencephalogr. Clin. Neurophysiol.,* 12:283–295.
73. Kendel, K., and Koufen, H. (1970): EEG Veränderungen bei cerebralen Gefäßinsulten des Hirnstamms. *Dtsch. Z. Nervenheilk.,* 197:42–55.
74. Blinn, K. A., and Noell, W. K. (1949): Continuous measurement of alveolar CO_2 tension during the hyperventilation test in routine electroencephalography. *Electroencephalogr. Clin. Neurophysiol.,* 1:333–342.
75. Morrice, J. K. W. (1956): Slow wave production in the EEG, with reference to hyperpnoea, carbon dioxide and autonomic balance. *Electroencephalogr. Clin. Neurophysiol.,* 8:49–72.
76. Gotoh, F., Meyer, J. S., and Takagi, Y. (1965): Cerebral effects of hyperventilation in man. *Arch. Neurol.,* 12:410–423.
77. Davis, H., and Wallace, W. McL. (1942): Factors affecting changes produced in electroencephalogram by standardized hyperventilation. *Arch. Neurol. Psychiatry,* 47:606–625.

13. Maulsby, R. L., Kellaway, P., Graham, M., Frost, J. D., Jr., Proler, M. L., Low, M. D., and North, R. R. (1968): *The Normative Electroencephalographic Data Reference Library*. Final Report, Contract NAS 9-1200, National Aeronautics and Space Administration, 172 pp.
14. Gastaut, H., and Broughton, R. (1972): *Epileptic Seizures: Clinical and Electrographic Features, Diagnosis and Treatment*. Charles C Thomas, Springfield, Illinois.
15. Creutzfeldt, O. D., Arnold, P-M., Becker, D., Langenstein, S., Tirsch, W., Wilhelm, H., and Wuttke, W. (1976): EEG changes during spontaneous and controlled menstrual cycles and their correlation with psychological performance. *Electroencephalogr. Clin. Neurophysiol.*, 40:113–131.
16. Engel, G. L., Romano, J., and Ferris, E. B. (1947): Variations in the normal electroencephalogram during a five-year period. *Science*, 108:600–601.
17. Rubin, M. A. (1938): The distribution of the alpha rhythm over the cerebral cortex of normal man. *J. Neurophysiol.*, 1:313–323.
18. Travis, L. E., and Gottlober, A. B. (1937): How consistent are an individual's brain potentials from day to day? *Science*, 85:223–234.
19. Chatrian, G. E., Petersen, M. C., and Lazarte, J. A. (1960): The blocking of the rolandic wicket rhythm and some central changes related to movement. *Electroencephalogr. Clin. Neurophysiol.*, 11:497–510.
20. Leissner, P., Lindholm, L-E., and Petersén, I. (1970): Alpha amplitude dependence on skull thickness as measured by ultrasound technique. *Electroencephalogr. Clin. Neurophysiol.*, 29:392–399.
21. Covello, A., De Barros-Ferreira, M., and Lairy, G. C. (1975): Etude telemetrique des rythmes centraux chez l'enfant. *Electroencephalogr. Clin. Neurophysiol.*, 38:307–319.
22. Gastaut, H., Terzian, H., and Gastaut, Y. (1952): Etude d'une activité électroencéphalographique méconnue: le "rythme rolandique en arceau." *Marseille Med.*, 89:296–310.
23. Hirt, H. R. (1968): Zur diagnostischen Bedentung der pathologischen Beta-Aktivität im EEG des Kindes und Jugendlichen. *Fortschr. Neurol. Psychiatr.*, 36:412–433.
24. Vogel, F. (1958): *Über die Erblichkeit des Normalen Elektroencephalogramms*. Thieme, Stuttgart.
25. Vogel, F., and Götze, W. (1962): Statistische Betrachtungen über die β-Wellen im EEG des Menschen. *Dtsch. Z. Nervenheilk.*, 184:112–136.
26. Dumermuth, G. (1965): *Elektroencephalographie im Kindesalter*. Thieme, Stuttgart.
27. Garsche, R. (1956): Die Beta-Aktivität im EEG des Kindes. I. Mitteilung Erscheinungsformen bei gesunden Kindern. *Z. Kinderheilkd.*, 78:441–457.
28. Garsche, R. (1956): Die Beta-Aktivität im EEG des Kindes. II. Mitteilung Erscheinungsformen bei cerebralen Erkrankungen. *Z. Kinderheilkd.*, 78:458–479.
29. Hirsch, W., Belitz, H., Geipel, G., Goetze, W., Kubicki, St., and Mex, A. (1958): Genetische-klinische Studien an abnormalen und cerebral geschädigten Kindern. *Monatsschr. Kinderheilkd.*, 106:209–221.
30. Simonova, O., Roth, B., and Stein, J. (1968): Veränderungen der physiologischen und pathologischen EEG-aktivität bei geistiger Tätigkeit und Aufmerksamkeit. *Arch. Psychiatr. Nervenkr.*, 211:460–469.
31. Vogel, F. (1970): The genetic basis of the normal human electroencephalogram (EEG). *Humangenetik*, 10:91–114.
32. Frost, J. D., Jr., Carrie, J. R. G., Borda, R. P., and Kellaway, P. (1973): The effects of Dalmane (flurazepam hydrochloride) on human EEG characteristics. *Electroencephalogr. Clin. Neurophysiol.*, 34:171–175.
33. Jung, R., Riechert, R., and Meyer-Mickeleit, R. W. (1950): Über intracerebrale Hirnpotentialableitungen bei hirnchirurgischen Eingriffen. *Dtsch. Z. Nervenheilk.*, 162:52–60.
34. Gibbs, E. L., Lorimer, F. M., and Gibbs, F. A. (1950): Clinical correlates of exceedingly fast activity in the electroencephalogram. *Dis. Nerv. Syst.*, 11:323–326.
35. Kellaway, P., and Fox, B. J. (1952): Electroencephalographic diagnosis of cerebral pathology in infants during sleep. I. Rationale, technique, and the characteristics of normal sleep in infants. *J. Pediatr.*, 41:262–287.
36. Kellaway, P. (1952): The development of sleep spindles and of arousal patterns in infants and their characteristics in normal and certain abnormal states. *Electroencephalogr. Clin. Neurophysiol.*, 4:369.
37. Gibbs, E. L., and Gibbs, F. A. (1962): Extreme spindles: correlation of electroencephalographic sleep pattern with mental retardation. *Science*, 138:1106–1107.
38. Wiener, J. M., Delano, J. C., and Klass, D. W. (1966): An EEG study of delinquent and nondelinquent adolescents. *Arch. Gen. Psychiatry*, 15:144–150.
39. Lairy, G. C. (1961): E.E.G. et neuropsychiatrie infantile. *Psychiatr. Enfant.*, 3:525–608.
40. Lairy, G. C. (1967): L'EEG comme moyen d'investigation des modalités individuelles d'adaptation aux situations de stress. *Electroencephalogr. Clin. Neurophysiol. (Suppl.)*, 25:282–298.
41. Igert, Cl., and Lairy, G. C. (1962): Intérêt pronostique de l'EEG au cours de l'évolution des schizophrènes. *Electroencephalogr. Clin. Neurophysiol.*, 14:183–190.
42. Cohn, R., and Nardini, J. E. (1958): The correlation of bilateral occipital slow activity in the human EEG with certain disorders of behavior. *Am. J. Psychiatry*, 115:44–54.
43. Werre, P. F. (1957): *The Relationships between Electroencephalographic and Psychological Data in Normal Adults*. Universitaire Presse Leiden, Leiden.
44. Garcia-Badaracco, J. (1953): EEG et psychisme: Les entretiens psychiatriques 1953. Collection Psyché, Arche, Paris, pp. 140–165.
45. Carels, G. (1959): Les ondes lentes postérieures de l'électroencéphalogramme

Russian scientists (139) interpret the findings as a measure of a "high level" of psychoemotional reactions during the early phases of the flight. Adey et al. (136) believe that more fundamental physiological substrates—concerned primarily with alerting and orientation—are involved. Whether the anterior theta rhythms in man are responsive simply as part of an alerting or orienting mechanism or are elements of a psychoaffective response has not been clearly established by experimental studies such as those of Walter (123,124) or Melin (140), who exposed young adults to shocking and horrifying movies and found increases in the theta and occasionally the delta components of the subjects' EEGs.

That the EEG patterns are indeed plastic and responsive to functional factors appears to be established; it has yet to be proved, however, that significant aberrations of the EEG of the child may be a consequence of prolonged emotional stress (e.g., chronic anxiety or frustration). Nordland (141) attempted to answer the question by comparing the EEGs of maladjusted children with histories of chronic psychological stress (e.g., conflict, insecurity, or anxiety) with a group in whom these factors were not significant. Her results indicated that "an abnormal EEG may be a symptom of protracted states of psychological tension"; but as Nordland herself points out, the study does not provide conclusive answers to the question. Nevertheless, the evidence is sufficient (142) to give pause to those who maintain the view that the dysrhythmic EEG is always evidence of organic dysfunction acquired through infection, injury, or other organic insult (143,144).

Extrinsic Factors

Extrinsic factors (drugs, trauma, infection, etc.) are considered in various other chapters of this book.

ACKNOWLEDGMENT

This work was supported in part by grant NS 11535 from the National Institute of Neurological and Communicative Disorders and Stroke, NIH, USPHS.

REFERENCES

1. Frey, T. S., and Sjögren, H. (1959): The electroencephalogram in elderly persons suffering from neuropsychiatric disorders. *Acta Psychiatr. Scand.*, 34:438–450.
2. Harvald, B. (1958): EEG in old age. *Acta Psychiatr. Scand.*, 33:193–196.
3. Obrist, W. D. (1954): The electroencephalogram of normal aged adults. *Electroencephalogr. Clin. Neurophysiol.*, 6:235–244.
4. Obrist, W. D., Busse, E. W., Eisdorfer, C., and Kleemeier, R. W. (1962): Relation of the electroencephalogram to intellectual function in senescence. *J. Gerontol.*, 17:197.
5. Obrist, W. D., Sokoloff, L., Lassen, N. A., Lane, M. H., Butler, R. N., and Feinberg, I. (1963): Relation of EEG to cerebral blood flow and metabolism in old age. *Electroencephalogr. Clin. Neurophysiol.*, 15:610–619.
6. Otomo, E. (1966): Electroencephalography in old age: dominant alpha pattern. *Electroencephalogr. Clin. Neurophysiol.*, 21:489–491.
7. Sheridan, F. P., Yeager, C. L., Oliver, W. A., and Simon, A. (1955): Electroencephalography as a diagnostic and prognostic aid in studying the senescent individual: a preliminary report. *J. Gerontol.*, 10:53–59.
8. Sulg, I. A., Cronqvist, S., Schuller, H., and Ingvar, D. H. (1969): The effect of intracardial pacemaker therapy on cerebral blood flow and electroencephalogram in patients with complete atrioventricular block. *Circulation*, 39:487–494.
9. Eeg-Olofsson, O. (1971): The development of the electroencephalogram in normal adolescents from the age of 16 through 21 years. *Neuropaediatrie*, 3:11–45.
10. Petersén, I., and Eeg-Olofsson, O. (1971): The development of the electroencephalogram in normal children from the age of 1 through 15 years—non-paroxysmal activity. *Neuropaediatrie*, 2:247–304.
11. Sem-Jacobsen, C. W., Petersen, M. C., Dodge, H. W., Lazarte, J. A., and Holman, C. (1956): Electroencephalographic rhythms from the depths of the parietal, occipital and temporal lobes in man. *Electroencephalogr. Clin. Neurophysiol.*, 8:263–278.
12. Gibbs, F. A., Gibbs, E. L., and Lennox, W. G. (1943): Electroencephalographic classification of epileptic patients and control subjects. *Arch. Neurol. Psychiatry*, 50:111–128.

epilepsy. In: *Basic Mechanisms of the Epilepsies,* edited by H. H. Jasper, A. A. Ward, Jr., and A. Pope, pp. 700–708. Little Brown, Boston.

112. Bray, P. F., and Wiser, W. C. (1964): A modified concept of idiopathic epilepsy. *Trans. Am. Neurol. Assoc.,* 89:140–142.
113. Bray, P. F., and Wiser, W. C. (1964): Evidence for a genetic etiology of temporal-central abnormalities in focal epilepsy. *N. Engl. J. Med.,* 271:926–933.
114. Bray, P. F., and Wiser, W. C. (1965): The relation of focal to diffuse epileptiform EEG discharges in genetic epilepsy. *Arch. Neurol.,* 13:223–237.
115. Bray, P. F., Wiser, W. C., Wood, M. C., and Pusey, S. B. (1965): Hereditary characteristics of familial temporal-central focal epilepsy. *Pediatrics,* 36:207–212.
116. Rodin, E. A. (1964): Familial occurrence of the 14 and 6/sec positive spike phenomenon. *Electroencephalogr. Clin. Neurophysiol.,* 17:556–570.
117. Vogel, F. (1965): "14 and 6/sec positive spikes" in Schlaf-EEG von jugendlichen ein- und zweierigen Zwillingen. *Humangenetik,* 1:390–391.
118. Petersén, I., and Åkesson, H. O. (1968): EEG studies of siblings of children showing 14 and 6 per second positive spikes. *Acta Genet. (Basel),* 18:163–169.
119. Barslund, I., and Danielsen, J. (1963): Temporal epilepsy in monozygotic twins. *Epilepsia,* 4:138–150.
120. Kellaway, P. (1957): Ontogenic evolution of the electrical activity of the brain in man and animals. Rapport du Premier Congrès International des Sciences Neurologiques, Bruxelles, pp. 141–154.
121. Lacy, J. R., and Penry, J. K. (1976): *Infantile Spasms.* Raven Press, New York.
122. Kellaway, P. (1959): Neurologic status of patients with hypsarhythmia. In: *Molecules and Mental Health,* edited by F. A. Gibbs, pp. 134–149. Lippincott, Philadelphia.
123. Walter, W. G. (1950): The function of the electrical rhythms in the brain. *J. Ment. Sci.,* 96:1–31.
124. Walter, W. G. (1959): Intrinsic rhythms of the brain. In: *Handbook of Physiology, Section 1: Neurophysiology,* Vol. I, edited by J. Field, H. W. Magoun, and V. E. Hall, pp. 279–298. American Physiological Society, Washington, D.C.
125. Kellaway, P. (1975): Afferent input: A critical factor in the ontogenesis of brain electrical activity. In: *Behavior and Brain Electrical Activity,* edited by N. Burch and H. L. Altshuler, pp. 391–420. Plenum Press, New York.
126. Kennard, M. A. (1969): EEG abnormality in first grade children with "soft" neurological signs. *Electroencephalogr. Clin. Neurophysiol.,* 27:544.
127. Bosaeus, E., Matoušek, M., and Petersén, I. (1977): Correlation between paedopsychiatric findings and EEG-variables in well-functioning children of ages 5–16 years. *Scand. J. Psychol.,* 18:140–147.
128. Matoušek, M., and Petersén, I. (1971): Objective measurement of maturation defects and other EEG abnormalities by means of frequency analysis. Fifth World Congress of Psychiatry Proceedings, Mexico City, pp. 759–765. Excerpta Medica Series No. 274 VII. Excerpta Medica, Amsterdam.
129. Lapouse, R., and Monk, M. A. (1958): An epidemiologic study of behavior characteristics in children. *Am. J. Public Health,* 48:1134–1144.
130. Lapouse, R., Monk, M. A., and Street, E. (1964): A method for use in epidemiologic studies of behavior disorders in children. *Am. J. Public Health,* 54:207–222.
131. Lapouse, R. (1965): The relationship of behavior to adjustment in a representative sample of children. *Am. J. Public Health,* 55:1130–1141.
132. Lapouse, R. (1966): The epidemiology of behavior disorders in children. *Am. J. Dis. Child.,* 111:594–599.
133. Harding, G. F. A., and Thompson, C. R. S. (1975): EEG rhythms and the internal milieu. In: *Handbook of Electroencephalography and Clinical Neurophysiology, Vol. 6: The Normal EEG Throughout Life, Part A: The EEG of the Waking Adult,* edited by G. C. Lairy, pp. 176–194. Elsevier Scientific, Amsterdam.
134. Passouant, P., editor (1975): *Handbook of Electroencephalography and Clinical Neurophysiology, Vol. 7: Physiological Correlates of EEG, Part A: EEG and Sleep.* Elsevier Scientific, Amsterdam.
135. Williams, R. L., Karacan, I., and Hursch, C. J. (1974): *Electroencephalography (EEG) of Human Sleep: Clinical Applications.* Wiley, New York.
136. Adey, W. R., Kado, R. T., and Walter, D. O. (1967): Computer analysis of EEG data from Gemini flight GT-7. *Aerospace Med.,* 38:345–359.
137. Burch, N. R., Dossett, R. G., Vorderman, A. L., and Lester, B. K. (1967): Period analysis of the electroencephalogram from the orbital flight of Gemini VII. Final report. National Aeronautics and Space Administration, Washington, D.C.
138. Sisakyan, N. M., and Yazdovskiy, V. I. (1964): First Group Flight into Outer Space. U.S. Department of Commerce, Joint Publications Research Service, Translation TT: 64–31567. Reference, p. 91.
139. Voskrenzenskiy, A. D., Gazenko, O. G., Izosimov, G. V., Kopanev, V. T., Maksimov, D. G., and Yazdovskiy, V. I. (1965): Working ability of cosmonauts during orbital flight. In: *Problems of Space Biology* (U.S.S.R.). U.S. Library of Congress, Aerospace Technology Division, Vol. 4, No. 91, p. 79.
140. Melin, K.-A. (1953): The EEG in infancy and childhood. *Electroencephalogr. Clin. Neurophysiol. (Suppl.),* 4:205–211.
141. Nordland, E. (1969): Conflict state and abnormal EEG: A study of boys with behavior disturbances and abnormal EEG. *Scand. J. Educ. Res.,* 13:199–221.
142. Ellingson, R. J. (1954): The incidence of EEG abnormality among patients with mental disorders of apparently nonorganic origin: a critical review. *Am. J. Psychiatry,* 111:263–274.
143. White, R. W. (1964): *The Abnormal Personality.* Ronald Press, New York.
144. Chess, S. (1969): *An Introduction to Child Psychiatry.* Grune & Stratton, New York.

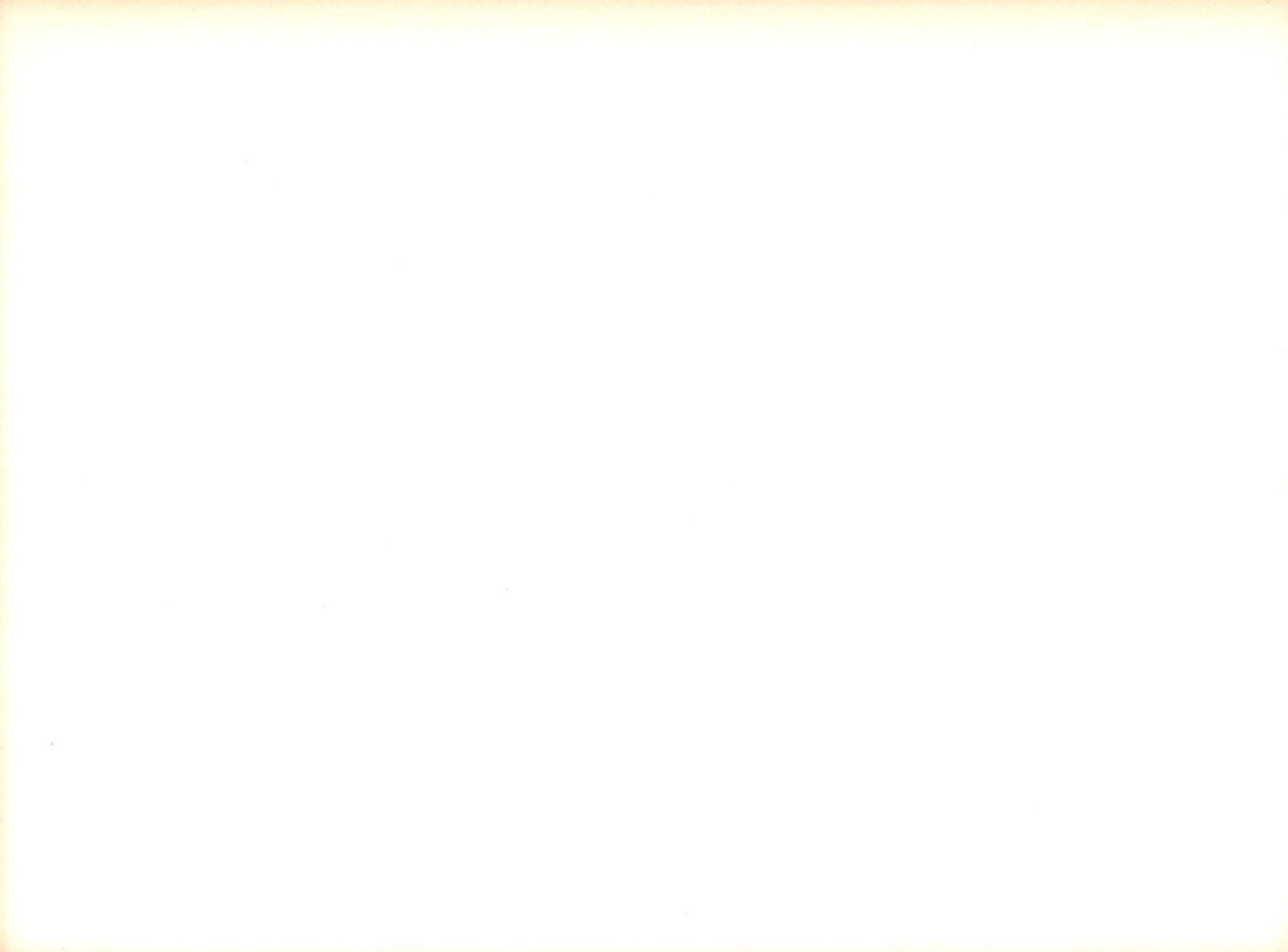

Chapter 6

EEGs of Premature and Full-Term Newborns

Robert J. Ellingson

Departments of Neurology and Psychiatry, University of Nebraska College of Medicine, Omaha, Nebraska 68105

Recording Technique	150
Electrodes	150
Electrode Arrays	150
Montages	151
Instrumental Control Settings	151
Recording Procedures	152
Artifacts	152
EEG of Prematures	153
Pattern A	153
Pattern B	155
Pattern C	155
Summary	157
Perinatal EEG Patterns	157
EEG of the Infant	161

Abnormalities in Newborns' EEGs 163
  Low-Voltage and Flat Tracings 163
  Burst-Suppression Pattern 166
  Spikes, Sharp Waves, and Slow Transients 166
  Rhythmic Patterns 168
  Seizure Activity 170
Deviations of Uncertain Significance 175
  Dysmature Patterns 175
  Poor Interhemispheric Synchrony 175
  Excessive Stage I 176
Conclusion 176
References 177

The interpretation of neonatal electroencephalograms (EEGs) is one of the most formidable tasks with which the clinical electroencephalographer has to cope. It is the purpose of this chapter to provide general electroencephalographers, who may not have had a great deal of training or experience with babies, with enough information so that their technicians can obtain satisfactory recordings and so that they can arrive at clinically sound judgments.

RECORDING TECHNIQUE

Electrodes

Because most babies move a good deal during recording, electrodes applied with collodion are preferred. The inverted saucer-shaped Ag-AgCl electrode with a small hole for the injection of electrolyte solution is best. In intensive care units or other places where fumes of acetone and ether are not permissible, disk electrodes with electrolyte paste may be used. Except for emergency situations where great speed is essential, needle electrodes are not needed and are not advised.

The often heard assertion that high interelectrode impedances are inevitable with babies is false. Impedances of less than 5,000 Ω can be attained regularly.

Electrode Arrays

The International 10–20 Electrode System (1) is strongly recommended. If the baby's ear lobes are too small, mastoid leads may be substituted and can be designated M1 and M2.

If the baby's head is very small or if time to apply a full set of electrodes cannot be allowed, the following electrodes can be used: FP1, FP2, C3, CZ, C4, T3, T4, O1, O2, A1 (or M1), and A2 (or M2).

Neonatal recordings consisting only of EEG tracings can no longer be considered acceptable. Recording other polygraphic variables is essential. These should include at least one channel each of electro-oculogram (EOG), electrocardiogram (EKG), and respirogram. A second channel of EOG may be useful for definitive identification of lateral eye movements. Electrodes for recording lateral eye movements should be placed at the left and/or right external canthi of the eyes and can be designated E1 and E2. Recording from infraorbital leads (IO1 and/or IO2) can be useful, as in adults, for distinguishing vertical eye movement signals from those of cerebral and other artifactual origin. A channel of submental electromyogram (EMG) may be used, if highly accurate staging of the wakefulness-sleep cycle is desired, but is usually not necessary for clinical purposes. Gross EMG electrodes may be used for recording seizure movements or other abnormal movements of the limbs or trunk. Finally, in infants with respiratory problems it may be valuable to devote three or four channels to respiration—abdominal and thoracic strain gauges and nasal and/or oral thermistors.

An obvious corollary of the necessity for devoting three or more channels to non-EEG variables is that it is very difficult, if not impossible, to do satisfactory neonatal electroencephalography on an 8-channel instrument.

Montages

If the full 10–20-system complement of electrodes is used, the same montages can be employed as for other patients in the laboratory. If a limited electrode array is used, special montages must be devised. In any case both scalp-scalp and reference montages should be used.

For recording non-EEG variables, the following derivations are recommended:

(a) For EOG (lateral eye movements), E1-A1 and E2-A1 (sic). If only one channel can be spared for EOG, E1-A2, E2-A1, or E1-E2.

(b) For distinguishing vertical eye movement, IO1-A1 and/or IO2-A2 in channels adjacent to FP1-A1 and/or FP2-A2.

(c) For respirogram, record from a strain gauge taped to the baby's ribs or installed in a pneumatic tube strapped to the baby's chest and/or abdomen, and/or from a thermistor taped under a nostril or in front of the mouth.

(d) For submental EMG, record between electrodes under the chin about 1 cm on either side of the midline.

(e) For EKG, lead 1 is preferred.

Instrumental Control Settings

For EEG, record at 7 μV/mm and at a time constant (TC) of 0.25 to 0.60 sec (not the commonly used 0.10 sec, unless it is necessary to eliminate very slow artifacts). The technologist should be prepared to increase or decrease amplification if unusually high or low voltages are encountered.

For lateral EOG (leads E1 and E2), record at 7 μV/mm and a time constant of 0.10 sec. For vertical EOG (leads IO1 and/or IO2), use the same settings as for the concomitantly recorded EEG tracings from FP1 and FP2.

For respirogram, adjust amplification to yield a clearly visible vertical deflection and use a relatively long time constant, 0.60 sec or longer, but not DC.

For submental EMG, record at 3 µV/mm (the tonic EMG of quiet sleep in the newborn may be of very low voltage) and a time constant of about 0.03 sec.

For recording EMG and movement from limbs or trunk, settings should be adjusted to yield deflections of reasonable height. No high frequency filtration should be used in EMG channels.

Recording Procedures

Allow extra time for a baby's EEG—one-half hour for preparation time and at least 1 hr for recording. Adequate information may be obtained in less recording time, but it is sometimes necessary to record longer.

In my laboratory the following scenario has been found satisfactory in most cases. The baby is prepared (electrodes applied,[1] checked, etc.) just *before* a feeding time. He is then fed, diapers are changed, he is put down in the crib, swaddled only if necessary, and recording is started. Ambient temperature should be that of a newborn nursery. If the baby is in an isolette, temperature should be allowed to return to an appropriate level before recording is started. The isolette heaters and fans cannot be on during recording, but if oxygen is in use, flow can and should be maintained. Using this procedure (varied as circumstances require) the baby should be ready, in the case of term or postterm babies, to fall asleep or, in the case of prematures not exhibiting a definite wakefulness-sleep cycle, to enter a period of quietude. Often no readable tracings can be obtained while the baby is awake, because of almost continuous movement. If the baby does not become quiet promptly, the technician must "wait him out" until a sufficient sample of relatively artifact-free recording is obtained. In very difficult cases it may be necessary to give up and try again later. It should be unnecessary to sedate newborns for the purpose of obtaining an EEG.

Continuous direct observation of the baby by the technician during recording is essential. The technician should make frequent notes concerning the baby's movements, including facial movements and eyelid position, on the recording paper, especially when unusual waveforms are observed in the EEG tracings. It is impossible to take too many notes. If a second technician is free at the time of recording a baby's EEG, it is a good idea to assign him/her as the observer and recorder of behavioral data, freeing the first technician to attend to other aspects of recording.

The question of how long to record is an important one. No pat answer can be given. If clear-cut abnormalities are seen frequently or continuously, it may not be necessary to record very long. When dubious phenomena are seen or when the EEG is apparently within normal limits, at least 1 hr of recording should be obtained, or more under some circumstances that are explained later.

Artifacts

The technician and the EEGer must beware of certain artifacts more or less peculiar to the newborn. Most of these are basically movement artifacts and include those associated with normal respiration, hiccoughing, sighing, sobbing, and sucking.

Newborns may breathe at rates of 100/min or more; the resultant artifact may look like monomorphic delta activity, especially during quiet sleep. Hiccoughing, sighing, and sobbing artifacts usually consist of short focal or generalized bursts of waves of mixed frequency.

---

[1] It is almost impossible to apply electrodes properly through the hand holes of an isolette. If the baby is in an isolette, it should be opened long enough to apply the electrodes as rapidly as good technique permits.

They may look obviously artifactual or they may not and can occur during sleep as well as wakefulness. If the respirogram is being recorded, there is usually little difficulty in identifying the nature of respiratory artifacts. If not, the observational efficiency of the technician is crucial.

Sucking may be continuous, producing rhythmic waves in the delta frequency band in one or more tracings, or it may be sporadic, producing spindle-shaped bursts of delta waves. Sucking artifacts are usually revealed in the submental EMG tracing, if used, even if a short TC is employed. They can usually be avoided by feeding before recording and by not using bottles and pacifiers that induce sucking behavior during recording. Even so, bursts of sucking-like movements of the mandible sometimes occur during quiet sleep. Sucking movements are *not* scored as movements in classifying sleep stages (see below).

EKG artifacts are more evident and persistent in newborns' EEGs than in those of older patients; they are usually present in reference montages.

EEG OF PREMATURES

The EEG patterns typical of the full-term newborn usually become established at 36 to 37 weeks conceptional age (CA).[2] Between 44 and 50 weeks CA (4 to 10 weeks after term birth), usually at 46 to 47 weeks CA, they evolve into the more familiar patterns of later infancy. EEG patterns typically seen between those age limits (36 and 44 to 50 weeks CA) are referred to here as "perinatal patterns," and are described later. This section is devoted to EEG patterns seen in prematures younger than 36 weeks CA.

Apparently nonpathological EEG activity of prematures, from the earliest ages at which babies survive long enough to have EEGs recorded (20 to 24 weeks CA) to approximately 36 weeks CA can be divided broadly into three patterns, which for convenience are referred to as "premature patterns A, B, and C." Each pattern is maintained for 1 to several weeks. The transition from one pattern to the next may occur relatively abruptly, often in less than 1 week. The developmental anatomical and physiological mechanisms responsible for these transitions are unknown.

Pattern A

Pattern A (Fig. 1) is seen in early nonviable and viable prematures. At what CA it first appears is unknown. It is certainly present at 22 weeks CA (2). The tracings show bursts of waves of mixed frequencies (< 1 to 15 Hz, but with dominance of the delta frequencies), often mixed with sharp waves and spikey waves, and usually of relatively high voltages. These bursts are separated by periods of more or less flat tracings lasting from a few to many seconds. The earlier the premature the longer the flat periods. Synchrony between hemispheres and between areas is poor. Approximate burst-for-burst interareal, and even interhemispheric, synchrony is sometimes observed; wave-for-wave synchrony rarely. The pattern is invariant; there is no change related to the activity cycle, if any, of the baby.

It is very tempting to call pattern A abnormal in a premature known to be in distress; it often strikingly resembles the pathological burst-suppression pattern (see for example 2, Chapters 5 and 12). The temptation must be resisted.

---

[2] CA as used here is the age of a fetus or a baby in weeks, dated from the first day of the mother's last menstrual period. Confirmation by other obstetric and pediatric data is desirable. After birth, CA equals gestational age plus age since birth. *Cf. chronological age,* which is age since birth regardless of length of gestation and is also sometimes abbreviated "CA," especially in psychometry.

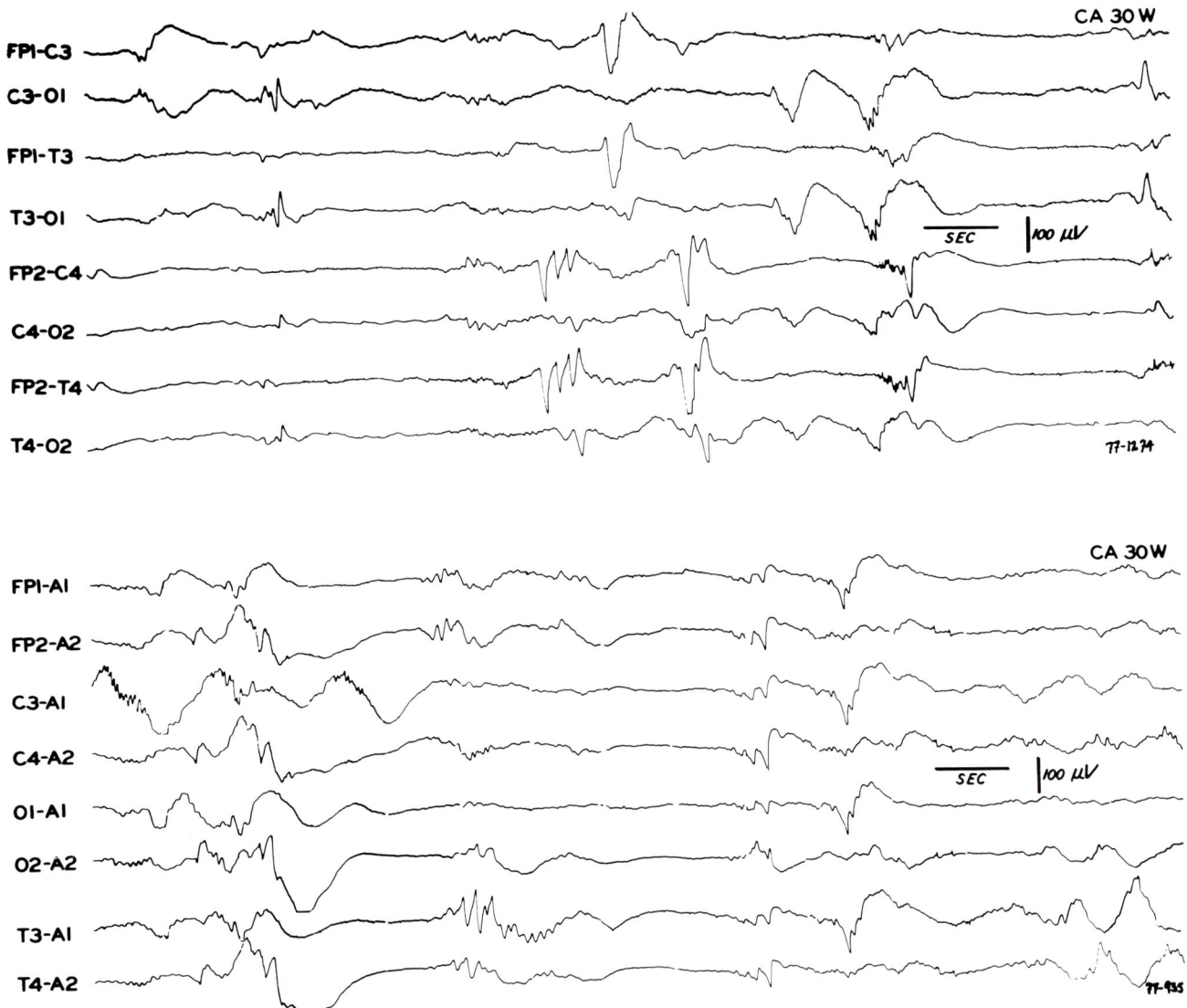

It has justifiably been asked, How do we know that this pattern is ever normal? May not the brains of all prematures born so early, even those later developing normally, be in a physiologically abnormal state when first subjected to the stresses of extrauterine life? The fact that no differences have been detected in premature pattern A between prematures displaying it who later develop normally and those who later develop abnormally, is not very strong evidence for a negative answer to the question. Stronger evidence comes from observations on animals (3). A number of species of mammals are normally born at earlier stages of physiological development than man. In some, for example, rat and mouse, there is no identifiable EEG activity at term birth. In all such species studied, the first activity to appear is an intermittent pattern. Early EEG development has also been studied in precocial species (born at a more mature stage of development than man), for example, the guinea pig, via early artificial parturition by cesarian section. In all of these species too, the earliest identifiable patterns are periodic. This evidence strongly suggests that premature pattern A reflects a universal early state of brain development, at least among mammalian species.

Pattern B

Pattern B (Figs. 2 and 3A) succeeds pattern A during the eighth lunar month of gestation, usually at about 30 weeks CA, but pattern A may be seen exceptionally as late as 33 weeks CA in babies who later develop normally. After tnat, pattern A may be considered abnormal. Activity becomes more continuous, although a tendency remains toward intermittent bursts of waves of mixed frequency (still delta dominant) against a background of lower voltage activity. The spike-and-sharp-wave components of the bursts are less prominent, whereas multifocal sporadic spikes and sharp waves become common. I prefer to call these spikes and sharp waves "multifocal transients" to avoid the pathological connotation of the former terms. They are rarely seen simultaneously in more than one area and are even more rarely bilaterally synchronous. They are the hallmarks of pattern B. Pattern B like pattern A may be invariant. Interhemispheric synchrony remains poor. Reversion to a more striking burst pattern (similar to pattern A) may be seen during quiet sleep as identified by non-EEG variables.[3]

Pattern C

Pattern C (Figs. 3B and 4) succeeds pattern B in roughly 2 or 3 weeks, most often at about 33 weeks CA. Multifocal transients diminish rapidly. The tendency toward intermittent bursting diminishes still further, and activity is more or less continuous during wakefulness and active sleep. The most easily recognizable feature of pattern

---

[3] Non-EEG evidence of the wakefulness-sleep cycle can usually be detected during the epoch when pattern B is observed or a bit earlier, although the latter point is controversial. Criteria include such features as alternating periods of the presence or absence of REMs, regular versus irregular breathing, the occurrence of body movements, and eye opening and closure.

FIG. 1. Top: EEG of a "normal" 12-day-old premature born at a gestational age (GA) of 28 weeks and a body weight of 910 g. Conceptional age (CA) 30 weeks at recording. Note the almost complete interhemispheric asynchrony. **Bottom:** EEG of a "normal" 10-day-old premature born at a GA of 28 weeks and a body weight of 960 g. Fair burst-for-burst, but virtually no wave-for-wave, interhemispheric synchrony. These strips are examples of the pattern referred to in the text as premature pattern A. In this and some of the following figures, the polygraph tracings have been omitted to simplify the illustrations.

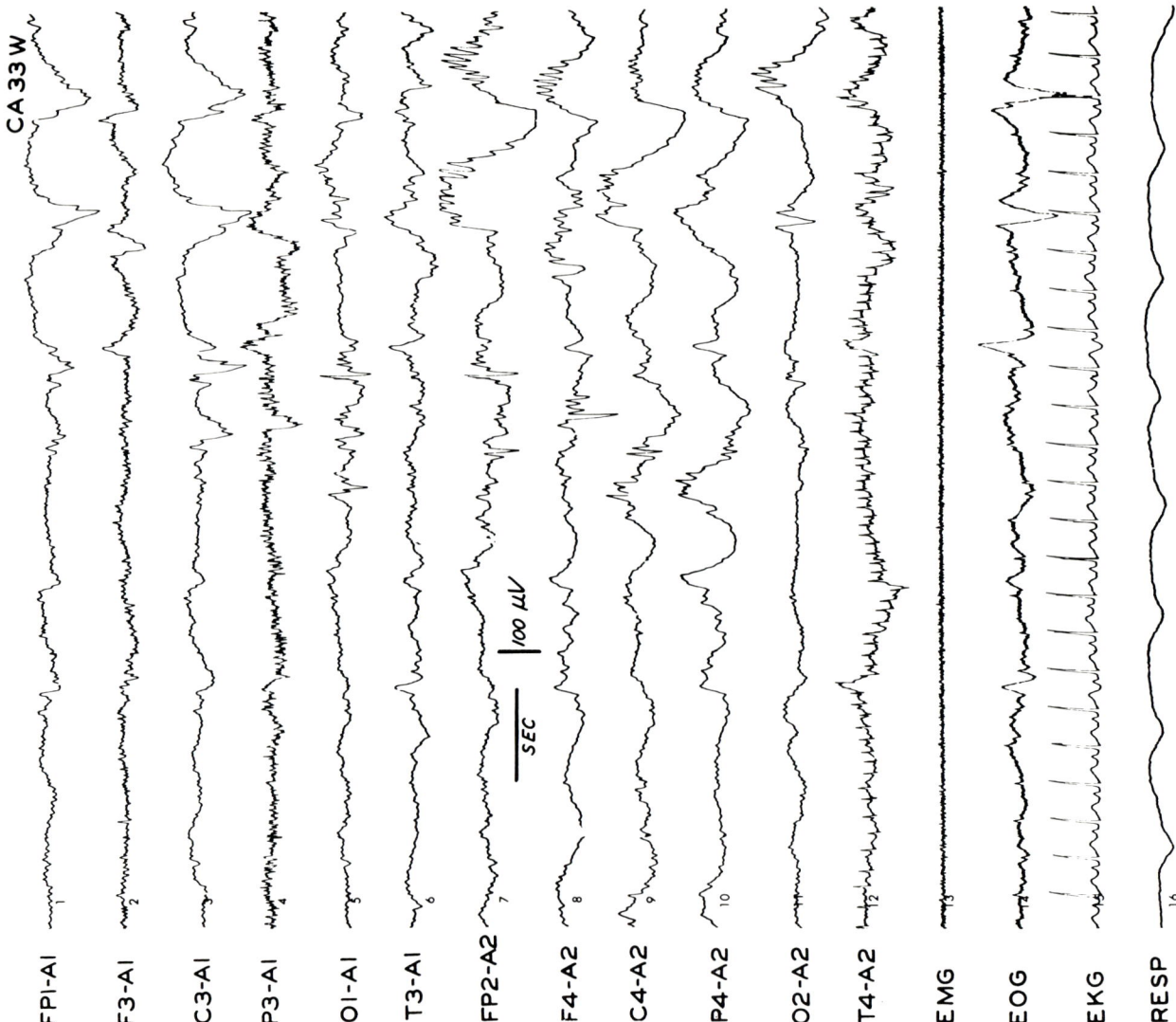

FIG. 2. EEG of a "normal" 6-day-old premature born at a GA of 32 weeks and body weight of 1,220 g. Quiet sleep. Note the multifocal transients; also the spindle-delta burst at the right. Possible frontal sleep transients on the left side apparently reflected in the EOG tracing as well. This is an example of the pattern referred to in the text as premature pattern B.

C is sequences of very slow (¼ to 1 Hz) delta waves (usually most prominent in the occipital and/or temporal areas), on which bursts of rhythmic faster waves are surcharged. These complexes have been called "spindle-delta bursts" by Lombroso (5).[4] The rhythmic fast components vary considerably in frequency (8 to 20 Hz) from baby to baby and have been called "brushes" (5) and "ripples." These superimposed waves tend to be sinusoidal, and the bursts tend to be spindle shaped. Although they have often been mistaken for classical sleep spindle bursts, especially when near 14/sec, they are *not*, nor are they forerunners of classical sleep spindles. The frequency range and topographical distribution are quite different, and these bursts usually disappear a number of weeks before sleep spindles first appear. Interhemispheric synchrony remains relatively poor in most infants, although the posterior slow delta waves are sometimes bilaterally synchronous.

EEG changes related to the wakefulness-sleep cycle become more definite at this epoch. These consist of increases in amplitude of the slowest components of the tracings, particularly of the posterior delta waves, during sleep, especially during what appears by other criteria to be quiet sleep. The quiet sleep pattern called *tracé alternant* (TA) emerges more definitely; at first, it still tends to resemble pattern A (Fig. 6A).

Summary

At least three more or less distinct stages of EEG pattern changes can be distinguished prior to the emergence of what we call here the "Perinatal Patterns." Identification of the successive patterns requires evaluation of the parameters of frequency and temporal and spatial distribution of waves and of the occurrence and distribution of transients and spindle-delta bursts. The most common rhythmic features are the ripples or brushes. Occasional short sequences of rhythmic theta waves may also be seen, especially in the rolandic region. The three patterns constitute a developmental sequence (6)—A succeeded by B succeeded by C. The transitions from one to the next, and from the last to the perinatal patterns, may be relatively abrupt (Fig. 3), but if one happens to record the EEG just when the transition is taking place, elements of both the earlier and later pattern will be observed and one may have difficulty classifying the EEG as belonging to one pattern or the other. The CA at which each transition occurs is variable, as is the duration of a given pattern. Such variability is very likely due at least in part to transient CNS and/or non-CNS disturbances (see section on dysmature patterns, below). Thus advancement or delay in maturation of the brain itself cannot be presumed on the basis of one or even two EEGs.

PERINATAL EEG PATTERNS

At about 36 weeks CA the EEG patterns characteristic of the full-term newborn usually succeed premature pattern C. The perinatal patterns have been described and illustrated in a manual for scoring states of sleep and wakefulness in newborn infants (7), based on the work of a committee of experts in neonatal electroencephalography. Four EEG patterns are distinguished (Fig. 5) and designated as the low-voltage irregular (LVI), mixed (M), high-voltage slow

---

[4] Spindle-delta bursts can be seen in patterns A and B, where they may be very striking and of high amplitude, but are usually single rather than in trains as they tend to be in pattern C.

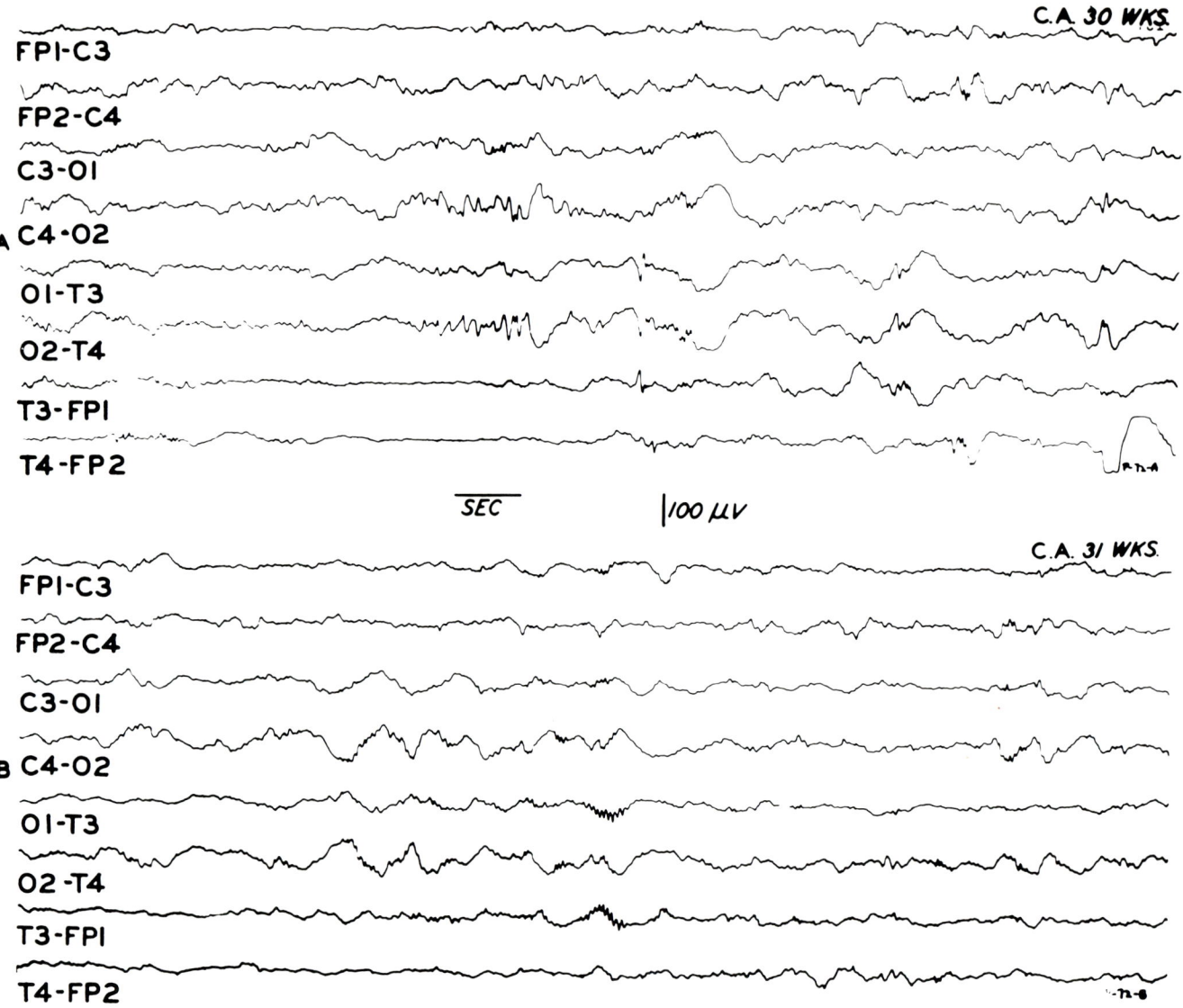

(HVS), and *tracé alternant* (TA) patterns.[5] The first three are actually variations of the same pattern: continuous diffuse arrhythmic irregular activity of mixed frequencies, predominantly delta. The difference is in the amplitude of the theta and especially delta components, relatively low in LVI, variably more prominent in M, generally of high amplitude in HVS. Spindle-delta bursts are relatively weak and infrequent or absent. It should be noted that the LVI pattern is by no means like the low voltage, predominantly beta, pattern associated with states of arousal and alertness in the adult. There is more theta and delta activity. It is "low-voltage-irregular" only relative to the M and HVS patterns.

The TA pattern (the French term tracé alternant[6] has stuck) in contrast consists of diffuse 1- to 3-sec bursts of delta and theta waves, sometimes with faster components and/or transients (spikes and sharp waves), separated by intervals of LVI activity, or even of flat tracings [Figs. 5(TA) and 6]. The pattern somewhat resembles premature pattern A, especially when it first appears (Fig. 6), but differs in that interburst intervals are on the average shorter (rarely over 10 sec and usually less) and there is usually good burst-for-burst interhemispheric and interareal synchrony.

---

[5] In contrast with what we are here calling premature patterns A to C, which evolve successively during preterm development, the four perinatal patterns are all present during the same developmental epoch, their manifestations varying with state, that is, the wakefulness-sleep cycle.

[6] *Tracé alternant* literally means "alternating tracing," designating an intermittent burst pattern. I prefer to reserve it in English to designate only the intermittent pattern seen in quiet sleep in the full-term newborn. The reader should, however, be aware that it is also used in other senses in French and by French writers as well as others when writing in English to refer to, for example, the alternating patterns of early prematurity and the pathological burst-suppression pattern.

The perinatal EEG patterns are related to the wakefulness-sleep cycle, as illustrated in the Anders et al. manual. Four stages of the wakefulness-sleep cycle are specified: W (wakefulness); D (drowsiness), analogous to stage 1 in the adult; A (active sleep), analogous to stage REM in the adult; and Q (quiet sleep), analogous to stages 2 to 4 in the adult. Five physiological criteria are used to specify the stages of the cycle: (a) EEG pattern, (b) respiratory regularity, (c) the presence or absence of tonic activity in the submental EMG, (d) the presence or absence of eye movements, particularly REMs, and (e) the occurrence or nonoccurrence of overtly observable movements (Table 1; Figs. 7 and 8).

EEG patterns are still not as useful in distinguishing stages of the wakefulness-sleep cycle as they become later. Patterns M and HVS may be seen at any stage of the cycle, although M is more common during stages W, D, and A, whereas HVS is more common during stage Q. The LVI pattern is not seen during quiet sleep. The TA pattern is seen only during quiet sleep.

For some purposes a fifth "stage" (not shown in Table 1) is used, namely, "indeterminate sleep" (stage I).[7] It is not really a separate stage of the wakefulness-sleep cycle but rather is defined as those periods of sleep that cannot be clearly classified as either stage A or stage Q. Transitional states between stages A and Q are classified as stage I. However, not all stage I is transitional sleep. Some newborns display more stage I than stages A and Q combined; for example, certain mental retardates tend to do so (8). However, an excess

---

[7] The term "indeterminate" is unfortunate, as it creates a logical inconsistency. Stage I is operationally defined, and its occurrence can therefore be determined. So how can it be indeterminate? However, the term has been widely used.

FIG. 3. EEGs of a "normal" premature born at a GA of 30 weeks and body weight of 1,560 g. **A:** EEG at 1 day of age; an example of premature pattern B. **B:** EEG at 8 days of age; weight 1,500 g; an unusually early appearance of premature pattern C. Note that the transition between the two patterns was completed within 7 days. (From Ellingson, ref. 4, with permission.)

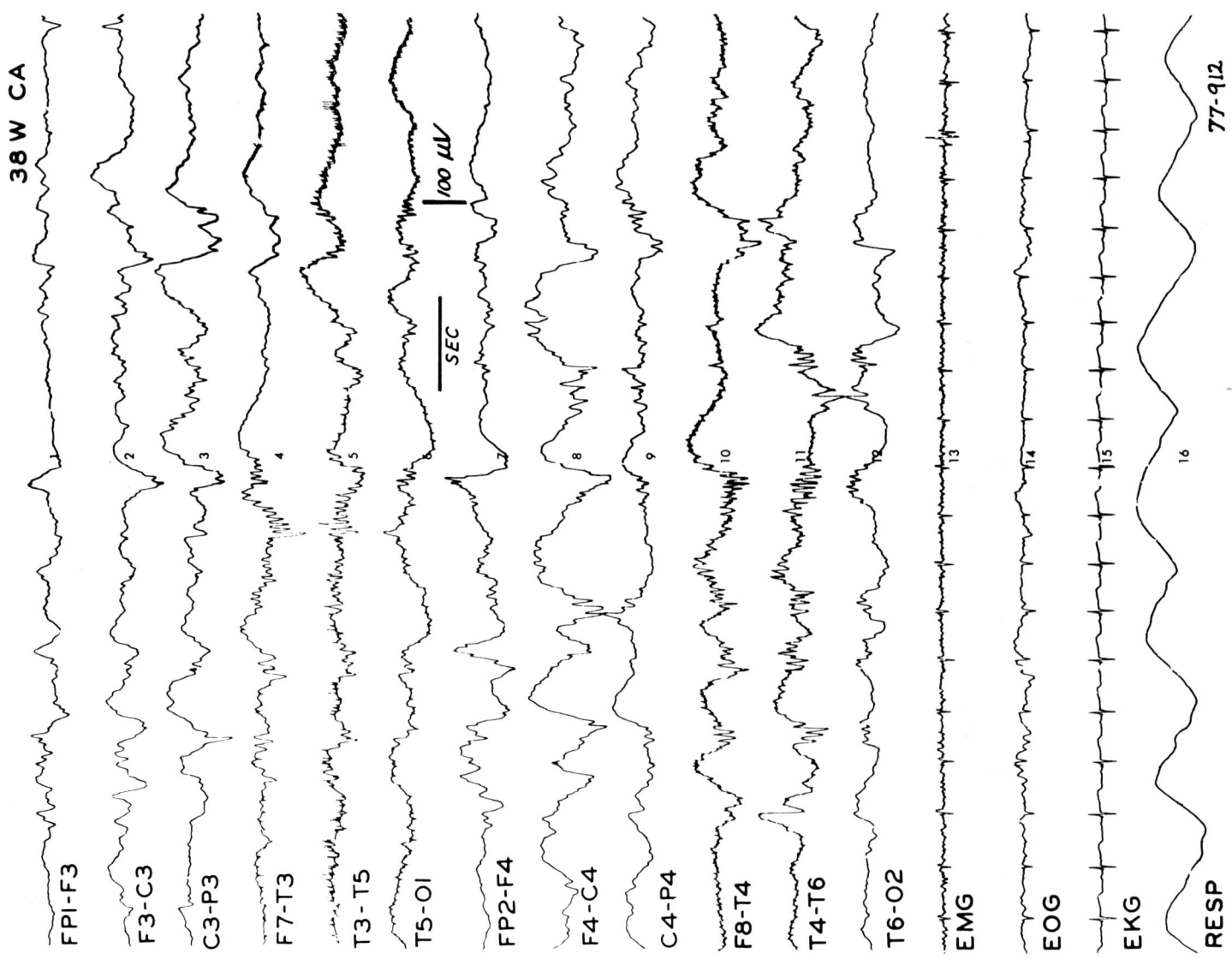

FIG. 4. EEG of a normal 15-day-old newborn born at a GA of 36 weeks and body weight of 2,700 g. Quiet sleep. Note the abundance of spindle-delta bursts. This is an example of the pattern referred to in the text as premature pattern C.

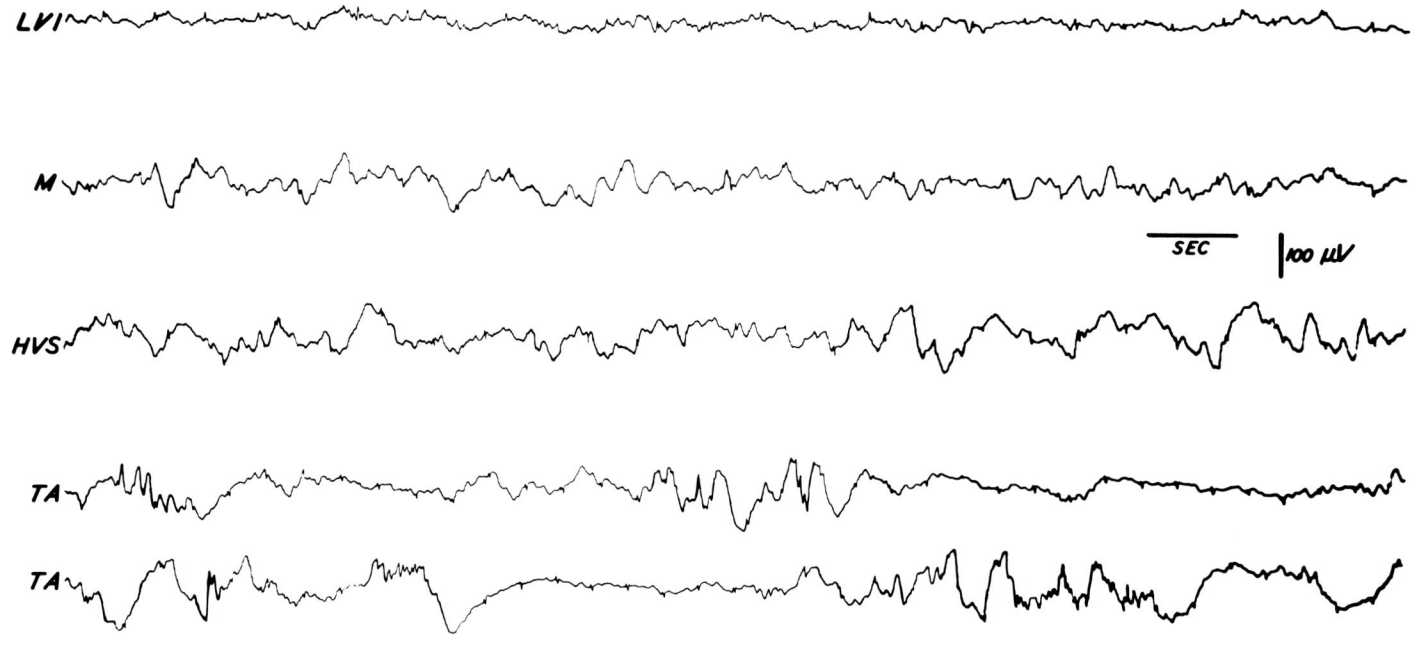

FIG. 5. Tracings of four EEG patterns of the perinatal period (roughly 40 ± 4 weeks CA) classified following Anders et al. (7): low-voltage irregular (LVI) pattern; mixed (M) pattern; high-voltage slow (HVS) pattern; *tracé alternant* (TA) pattern *(see text)*. The two TA tracings are continuous.

of stage I in a single EEG can be considered no more than a suspicious finding; all sorts of circumstances that temporarily upset a baby might cause such a result.

A salient feature of the perinatal sleep EEG is that the infant tends to pass from drowsiness into stage A, in contrast with the adult in whom the initial sleep stage is normally slow-wave (quiet) sleep. Further, the percentage of sleep time spent in stage A is approximately 50% at term and greater than that before term (9). Active (REM) sleep time as a percentage of total sleep time decreases to close to the adult level of approximately 20% by the end of the third year of life; slow-wave sleep time increases correspondingly.

EEG OF THE INFANT

Between 4 and 10 weeks postterm (44 to 50 weeks CA), most often at 6 to 7 weeks, the perinatal patterns evolve into what are referred to for present purposes as the "infantile patterns." The transition usually takes place in 2 weeks, but may require 3 or 4 weeks

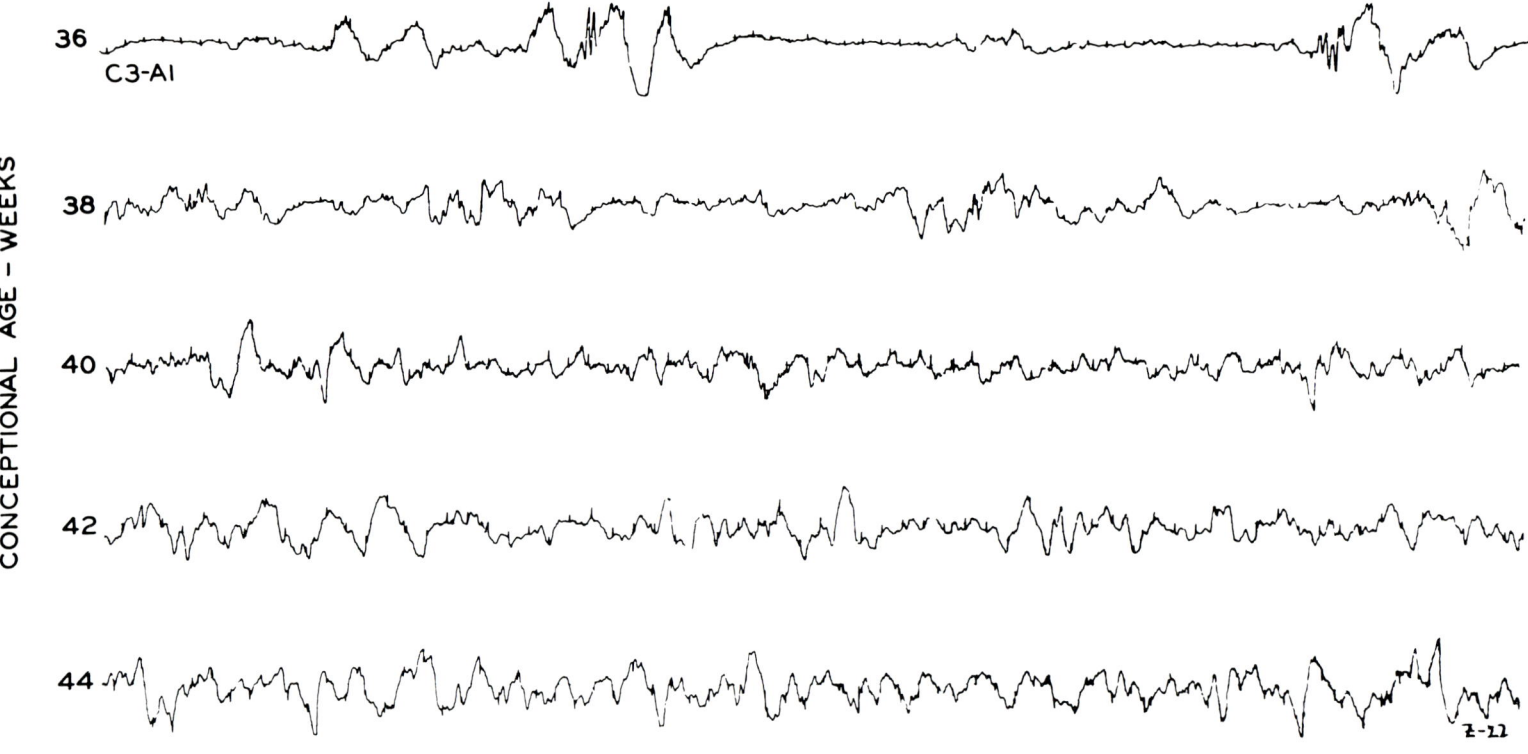

FIG. 6. Evolution of the TA pattern of quiet sleep in a "normal" premature born at a GA of 32 weeks and with a body weight of 1,450 g. The tracings represent the "best" TA patterns seen in the C3-A1 derivation in 2- to 3-hr-long EEGs recorded at 2-week intervals at CAs of 36 to 44 weeks. By 44 weeks in this baby the presence of the TA pattern is doubtful.

in occasional normal infants (10). Infantile sleep patterns approximate those of the adult.[8]

---

[8] After the transition to the infantile patterns the classification systems of Davis et al. (11) or Dement and Kleitman (12,13) become appropriate for delineating the stages of the wakefulness-sleep cycle.

The transition is primarily characterized by three changes: (a) active (stage A; REM) sleep onset is replaced by quiet (slow-wave) sleep onset, that is, the first stage of sleep following drowsiness is quiet or slow-wave sleep rather than active (REM) sleep; (b) the TA pattern, as a characteristic of quiet sleep, disappears (Fig. 6),

TABLE 1. *Criteria of the stages of the wakefulness-sleep cycle*

	Stage			
	W	D	A	Q
EEG pattern	LVI/M/rarely HVS	LVI/M/rarely HVS	LVI/M/rarely HVS	M/HVS/TA
Respiration	Irregular	Irregular	Irregular	Regular
Submental EMG pattern	Usually phasic	Usually phasic	Phasic	Tonic
Eye movements	Usually present variable/eyes open, "bright"	Few or none/eyes open or half closed, "glassy"	REMs present/eyes closed	None/eyes closed
Body movements	Usually present/vocalization, crying	Occasional	Present	Rare or absent

The indeterminate stage of sleep is omitted.
After Anders et al., ref. 7.

and the HVS pattern becomes characteristic of the deepest sleep (stages 3 and 4); and (c) the sleep spindle burst becomes a prominent characteristic of slow wave or quiet sleep (14). Weak and evanescent sleep spindle bursts may be seen in the EEGs of some babies as early as 38 weeks CA, but they do not become a prominent feature until the transition to the infantile patterns occurs.

Stage W is still characterized by continuous arrhythmic irregular activity of mixed frequencies, mostly theta and delta, until the "alpha rhythm" appears at 3 to 4 months postterm (15).

Thus, sometimes as early as the end of the first month, usually by the end of the second month, and almost always before the end of the 10th week after term birth, the EEG has assumed most of the characteristics familiar to the electroencephalographer. Many developmental changes are still to occur, but the relatively bizarre patterns of the premature and perinatal periods are in the past.

ABNORMALITIES IN NEWBORNS' EEGs

Up to this point we have described the normal evolution of the EEG through the end of the neonatal period. EEG phenomena that can be considered abnormal are the subject of this section. They are divided into five groups.

Low-Voltage and Flat Tracings

The gravest EEG abnormality in the newborn is the EEG that is diffusely "flat" at standard gains and shows no activity of cerebral origin[9] or only very low-voltage activity at advanced gains.

Less grave is the diffusely low-voltage EEG (no activity > 20 μV; that is, some activity visible at 7 μV/mm and activity of otherwise normal appearance clearly visible at advanced gains). The recording must of course be continued long enough (at least 1 hr) to make sure that the pattern is invariant and not just an usually low-voltage

---

[9] The criteria of cerebral death in newborns are the same as for older patients; electrocerebral inactivity alone is not sufficient evidence upon which to diagnose death. It should be noted that reservations have been expressed by some investigators concerning the strict applicability of the criteria in infants and even in young children. The most comprehensive study on cerebral death, the NINDS collaborative study, excluded infants under 1 year of age, and data on that age group are less extensive than for older subjects.

Procedures for recording EEGs in cases of suspected cerebral death in newborns are identical with those for older patients.

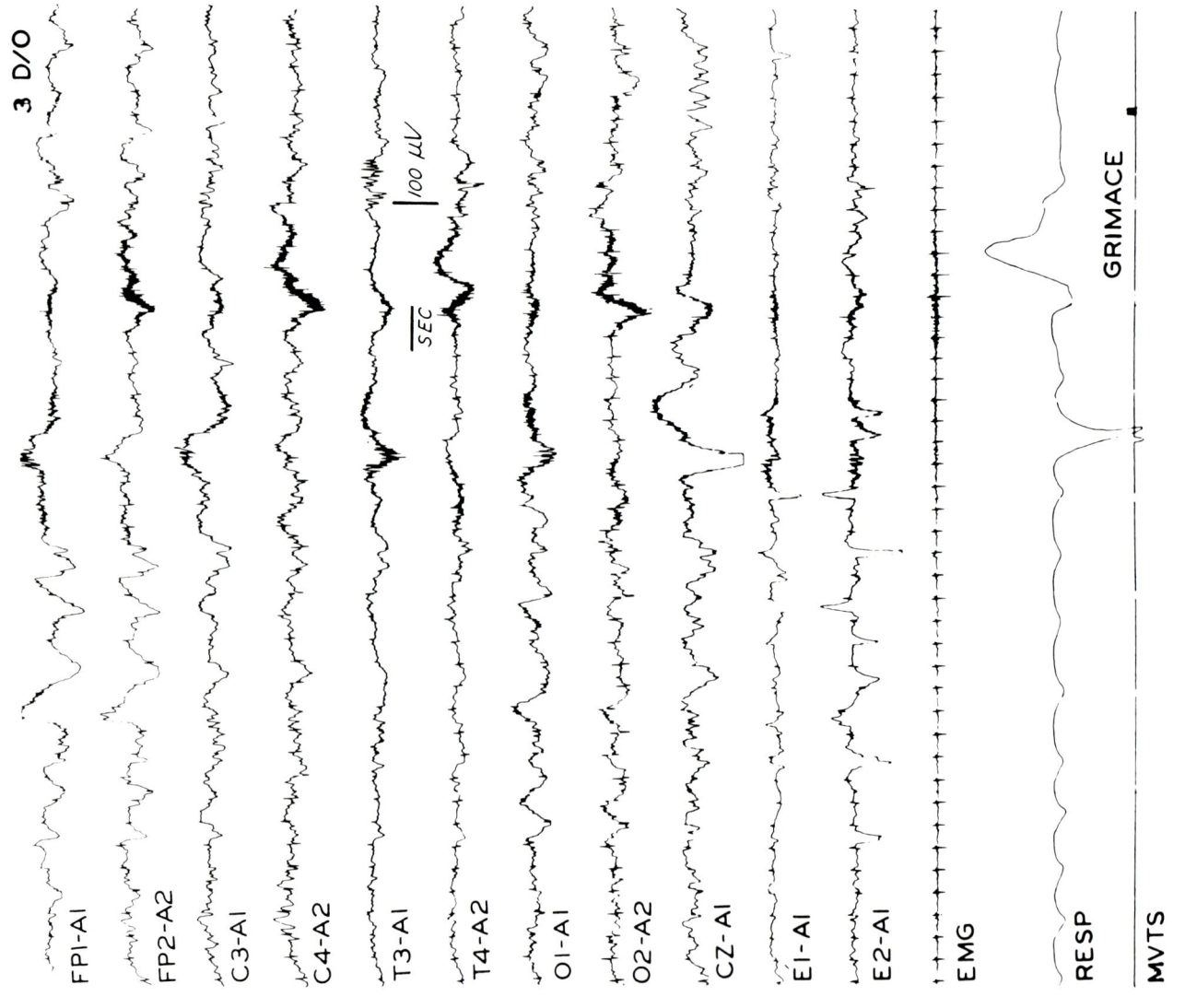

FIG. 7. EEG-polygraph recording of active sleep (stage A) in a normal full-term 3-day-old infant. The EEG tracings are of the M pattern; clear REMs are seen in the EOG tracings (E1-A1 and E2-A1); respiration (RESP) is irregular; the movement code mark (MVTS) indicates a facial movement observed. Recording paper speed was 15 mm/sec.

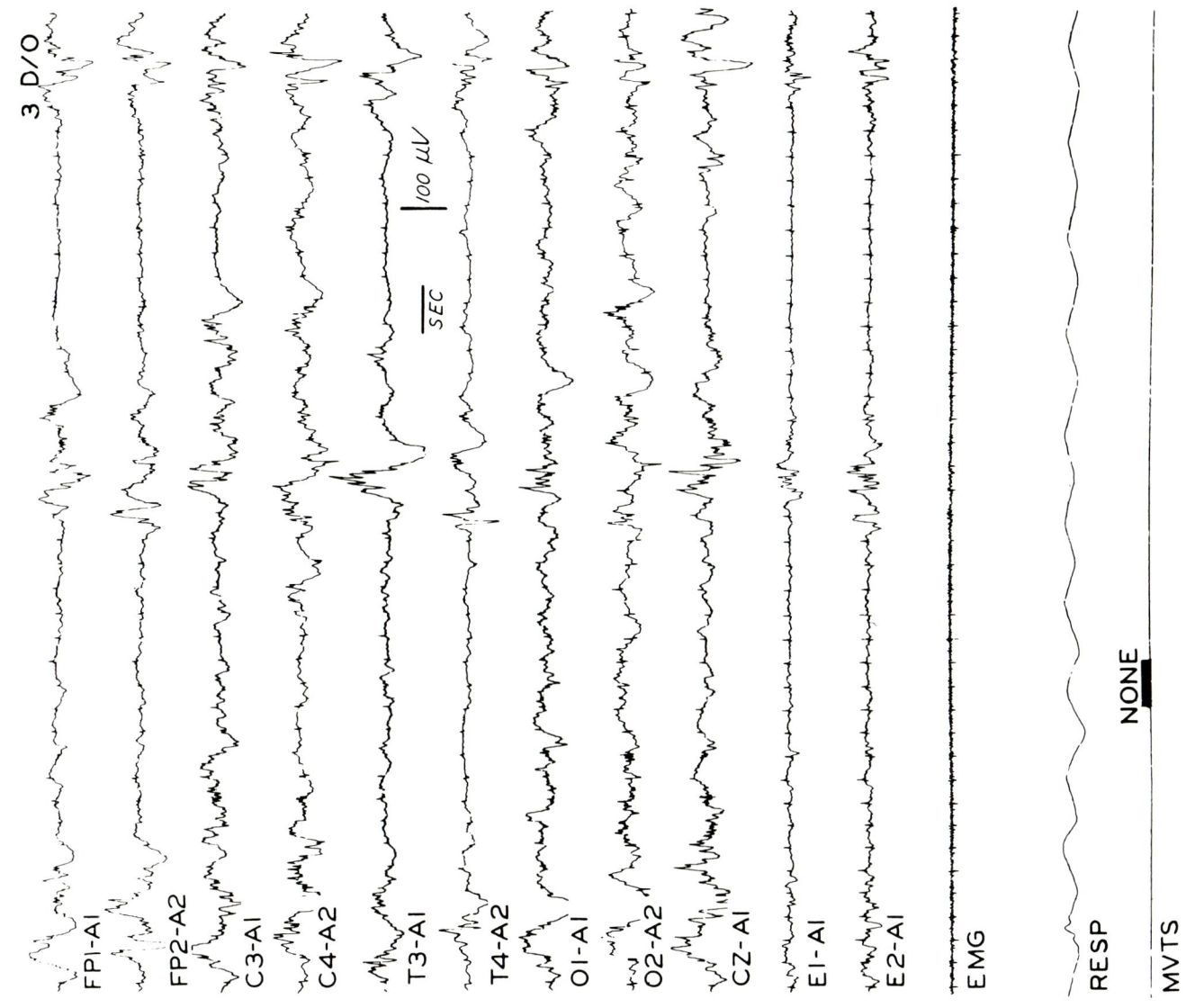

FIG. 8. Recording of quiet sleep (stage Q); same recording session as Fig. 7. EEG tracings are of the TA pattern; no REMs; respiration is regular; the movement code mark indicates no movement observed. Recording paper speed was 15 mm/sec.

LVI episode destined to alternate with M, HVS, and/or TA patterns. If the low-voltage pattern is invariant, the EEG should be repeated. Occasional normal premature and full-term newborns will yield invariant low-voltage tracings for 1 to a few days after birth. If the low-voltage pattern persists for a week or more, concern is warranted (Fig. 9).

Although moment-to-moment amplitude symmetry between homologous areas of the two hemispheres is very often poor in the neonate, if one considers periods of a minute or longer the neonate's EEG is remarkably symmetrical (16). At present, it is probably best to adhere to the 2:1 rule of thumb. In the absence of other abnormalities, asymmetry should not be considered abnormal unless the amplitude on one side is at least twice that on the other consistently throughout a recording (and not just in one montage), technical causes having been eliminated. Even then it is best to verify the finding in a second recording before making much of it (Fig. 10).

Focal flattening is almost always a significant abnormality (Fig. 11), suggesting focal lesions such as porencephaly and effusions. If there is any question at all concerning the technical adequacy of the recording, it should be repeated for verification.

Burst-Suppression Pattern

The burst-suppression pattern (Figs. 12 and 13) is of clinical significance only less grave than electrocerebral inactivity. It is of prime importance to differentiate the true burst-suppression pattern from the intermittent patterns of prematurity (especially premature pattern A) and from the perinatal TA pattern. On the basis of the configuration of the activity in the bursts alone the differentiation is often difficult to make (Fig. 12). Evidence of consciousness or arousability is important in making the differentiation.

Differentiation of the TA pattern is not usually very difficult. TA episodes usually last 15 to 20 min (rarely as long as 30 min), are associated with the non-EEG characteristics of quiet sleep (Table 1), and will be replaced by normal LVI, M, or HVS patterns. The EEG must of course be of sufficient length to allow cyclic variations to be identified.

In the premature, especially under 33 weeks CA, differentiation of intermittent patterns of prematurity may be very difficult. Like the burst-suppression pattern the intermittent patterns of early prematurity are usually invariant, and the bursts may contain many spikes and sharp waves. If the differentiation cannot be made, it should be admitted and serial EEGs ordered, or recommended, in order to resolve the question. At later ages (34 weeks CA and beyond), the invariant intermittent burst pattern is abnormal.

Spikes, Sharp Waves, and Slow Transients

Sporadic multifocal spikes, sharp waves, and slow transients (periods < 70 msec, 70 to 200 msec, and > 200 msec, respectively) are common in early prematurity (premature patterns A and B). They are common enough in late prematurity and around term (36 to 40 weeks CA) that they cannot be considered definite abnormalities. Beyond 40 weeks CA they should not be seen during wakefulness but may still be present during sleep, especially in the TA pattern of quiet sleep.

Unifocal sporadic spikes and other unifocal sporadic transients can be considered abnormal at any age, save for prominent unilateral or bilateral frontal sharp transients *(encoches frontales),* which are common from 30 weeks CA through the first and even into the second month postterm (Fig. 14). These must not be confused with pathological transients, even when they are the only transients evi-

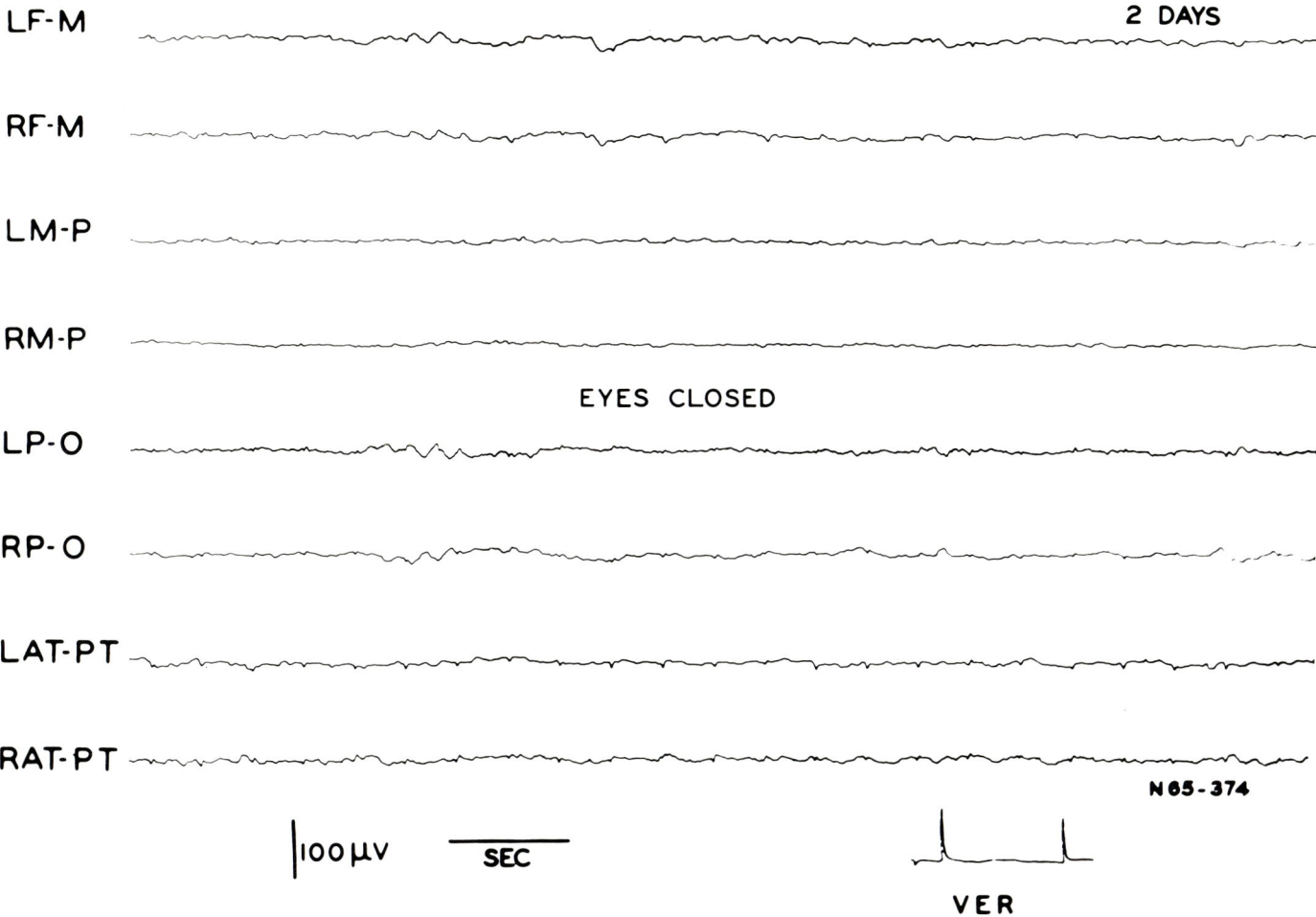

FIG. 9. EEG of a 2-day-old full-term newborn showing invariant low-voltage tracings; almost all activity below 20 μV. A probable diagnosis of cytomegalic inclusion disease had already been made on the basis of a radiograph showing intracranial calcification typical of the disease and was later confirmed immunologically. Visual evoked potentials could not be demonstrated; the write out of an average of 100 (VER) shows no response (the first spike artifact is the stimulus artifact; the second is a time marker 500 msec later). EEGs over the subsequent 4 weeks showed no change. An EEG at 5 months showed intermittent multifocal seizure activity. At 8 months hypsarrhythmia was seen. The child survived for several years in an institution for the retarded. L, left; R, right; F, prefrontal; M, precentral; P, parietal; O, occipital; AT, anterior temporal; PT, posterior temporal.

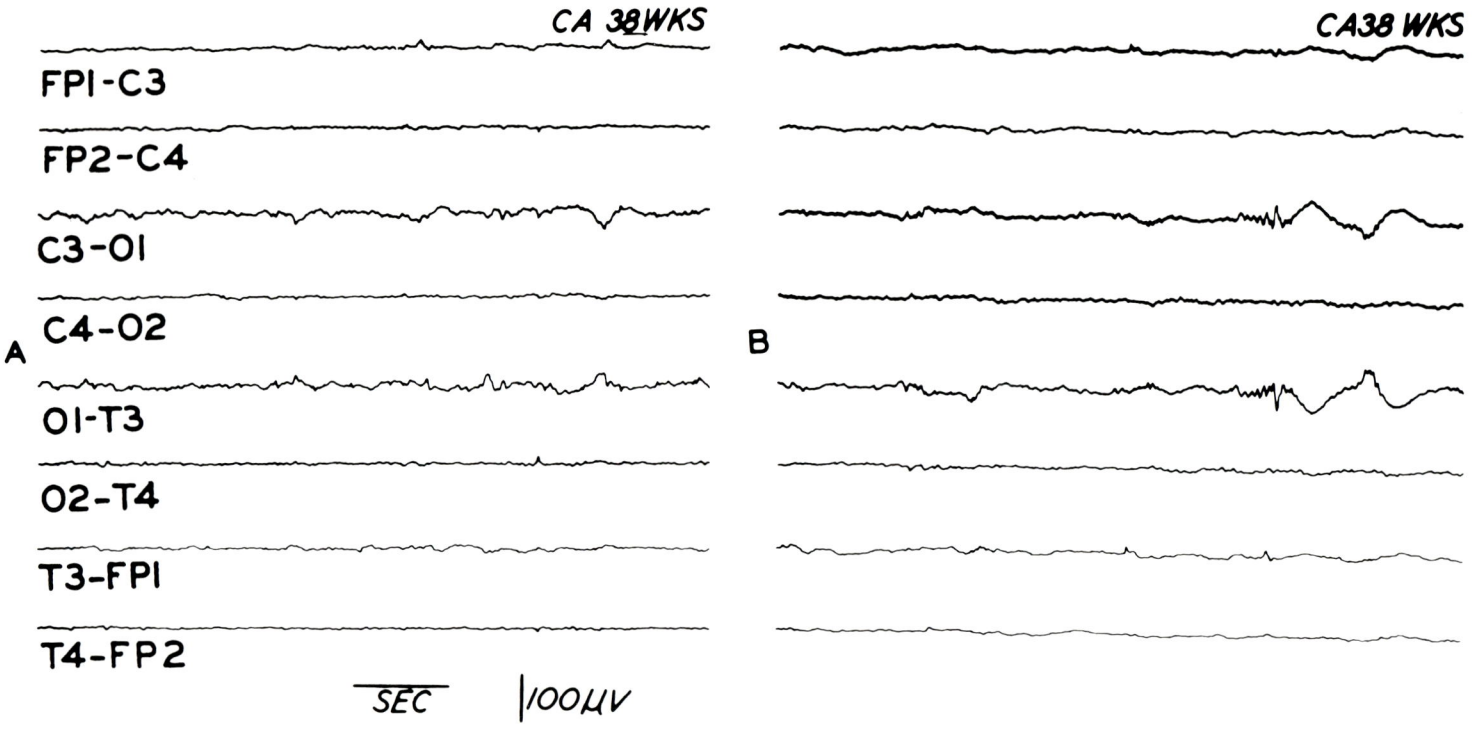

FIG. 10. EEGs of monozygotic 1-day-old twin boys born at a GA of 38 weeks. Note the remarkable similarity of the recordings, especially the amplitude asymmetry (relatively flat tracings over the right hemisphere). The boys developed normally. They were last seen at 6 years of age.

dent. Repetitive spikes are always pathological, but frontal sharp transients may normally occur in *short* sequences. Spikes, sharp waves, and slow transients are not infrequently surface positive in newborns in contrast with older patients in whom true positive spikes are rare. Positive slow transients, especially in the rolandic region, suggest intraventricular hemorrhage.

Rhythmic Patterns

Sustained rhythmic activity is unusual in newborns' EEGs (Fig. 15). The principal exceptions are the ripples or brushes of the delta-spindle burst (the characteristic feature of premature pattern C). Less commonly, semirhythmic or rhythmic 4 to 5/sec activity may

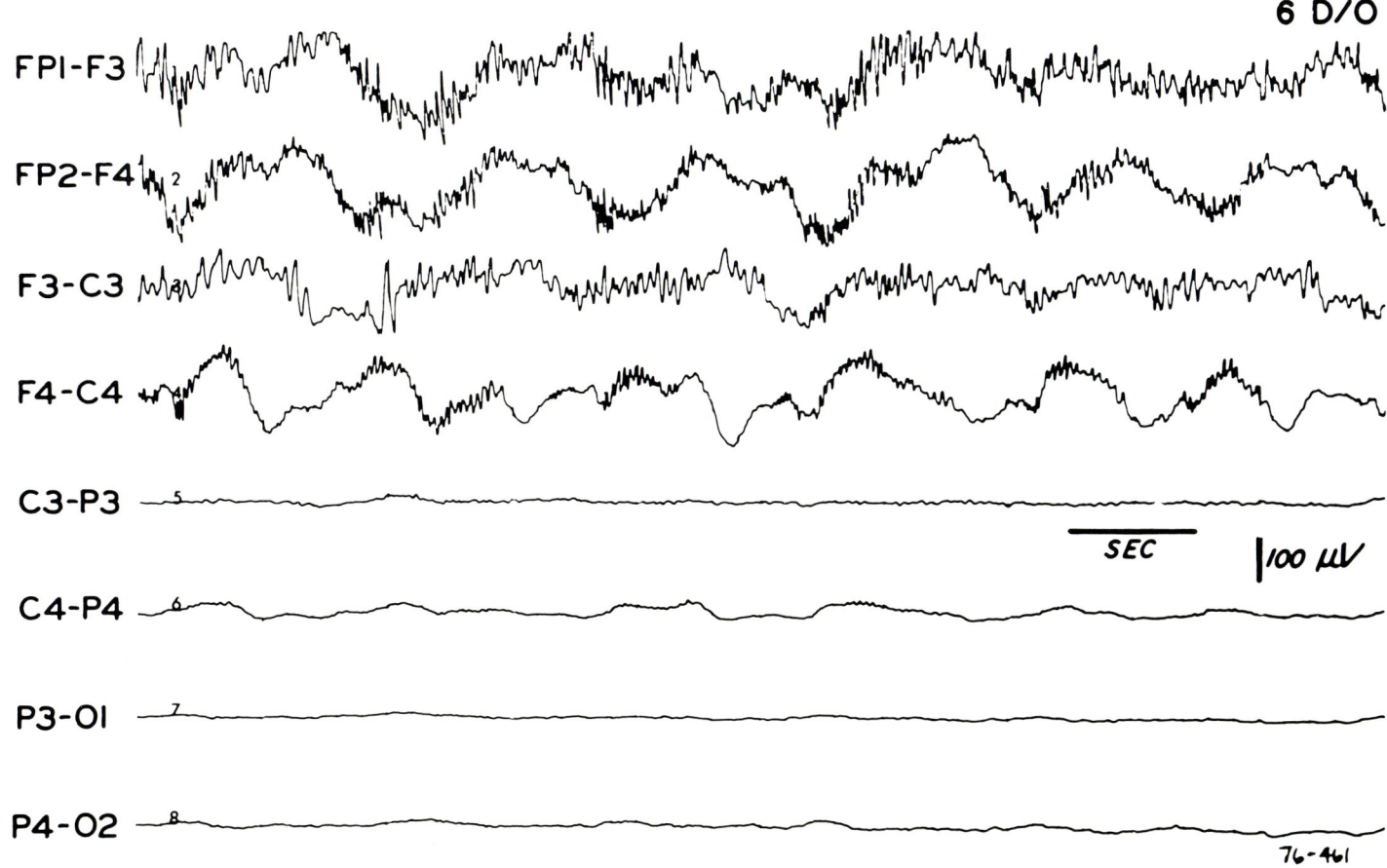

FIG. 11. Bilateral posterior quadrant flat tracings in a 6-day-old newborn born at a GA of 42 weeks and birth weight of 5,020 g. Holoprosencephaly. The topographical distribution of activity and inactivity is typical. The anterior fast activity on the left side is a mixture of fast waves induced by anticonvulsant medication and a little muscle potential artifact. Bursts of seizure activity on a slow background are seen on the right side. The strip is from the end of a clinical seizure manifested by rhythmic mandibular movements and synchronous bilateral flexor movements at the wrists. Several identical seizures occurred during the recording.

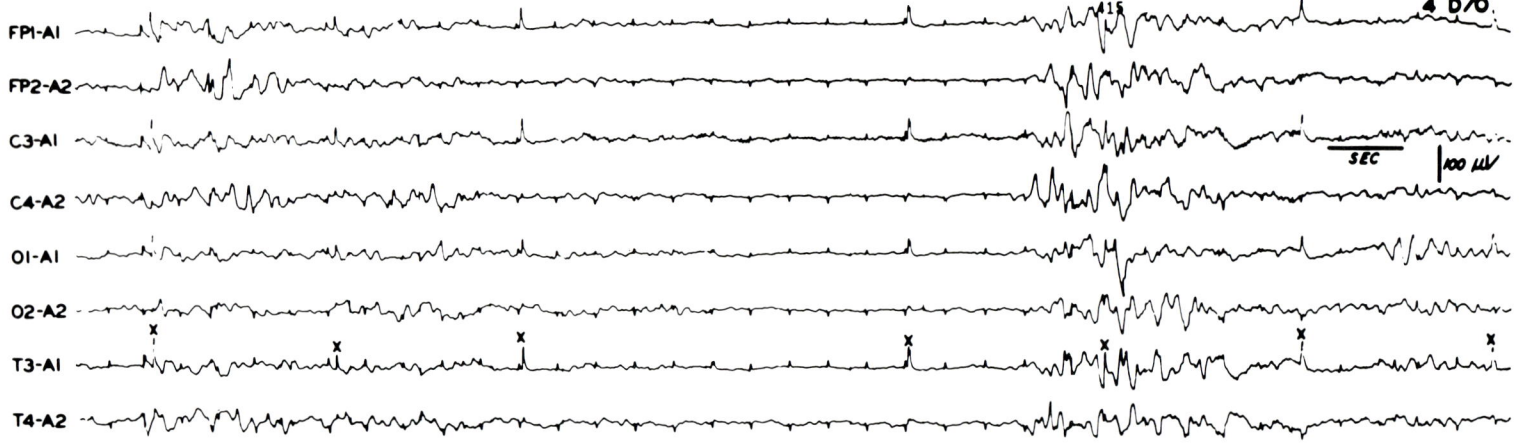

FIG. 12. Invariant burst-suppression pattern in a comatose 4-day-old full-term newborn. The baby had been delivered into the bath water by an obese mother who claimed she did not know she was pregnant. The baby was drowned, but resuscitated. He subsequently experienced several seizures. At the time of recording he was seizure free. The Xs mark artifacts produced by an intravenous infusion pump. EKG artifact is obvious. The child subsequently recovered and has developed normally to 6 months of age.

be seen in the rolandic areas of the full-term newborn, and still less commonly bursts of rhythmic 8/sec waves in the same areas. Finally, evanescent sleep spindle bursts may be seen at term. All of these activities normally either occur in short bursts or, when sustained, tend to be semirhythmic at best.

Apart from these phenomena, rhythmic activity in the alpha and theta frequency bands may be considered abnormal, especially if in areas other than rolandic (2), but it must be sustained and monomorphic to be considered abnormal.[10] Such activity is usually associated with other more obvious types of EEG abnormality (Fig. 15) and in some instances actually constitutes the electrical signs of a seizure (17).

Monomorphic delta activity (17) is also an abnormal finding. Again the only electrical sign of a seizure may be a sequence of monomorphic delta waves (Fig. 16D).

Seizure Activity

The electrical signs of seizure in the newborn are much more varied than in older patients, not only between seizures, but also within a single seizure (Fig. 16). The wave forms often appear bizarre to those accustomed only to the seizures of childhood and adulthood.

---

[10] Beware: highly rhythmic activity may be artifactual, for example, the result of a loose electrode.

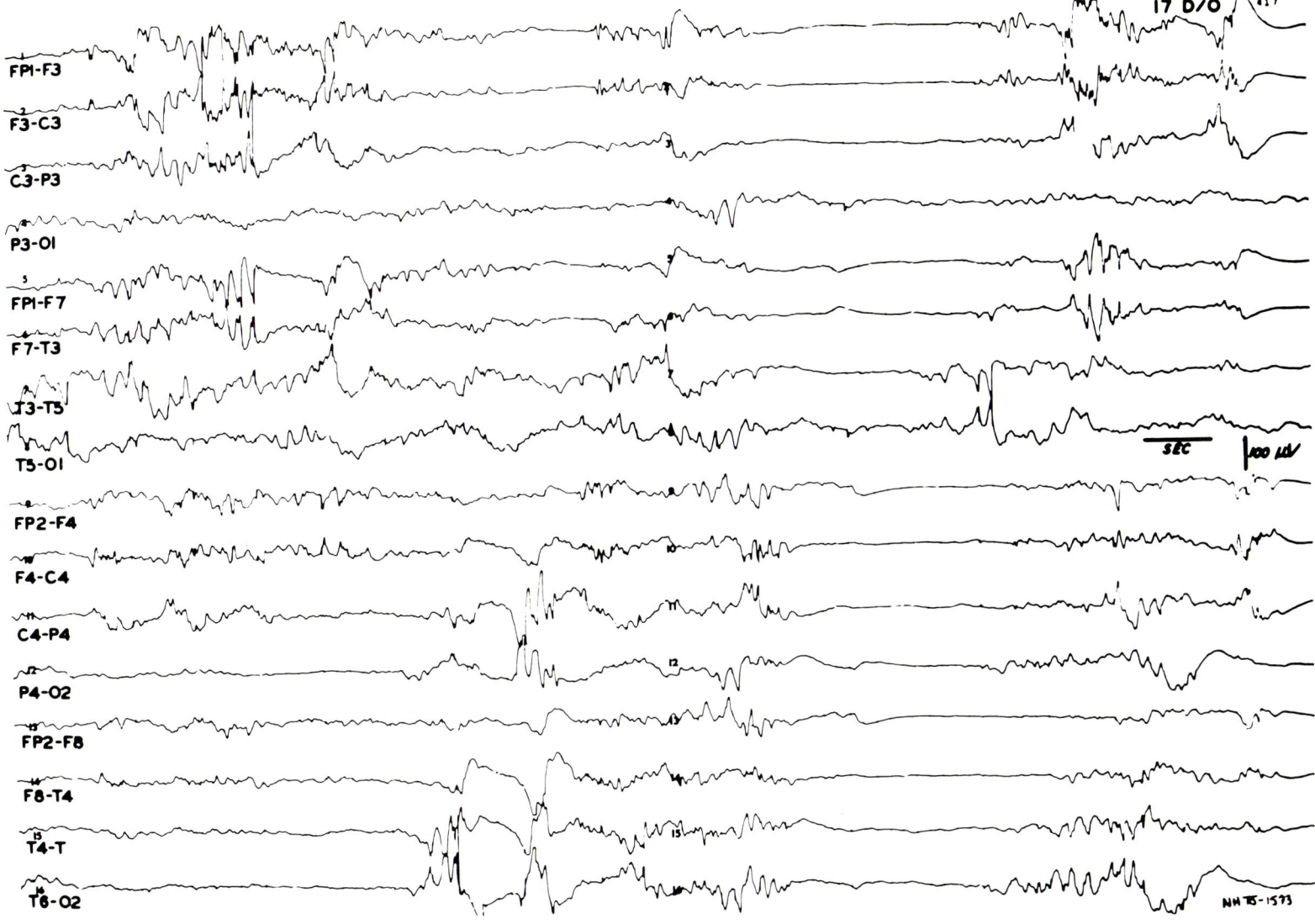

FIG. 13. Burst-suppression pattern with epileptiform features in a 17-day-old full-term newborn suffering from myeloschisis and seizures. In this interictal EEG note the poor *intra*hemispheric and *inter*hemispheric synchrony of the bursts, a feature which is common in burst-suppression in newborns, both prematures and full-term. Lost to follow-up.

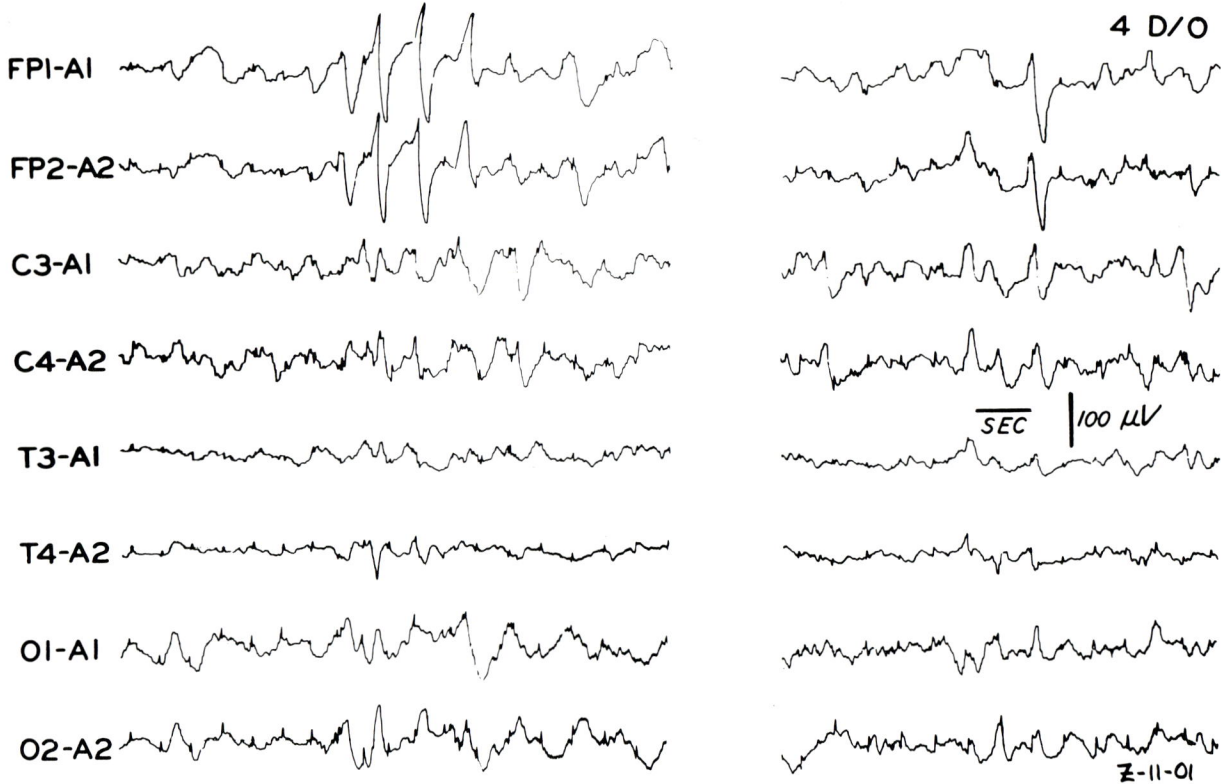

FIG. 14. Frontal sharp transients *(encoches frontales)* in the EEG of a normal 4-day-old full-term newborn. They may be unilateral or, as here, bilateral and may occur in sequences *(left)* or singly *(right)*. They are often very prominent at F3 and/or F4 and can frequently be detected as far back as the C3 and C4 electrodes *(right)*. Their manifestation is variable. This is a particularly striking example. They must not be confused with pathological transients. Recording paper speed was 15 mm/sec.

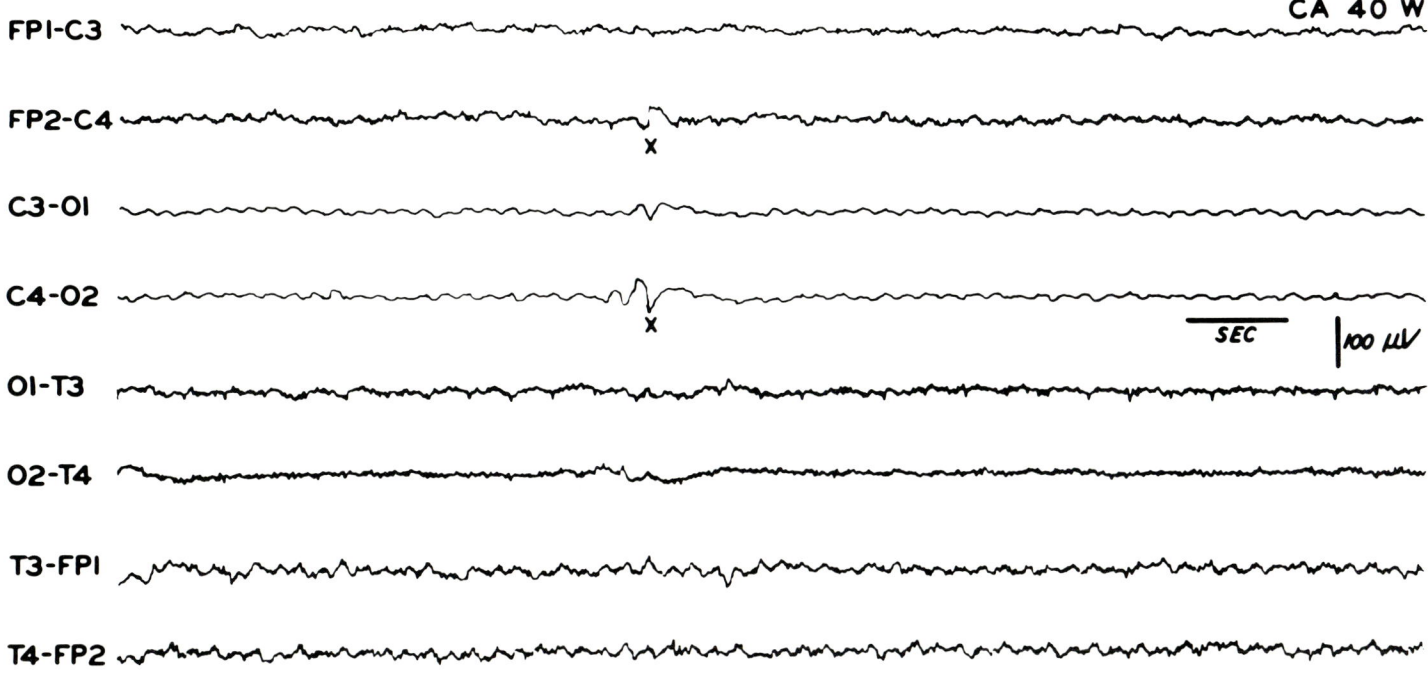

FIG. 15. Low-voltage generalized 4½ per sec rhythm during an interictal period in the EEG of a 2-day-old full-term newborn. X marks an infusion pump artifact.

The only consistent features of neonatal electrical seizure activity are that they are virtually always focal (not generalized) and highly repetitive. The foci are usually not topographically consistent from seizure to seizure; in status epilepticus a focal seizure in one area may in fact begin before a seizure in another area has come to an end.

Hypsarrhythmia is extremely rare in the neonatal period. Classical generalized spike-and-wave activity is never seen.

One of the few areas in which the EEG has proved to be of significant prognostic value is in neonatal sporadic seizures and neonatal status epilepticus (18–20). Allowing that the occurrence of neonatal seizures in itself is not a favorable sign, the prognosis is much im-

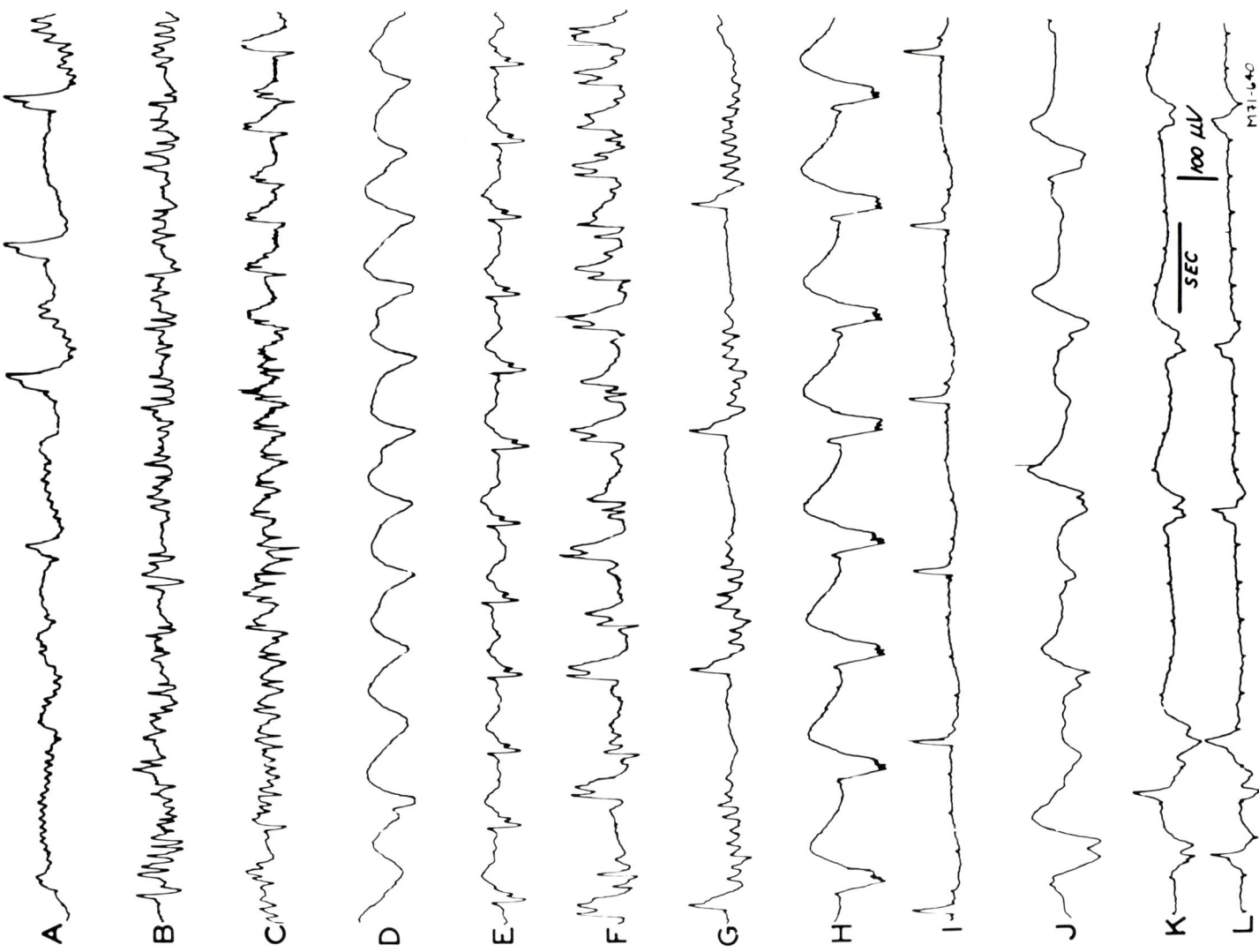

FIG. 16. Seizure activity. All strips are tracings of various derivations from the same recording, in which a series of focal seizures occurred, in a 2-day-old premature born at a GA of 34 weeks. None of the activity shown is artifactual save for the weak EKG artifact in tracings I, K, and L. Tracing A shows the beginning of a seizure; B and C are early during seizures; D to I are from the middles of different seizures; J to L are recorded during seizures. K and L are simultaneous tracings from O1-A1 and O2-A2 derivations.

proved if the interictal EEG is normal. The prognosis is most grave if the interictal EEG is flat or nearly flat and hardly less grave in the presence of a burst-suppression pattern. Other interictal abnormalities bear an intermediate prognosis. If the interictal EEG is abnormal, rapid resolution to a normal pattern (in a matter of a few days) is prognostically better than persistence of the abnormality. [For a more comprehensive summary of the pertinent literature, see (2), Chapter 9.]

DEVIATIONS OF UNCERTAIN SIGNIFICANCE

Dysmature Patterns

It has frequently been asserted that the EEG pattern of the premature and full-term newborn is a function of CA and is independent of gestational age at birth, chronological age since birth, and other factors (21,22). By and large this is true, but there are some exceptions. What does one make of it when the EEG pattern is not appropriate to a baby's well-established CA? Three types of such anachronistic deviations can occur: (a) in simple *immaturity,* the EEG pattern is consistently immature for the baby's CA over a period of time; (b) in *regression,* the EEG pattern is appropriate to the baby's CA, but a subsequent EEG shows reversion to less mature patterns,[11] and (c) in *heterochronism,* both mature and immature patterns for the baby's CA occur within a single recording, for example, a mature pattern for age in stages W, D, and A and an immature pattern in stage Q. There must be a distinct difference in the levels of maturity.

Remember that if one happens to record an EEG in a transitional phase between one pattern and the next more mature pattern, elements of both will be seen in the tracings; this is not heterochronism.

Some data (6) suggest that anachronistic patterns in the newborn period occur more frequently in infants who later develop abnormally than in those who develop normally, but the evidence is too fragmentary to warrant firm conclusions. Lombroso (5) has shown that almost any illness, including one without any manifest CNS symptoms or signs, may cause a transient regression in EEG pattern in the newborn.

In summary, a clearly dysmature EEG suggests that the baby is ill or disordered in some fashion, but the illness may be temporary and may not even directly involve the CNS.[12]

Poor Interhemispheric Synchrony

In the absence of any other deviation in EEG pattern, poor interhemispheric synchrony may be an abnormal sign in the postneonatal period; it is common in hydrocephalus and some other disorders. In the premature, interhemispheric asynchrony is the rule. At term, most normal babies will show a tendency to fair or even good interhemispheric synchrony between homologous areas of the right and left hemispheres over the convexity with persisting poor synchrony between the temporal areas. Nevertheless at present poor interhemispheric synchrony in all areas should not by itself be considered abnormal until later in the first year of life. Further studies are needed to clarify the significance of such deviations.

---

[11] Determination of regression requires serial electroencephalography. If one has only a single immature EEG in hand, there is no way of knowing whether it represents simple immaturity or regression.

[12] These remarks refer to EEGs in which dysmaturity is the only deviation from expected normal patterns. Dysmature background activity is common in EEGs showing more definite abnormalities (above) and, when present, adds to the overall degree of abnormality.

Excessive Stage I

As stated earlier, elevated percentages of sleep stage I have been observed in Down's syndrome babies and in some other abnormal conditions. More simply, this means that cycling between active and quiet sleep is less regular and clear-cut than normally. Reliable determination of sleep stages and their proportional durations, however, requires (a) at least 3 to 4 hr of recording, (b) recording of non-EEG as well as EEG variables, and (c) careful ratings of the five criterion variables (Table 1). These requirements are beyond the capacity of most clinical EEG laboratories, for reasons of time if nothing else. Unless the determinations can be properly made, it is best not to undertake them. In any case, it must be remembered that non-CNS illness and even upsetting events occurring on the night or day before the recording can result in transient disturbances of the sleep cycle in anyone.

CONCLUSION

In an exposition of this length it is impossible to include all of the details to be found in the extensive literature on neonatal electroencephalography. For example, some electroencephalographers with a great deal of experience with neonates have been able, from more detailed knowledge of the EEG patterns (21), to estimate CA within ±1 or 2 weeks. This author has not often been able to do that well, especially in the presence of moderate-to-severe EEG abnormality, but that may be his fault.

It has also been necessary here to indulge in a certain amount of simplification and perhaps overgeneralization. Therefore, the reader is warned not to hold to the generalizations presented too rigidly. For example, the age limits given for the manifestation of the various EEG patterns should not be rigidly followed in judging whether a given patient's recording is normal or abnormal.

There is no uniform or accepted nomenclature for phenomena peculiar to the EEG of the neonate. Such terms as "spindle-delta bursts" are not widely used or understood. The designations of premature patterns A, B, and C, neonatal patterns, and infantile patterns in this chapter are idiosyncratic; do not expect to find them elsewhere. They are intended as approximate guidelines. Other workers may distinguish a greater number of developmental stages. A real need exists for a standard nomenclature for neonatal electroencephalography. It is hoped that one will be produced soon.

It is also hoped that the importance of differentiating between invariant EEG patterns and cyclic pattern variations has been sufficiently emphasized so that the importance of obtaining EEGs of adequate length is appreciated; 20- to 30-min recordings are usually inadequate.

Likewise, serial recordings are as important in neonatal electroencephalography as in any area of electroencephalography, or even more so. Not infrequently more than one EEG is required just to decide whether observed phenomena are normal or abnormal. Even when that basic decision is not in question, the evolution of EEG patterns may be more important in prognosis than the patterns of any single recording.

It must be evident that a great deal remains to be learned about the rapidly evolving EEG of the neonatal period. It is therefore natural to feel somewhat uncomfortable when confronted with EEGs of newborns. They are difficult to evaluate, and there is no disgrace

Note: The *Atlas of Neonatal Electroencephalography* (23) was published after the completion of this chapter. I have reviewed it in detail and recommend it. It is a valuable reference for any laboratory in which more than occasional neonatal EEGs are recorded.

in sometimes having to equivocate. Less harm is done in confessing ignorance or indecision than in jumping to wrong conclusions.

REFERENCES

1. Jasper, H. H. (1958): The ten twenty electrode system of the International Federation. *Electroencephalogr. Clin. Neurophysiol.*, 10:371–375.
2. Engel, R. C. H. (1975): *Abnormal Electroencephalograms in the Neonatal Period.* Charles C Thomas, Springfield, Illinois.
3. Ellingson, R. J., and Rose, G. H. (1970): Ontogenesis of the electroencephalogram. In: *Developmental Neurobiology,* edited by W. A. Himwich, pp. 441–474. Charles C Thomas, Springfield, Illinois.
4. Ellingson, R. J. (1964): Studies of the electrical activity of the developing human brain. In: *Developing Brain, Vol. 9: Progress in Brain Research,* edited by W. A. Himwich and H. E. Himwich, pp. 26–53. Elsevier, Amsterdam.
5. Lombroso, C. T. (1975): Neurophysiological observations in diseased newborns. *Biol. Psychiatry,* 10:527–558.
6. Ellingson, R. J., Dutch, S. J., and McIntire, M. S. (1974): EEG's of prematures: 3–8 year follow-up study. *Dev. Psychobiol.,* 7:529–538.
7. Anders, T., Emde, R., and Parmelee, A., editors (1971): *A Manual of Standardized Terminology, Techniques and Criteria for Scoring of States of Sleep and Wakefulness in Newborn Infants.* UCLA Brain Information Service, NINDS Neurological Information Network, Los Angeles.
8. Petre-Quadens, O. (1972): Sleep in mental retardation. In: *Sleep and the Maturing Nervous System,* edited by C. D. Clemente, D. P. Purpura, and F. E. Mayer, pp. 383–417. Academic Press, New York.
9. Roffwarg, H. P., Muzio, J. N., and Dement, W. C. (1966): Ontogenetic development of the human sleep-dream cycle. *Science,* 152:604–619.
10. Ellingson, R. J. (1975): Ontogenesis of sleep in the human. In: *The Experimental Study of Human Sleep: Methodological Problems,* edited by G.-C. Lairy and P. Salzarulo, pp. 129–149. Elsevier, Amsterdam.
11. Davis, H., Davis, P. A., Loomis, A. L., Harvey, E. N., and Hobart, G. (1938): Human brain potentials during the onset of sleep. *J. Neurophysiol.,* 1:24–38.
12. Dement, W., and Kleitman, N. (1957): Cyclic variations in EEG during sleep and their relation to eye movements, body motility, and dreaming. *Electroencephalogr. Clin. Neurophysiol.,* 9:673–690.
13. Rechtschaffen, A., and Kales, A., editors (1968): *A Manual of Standardized Terminology, Techniques and Scoring System for Sleep Stages of Human Subjects.* Public Health Service, U.S. Government Printing Office, Washington, D.C.
14. Metcalf, D. R. (1969): EEG sleep spindle ontogenesis. *Neuropädiatrie,* 1:428–433.
15. Lindsley, D. B. (1939): A longitudinal study of the occipital alpha rhythm in normal children: Frequency and amplitude standards. *J. Genet. Psychol.,* 55:197–213.
16. Varner, J. L., Ellingson, R. J., Danahy, T., and Nelson, B. (1977): Interhemispheric amplitude symmetry in the EEGs of full-term newborns. *Electroencephalogr. Clin. Neurophysiol.,* 43:846–852.
17. Dreyfus-Brisac, C., and Monod, N. (1972): Neonatal status epilepticus. *Handbook Electroencephalogr. Clin. Neurophysiol.,* 15B: 38–52.
18. Monod, N., and Dreyfus-Brisac, C. (1972): Prognostic value of the neonatal EEG in full-term newborns. *Handbook Electroencephalogr. Clin. Neurophysiol.,* 15B:89–112.
19. Monod, N., Dreyfus-Brisac, C., and Sfaello, Z. (1969): Dépistage et pronostic de l'état de mal néonatal. *Arch. Franç. Pediatr.,* 26:1085–1102.
20. Rose, A. L., and Lombroso, C. T. (1970): Neonatal seizure states. *Pediatrics,* 45:404–425.
21. Dreyfus-Brisac, C. (1962): The electroencephalogram of the premature infant. *World Neurology,* 3:5–15.
22. Dreyfus-Brisac, C. (1975): Neurophysiological studies in human premature and full-term newborns. *Biol. Psychiatry,* 10:485–496.
23. Werner, S. S., Stockard, J., and Bickford, R. (1977): *Atlas of Neonatal Electroencephalography.* Raven Press, New York.

Chapter 7

Optimal Display of EEG Activity

Charles E. Henry

The Cleveland Clinic Center, Cleveland, Ohio 44106

Montages 179
Instrumental Controls... 197
    Sensitivity... 197
    Frequency Controls.. 199
    High Frequency Filters.. 201
    Low Frequency Filters 202
Determination of Electrocerebral Inactivity 204
References 220

The previous chapters dealing with minimal technical requirements, polarity, and localization of electrical fields are important for the understanding and appreciation of the contents of this chapter. Here we tackle the problem of putting all these components together in the form of an *intelligible* electroencephalogram (EEG).

MONTAGES

The EEG, the ink-written display of the electrical activity of the brain as a temporal sequence of frequency and voltage output, may take many forms. Let us assume that the 21 electrodes of the International, or 10–20, system constitute the basic minimum for adequate head coverage. And let us recognize 48 years after Berger's original work with 1- or 2-channel units, and 30 years following the introduction of the 8-channel Grass Model 3 "workhorse," that 16-channel instruments now constitute a reasonable minimum standard. Thus, given 21 leads and 16 channels (each of which has two inputs), we have a very large number of ways in which these can be combined to display the EEG.

The cardinal criterion for a good montage is that the EEG features, normal and abnormal, are displayed in an unambiguous fashion, and thus are easy to see. The EEGer's need for this is obvious. Equally important is that the recording technologist, who has only 10 to 20 sec to scan each portion of the record as it evolves, should be able to appreciate its features. Without such understanding there is little chance for an orderly, logical, and efficient EEG examination. A further reason for effective and easy-to-learn montages is apparent when we consider technician trainees, neurology residents, laboratory visitors, and all those who see illustrations and lantern slides of EEG tracings.

Consideration of such figures and slides indicates that we still suffer from a great diversity of montages. It suggests that few have read the expanded definition of this word in *Webster's Unabridged Dictionary*. This definition implies that a good montage is more than merely the sum of its individual derivations. Many electroencephalographers, however, do not consider construction of montages carefully enough, a neglect often stemming from uncritical acceptance of montages they had been exposed to in their training laboratories. As these montages became familiar, they were adopted as somehow the "right" way to display the EEG. Few change, and even years later one can often identify the places where EEGers have trained by the montages they still cling to. Nowhere, unfortunately, is this more obvious than for those electroencephalographers who have a myopic devotion to the alleged virtues of exclusive "monopolar" *or* bipolar recording, of which more later.

Some things are best illustrated by examples of how *not* to do EEG, or of how to do EEG the hard way. Figure 1 shows many examples of such 8-channel montages. All these are from records and montage sheets that we have seen in the past decade. For relative simplification only half of the head is shown, although the complexity of the Fig. 2 sequences requires the full display.

Space does not permit discussion of the pitfalls and the potentials for error and misinterpretation inherent in these idiosyncratic curios. Most, perhaps all, are still in use. We use them occasionally in teaching sessions to demonstrate the folly of open-ended derivations and the snares of tiny triangles. To a considerable degree they reflect the great difficulty in getting adequate head coverage with only 8 channels. Their critical and careful study is recommended.

The capacity for such literal nonsense is expanded with the addition of more channels. The logical and the sensible approach would be to evolve whole new sets of montages. More often, unfortunately, 16 channels have been used for the simultaneous running of two old 8-channel montages. At times this arrangement has led to duplication, with some channels turned off! Only rarely are 16 channels used to create a logical display, such that the EEG features are easily transposed to or fitted over the head.

Consider the following. The output of 21 electrodes in 16 channels could be recorded as in Fig. 3. The EEG of this boy with cerebral palsy and seizures is focally abnormal. As shown on the derivations at the left, every lead is sampled at least once. Although it is generally easier to grasp a sketched montage, the complexity is such that this is not feasible here. Some of the derivations are from the left to the right and vice versa. Some are from the anterior to the posterior region, and vice versa. Some derivations are in angled chain sequence and some are open-ended. This montage, in effect, incorporates many

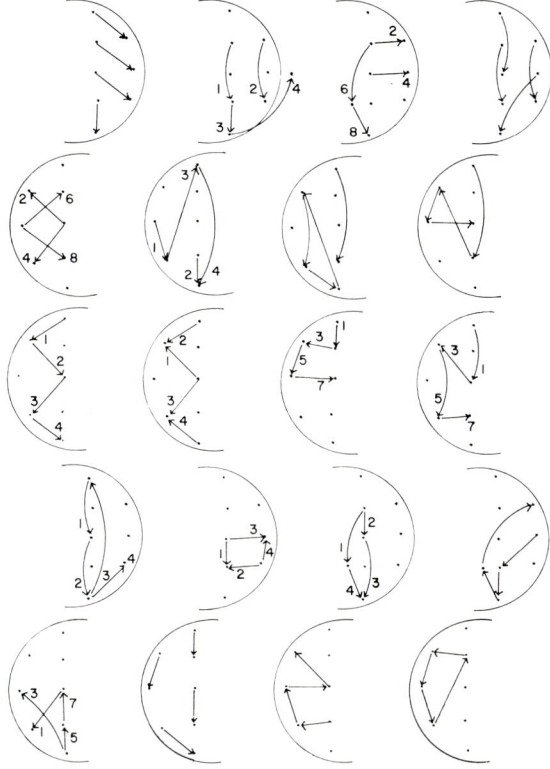

FIG. 1. Twenty examples of 8-channel montages, the contralateral hemisphere having symmetric derivations. Arrows indicate grid I–grid II sequences; numbers indicate channel.

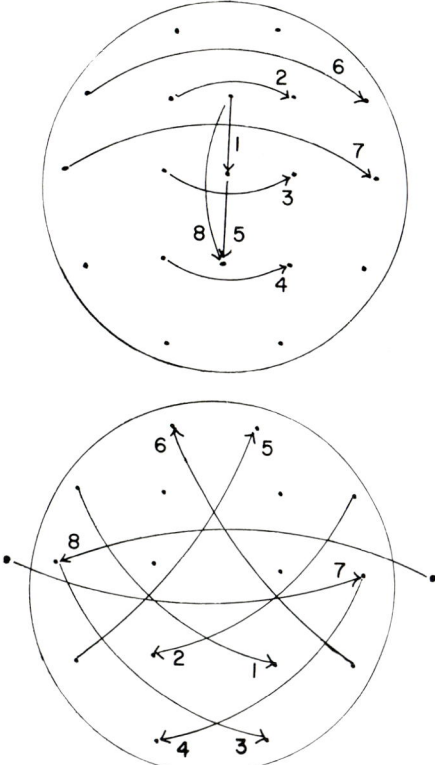

FIG. 2. Complex 8-channel montages illustrating nonsensible and illogical EEG montage technique. Notations are the same as in Fig. 1.

of the bad features illustrated in Figs. 1 and 2. Careful study reveals a predominantly right-sided discharge, although it is difficult to be certain of any more focal features.

Figure 4 shows the same patient recorded with an ear reference system, but the reference is on either the first or the second grid. There is no logic in the array, neither left versus right nor anterior versus posterior. Since this is made with ipsilateral ear reference technique, one can readily see the lateralization and, from channels

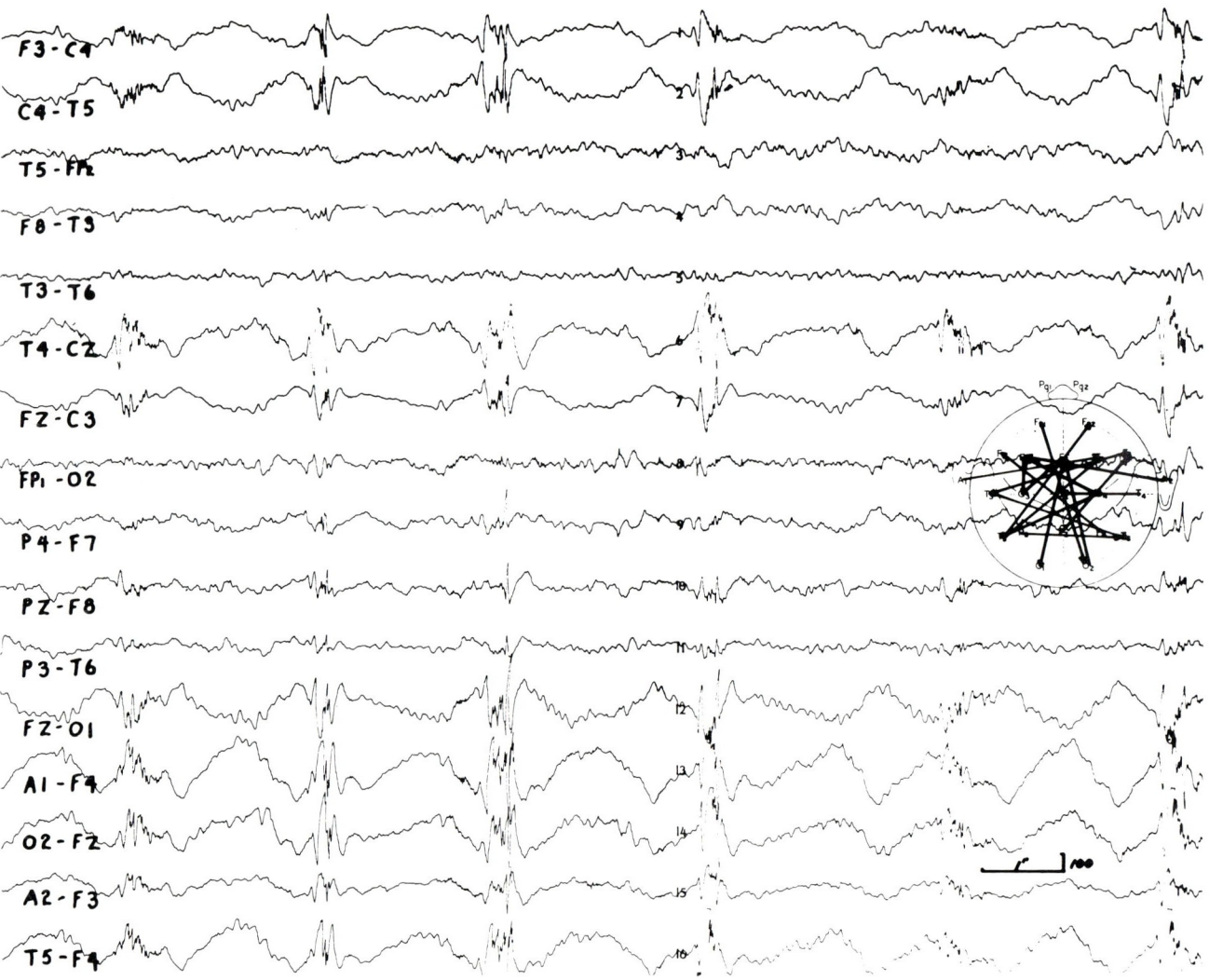

FIG. 3. Focally abnormal record as displayed with a scrambled chaos montage.

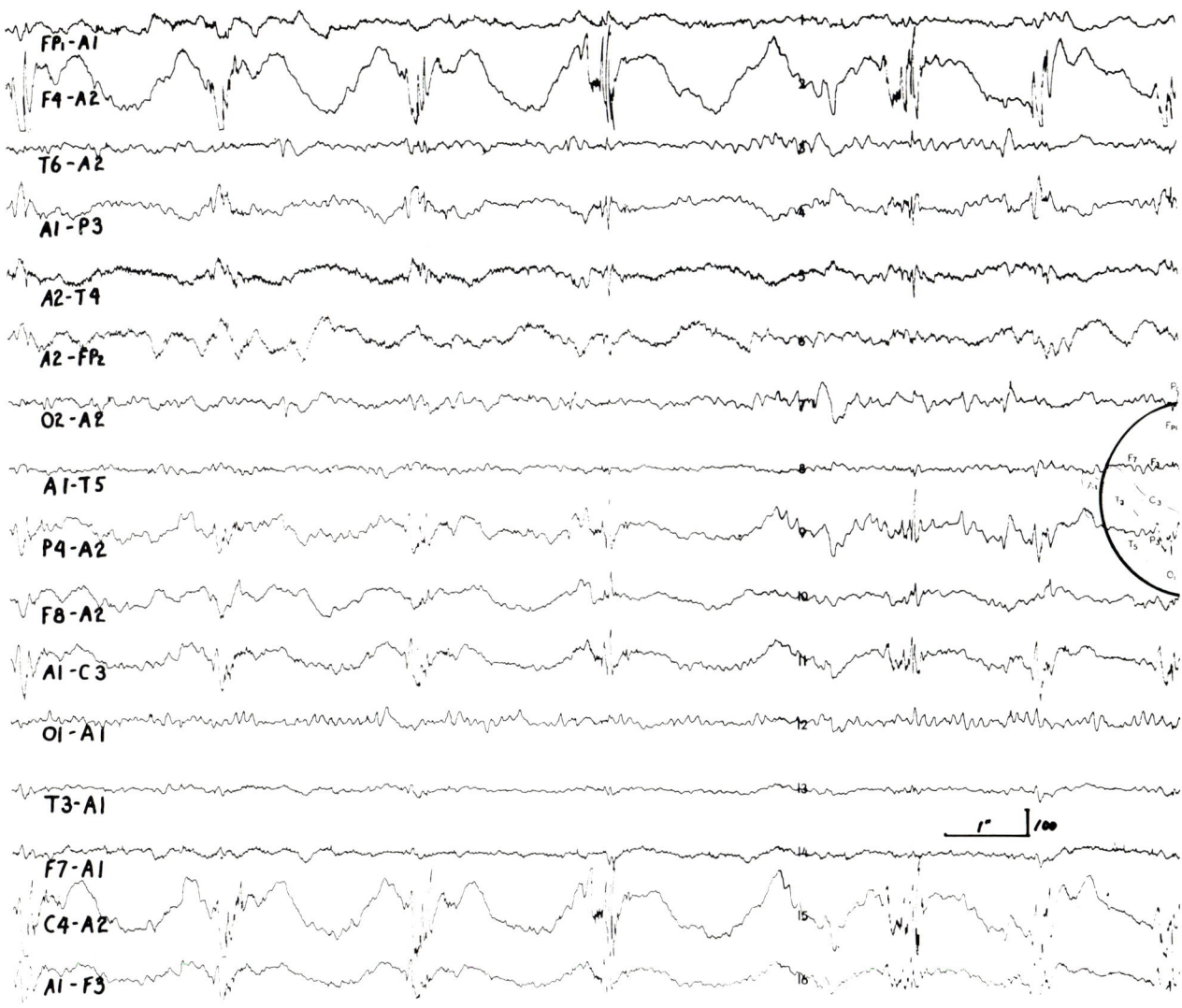

FIG. 4. EEG from same patient as Fig. 3, recorded with scrambled ear reference montage.

2 and 15, even the focal emphasis. The voltage spread and polarity are not readily appreciated.

Figure 5 incorporates a more orthodox procedure. Each derivation is in the usual anterior-posterior (A/P) arrangement, and each electrode is connected to an immediately adjacent lead. Nonetheless, the lack of any systematic arrangement makes it very difficult to utilize phase reversal for localization.

Although the activity in Figs. 3, 4, and 5 is genuine, it would be difficult to write a definitive report of findings based on these samples. With only these three montages, it would be awkward to show the abnormality to the interested referring pediatric neurologist. If used to illustrate a case report, a journal editor would be justified in suggesting more intelligible figures. As lantern slides at a meeting, they would be a catastrophe.

The identical derivations of Fig. 5 are rearranged and shown in Fig. 6 in a logical montage. Indeed, this is *the* logical and *the* sensible arrangement for such derivations in a 16-channel display. Phase reversal and polarity are unambiguous. The degree of spread into the adjacent right temporal and contralateral frontocentral is immediately apparent. The montage is thus superior to the version that looks first at the parasagittal distribution on channels 1 to 8, and the temporal distribution through channels 9 to 16.

Finally, the data from the reference recording of Fig. 4 are rearranged and shown in Fig. 7 in a montage which is easier to grasp. The ipsilateral ear lead is always on the second grid, and the sequence is systematically left/right. Again, the principle of homotopic adjacent electrodes in close channel proximity is utilized. This is superior to a system with capricious separation of head regions widely in the 16 channels of recording.

The preceding progression from idiosyncratic 8-channel montages, to awkward 16-channel displays, to logical and easy-to-understand and easy-to-learn montages, illustrates the progression from difficult to easy EEG. The increasing availability of 18-channel equipment further increases the capacity for logical and complete coverage of the head. Thus, the montage of Fig. 6 on 16 channels is expanded to include the often neglected midline placements with 18 channels (Fig. 8). The logical place for these is in channels 9 and 10, as shown, not added on in channels 17 and 18.

Before we deal with the important matter of the appropriate montage for individual problems further comment about other montage principles is in order. The situation is needlessly complicated when a diversity of grid I inputs is employed for different reference montages. As indicated from the data sheet montage summation (Figs. 15 and 16), the first grids are largely the same for all reference systems. All personnel benefit from this. Minor modification is necessary with 18 channels. For ear reference it is simpler to preserve the basic 16-channel array, and use channels 17 and 18 for FZ and PZ to A2. It is understood that CZ would be substituted for either FZ or PZ as appropriate. For CZ reference the ears are used as grid I inputs to channels 17 and 18. The same principles apply when using average, chin, or low neck reference.

There has been prolonged and quite needless controversy regarding the preferential right/left or left/right montage display. In 1957 a committee of the International Federation (eight of 11 being Europeans) recommended a right/left (R/L) sequence. In general, European laboratories follow this custom. With numerous exceptions, others do not. The committee of the American EEG Society that formulated the Guidelines for Technique (No. 2) (see Chapter 2 and Appendix) found that the majority of laboratories in North America favored a left/right (L/R) sequence. The first EEG figures in Volume I #1 of the *EEG Journal* used a L/R display. In truth, it matters little. We are, by and large, an overwhelming L/R culture as reflected in our writing and our printed pages. Similarly, the A/P sequence seems more natural. Thus the basic display of Fig. 8 falls easily

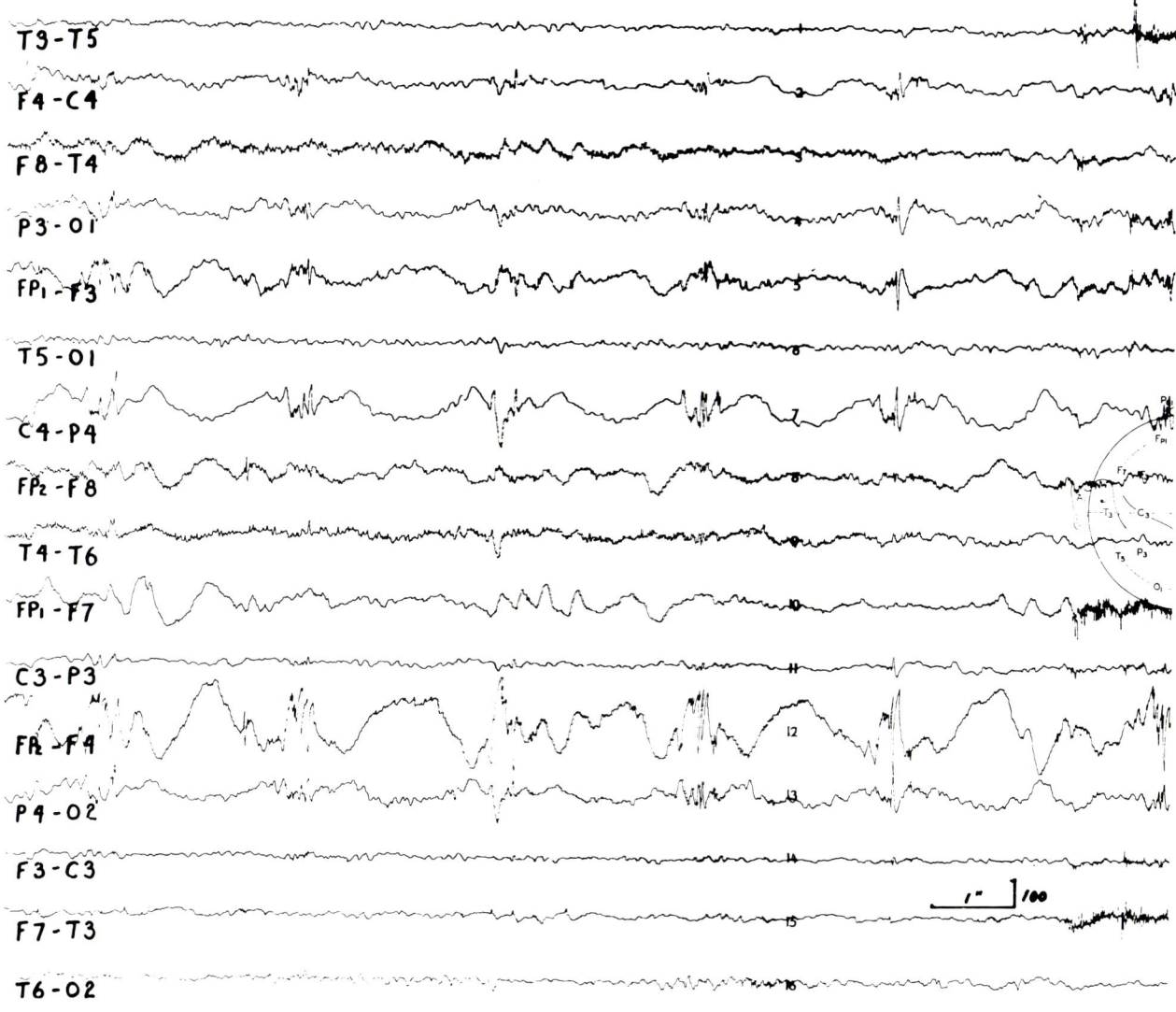

FIG. 5. EEG from same patient as Figs. 3 and 4, recorded with scrambled nonsequential bipolar derivations.

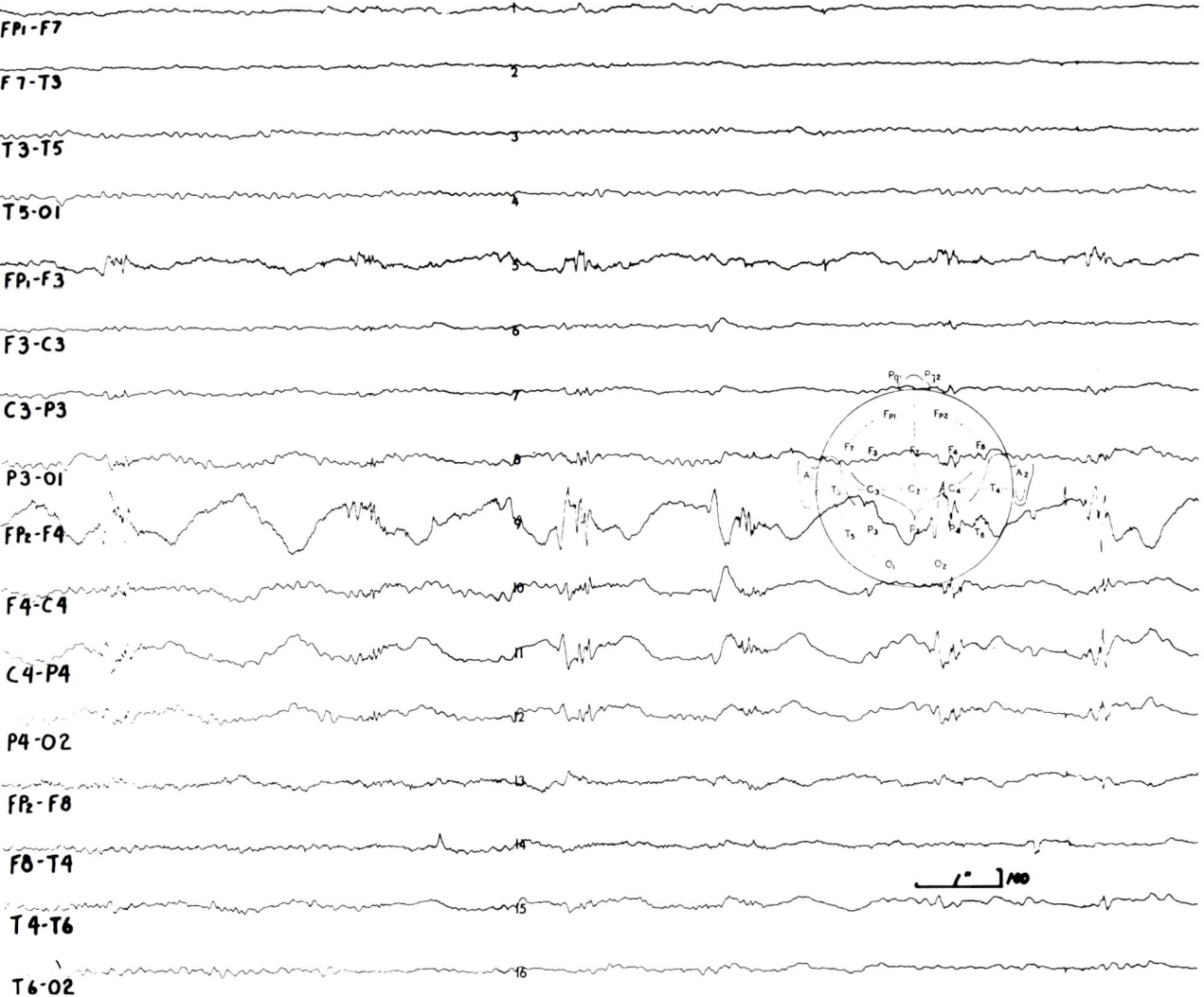

FIG. 6. EEG from same patient as Figs. 3, 4, and 5, recorded with simple logical bipolar chain sequence.

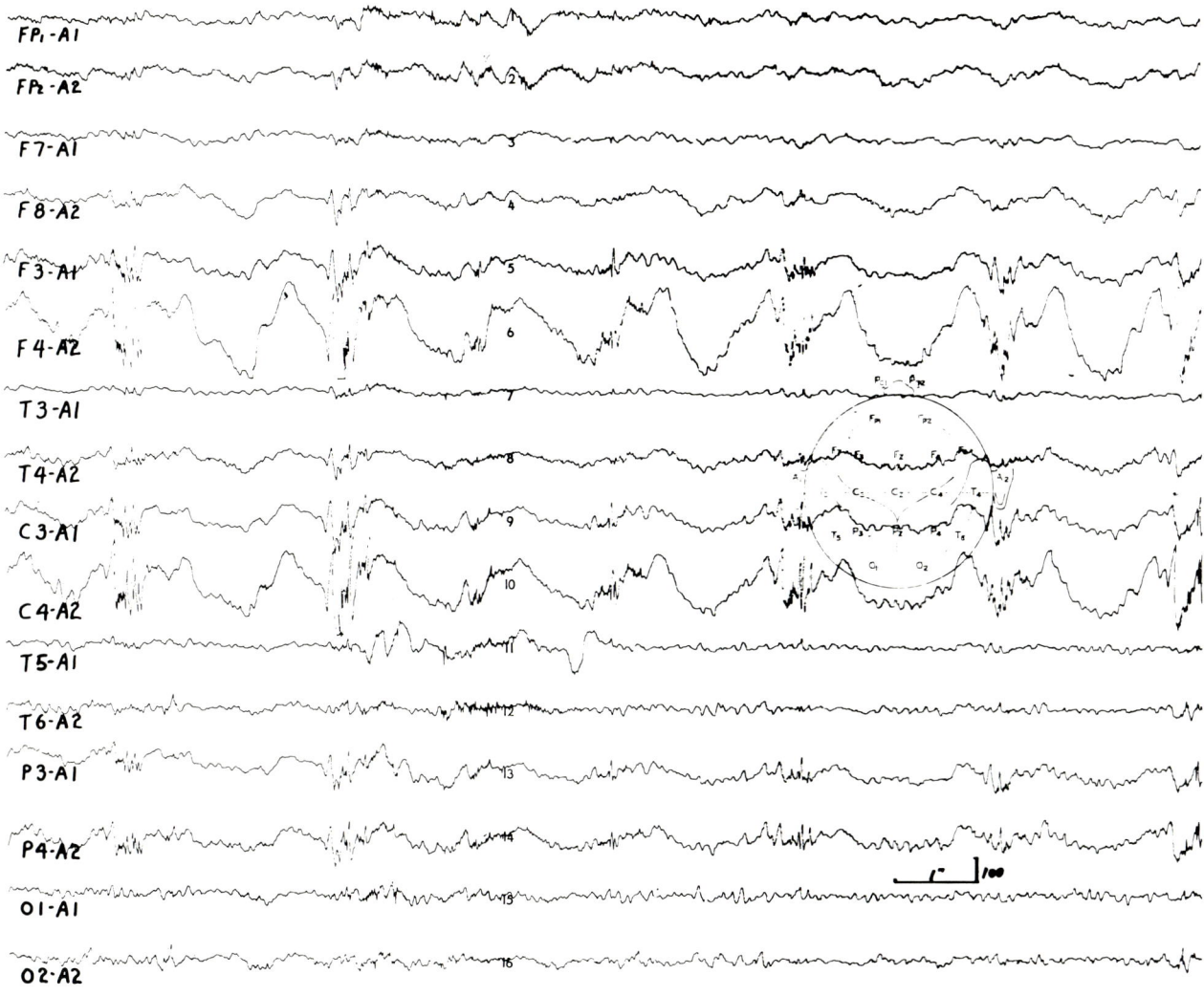

FIG. 7. Same patient as Figs. 3–6, recorded with simple logical ear reference montage.

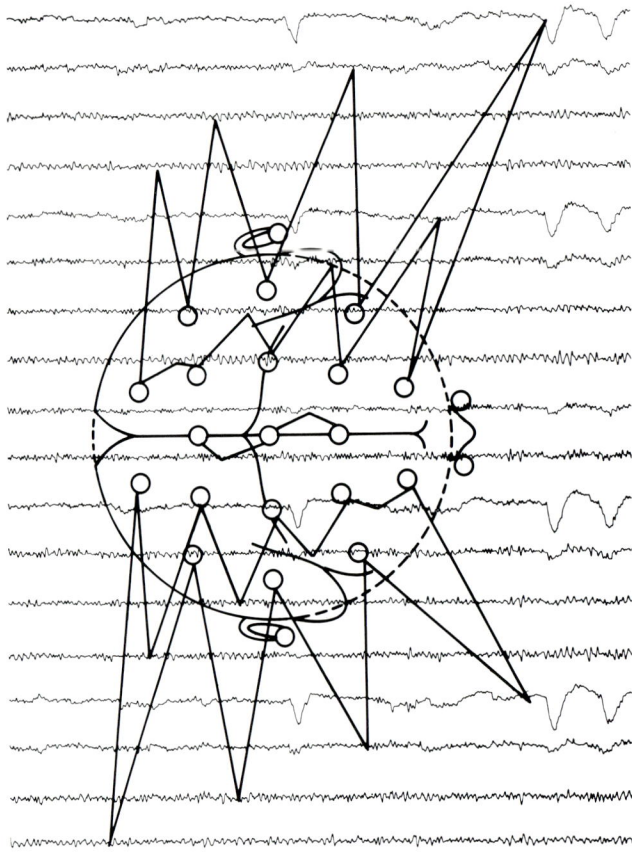

FIG. 8. The 16-channel montage of Fig. 6 as expanded to 18 channels. The montage is the same as montage A seen in Fig. 16.

into place as the head diagram is turned through 90 degrees, with nose to the right. The upper channels survey the left lateral regions, the medial channels sweep the left, the midline and then the right parasagittal distribution, and close with the right lateral display at the bottom.

The value of such a basic scan or survey run, involving nearly all electrodes, is largely lost, particularly with 16 or 18 channels, when the sequential block linkage system is not used. Although there is advantage in immediate juxtaposition of homologous derivations, for example, Fp1–F7, Fp2–F8 . . . C3–P3, C4–P4 . . . etc., etc., with practice one can readily make such comparisons with the degree of channel separation in the A montage (see Figs. 15 and 16). Because this largely involves close scrutiny of background fast activity, most important for parasagittal regions, an opportunity to see this is offered by the bottom 6 channels of montage C (Fig. 9). Intruding channels, of course, yield a considerable (though not impossible) complication in the evaluation of polymorphic, very slow activity. As a sign of a destructive lesion, this is usually lateralized, or relatively focal. Hence, the easy comparison of medial and lateral regions of the *same* hemisphere, including midline spread, is sometimes more important than easy comparison of left and right sides.

Abnormalities involving frontal and occipital polar emphasis, especially when shifting or partially lateralized, may require a display that includes transverse derivations. This is readily accomplished with 16 or 18 channels (Fig. 9). Many laboratories use some variation of the sequence shown in channels 1 to 10 (Fig. 9C) often starting with Fp1–F7 on channel 1 and completing the circle with Fp2–Fp1 on channel 10. Since statistically, the left frontotemporal is the most common region of abnormality, it is more useful to start the sequence elsewhere. The arrangement in (Fig. 9C) preserves the frontotemporal sequence in an unbroken chain. The competent technologist will alter as needed to preserve the posterior sequence, often

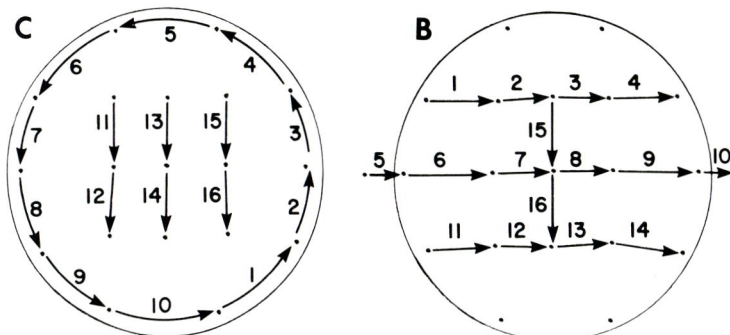

FIG. 9. Sketched montages such as these seen here are more quickly comprehended than when the derivations are written out. (Montages B and C can be found in their written form in Fig. 15.)

desirable with children. The shorter parasagittal midline cuts, which again the resourceful technologist will adjust to more frontal or occipital coverage as appropriate, serves to identify the degree of spread. As noted, this montage is also useful for convenient evaluation of background activity through the frontal, central, and parietal regions, all closely grouped into 6 adjacent channels, 11 to 16. With 18 channels there is an ear-ear sample, as well as a chest-ear EKG monitor, the latter well worth sampling on *every* patient.

Another transverse montage, crossing through the midline or Z electrode positions, is shown in Fig. 9B. Channels 15 and 16 tend to be redundant and are often changed to sample the frontal or occipital poles.

The preceding montages, with some variations, are in common use through many laboratories. With only minor concessions, and ignoring the basically unimportant L/R habit patterns, we could have communality of basic montages with resulting obvious benefits. The universal use of a few standard montages would in no way inhibit the remainder of the EEG examination. It would be appropriate to have an *ad hoc* committee prepared to report on this at the time of the next International EEG Congress.

An enduring interest in montages has resulted in some informal and quasi-experimental studies. The same patients have been recorded with a very wide variety of montage techniques, including some of those in Fig. 1. Sixteen or more channels permits the simultaneous use of the same electrodes in various combinations. For example, it is highly instructive to record 3-Hz spike-and-wave activity on the 18-channel montage designated K in Fig. 16. The simultaneous display of this familiar pattern in bipolar and reference recording demonstrates the superiority of the latter *for this specific problem*. In another example, the double electrode distance derivations of the J montage (Fig. 16), useful for cerebral death studies, have not been very helpful for the detection of focal slow activity. This has taught us that the omission of the T5, T6, P3, P4, and Pz electrodes may result in missed focal abnormality, especially in children. We have preserved those montages that have been maximally useful for optimal visual display, not neglecting the ease with which these may be learned and understood by the tyro as well as the sophisticate in EEG, and we continue to change as needed. Thus, the overly complex F run (Fig. 16), an efficient trap for positive bursts, was found to be too restrictive and was modified, but the modification (Fx) in turn became a little-used montage.

There remain at least two basic problems, the first of which is inherent in preselected montages. The convenience and speed of selection plus the absolute absence of error make these montages an imperative choice for all laboratories. Each montage may be thought of as a sieve or trap, variably useful for the detection and optimal display of certain features of the EEG, both normal and abnormal. They are, or should be, designed for particular problems and hence not all are equally useful. In fact there are times when no preselected montage is adequate for rare, complex, multiple, and atypical abnormalities. The alert and knowledgeable technologist recognizes such unusual features, including problems posed by activation procedures. Appropriate selection, modification, and change is not just an option. It is an obligation.

A second and related problem is that none of the preceding more or less standard montages is effective in the display of certain temporal lobe abnormalities. Whether sharp and paroxysmal or slow, when these abnormalities are of low voltage with a broad field invading the ear, they may be very difficult to detect. The problem is compounded when they are, as happens not uncommonly, shifting or bilateral in distribution. They may occur unexpectedly and only in sleep, with no ready opportunity for nasopharyngeal or other additional leads.

We have evolved a system of sequential coronal triangular cuts through the temporals, illustrated in Fig. 10. These are vastly more effective with at least 16 channels. The montage is difficult to sketch in a two-dimensional flat plane, but easy to visualize in three dimensions. The wide and equal lead separation of this bipolar sequential closed chain gives increased recorded voltage (physiological amplification). The distribution of such values independently through anterior, mid- and posterior temporals, as well as from the ear, is easily determined. The instrumental phase reversal from a successive grid I–grid II overlap (FZ–F8, F8–F7, F7–FZ) multiplies the visual cues such that even low voltage spikes and their polarity are easily detected. Midline activity, especially in sleep, is readily identified and scarcely appears in the transtemporal linkage derivations. Perhaps even more important is the ease, and the confidence, with which even very slow activity of low voltage (0.3 Hz at 25 μV) may be seen. Some trace of EKG is generally present in the A2–A1 derivation in channel 16, often supplemented by an EKG monitor recorded independently. Finally, the rapid scan of such a recording is very

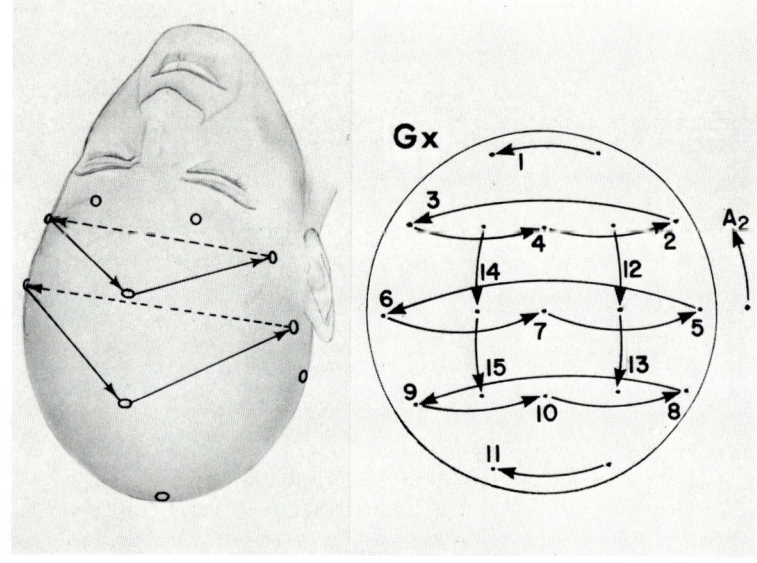

FIG. 10. Sequential triangle montage for detection of temporal lobe abnormality.

simple; channels are quickly grouped into sets of three, with easy orientation even with 18-channel display (Fig. 11).

The use of short distance derivations to yield small triangles for fine localization is fraught with danger. The misinterpretation comes from reliance on the point of phase reversal to indicate the focal abnormality. Figure 12 shows several simple 3-channel montages. In A the negative sharp discharges present no problem. In B the eye blink is emanating from Fp1, but activity that is equipotential at F7 and F3 could give a similar picture. What about the theta and rather ill-defined sharp transients from channels 2 and 3 in C?

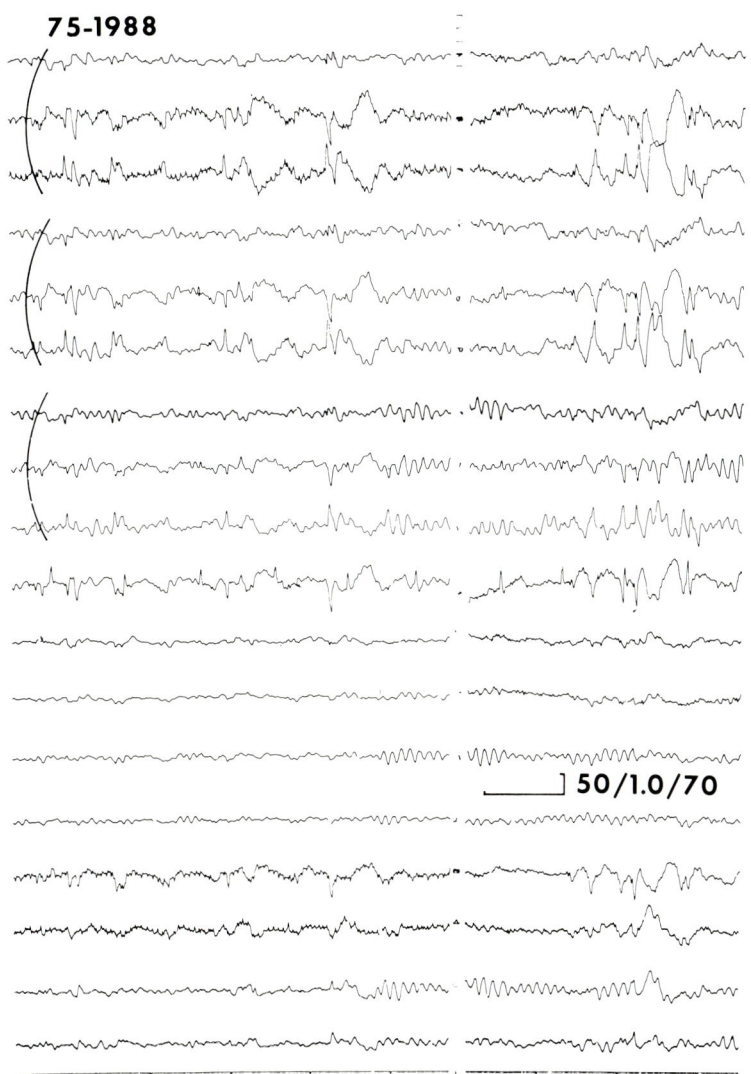

FIG. 11. Eighteen-channel EEG from 39-year-old patient with 3-year history of loss of contact with environment and olfactory hallucinations. (See montage I, Fig. 16.) The abnormality is so abundant that the traditional serial chain linkage through the temporals (lower 8 channels) is adequate. Note, however, the left margin where negative sharp waves are scarcely detectable except in the circular triangles, and the involvement of A1. Recorded voltage is lower, regional gradient is less clear, and overall complexity is reduced in the traditional montage.

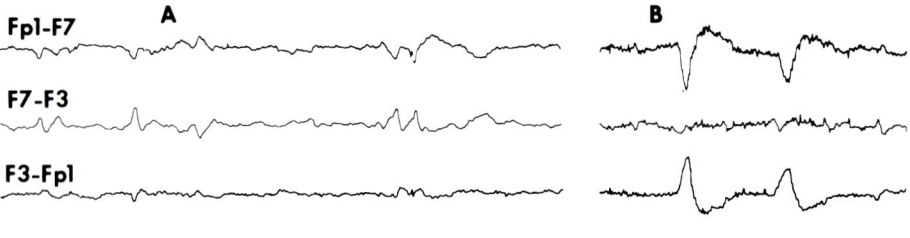

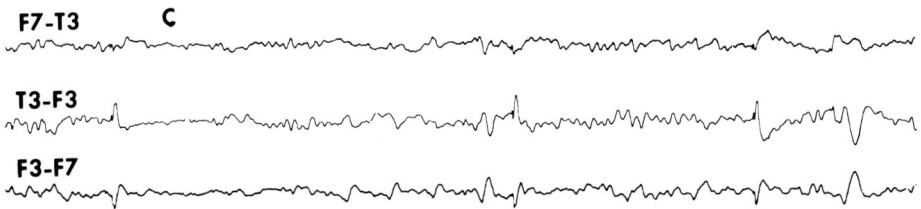

FIG. 12. Tiny triangle montages may yield false localization.

The phase reversal is mostly from F3, and if one disregards polarity, often explicably positive, F3 might be considered the focus. Much more often, however, the focus will be broadly F7 and T3, with near cancellation of abnormality.

This is even more likely to occur with slow activity shown in Fig. 13. On the left, the small triangle at the bottom localizes the delta activity to F3. Yet the serial parasagittal chain shows virtual absence of slow activity from F3. The top four channels indicate an unambiguous focus at F7 and T3, with the familiar cancellation of slow activity in the F7–T3 derivation. When either of these is run against an uninvolved lead, the delta is recorded along with the misleading phase reversal, due to the involved leads being on opposite grids.

The same phenomenon is illustrated on the right in Fig. 13. Again there is apparent localization to F3 in the bottom three channels, the false focus made more plausible from the instrumental phase reversal. These same three leads seen against the distant A2 reference prove the F7 and T3 focus with minimal abnormality from F3. The superiority of the coronal triangle montage is demonstrated in the upper six channels. The higher voltage slow activity is even more clearly disclosed, maximal at F7.

These simple montage experiments are recommended as supplements to the usual lecture-and-record-reading teaching sessions. They are also beneficial to the technologist who thereby learns practical aspects of principles of localization. They help to counteract the static and stereotyped approach to EEG, so comforting to the beginner and so reassuring to the senior EEGer. The leavening of doubt and skepticism is important for all levels of EEG.

There are, in fact, occasions when even the generally useful and reliable circular triangle display may lead to error (Fig. 14). Thus,

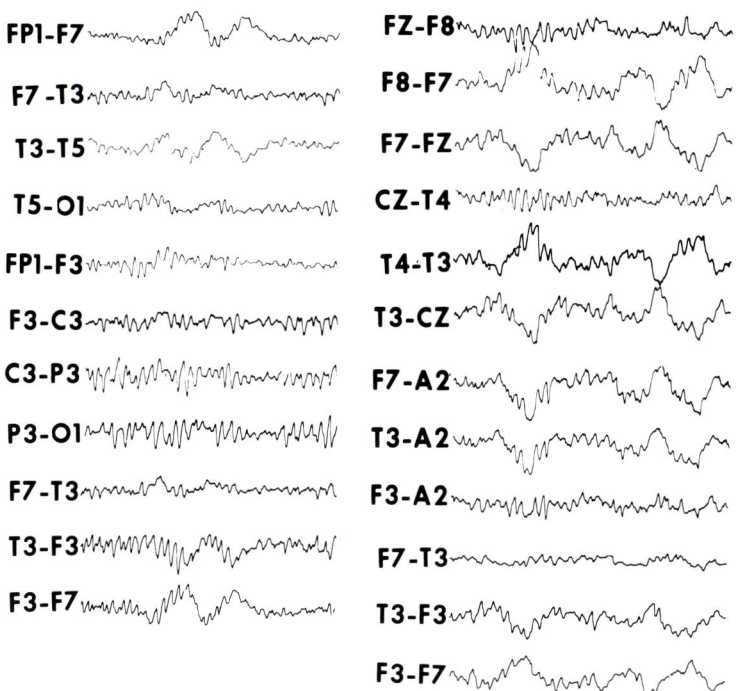

FIG. 13. The small triangle montage in the lower three channels of each tracing yields false localization to F3.

a right frontotemporal destructive lesion that involves, even somewhat unequally, F8 and F4 would tend to show less abnormality in the FZ–F8 derivation. FZ, also in the field, would be more active than F7, as would F8. The result would be out-of-phase abnormality *apparently* from the uninvolved F7 electrode. Although there will be helpful inconsistencies in other channels (note the right temporal negative spike) which should alert one to this possibility, the simplest solution is to simultaneously monitor the activity from the parasagittal regions. Preselected arrangements generally useful for this are shown in Gx (16-channel) (Figs. 14 and 15), and H (18-channel) (Fig. 16). Again, the supplementary coverage is adjusted for anterior or posterior regions as may be needed.

This discussion of montages would be incomplete without yet another attempt to lay to rest the twin ghosts of monopolar recording and the inactive reference electrode. Monopolar recording in EEG is a literal impossibility; amplifiers have two inputs. It is now rare to find a true believer in the (fictitious) inactive ear. Nevertheless the very word monopolar encourages a faith that the input to grid I is somehow more important than the input to grid II. The latter is very often not even specified. This overwhelming emphasis on grid I is responsible for much of the persisting confusion about polarity: upward pen deflection is interpreted as negative, downward as positive. This is true (see Chapter 2) *only* for events on grid I. Even the most famous monopolarists made this misinterpretation. Thus, it was not correct in 1948 (Gibbs et al., 6) nor later when reiterated in the Atlas (Gibbs and Gibbs, 7) to describe psychomotor (temporal lobe) spiking as negative in the temporal region and positive in all other regions of the head. The active ear was acknowledged but its responsibility for the apparent diffuse "positive" (actually negative) discharge was not understood. Nor are the statements equivalent that either the temporal region goes negative or the rest of the brain goes positive. In this instance it is only the temporal region that has the negative spike; the rest of the body is not involved. This same preoccupation with grid I led to a similar error in the interpretation of positive spikes with "reversed polarity" in the nasopharyngeal leads (7). Again, it is a case of grid II (the ear) being the source of the discharge; the polarity remains positive and the spikes are not present in the nasopharyngeal leads.

One might elect to study a posterior spike-wave discharge using

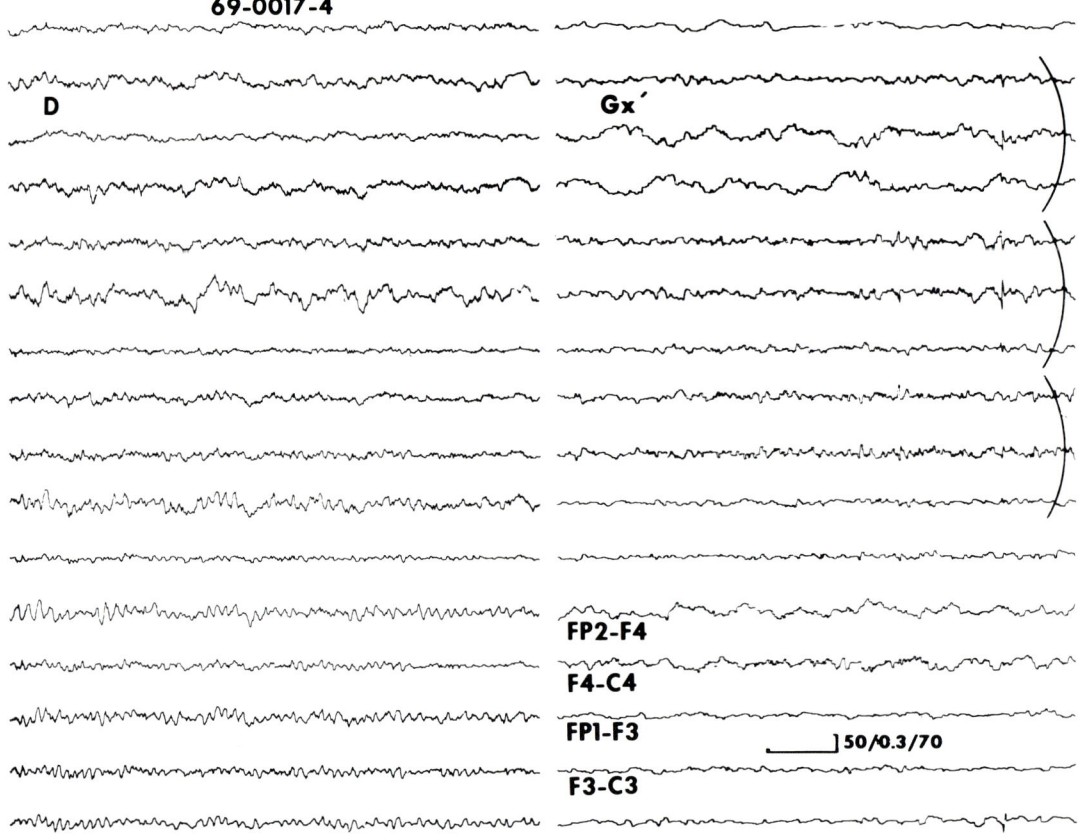

FIG. 14. False lateralization from circular triangle montage *(segment on right)* resulting from widespread frontotemporal slow activity (derivations for upper 12 channels as in Galt montage, Fig. 15). Correct lateralization is proven in channels 12 to 15 *(segment on right)* and by reference recording *(segment on left,* see run D, Fig. 15).

the distant frontal lead as a reference. With eye opening, this grid II reference would inject the characteristic negative potential as a downgoing pen deflection in all channels. It would be incorrect to say the events were caused by the rest of the brain being driven positive by the eye movement. The potential remains negative and is (largely) confined to the frontal leads.

A chest-to-ear derivation yields a clean QRS complex of several millivolts. An ear–chest derivation shows an identical pattern in mir-

EEG # ______ Name ______

Date ______ Age ______ Sex ______ Hand ______ Food ______

Time ______ Room # ______ CC # ______

Model ______ Ref. Dr. ______

INTERNATIONAL ELECTRODE PLACEMENT

MONTAGES

A	B	C	D	E	F	Falt	G	Galt
Fp_1-F_7	F_7-F_3	O_2-T_6	Fp_1-A_1	Fp_1-Cz	T_3-A_2	T_3-A_2	$Fz-Fp_2$	Fp_2-Fp_1
F_7-T_3	F_3-Fz	T_6-T_4	Fp_2-A_2	Fp_2-Cz	T_5-A_2	T_5-A_2	Fp_2-Fp_1	$Fz-F_8$
T_3-T_5	$Fz-F_4$	T_4-F_8	F_7-A_1	F_7-Cz	T_5-A_1	T_5-A_1	Fp_1-Fz	F_8-F_7
T_5-O_1	F_4-F_8	F_8-Fp_2	F_8-A_2	F_8-Cz	T_5-Cz	T_5-Cz	$Fz-F_8$	F_7-Fz
Fp_1-F_3	A_1-T_3	Fp_2-Fp_1	F_3-A_1	F_3-Cz	O_1-A_2	O_1-A_2	F_8-F_7	$Cz-T_4$
F_3-C_3	T_3-C_3	Fp_1-F_7	F_4-A_2	F_4-Cz	T_4-A_1	T_4-A_1	F_7-Fz	T_4-T_3
C_3-P_3	C_3-Cz	F_7-T_3	T_3-A_1	T_3-Cz	T_6-A_1	T_6-A_1	$Cz-T_4$	T_3-Cz
P_3-O_1	$Cz-C_4$	T_3-T_5	T_4-A_2	T_4-Cz	T_6-A_2	T_6-A_2	T_4-T_3	$Pz-T_6$
Fp_2-F_4	C_4-T_4	T_5-O_1	C_3-A_1	C_3-Cz	T_6-Cz	T_6-Cz	T_3-Cz	T_6-T_5
F_4-C_4	T_4-A_2	O_1-O_2	C_4-A_2	C_4-Cz	O_2-A_1	O_2-A_1	$Pz-T_6$	T_5-Pz
C_4-P_4	T_5-P_3	F_3-C_3	T_5-A_1	T_5-Cz	T_3-T_5	Fp_1-F_3	T_6-T_5	O_2-O_1
P_4-O_2	P_3-Pz	C_3-P_3	T_6-A_2	T_6-Cz	T_5-O_1	F_3-C_3	T_5-Pz	F_4-C_4
Fp_2-F_8	$Pz-P_4$	$Fz-Cz$	P_3-A_1	P_3-Cz	T_4-T_6	C_3-P_3	$Pz-O_2$	C_4-P_4
F_8-T_4	P_4-T_6	$Cz-Pz$	P_4-A_2	P_4-Cz	T_6-O_2	Fp_2-F_4	O_2-O_1	F_3-C_3
T_4-T_6	$Fz-Cz$	F_4-C_4	O_1-A_1	O_1-Cz	T_5-T_6	F_4-C_4	O_1-Pz	C_3-P_3
T_6-O_2	$Cz-Pz$	C_4-P_4	O_2-A_2	O_2-Cz	A_1-A_2	C_4-P_4	A_2-A_1	A_2-A_1

Remarks:

Cooperation:

Drowsy ______

Sleep ______

Sedation ______

HV ______

PS ______

Other ______

Medication ______

Previous EEG ______

Last seizure ______

Probable DX ______

Rating N ______ Technician ______

FIG. 15. Basic data sheet which identifies all preselected 16-channel montages and helps insure availability of clinical and EEG data.

ror image; the polarity and source do not change. The QRS does not arise in the ear, and it is not helpful to conceptualize the EKG in terms of electrical events in the lobe of the ear.

Take another example—the case of reference recording to joined leads on both ears. A bad lead on either ear will show an identical artifact on all channels. It is nonsense to describe this phenomenon as the brain being driven in opposite polarity to the ear artifact. There is no change in the brain; the artifact is restricted to its point of origin.

A delta focus at T3, as may occur with a neoplasm, usually spreads to involve A1. Ipsilateral ear reference recording will show delta activity widely in the channels recording from the left hemisphere. Recording to joined ears will show the delta activity in all channels. In these cases the lowest voltage will be in the T3–A1 or T3–A1 + A2 derivation. What would the neurosurgeon do with a report that relative to the left temporal the rest of the brain shows higher voltage diffuse delta activity? The delta activity is not diffuse; the surgeon needs to know that the delta activity is left temporal.

We have considered the problems of reference recording in some detail. Although these are not unique to this technique, misinterpreta-

A	B	C	D	E	F	G	H	I	J	K
Fp1-F7	F7-F3	O2-T6	Fp1-A1	Fp1-Cz	F7-A2	Fz-Fp2	Fp2-Fp1	Fz-F8	Fp1-T3	Fp1-F3
F7-T3	F3-Fz	T6-T4	Fp2-A2	Fp2-Cz	T3-A2	Fp2-Fp1	Fz-F8	F8-F7	T3-O1	F3-C3
T3-T5	Fz-F4	T4-F8	F7-A1	F7-Cz	T5-A2	Fp1-Fz	F8-F7	F7-Fz	F7-T5	C3-P3
T5-O1	F4-F8	F8-Fp2	F8-A2	F8-Cz	Fz-F8	F7-Fz	F7-Fz	Cz-T4	Fp1-C3	P3-O1
Fp1-F3	A1-T3	Fp2-Fp1	F3-A1	F3-Cz	T5-Cz	F8-F7	Cz-T4	T4-T3	C3-O1	Fp2-F4
F3-C3	T3-C3	Fp1-F7	F4-A2	F4-Cz	O1-A2	F7-Fz	T4-T3	T3-Cz	F3-P3	F4-C4
C3-P3	C3-Cz	F7-T3	T3-A1	T3-Cz	F8-A1	Cz-T4	T3-Cz	Pz-T6	Fz-Pz	C4-P4
P3-O1	Cz-C4	T3-T5	T4-A2	T4-Cz	T4-A1	T4-T3	Pz-T6	T6-T5	Fp2-C4	P4-O2
Fz-Cz	C4-T4	T5-O1	C3-A1	C3-Cz	T6-A1	T3-Cz	T6-T5	T5-Pz	C4-O2	Fp1-A1
Cz-Pz	T4-A2	O1-O2	C4-A2	C4-Cz	T6-A2	Cz-T4	T5-Pz	A2-A1	F4-P4	Fp2-A2
Fp2-F4	T5-P3	F3-C3	T5-A1	T5-Cz	T6-Cz	A2-A1	O2-O1	Fp2-F8	Fp2-T4	F3-A1
F4-C4	P3-Pz	C3-P3	T6-A2	T6-Cz	O2-A1	A1-Cz	A2-A1	F8-T4	T4-O2	F4-A2
C4-P4	Pz-P4	Fz-Cz	P3-A1	P3-Cz	Fp1-F3	Pz-T6	F4-C4	T4-T6	F8-T6	C3-A1
P4-O2	P4-T6	Cz-Pz	P4-A2	P4-Cz	F3-C3	T6-T5	C4-P4	T6-O2	F7-Fz	C4-A2
Fp2-F8	Fz-Cz	F4-C4	O1-A1	O1-Cz	C3-P3	T5-Pz	P4-O2	Fp1-F7	Fz-F8	P3-A1
F8-T4	Cz-Pz	C4-P4	O2-A2	O2-Cz	Fp2-F4	Pz-O2	F3-C3	F7-T3	T5-Pz	P4-A2
T4-T6	Fp1-A1	A1-A2	Fz-A2	A1-Cz	F4-C4	O2-O1	C3-P3	T3-T5	Pz-T6	O1-A1
T6-O2	Fp2-A2	Pg1-A2	Pz-A2	A2-Cz	C4-P4	O1-Pz	P3-O1	T5-O1	A1-A2	O2-A2

FIG. 16. Eighteen-channel data for preselected montages.

tions have been ubiquitous. This is especially so for those trained on, and using only, this procedure. We must remember that our differential amplifiers are just that. They react to the difference in voltage between the two input grids. Almost never, in any system, is this voltage precisely equal in amount and phase, and the differences are ceaselessly changing on each grid. The experienced EEGer and technologist will be able to use and interpret any type of reference or bipolar technique. The protean features of the EEG should not be forced into a preconceived Procrustean bed. The discussion by Magnus (14) and especially Osselton (18,19) will be helpful. Even better is the extensive modern treatment of these and other problems in the *Handbook of EEG and Clinical Neurophysiology* (13).

Nevertheless, there is no substitute for personal experience. The montages given in this chapter, particularly those for 18 channels (Fig. 16), utilize all four "types" of study: short distance bipolar; long distance bipolar; common reference; and average reference. Furthermore, the apparent redundancy in runs I and K is deliberate to allow the *simultaneous* comparison of different techniques. The use of run I for subtle temporal lobe abnormality is instructive. As previously noted, run K discloses important variations in the morphology, voltage, and distribution of diffuse spike-and-wave activity. An extended experience with this approach has led us to agree with Fischgold et al. (in ref. 14): "There are no infallible methods; there are only men who believe themselves infallible." The matter was summarized succinctly by Osselton in 1964 (17) when he said, "Why look with one eye when two are available?" There are, in fact, few monocular EEG laboratories in 1978.

Despite the injunctions of the *Guidelines in EEG* (Appendix), the deplorable practice of cryptic EEG continues: montage identification only as run A, run #3, etc., with no further data. No better is the equally arcane procedure where derivations are given in symbols (as 1–3, 3–9, 9–7, etc.) with no data on electrode location. One solution is a stamp or map showing lead placement (Fig. 18). Stamps may be used to show each montage. Or, the technologist may write in the derivations for each channel of each montage.

However, stamps often tend to be unclear or smudged. The busy technologist, bored with endless repetition of writing or sketching montages, tends to scribble, and the notations are often unclear.

The useless work involved is perhaps tolerable with 8-channel, but not with 16- or more channel equipment. Consider the "bits" of information that must be transcribed. A simple parasagittal montage with the 10–20 system (FP1–F3, etc.) requires 32 bits. The addition of the needed data on sensitivity and filters, and perhaps time of day, yields some 40 to 50 bits per montage. If this is written only once for each of seven montages (a common number) and each montage is used only once, the technician still contributes 300 to 350 bits of make-work. The numbers resulting from five records per day, etc., and doubled for 16-channel units are appalling. Good technologists have better things to occupy their time.

A simple and inexpensive solution is the use of a basic data sheet (Fig. 15) which becomes a permanent part of each EEG. All montage ambiguity is eliminated. The technologist need only note montage modification and recording parameters. Records are readily interpreted even by those with no knowledge of English. Procedures and notations in use 20 years ago, or hence, will still be clear instead of cabalistic, not unimportant in the present legal climate. Pertinent clinical data, including medication, are incorporated into the record where they belong. In summary, electroencephalography is downgraded when these most elementary aspects of good laboratory practice are ignored. The solution is not only easy, but it saves technologist time and provides some degree of legal protection.[1]

INSTRUMENTAL CONTROLS

Virtually all modern electroencephalographs and even most of the very early units have four instrumental controls. A knowledge of their function and the ability to actively utilize them appropriately is necessary for the practice of high quality EEG examination. These controls involve sensitivity, high and low frequency filters, and paper speed. Although each is independent of the others, in combination they may be used to reveal—or to mask—EEG abnormality.

It is worth recalling that all of the electronic controls (sensitivity and filters) tend to *degrade* amplifier performance. Thus, the sensitivity control progressively reduces the inherent total gain of the system. The filter controls reduce the band width of the amplifier. For obvious reasons the electrical engineer uses a sine wave input for the determination of amplifier performance. The EEG is not composed of such waves, and for the most part we shall use the more complex actual EEG signals in this section.

The EEG technician trainee and the beginning EEGer are already familiar with instrumental controls on day 1 in the laboratory. The volume or the loudness (sensitivity) control on TV, radio, and phonograph systems has the precise function of that control on the EEG. Even the direction of turn, clockwise to increase, is identical. The bass and treble controls, present on even budget quality hi-fi equipment, are merely low and high frequency filters. And for the treble (high frequency) control, the direction of turn is again identical—clockwise for high frequency passage. What a paradox that this available experience is not more universally used in the EEG laboratory. Let us see what happens when these are neglected.

Sensitivity

All channels in Fig. 17 are made from the same P4–A2 derivation. As indicated, the sensitivity is decreased progressively from 7 to 150 μV/mm. The distorted morphology in the upper channels is familiar to all who read the EEG literature. There is severe overload at the "standard" sensitivity of 7 μV/mm as the pens are driven

---

[1] A Montage Symposium was held at the 1976 joint meeting of the American EEG Society and the American Society of EEG Technologists. The seven papers presented at that time have already been published in the March and June, 1977 issues of *Am. J. EEG Technol.* They are required reading for all workers in EEG.

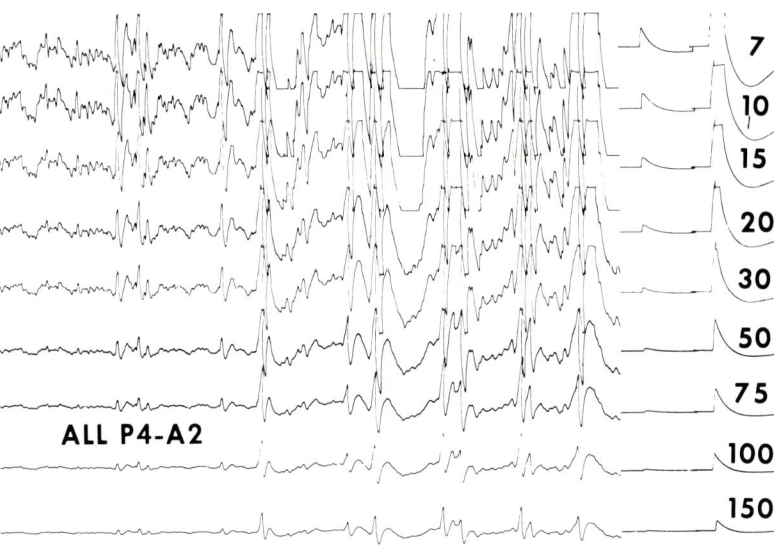

FIG. 17. "High voltage" paroxysmal discharge from P4–A2 recorded at various different sensitivity settings as indicated at the right. The first calibration signal is 50 μV, useless for channels with low sensitivity. The second calibration signal is 500 μV, useless at higher gain but necessary for adequate calibration at a sensitivity (S) of 75 or 100. Thus, the value of the calibration voltage should be in the range of the EEG signals obtained in that record.

beyond their linearity, with confusing overlap of tracing between channels. Adequate recording of such discharges, which may exceed 1.5 mV, needs a sensitivity of about 75 μV/mm. This allows a confident assessment of voltage and wave form and laterality difference. It is perfectly true that background rapid activity is not detectable at such sensitivity; this is no problem. Previous and subsequent recording at higher sensitivity establishes any differences; on occasion, simultaneous recording of derivations at different sensitivities may be useful.

Although voltage is actually the easiest parameter to measure, it is rare to find numeric values in EEG reports. This despite the fact that it is an economy of words to state "250 μV" rather than "moderate to high voltage." Voltage, which is not the same as amplitude, may be an important feature in serial studies of patients with destructive central nervous system disease and in patients with epilepsy. A qualitative estimate of changes would be possible if all studies were made in the same laboratory; this would not be possible for records made in different laboratories, hence the need for numbers.

A brief description of sensitivity determination may be helpful.[2] This is not necessarily the number indicated on the index dial. Vacuum tubes gradually lose efficiency, and after some years an initial 7-mm pen deflection to a 50 μV signal may have dropped to 6- or even 5-mm. Since sensitivity is the number resulting from the microvolt input divided by the pen deflection in millimeters, this could be changed from 7.1 to 8.2 or 10.0 μV/mm. Furthermore, this substantial *decrease* in sensitivity is unequal on all channels. The hazards and errors resulting from inaccuracies may be easily eliminated by readjustment of an equalizer control. Another aspect of calibration is discussed in the section dealing with electrocerebral silence.

Figure 18 is another example of the need for sensitivity control. This diffuse spike-and-wave discharge is initially displayed at sensitivity (S) 20 (or minus 3 on the all channel control of the Grass Model 6). The next section is recorded at an appropriate sensitivity of 75 μV/mm, or one-tenth of the standard sensitivity. The overlay represents the theoretical size of a single spike-wave complex from the frontal regions (ear reference) at the standard sensitivity of 7 μV/mm. No pen writing units can do this. It would be possible with an ink jet system, but the pens would require 7 to 8 inch spacing. The sheer bulk of equipment and very wide paper (5 feet for 8 channels) make this quite impractical. The easy solution is sensitivity control, a familiar principle to all who use audio (for loudness) and visual (for size) equipment. Some very old electroencephalographs had a nonlinear pen excursion. Thus, sensitivity might be, for example, at 10 μV/mm near the baseline and at some unknown, but much lower, sensitivity near the limits of pen excursion. The use of "compression amplifiers" to avoid gain control is now rare.

It is not uncommon for spike-wave paroxysms to exceed 1 mV and we have recorded other discharges well in excess of 2 mV. Nevertheless, there is more to sensitivity control than reduction of amplification. Equally important are the patients with such low voltage that little activity is detectable, and laterality differences not determinable, at S7. In Fig. 19 at S7, there are only uncertain laterality differences. At S3 (Fig. 20), a polymorphic slow pattern is detectable from the right frontal region at less than 25 μV. Fast activity is ill-defined on either side but relatively reduced on the right. The record on this patient seen for depression versus brain tumor, neurologically negative, was correctly interpreted as consistent with a destructive right frontal process; this was a glioblastoma grade IV.

There are occasions when a combination of pharmacological and EEG techniques are required to achieve a useful recording. The bedside tracing in Fig. 21 was made 3 days following a brainstem (pontine) infarct. Vertebral artery occlusion was demonstrated by angiography. EMI scan was negative. The EEG at S7 is virtually obliterated by EMG activity except for a possible periodic frontal slow transient. After 4 mg pancuronium bromide (Pavulon ®), which nearly eliminated the EMG artifact, the record at S2 allows confident identification of a periodic sharp transient of about 30 μV (maximal in the frontal regions, remarkably independent between sides) and virtual absence of background activity.

Frequency Controls

The fact that these frequency controls have been described in such pejorative terms as "muscle filters" and "sway filters" is an index of how these controls are misunderstood. It reveals that they are regarded as ways of *removing* something from the EEG. Unfortunately, amplifiers are unable to discriminate between the activity

---

[2] We shall use the Grass Models 6 and 8 as the instrumental prototype. The principles are applicable to all brands of EEG equipment, and actual sensitivity and filter values have only minor differences among brands. The manufacturers' instruction manuals are explicit; these make good reading.

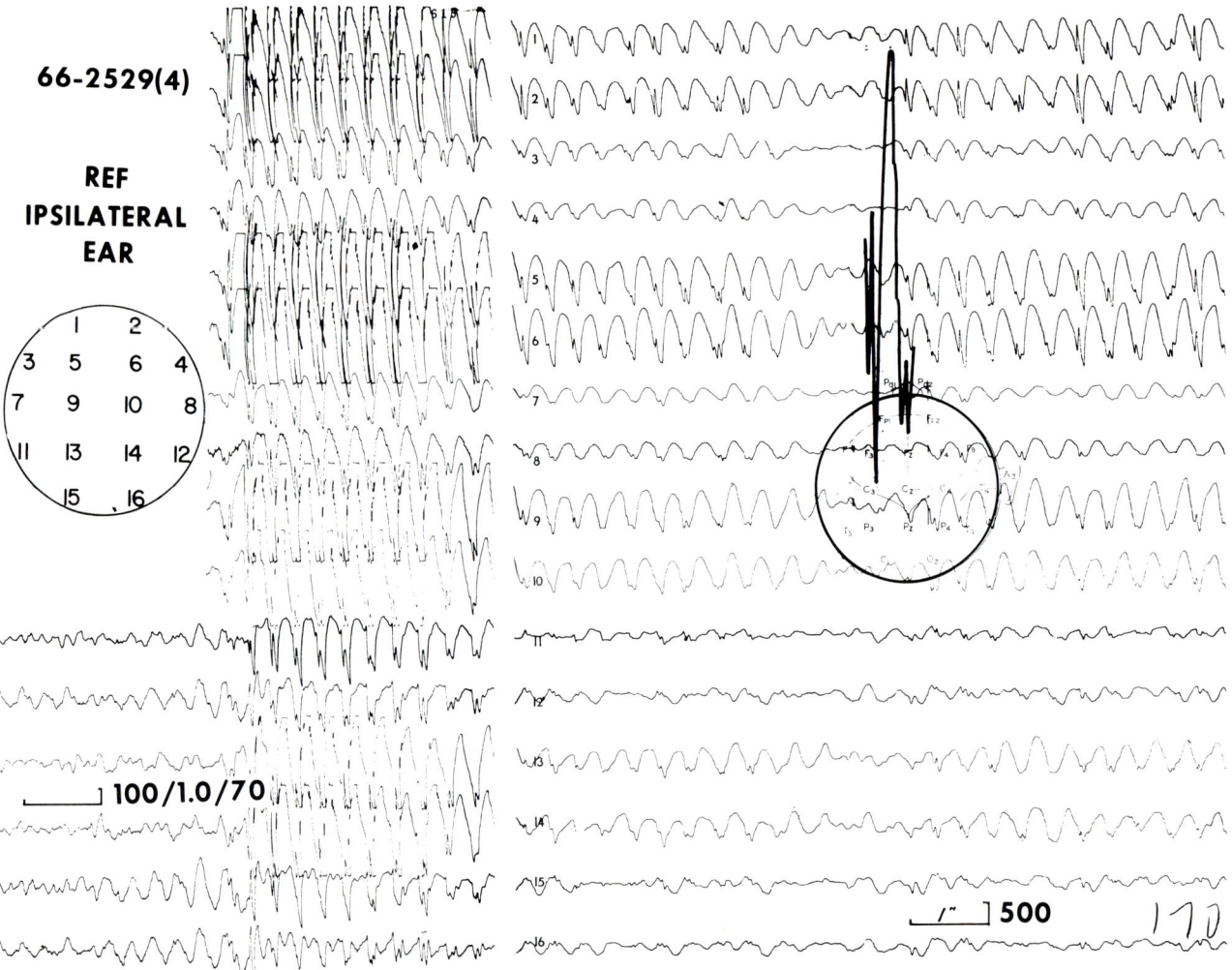

FIG. 18. Badly distorted spike-wave discharge even at S20; this is the sensitivity resulting from full use of the "emergency" gain control on the Grass Model 6, too often assumed to be the lowest sensitivity available. S75, obtained by use of the individual amplifier sensitivity controls, yields a better record.

of brain and muscle, or between delta and sweat activity. As with montages and sensitivity, such controls should be, and can be, used to *increase* the information made readily available.

Frequency response data are usually presented as in Fig. 22, but with a smoothed curve based on a limited number of point values. The data in this figure were derived as follows. Four Model 6 amplifiers were adjusted to yield identical 20-mm pen deflections at 10 Hz. On one channel controls were set with longest time constant and least high frequency (HF) filtering, and with no notch (60-Hz) filter in operation. The next channel had only notch filtering. The next had low frequency (LF) filter setting 1.0 and HF 35 filtering, and the last channel had a combination of LF 5.0 and HF 15. The 60–Hz filter was also used on these last two channels. Pen excursion was measured for a large number of frequencies between 0.1 and 100 Hz, and the values plotted as shown.

Such frequency response curves yield a precise index of the amplitude at which various frequencies are recorded at the different control settings. It is our experience that relatively few technologists and EEGers readily translate such curves into the effects on the EEG. The implication of filtering both ends of the frequency band to yield a "nice clean record" needs emphasis. Not even the alpha rhythm is recorded without some reduction, and the amplitude reduction is progressively severe for all activity on either side of this range.

High Frequency Filters

The effect of high frequency filtering on the actual EEG is shown in Fig. 23. The samples include both reference and bipolar-deriva-

FIG. 19. EEG from patient without neurological abnormality, referred for depression vs brain tumor. (See run A, Fig. 16, at S7.) Low voltage record with no convincing abnormality.

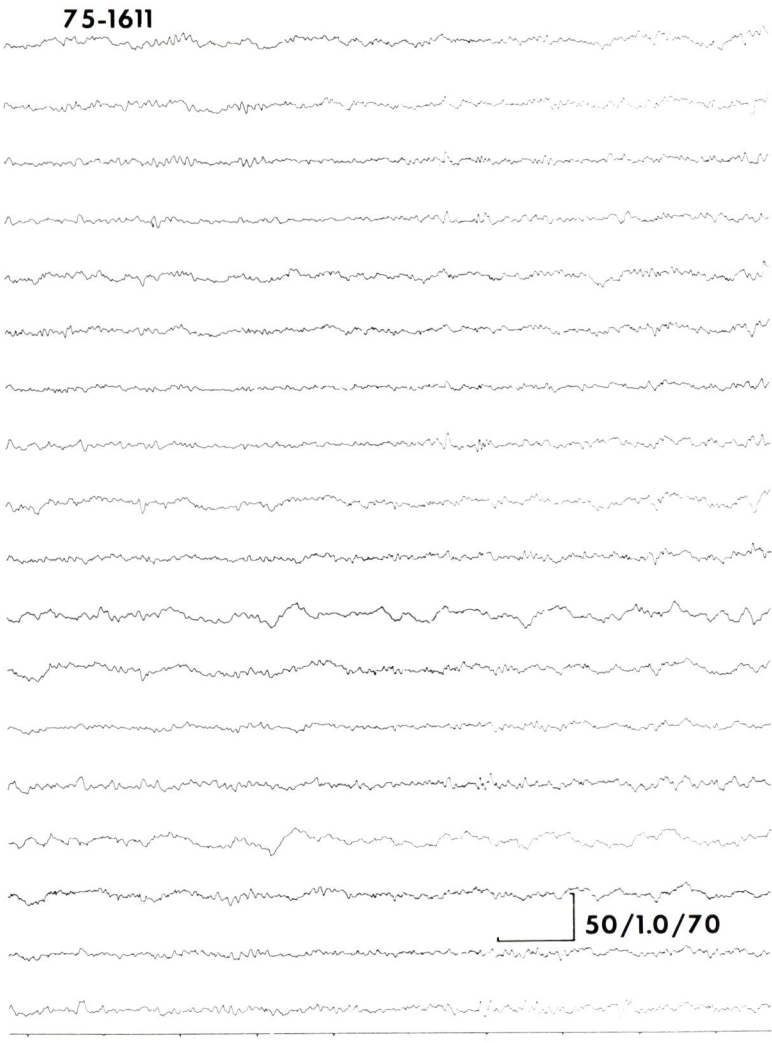

tions. They were recorded at three different high frequency filter settings as indicated, with the top channel (only) having the notch filter in use. The HF 70 setting records the spike of the spike-wave complex at 270 μV. This is reduced to 240 μV at HF 35 and 180 μV at HF 15, and the morphology of the discharge is altered. High frequency filtering, of course, does not affect the slow components; the slanted line indicates the change in amplitude of the spike relative to wave. The identified spike from F3–A1 is similarly reduced by filtering, including use of the notch filter.

The choice of such obvious and discrete phenomena as illustrated is dictated by didactic considerations. In practice lower voltage spikes and fast activity, already partially masked by other activity, may be even more effectively decreased by injudicious filtering. Indeed, *judicious* is the word that should govern the use of such controls. The "muscle filter" is the one first used, and too often overused, by the technologist. Competent EEGers should be able to read through records with some myogenic contamination, but the identification of myogenic activity may be very difficult when the EMG potentials are smoothed and distorted by filtering. Prevention by reassurance, and alleviation by relaxation of the patient, is a better way to go.

Low Frequency Filters

In marked contrast to high frequency filtering, this control is likely never to be used. Some laboratories even prefer equipment manufactured with the absence of such a filter! It could be argued that this

FIG. 20. EEG from same patient and with same montage as Fig. 19, but recorded at S3. This reveals polymorphic right frontal delta activity, less than 25 μV, with local relative reduction of very low voltage rapid background activity.

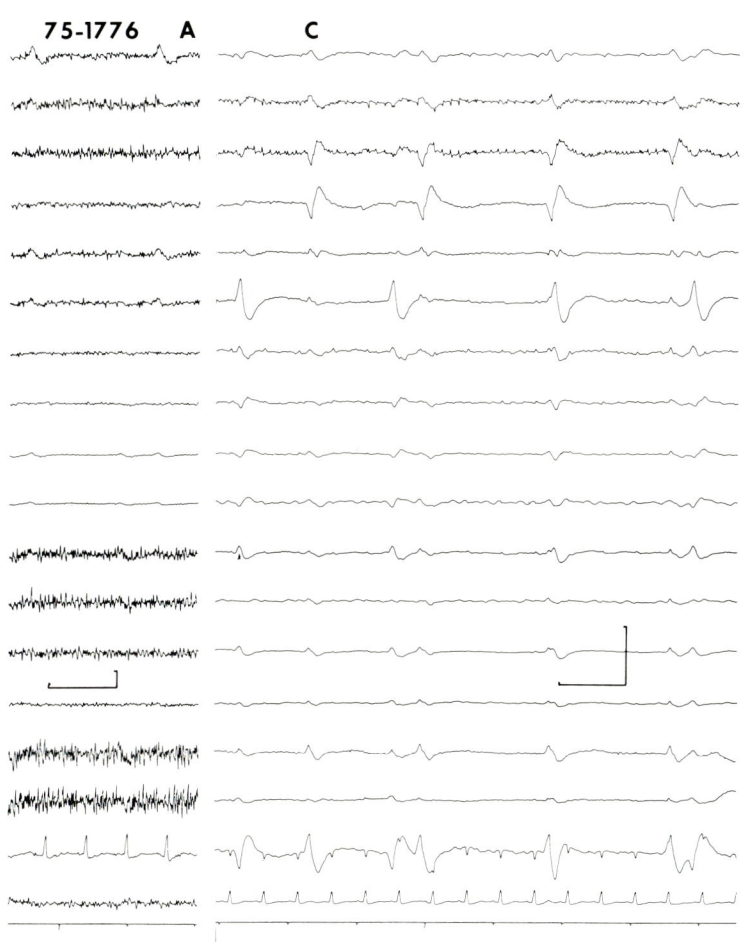

would at least prevent the misuse of low frequency filtering, which can have such a disastrous effect on slow activity. The penalty for its absence, or its non-use, is that very slow delta activity of destructive lesions may not be seen at all.

Figure 24 shows the same 4-channel montage in triplicate, each at S10 and HF 70. Delta activity is virtually absent in the lowest block recorded with LF 5.0. Much of it is detectable at the "standard" setting of LF 1.0. Nevertheless, the top four channels recorded at LF 0.3 show higher amplitude slow activity as well as slower delta components.

The difference in recorded activity at the standard and at the longer time constant settings is even more apparent in Fig. 25 because the activity is slower. The delta contribution is in the range of 0.3 Hz, and its true amplitude is not recordable even at LF 0.3. The same patient's tracing is shown in Fig. 26 recorded at slower (15 mm/sec) chart speed. This maneuver is of substantial assistance in the visualization of such very slow activity. It is not only simple to do, but saves on paper costs.

Again, the proper use of low frequency filter controls is to *add* something to the EEG by permitting inherent abnormality to be recorded. This is even easier to do with more modern equipment which has ganged controls on all channels and a more extended low frequency response.

These and other simple demonstrations of the importance of filter controls are readily carried out in any laboratory. For teaching purposes they are more effective than the rote learning of frequency-response curves and the definition of time constant. For indoc-

FIG. 21. EEG of patient with probable brainstem infarct 3 days earlier. Run A from Fig. 16 is shown at left, with S7 and severe electromyogram (EMG) contamination, showing trace of left frontal slow activity. At right, run C from Fig. 16 following 4 mg pancuronium bromide, and with S2, shows absence of normal physiological activity and independent 30-μV frontal periodic sharp transients.

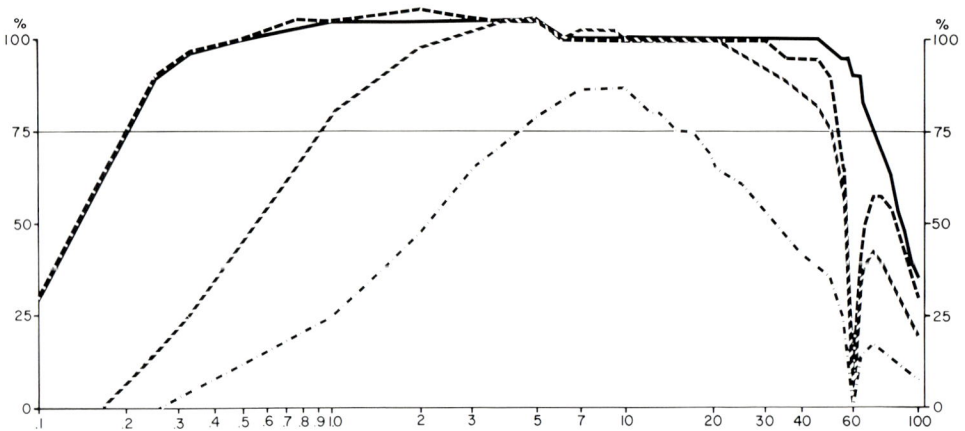

FIG. 22. Frequency response of four Grass Model 6 amplifiers with progressively restrictive filtering at each end of the scale. Not shown are the changes in the square wave calibration signals resulting from *simultaneous* high and low frequency filterings. It is recommended that readers carry out this simple exercise using their own gear. The resulting calibrations may be displayed, with benefit in the recording and record reading areas of the laboratory.

trination of good technique, they are better than pages of recommendations.

DETERMINATION OF ELECTROCEREBRAL INACTIVITY

This section heading represents a deliberate choice of words. It excludes consideration of quality of survival and what constitutes life or death. We shall consider only the problem of the presence or the absence of electrical activity from the brain.

Unfortunately, it is more difficult to prove the absence than the presence of anything. Failure to find may reflect searching in the wrong places or using the wrong tools. More powerful and different types of telescopes revealed unsuspected stars. The absence of virus particles cannot be proved by optical microscopy. The absence of EEG activity can *not* be determined with routine laboratory sensitivity of 7 μV/mm.

The inherent noise level of even well-maintained EEG gear is in the range of 1 to 2 μV, which sets the limit for the detection of cerebral activity. The term for the absence of such activity is electrocerebral inactivity or electrocerebral silence (ECS). The American EEG Society Guidelines for this determination are included in the Appendix. If these 12 recommendations are unfamiliar to the reader they should be reviewed. Comment on the evolution of some of these standards, and the degree to which they have been achieved, is appropriate.

The initial recommendation of a 1-hr recording with repeat study is analogous to the search for paroxysmal discharges in the suspected epileptic patient. Transient events may not appear in a brief examination. The 60-min search for any activity is a conservative measure. Increased experience suggests that a 30-min study, without technical complications, is probably adequate, being accepted as the minimal time in the 1976 revision of the above Guidelines. None of the 211 patients recorded at the Cleveland Clinic with ECS during the first

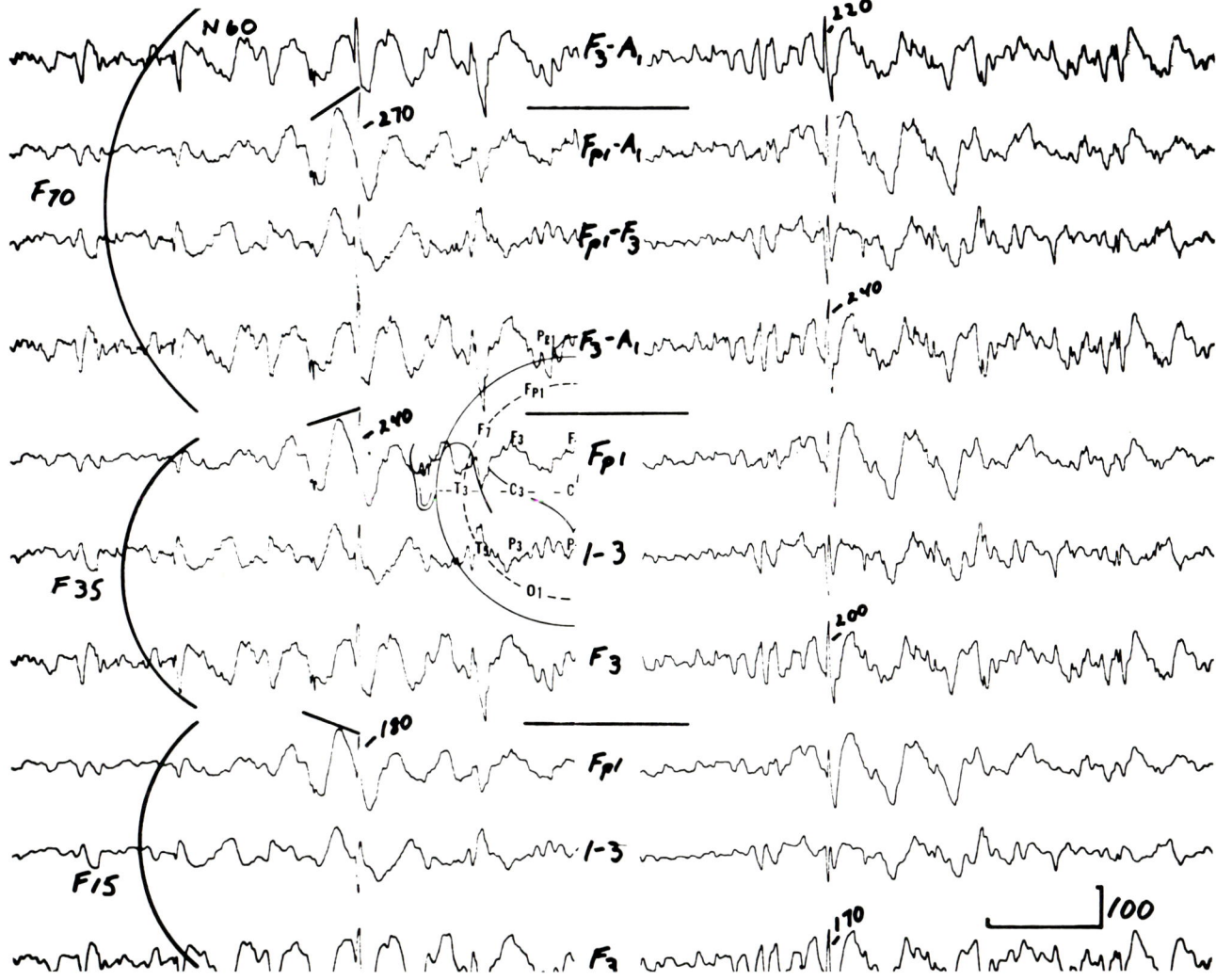

FIG. 23. The effect of high frequency filtering on spike activity. Montages are replicated at same sensitivity. Note progressive decrease in recorded voltages with increased HF filtering. Unretouched photographs may fail to reproduce the thin faint trace from very rapidly moving sharp pens.

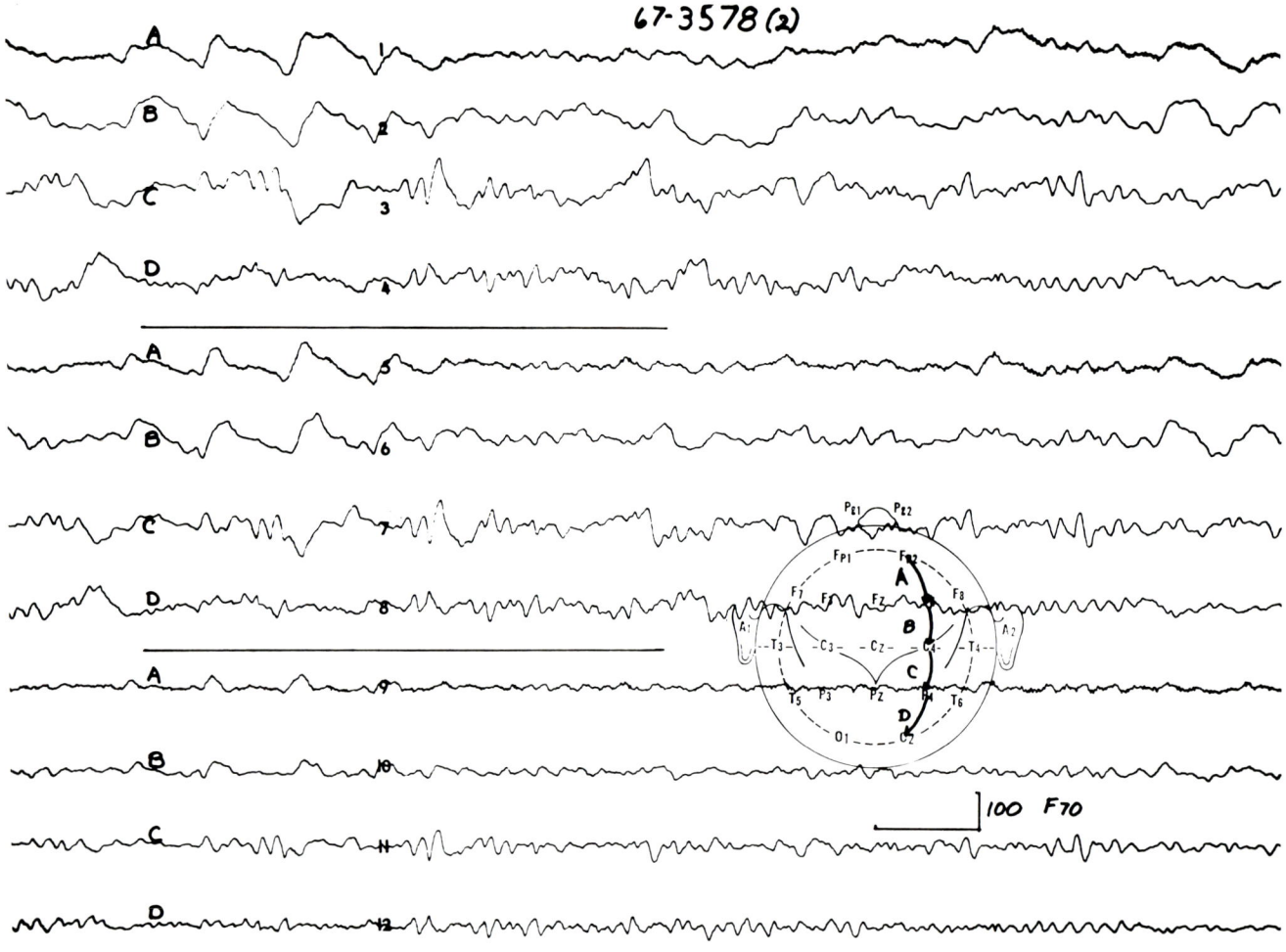

FIG. 24. Slow activity from right frontoparietal metastatic lesion. Right parasagittal serial chain montage in triplicate. The center bloc is made with the standard LF setting of 1.0. Slow activity is of higher voltage with better definition of slower delta components at LF 0.3 *(top four channels)*, and virtually absent at LF 5.0 *(bottom four channels)*.

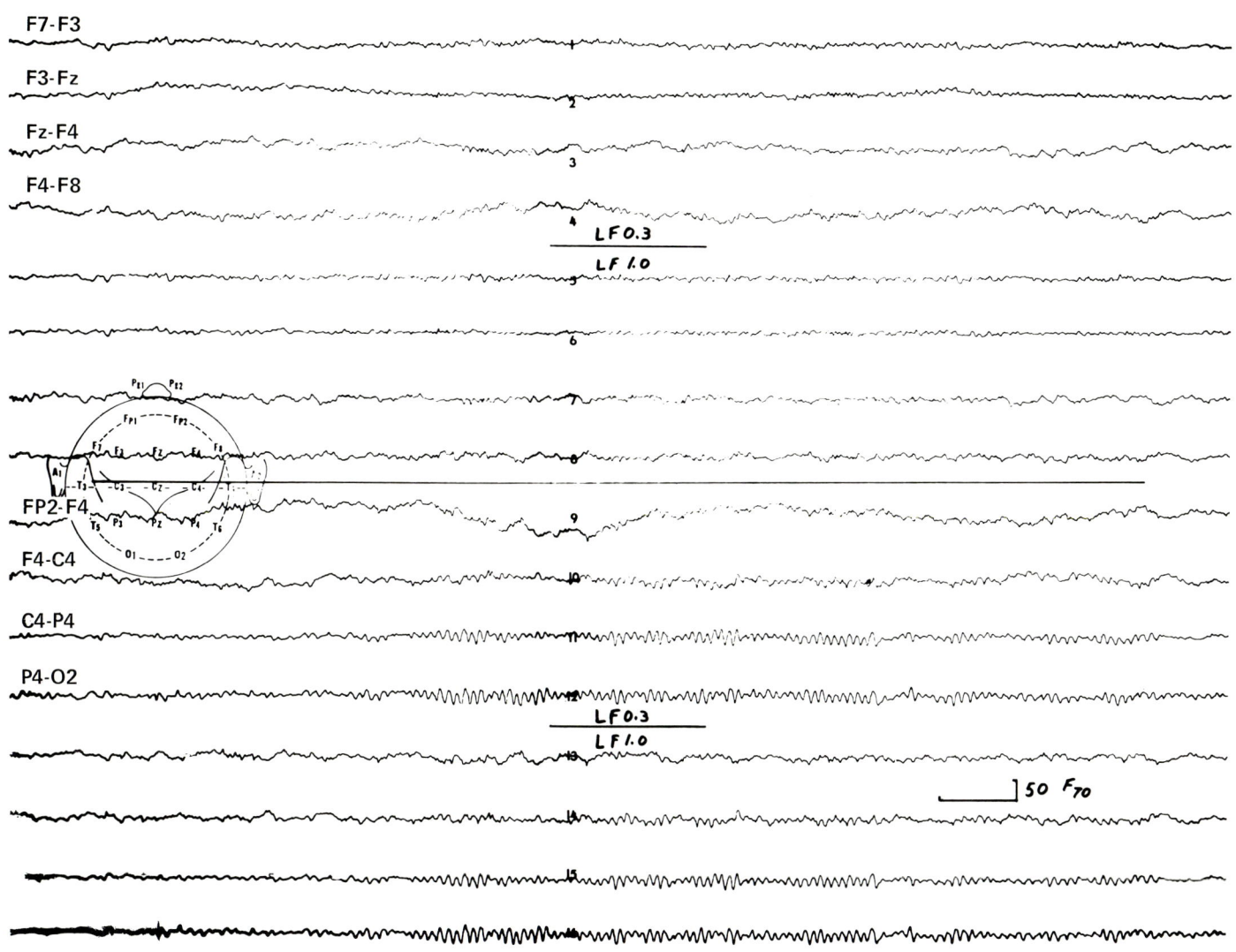

FIG. 25. Posttraumatic delta focus at F4. Duplication of frontal transverse montage (channels 5 to 8), and right parasagittal montage (channels 13 to 16). Focal very slow activity is well defined only at LF 0.3.

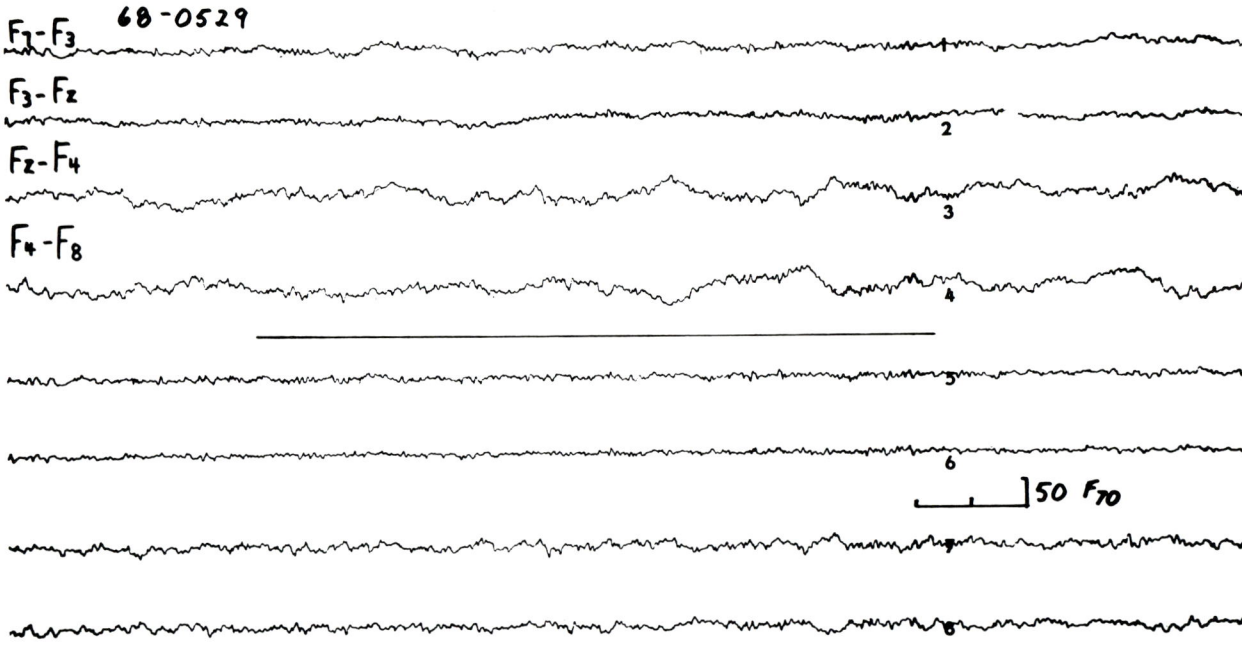

FIG. 26. EEG from same patient as Fig. 25. Frontal transverse montage duplicated at LF 0.3 *(upper four channels)*, and LF 1.0 *(lower four channels)*. Chart speed of 15 mm/sec is helpful in further identification of delta activity in the range of 0.3 Hz.

30 min showed any activity in the next 30 min, or on repeat study. This agrees with the findings at the University of Iowa (J. R. Knott, *personal communication*, 1977). Thus, the likelihood of finding activity on repeat examination in 6 to 24 hr is remote, and any such repeat study may be governed by clinical considerations.

There is more to ECS recording than sensitivity *per se,* but since any record may be made "flat" by simply reducing the sensitivity, it is imperative that adequate gain be employed. A definition of irreversible coma was published in 1968 (1) by 13 members of an *ad hoc* committee of the Harvard Medical School. This stated that "the apparatus should be run at standard gains 10 μV/mm, 50 μV/5 mm. Also it should be isoelectric at double this standard gain which

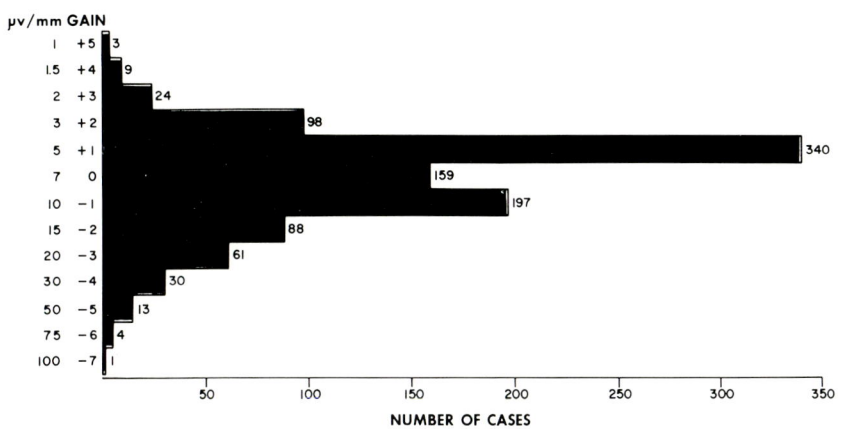

FIG. 27. Gain changes, 1,000 cases Cleveland Clinic 1971. Distribution of maximum and minimum sensitivity used in routine consecutive series of patients. Although most records start at S7, 340 patients were run with S5 maximum at some time, another 98 at S3, etc. S1 on the Model 6 Grass unit was achieved by removing the reduction from the equalizer control, not always feasible or helpful. Total range involves 13 gain settings, from 1 to 100 μV/mm.

is 5 μV/mm or 25 μV/5mm." Such sensitivity standards were and are permissively inadequate. Few laboratories use S10 as a standard for adult patients. Doubling the sensitivity to 5 μV/mm only achieves a level equal to the most often used routine value in this laboratory (Fig. 27) and some other major laboratories. The *ad hoc* report referred to above also suggested that full gain (level not specified) be utilized for 5 to 100 sec, although artifacts usually predominate. The Guidelines of the American EEG Society now recommend a sensitivity of 2 μV/mm as the absolute minimal standard. It is further recommended that virtually all of the tracing be run with at least that much sensitivity. Since virtually all equipment manufactured over the past 15 years readily allows a further doubling of even this sensitivity, the reluctance to use all available gain is difficult to understand.

Evidently much of the problem is due to electrodes. All bedside studies, including those done in the intensive care units, require the best electrodes and the best equipment available.[3] We have found no substitute for collodion-attached leads with provision for injecting electrode contact jelly to lower and equalize impedances. Such leads are stable, less vulnerable to the wide variety of artifacts that plague such recordings, and may be left in place for several days. Collodion technique is easily mastered; there is no excuse for electrode trouble in any laboratory.

Other instrumental controls also have their use in the determination of ECS. The 60-cycle (notch) filter may be used without hesita-

---

[3] At the time of the meeting of the American EEG Society in July 1974, there was a consensus that telephone-transmission-EEG from a patient prepared by a superficially trained technician, with no primary ink tracing at the sending end of the system, was not acceptable. The hazards and deficiencies are multiplied for bedside and ECS recordings. The use of makeshift single channel recorders, as from EKG machines, and other systems with no direct written record, are similarly to be deplored. A pertinent question is—would you accept such procedures for use on yourself or your family?

tion, and considerable high frequency filtering of HF 30 or 35 may be necessary. It is rather more difficult to use the longest time constant settings in such studies, but this is generally possible with bipolar recordings. The technologist records, or otherwise logs in, respiration cycles. Very slow delta activity is not common in records from near-ECS patients, but slower chart speed may assist in the identification of any such activity.

There is divergence of opinion regarding the number of scalp electrodes needed for ECS studies. The Guidelines give 8 as the minimum. Put simply, we feel that it is inconsistent to use 19 leads for the patient referred with the question of whiplash injury and only 8 leads where there is quite literally a question of life or death. Furthermore, when first seen, one does not know whether or not the patient will show ECS. If not, a full set of leads is necessary for evaluation of possible focal abnormality. Figure 28 demonstrates that even such standard coverage gives by no means a complete survey; there are generous expanses of brain not sampled.

Another reason for the full 10–20 system is the increased recording options made available when widely spaced derivations are used (see run J, Fig. 16). Ear reference technique invariably yields increased EKG contamination, compounded if the reference is the contralateral ear. Occipital pole leads, 01 and 02, are more difficult to attach and are particularly vulnerable to slight head movement associated with mechanical respiration. The F3–P3 and F4–P4 derivations, and the use of CZ as a common reference, often give a cleaner tracing. It is not safe to rely on a few closely spaced leads as was done in a much-quoted paper dealing with recovery after alleged ECS (3). A montage of F4–C3/C3–Fz/F4–FZ at a sensitivity of 6 μV/mm is inconclusive.

There has been some anxiety that a record might be incorrectly interpreted as ECS due to instrument failure or technologist error. An absolutely linear straight line pen output would indeed raise

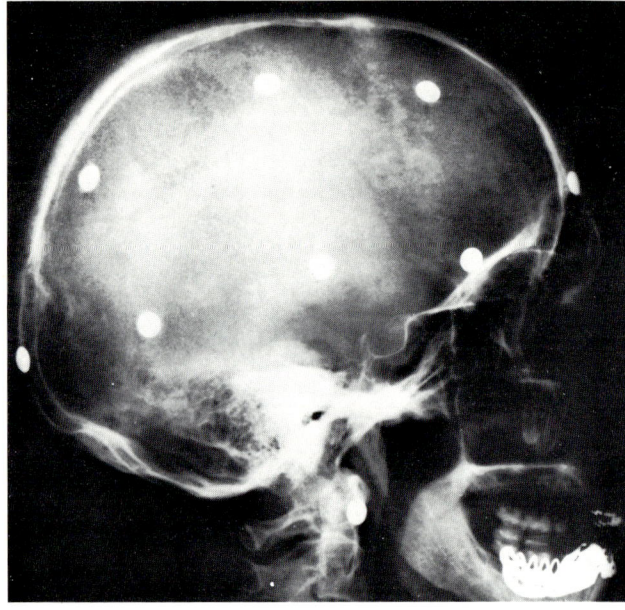

FIG. 28. Skull X-ray showing carefully measured electrode placement, right side, 10–20 system.

such a suspicion. System integrity is easily determined by gently touching the electrodes to induce artifact. If intact, there is *never* an absolute lack of activity (Figs. 29 and 33–35). This may be inherent in the amplifiers at 1 to 2 μV. Some EKG activity is almost invariably present. Recording during nursing procedures also detects useful artifact. There are occasions when the recommended noncephalic monitor will be useful. It should be remembered that the purpose of such studies is to evaluate the EEG. To the extent that one-fourth or more of the channels are devoted to other measures, the EEG

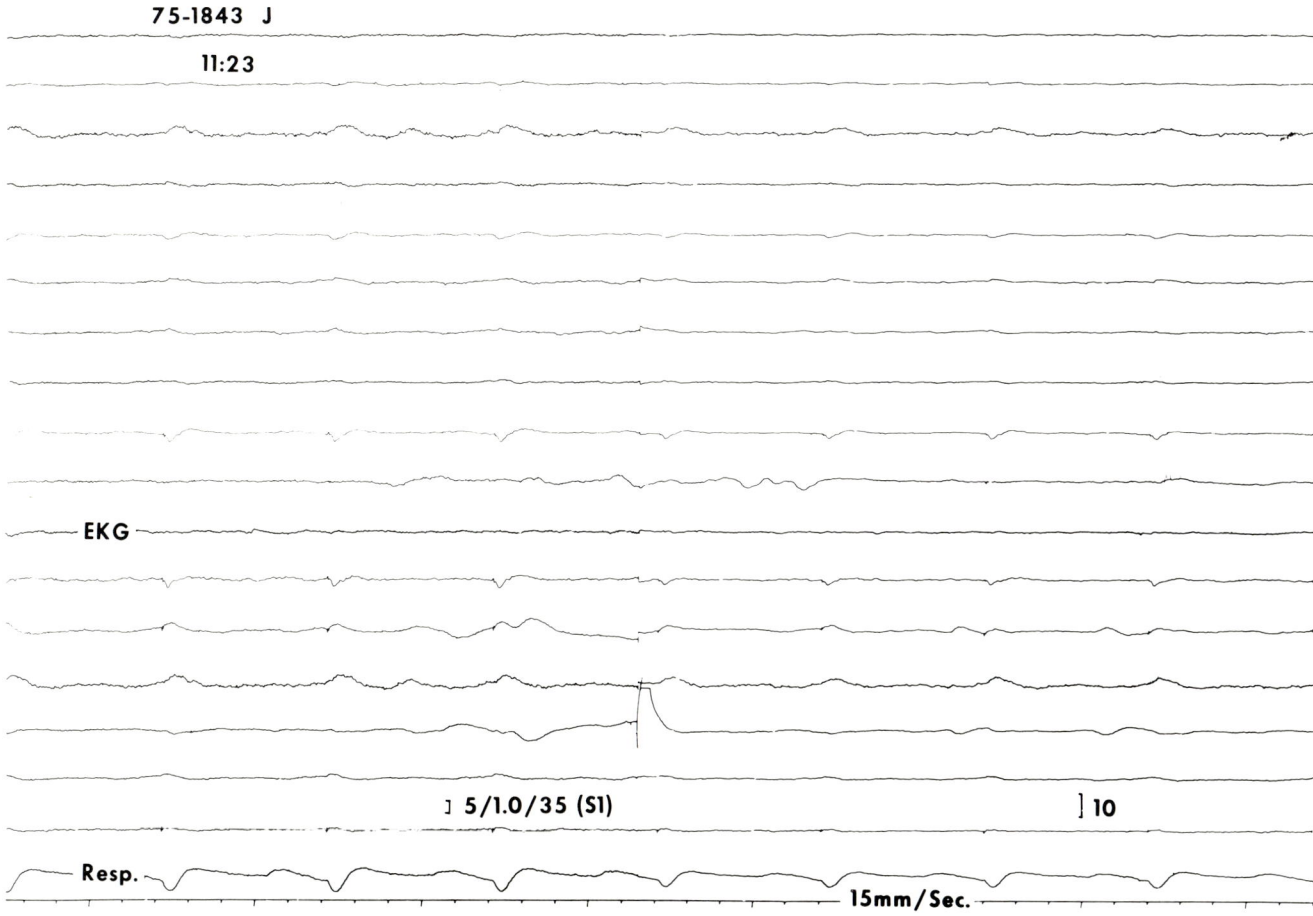

FIG. 29. ECS record from 14-year-old boy after severe abdominal and chest trauma. A second cardiopulmonary arrest occurred 7 hr earlier. The last EKG complex occurred 23 min before this sample. J montage (as seen as in Fig. 16) with wide spaced derivations; chart speed 15 mm/sec. The 20 sec of record at the left is made with S1. The sample at the right, following gain change artifact, is at S1.5. Some artificial respiration artifact is detectable. Note that the tracing, with no EKG activity, is not an absolutely straight flat line.

is neglected. Judicious sampling as needed is usually adequate. Artifact identification is critical, but elimination is superior.

The use of EEG in the evaluation of brain death is merely an extension of the rapidly growing use of EEG for the bedside study of patients who are too ill to come to the laboratory. All electroencephalographs are portable, and given elevators and corridors no hospital patient should be inaccessible. The technologist plays an important role, and the combined experience of a number of these experts is available from an International Roundtable (21). To be sure, new problems are encountered, and there is no substitute for local personal experience. Various types of new and unexpected artifacts soon become familiar. The periodic "suppression-burst" artifact pattern induced by mechanical respirators may be difficult to eliminate. Some EMG activity is not inconsistent with ECS. Patients with indwelling thoracic catheters are subject to increased shock hazard. Adequate patient grounding is necessary but multiple grounds should be avoided. It is not safe to assume that existing AC wiring is correctly polarized and grounded, even in modern intensive care units. Verification and correction as needed is imperative (9). Some ground fault detection systems may induce line artifact as a submultiple of the 60-cycle current. "Cheater plugs" to couple to a two-prong AC outlet are absolutely forbidden. The article by Montoya and Hill (15) gives many practical suggestions for coping with both environmental and physiological artifact.

The EKG is the most ubiquitous of these physiological artifacts and may be a serious problem in the near absence of any cerebral activity. Such unwanted signals are actually present to some degree in all EEGs. They are much less obvious when the signal-to-noise ratio permits a sensitivity of 5 μV/mm or less, and when there is ongoing rhythmic activity to mask the EKG. (It is sobering to realize that had EEG voltages been of the order of only one log unit less—not a big difference in physiologic systems—they could not have been detected by Berger and conventional EEG would be virtually impossible.) When the EEG is markedly reduced in voltage the EKG contamination is then more obvious and of course is increased, along with any EEG activity, at the necessarily high sensitivity used in such studies. Change in head position (22) and montage may be helpful. Few laboratories have computer assistance (2) available; to some degree, a variation of such template subtraction technique may be done by visual means. The transillumination of superimposed pages of record will identify stable and repetitive electrical and ballistocardiographic signals, leaving the more random EEG activity, if there be any, apparent to the eye.

It is advisable for the EEGer to participate personally in some of the bedside EEG studies, and many prefer to be present during a portion of ECS recording. Authorization of the use of succinylcholine or, in our experience, the superior drug pancuronium bromide may be needed to eliminate myogenic activity. We elect to accept some predictable artifact and continue to record during stimulation and nursing procedures. Lateral eye movement is readily detectable from F7 and F8 if evoked by caloric stimulation. Suction is a potent stimulus that may elicit some arousal not present to pain. For the latter, we are indebted to Spanish-trained Dr. Antonio Culebras for a simple way of inducing severe pain, without artifact and without disfiguration: the flat handle of a reflex hammer, or the smooth blades of closed scissors, are inserted and turned between fingers which are held together.

Photic stimulation should always be accomplished. If the stimulator is bolted to the EEG chassis it can't be left behind and can't be damaged by dropping. It is easy to differentiate occipital photic driving from retinal response or a photosensitive electrode.

It is impossible to illustrate the range and complexity of ECS recording by a few single page figures. The 115 well-documented cases of acute cerebral anoxia, not all of whom progressed to ECS, described by Prior are the best published source of illustrations (20) to date. These are almost unique in that artifacts have not been edited out and there is full disclosure of filter and sensitivity data. For the latter this reached 2 μV/mm, much safer than the 5 μV/mm criterion of "absolutely isoelectric" EEGs in the series by Juul-Jensen (11).

The results of a large prospective collaborative study of the EEG in coma and cerebral death published in 1976 (1*a*) and 1977(25) establish the degree to which ECS tracings are reliably predictive of death or survival.

We have occasionally studied a patient immediately before, during, and subsequent to cardiac and/or respiratory arrest. Figures 30 to 35 illustrate this sequence in a 31-year-old patient with terminal hepatic coma and recent repeated arrests with hopeless prognosis. Her respiration rate decreased to 4/min when half of the electrodes had been applied, so recording was begun with only the available right-sided coverage. Respiration had ceased by 1:53 P.M. (Fig. 30), and the EKG had become intermittent. The sample at 1:56 P.M. (Fig. 31) shows the agonal EKG complex. Some brain activity is still detectable at S1.3, and further reduced in amount at 1:58 P.M. (Fig. 32). Such activity underwent gradual dissolution during brief samples obtained as the remainder of the electrodes were attached. The samples at 2:15 (Fig. 33), 2:36 (Fig. 34), and 2:41 P.M. (Fig. 35) show no organized activity and nothing over approximately 2 μV, even with widely spaced derivations (Figs. 34 and 35), the actual montage being unimportant. Nevertheless, the record is never totally and absolutely devoid of some irregularity. The pen drift is more apparent with longer time constant (0.4 seconds). There is no response to photic stimulation (Fig. 35). The effect of different sensitivity is shown in Fig. 33. The same pair of derivations is repeated at S7, 5, 3, 2, and 1.3 μV/mm, and the vertical bars indicate the size of a 50-μV signal at each sensitivity.

There are both ancient and modern verified reports of patient recovery after being pronounced dead. The newspaper accounts evoke anxiety and public mistrust, with understandable reluctance to participate in organ donor programs. Such tragic comedies of errors should be impossible with EEG studies to establish ECS. Nonetheless, just such a case was reported again in 1975. The alleged ECS patient "revived" during preparation for organ removal. What can be done to prevent such embarrassments and avoid even more tragic errors?

The sensible physician will bear in mind that the EEG data are only one aspect of the problem of cerebral death. The sagacious EEGer and his technologist colleagues will equally bear in mind the importance of the word *data*. A perfunctory EEG report of "flat EEG" or "no activity at maximal gain" is insufficient and inadequate. In some laboratories this has meant only 5 μV/mm (+1 on the all channel sensitivity control) on the Grass Model IV and Model 6 units. In others the actual sensitivity may be indeterminable. This may result from lack of information about switch settings and/or absence of adequate calibration data. This even occurs in publications dealing with ECS (12,24). There is a simple solution—write everything down on the actual tracing and calibrate with an appropriate signal. The principle is illustrated in Fig. 17. The square wave calibration deflection must be large enough to measure with some accuracy yet not so large as to overload the system. A 50-μV signal at S1 or S2 is useless (Fig. 33); 5 or 10 μV is required. There is a discussion of calibration technique and a useful table of voltages in a paper by Grass (8).

Good EEG practice does not end with high quality recording. The laboratory findings may be correct but essentially useless if they are not reported adequately. The fundamental features of the EEG, normal and abnormal, awake and asleep, spontaneous and provoked, should be described. Some degree of quantification may be necessary. To be useful, all this must be directed to the clinical problem(s)

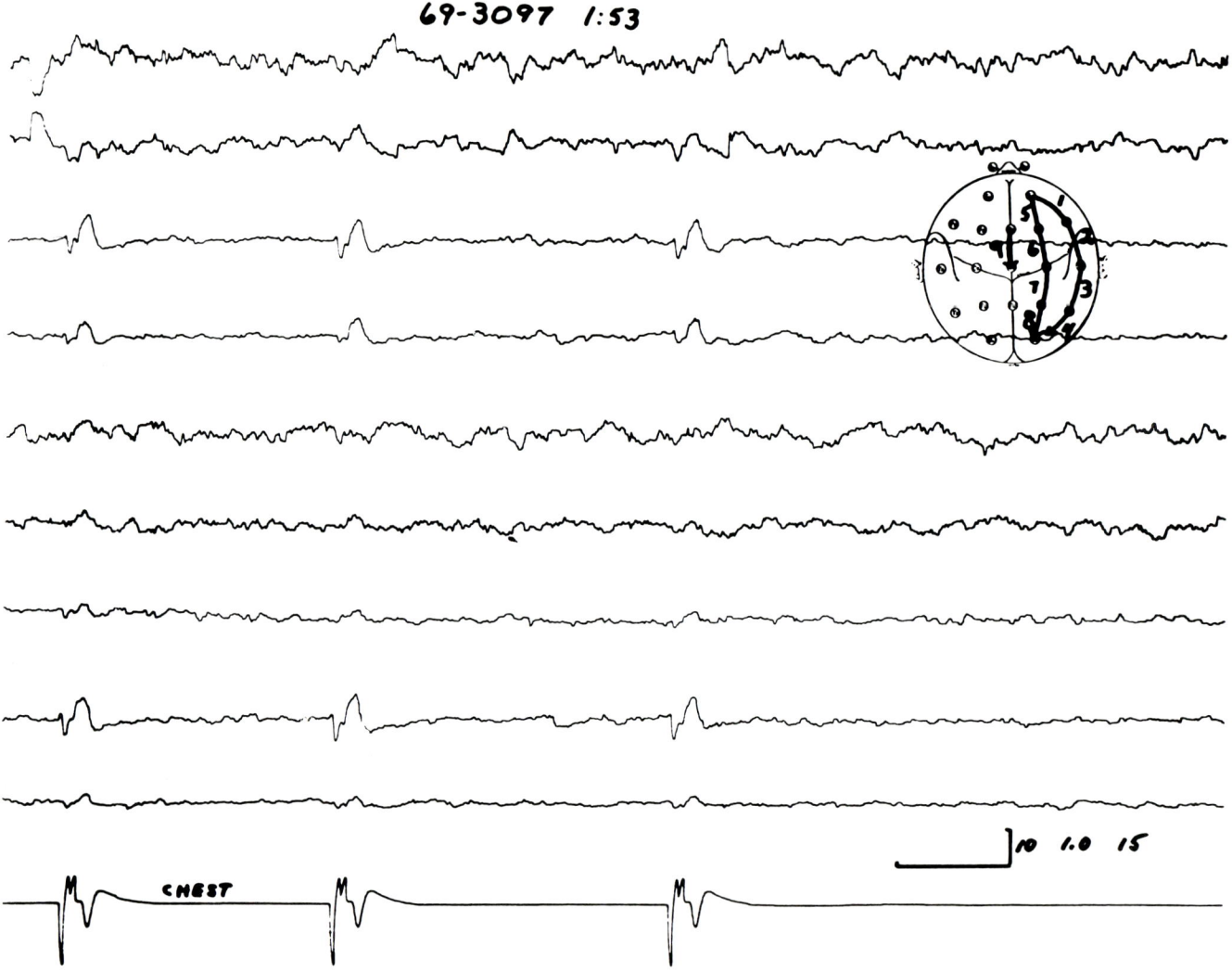

FIGS. 30–35. *(pp. 214–219.)* Gradual disappearance of EEG activity as EKG ceases. There is never total absence of pen movement (see text for details). Horizontal line indicates 1 sec.

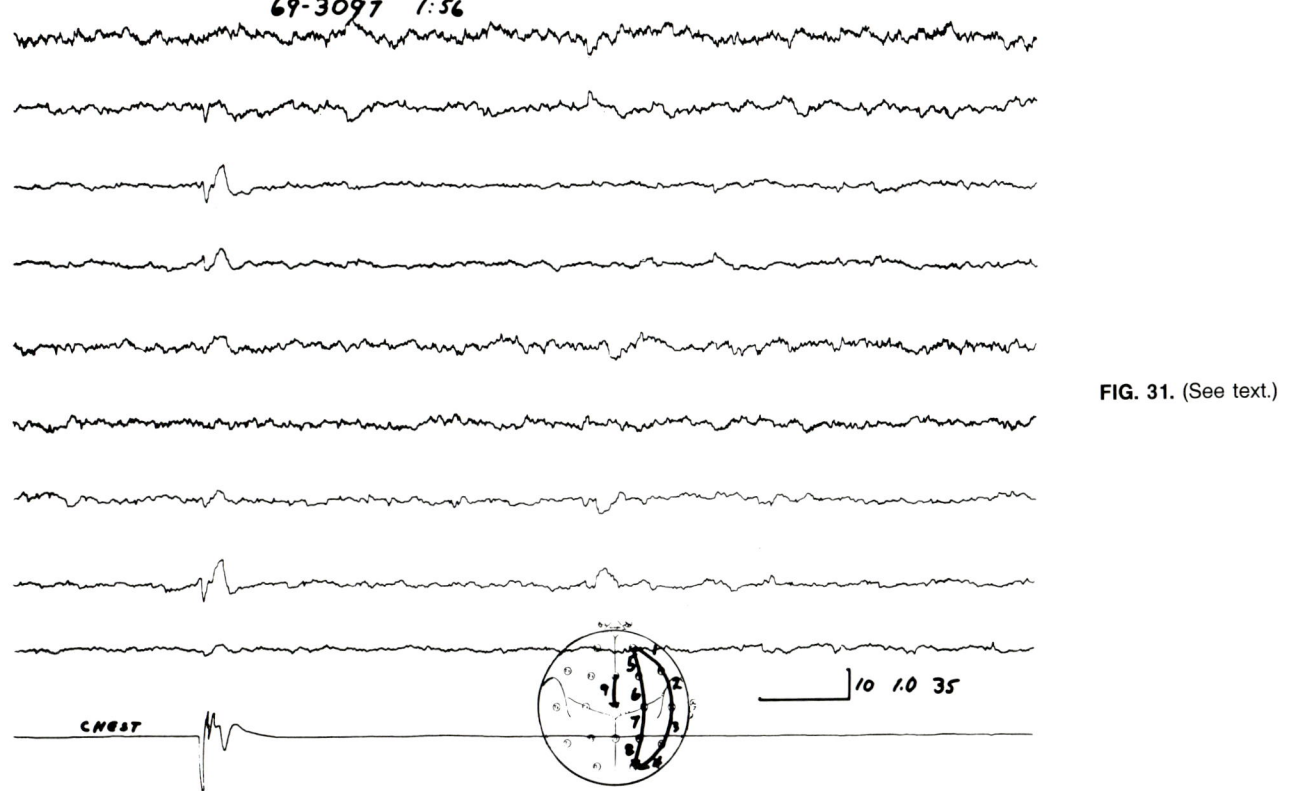

FIG. 31. (See text.)

and be presented in a form understandable to the referring physician [see the preface by Krayenbuhl in Hess (10)]. Nowhere is this more important than in the report of findings with respect to the question of cerebral death. Given the sensitivity and other parameters of the recording the EEGer can state the evidence on which a conclusion is based. It is mandatory that these facts become a part of the medical—and potentially legal—record of the patient.

It is suggested that a prudent approach is somewhat as follows: first, document your understanding of the clinical problem; second, document the clinical state of the patient at the time of examination;

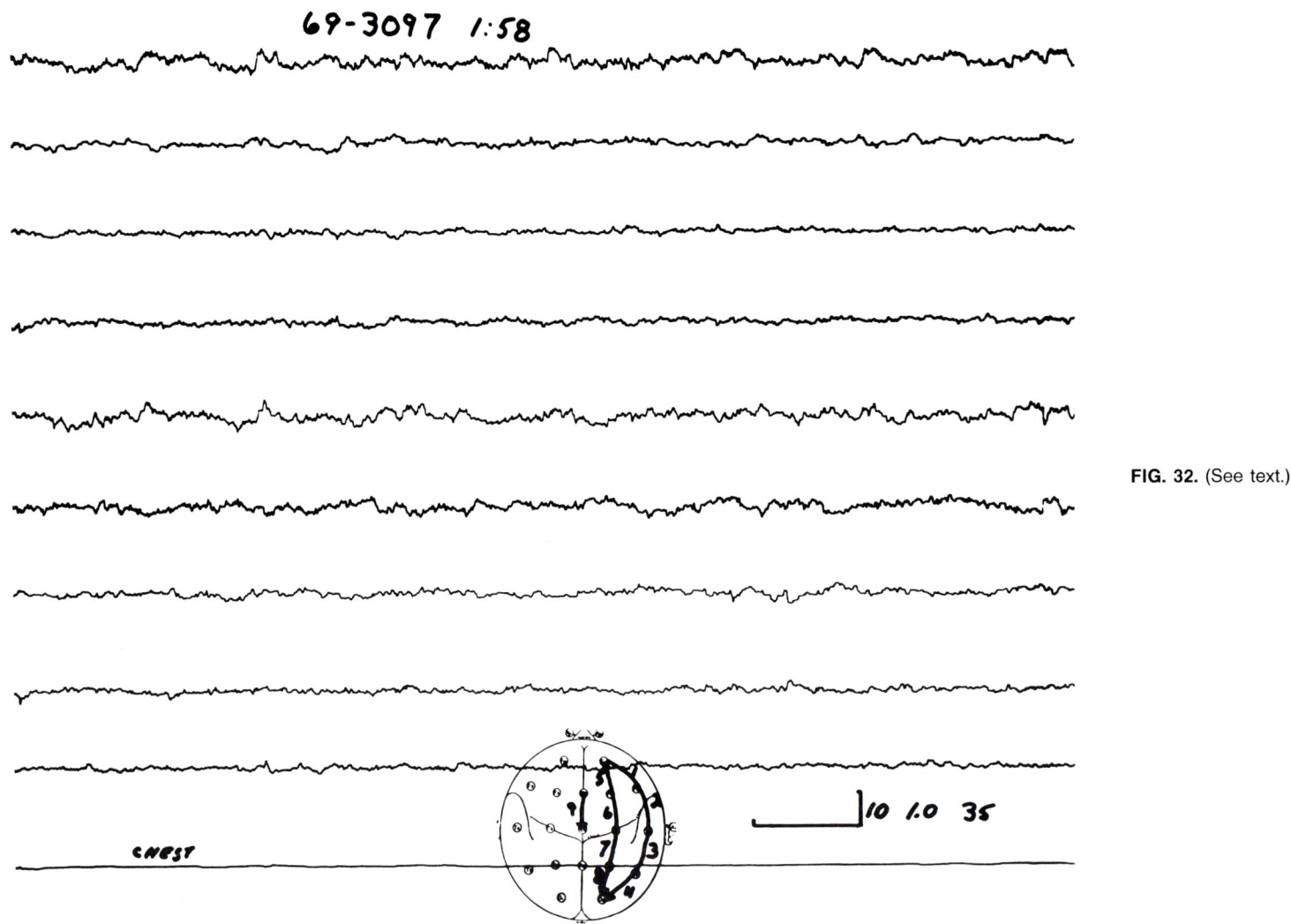

FIG. 32. (See text.)

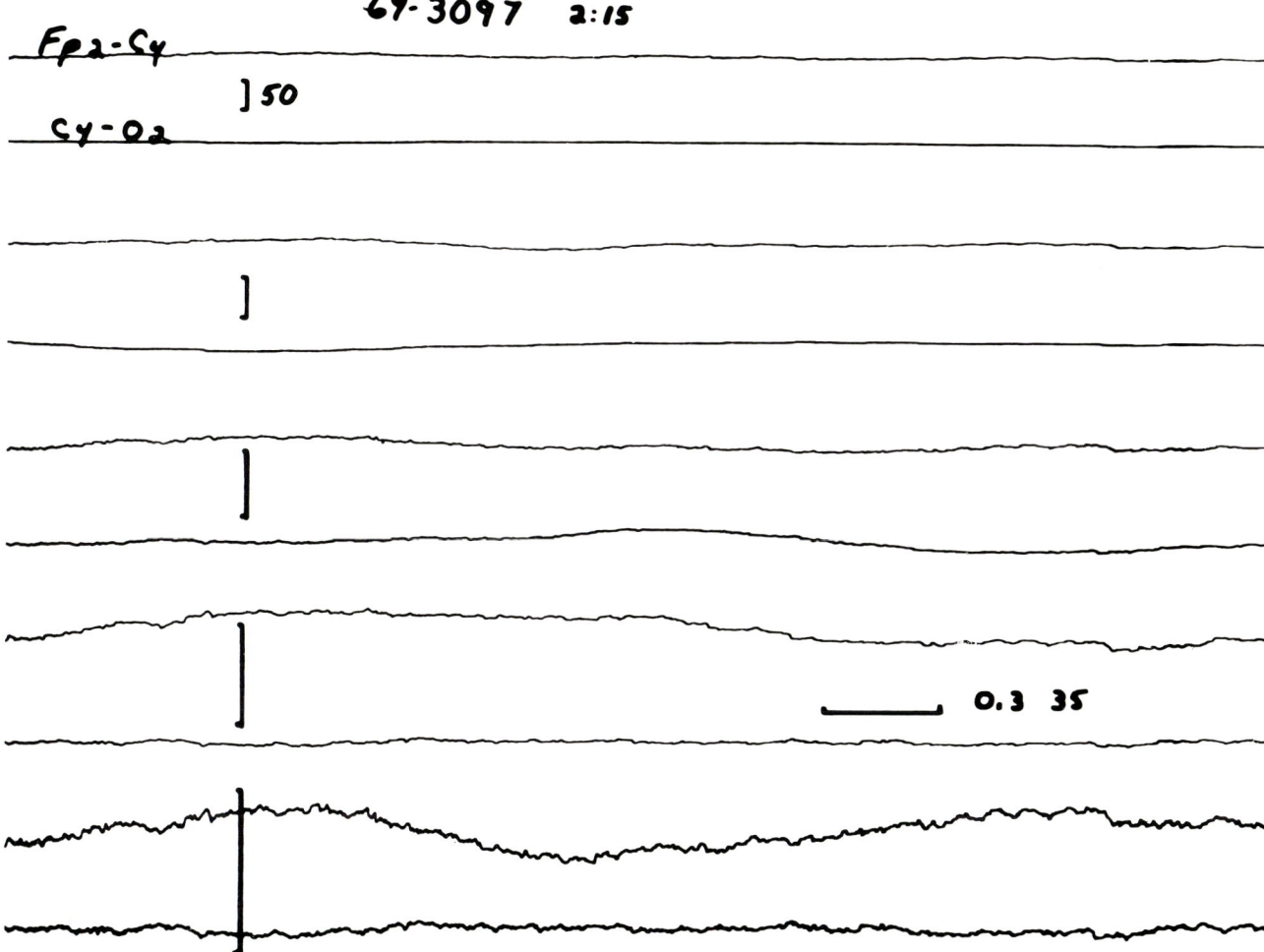

FIG. 33. Actual and theoretical size of 50-μV calibration signals *(vertical lines)* at sensitivity 7, 5, 3, 2, and 1.3 μV/mm from above downward (compare with Fig. 17).

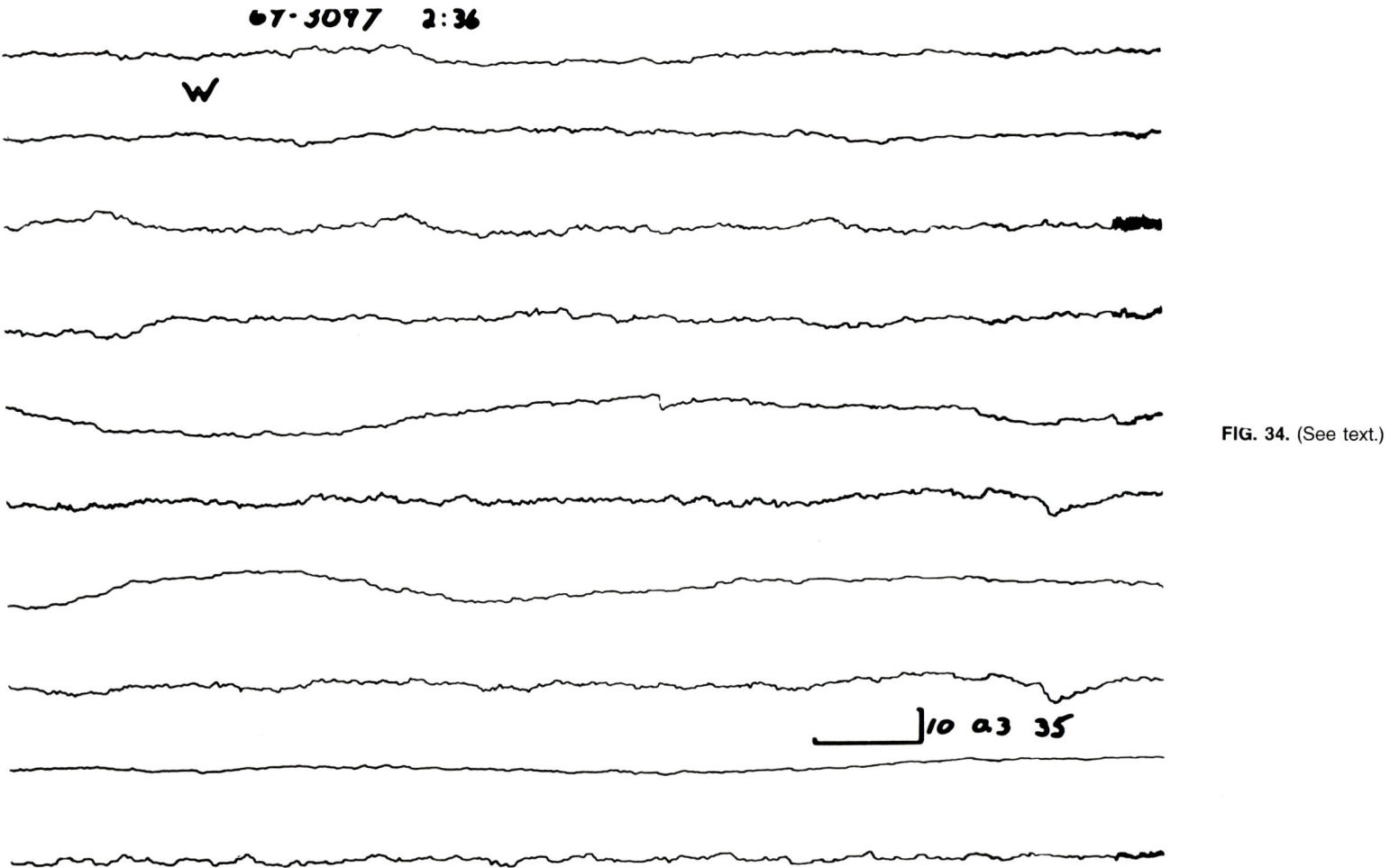

FIG. 34. (See text.)

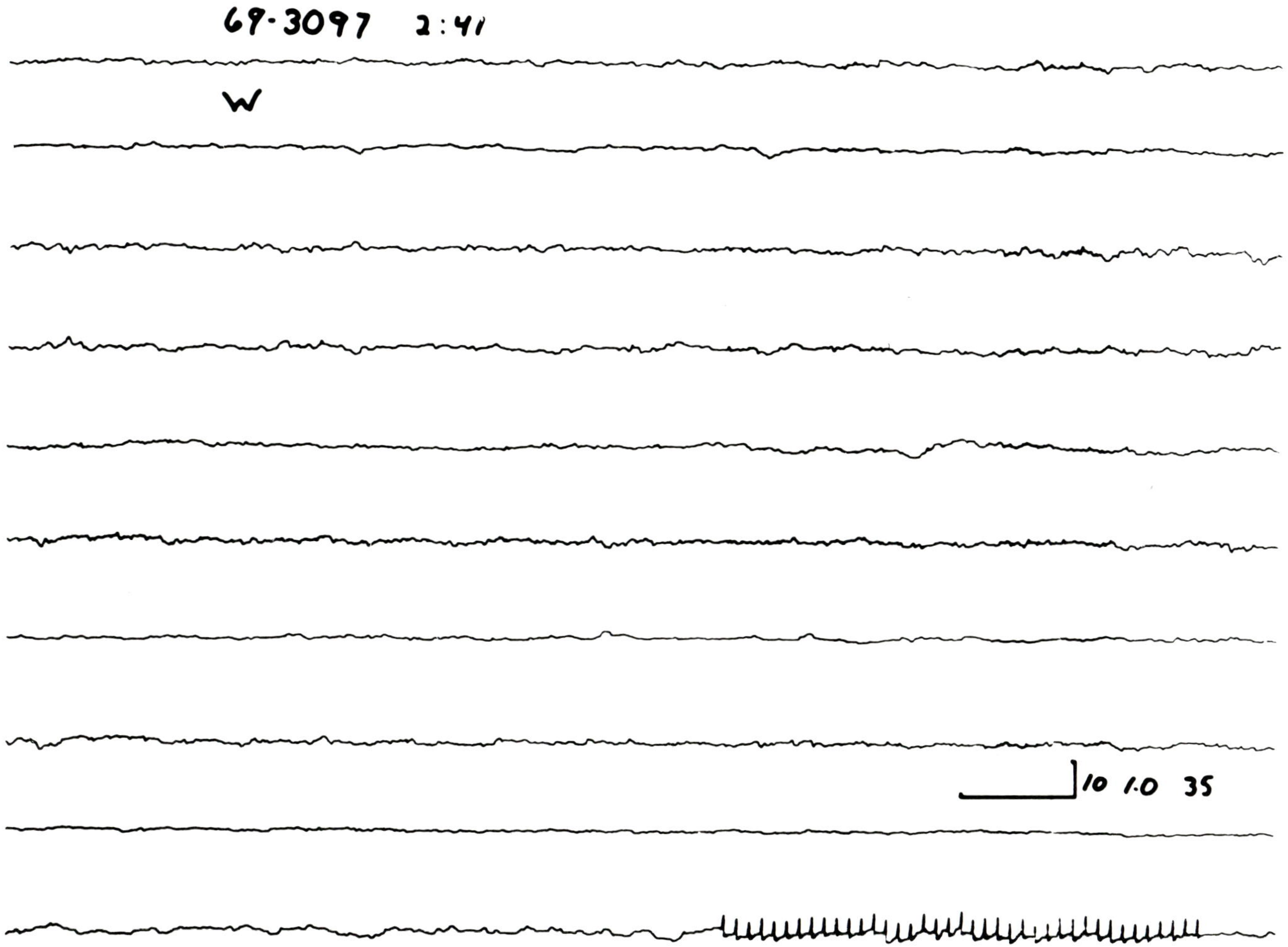

69-3097 2:41

W

FIG. 35. (See text.)

10 1.0 35

and third, clearly and specifically document what was done during the recording, and identify the technologist.

Thus:

CVA on _____ followed by progressively deep coma, now unresponsive to pain. Pupils fixed and dilated, no spontaneous respiration, no brain stem reflexes. Electrolytes satisfactory, T 99, BP 70/52. Bedside EEG in room _____.

This EEG was made on a Grass Model 6 16-channel instrument with a full complement of 10–20 electrode placements. It was started at 1:17 P.M. and concluded at 2:20 P.M. Most of the tracing was made at the maximal available sensitivity of 1.5 or 1.0 μV/mm, including some with extended time constant of 0.4 sec and with increased interelectrode distance derivations.

There is no trace of electrical activity from the brain. There is no response to painful stimulation, to passive eye opening and closing, to intermittent photic stimulation, or when the respirator is disconnected for 15 sec.

Impression: electrocerebral silence at sensitivity of 1 μV/mm.

REFERENCES

1. Ad Hoc Committee (1968): A definition of irreversible coma. *JAMA*, 205:337–340.
1a. Bennett, Donald R., Hughes, John R., Korein, Julius, Merlis, Jerome K., and Suter, Cary (editors) (1976): *Atlas of Electroencephalography in Coma and Cerebral Death.* Raven Press, New York.
2. Berger, E. L., Stockard, J. J., Aung, M. H., and Bickford, R. G. (1974): Removal of EKG artifact from EEG in brain death and other recordings. *Electroencephalogr. Clin. Neurophysiol.*, 37:202–203.
3. Bird, T. D., and Plum, F. (1968): Recovery from barbiturate overdose coma with a prolonged isoelectric electroencephalogram. *Neurology (Minneap.),* 18:456–460.
4. Cooper, R., Osselton, J. W., and Shaw, J. C. (1974): *EEG Technology,* 2nd ed., p. 272. Butterworths, London.
5. Craib, A. R., and Perry, M. M. (1975): *EEG Handbook,* 2nd ed. Beckman Instruments Inc.
6. Gibbs, E. L., Gibbs, F. A., and Fuster, B. (1948): Psychomotor epilepsy. *Arch. Neurol. Psychiatr.,* 60:331–339.
7. Gibbs, F. A., and Gibbs, E. L. (1952): *Atlas of Electroencephalography: Vol. 2; Epilepsy,* p. 422. Addison-Wesley, Reading, Mass.
8. Grass, E. R. (1969): Technological aspects of electroencephalography in the determination of death. *Am. J. EEG Technol.,* 9:77–90.
9. Grass, E. R., and Grass, A. M. (1972): *Electrical Safety.* Grass Instrument Co.
10. Hess, R. (1966): *EEG Handbook,* p. 148. Sandoz.
11. Juul-Jensen, P. (1970): *Criteria of Brain Death.* Munksgaard, Copenhagen.
12. Levin, P., and Kinnell, J. (1966): Successful cardiac resuscitation despite prolonged silence of EEG. *Arch. Intern. Med.,* 117:557–560.
13. MacGillivray, B. B. (editor) (1974): Traditional methods of examination in clinical EEG. In: *Handbook of EEG and Clinical Neurophysiology,* Vol. 3, Part C, p. 126. Elsevier, Amsterdam.
14. Magnus, O., Storm Van Leeuwen, W., and Cobb, W. A. (editors) (1961): Electroencephalography and cerebral tumors. Suppl. 19. *Electroencephalogr. Clin. Neurophysiol.*
15. Montoya, M. L., and Hill, G. (1968): EEG recording in intensive care units. *Am. J. EEG. Technol.,* 8:85–95.
16. Oliver, S. (1967): Artifacts in EEG recordings in intensive care units. *Spike and Wave,* 18:1–18.
17. Osselton, J. W. (1964): Letter to the editor. *Am. J. EEG. Technol.,* 4:28.
18. Osselton, J. W. (1966): Bipolar, unipolar and average reference recording methods. I. Mainly theoretical considerations. *Am. J. EEG. Technol.,* 6:129–141.
19. Osselton, J. W. (1969): Bipolar, unipolar and average reference recording methods. II. Mainly practical considerations. *Am. J. EEG. Technol.,* 9:117–133.
20. Prior, P. F. (1973): *The EEG in Acute Cerebral Anoxia,* p. 314. Excerpta Medica, Amsterdam.
21. Round Table Discussion (1974): Bedside electrophysiological study of acutely ill patients. *Am. J. EEG. Technol.,* 14:95–132.
22. Sims, J. K., and Billinger, T. W. (1971): Types of EKG artifact seen during EEG electrocerebral silence. *West Wind,* 11:89–94.
23. Snodgrass, L. and Knott, J. R. (1962): Some effects produced by three sets of EEG controls: Amplification, low frequency filters and high frequency filters. *Am. J. EEG. Technol.,* 2:65–81.
24. Tentler, R. L., Sadove, M., Becka, D. R., and Taylor, R. C. (1957): Electroencephalographic evidence of cortical "death" followed by full recovery. *JAMA,* 164:1667–1670.
25. Walker, A. E. (1977): *Cerebral Death.* Professional Information Library, Dallas, Texas.

Chapter 8

Use of the EEG for Diagnosis and Evaluation of Epileptic Seizures and Nonepileptic Episodic Disorders

David D. Daly

Department of Neurology, The University of Texas, Health Science Center at Dallas, Dallas, Texas 75235

Introduction	222
Recording Methodology	225
Interictal Abnormality	225
Localized Paroxysmal Abnormality	225
Spikes and Sharp Waves	227
Periodic Discharges	233
Localized Continuous Abnormality	235
Multifocal Paroxysmal Abnormality	235
Multifocal Spikes	235
Hypsarrhythmia	237
Generalized Paroxysmal Abnormality	239
Three-Hz Spike-and-Slow-Wave ("Classical") Complexes	239
Multiple-Spikes-and-Slow-Wave Complexes	245

Sharp-and-Slow-Wave Complexes ("Slow Spike-and-Wave") 248
Secondary Bilateral Synchrony 250
Generalized Periodic Discharges 252
Nonspecific Paroxysmal Discharges 253
Normal EEG 253
Activation Procedures 256
    Sleep Recording 256
    Hyperventilation 258
    Photic Stimulation 260
Syncope 262
Narcolepsy 264
References 264

INTRODUCTION

Electroencephalography constitutes the single most valuable laboratory test in the evaluation of patients with epilepsy. It is a safe, noninvasive, readily repeated procedure to evaluate the electrophysiological state of the patient in the interictal period and occasionally during a seizure. Despite this statement it is an unfortunate fact that the results of an electroencephalogram (EEG) are frequently misinterpreted or misunderstood. Many laboratories continue to receive meaningless requests to "rule out seizure disorder" or "exclude febrile convulsions." Regrettably some laboratories produce nonsensical interpretations such as, "This normal EEG is typical of grand mal epilepsy under treatment." The fact that this patient eventually was found to have a brain tumor caused no little distress to his attending physician.

Much of this confusion dissolves after consideration of certain semantic problems involving the definitions and classifications of seizures and epilepsy. Hughlings Jackson defined a seizure as the result of occasional, excessive, and disorderly discharge of gray matter; this prescient description accords with contemporary electrophysiological studies with microelectrodes (9,68). Behaviorally, seizures are paroxysmal, in the sense of interrupting ongoing behavior, brief, usually lasting no more than a minute or two, and stereotyped. In turn, epilepsy may be defined as a chronic disorder characterized by recurring seizures.

In the past attempts at classification have often failed to make this distinction between seizures and epilepsy with resulting semantic confusion. For example, the terms "psychomotor epilepsy" and "temporal lobe seizures" have been used synonymously and interchangeably to refer to automatisms. However, depth electrode studies have made it clear that automatisms may arise entirely extratemporally in association with discharge originating in the orbital surface of

TABLE 1. Classification of seizures

I. Partial seizures		II. Generalized seizures	III. Unilateral seizures
Elementary	Complex		
1. Motor symptoms (jacksonian) 2. Special sensory or somato-sensory symptoms 3. Autonomic symptoms	1. Impairment of consciousness only 2. Cognitive symptomatology 3. Affective symptomatology 4. "Psychosensory" symptomatology 5. "Psychomotor" symptomatology (automatisms)	1. Absences (petit mal) 2. Bilateral massive epileptic myoclonus 3. Infantile spasms 4. Clonic seizures 5. Tonic seizures 6. Tonic-clonic seizures (grand mal) 7. Atonic seizures 8. Akinetic seizures	
Partial seizures secondarily generalized			

Proposed by the International League Against Epilepsy. (From Gastaut, ref. 48.)

the frontal lobe (53,89). The classification of seizures proposed by the International League Against Epilepsy (48) rests on behavioral descriptions of seizures buttressed by data on the interictal and ictal EEG. The classification divides the large majority of seizures into two general groups: partial or focal seizures and seizures generalized from onset (Table 1).

Partial seizures may have elementary symptomatology, for example, somatomotor seizures involving the hand (jacksonian seizures). Elementary partial seizures may subsequently undergo "generalization" resulting in a so-called secondarily generalized convulsion. Complex partial seizures involve more intricate subjective experiences, for example, feelings of familiarity or a sense of fear. Complex partial seizures may likewise undergo secondary generalization into tonic-clonic convulsions. However, they may also undergo a less extensive nonconvulsive "generalization" with the temporolimbic system to produce the confusional states called automatisms (34). In each of these types of partial seizures the interictal EEG abnormality may have identical morphology and differ only in the location of the abnormality. Hence, earlier attempts to ascribe a characteristic interictal EEG abnormality to a particular type of seizure, for example, "psychomotor waves," were doomed to failure.

Seizures generalized from the onset include several types (Table 1). These differ widely in their manifestations but have in common a lack of focal onset and a lack of postictal focal residual behavioral deficits. Included in this category are absence (petit mal), bilateral epileptic myoclonus, infantile spasms, and tonic-clonic convulsions. The old term "grand mal" has been dropped since it did not distinguish between tonic-clonic convulsions generalized from the onset and those secondarily generalized.

Unilateral seizures occur primarily in children (1,50) whereas anarchic or "wandering" seizures are limited to the newborn period. In newborns and younger children the form of the seizure is dictated in part by the immaturity of the brain, and hence as maturation progresses the character of seizures may change and evolve.

Although major questions remain concerning pathophysiological mechanisms implicit in this concept of classification (5), it constitutes a significant advance and a clinically usable classification. The proposed classification of the epilepsies (95), for various reasons remains much less complete (92). It classifies the epilepsies on the bases of seizure type, the presence or absence of clinical evidence of brain pathology, the age at onset, and the etiology. The ictal and interictal EEGs supply additional information as they do in the classification of seizures. Hence, two patients might have identical seizures, for example, complex partial seizures with automatisms, yet have totally different types of epilepsy. Thus, one patient might have complex partial seizures with automatisms, no neurological deficit, onset at age 12 years, etiology of mesial temporal sclerosis, and an interictal EEG with sporadic focal spikes. Another patient with complex partial seizures with automatisms might have evidence of interictal aphasia, onset at age 45 years, etiology of glioma, and interictal EEG abnormality in the form of persistant polymorphic delta activity. Nevertheless, the classification of the epilepsies remains largely a catalog of causes—some focal, some multifocal, some diffuse, some with presumed genetically determined neurochemical derangements, such as the epilepsies with absence beginning in childhood and ictal EEG abnormalities consisting of 3-Hz spike-and-slow-waves. And major questions remain unanswered: why are some tumors and cerebral scars epileptogenic and others not? Age of the patient, indolence, and location of the lesion are obviously all factors. Thus, this classification must be regarded as not yet definitive but "in evolution."

Given a recording, the electroenceophalographer can usually make a reasonably accurate description of interictal abnormality, including its morphology, location, and reactivity to state changes. Problems begin when the EEGer must interpret the significance of these findings to the clinician. Serious problems can be avoided if several points are kept in mind.

1. Since the classification of the epilepsies emphasizes the multiple causes of epilepsy, not surprisingly *no* electrical event is pathognomonic of epilepsy, and *no* electrical event is unique to a particular type of seizure. Thus *no* report should refer to an interictal spike as a "seizure discharge." Electroencephalographers even differ over the propriety of the term *epileptiform* discharge. Properly used the term is acceptable (129); this is discussed subsequently.

2. We lack adequate "transfer functions" relating interictal EEGs and seizures, and interictal and ictal EEGs. Given a child with 3-Hz spike-and-slow-wave complexes in the EEG, does this child have no seizures, absences only, or absences and tonic-clonic convulsions? Does the interictal EEG abnormality transform into ictal abnormality by "prolongation" (62)? Is the transformation by the disappearance of interictal discharges as in the case of some temporal spike foci (75) or by the "electrodecremental" seizures of hypsarrhythmia? Or is the seizure heralded by the appearance of 10-Hz "epileptic recruiting rhythms" (49)?

3. We also lack transfer functions between the ictal EEG and the behavioral state. Thus, a patient exhibiting a behavioral automatism with mastication may show 3-Hz spike-and-slow-waves (107), diffuse theta activity, or no change at the scalp (49,75). Clearly to refer to trains of rhythmically repeating temporal spikes or to 4-Hz "flat-topped" waves as "larval psychomotor discharges" is totally unjustified.

Bearing these caveats in mind, what should the electroencephalographer say? First, a diagnosis of epilepsy can be *confirmed only* if a seizure is recorded during an examination. Abnormalities or their absence should be interpreted in the light of clinical findings. For example, the finding of a focus of polymorphic delta activity would cast serious doubt on a diagnosis of syncope due to cardiac arrhythmia and would raise the question of an intracranial cause for the episode of unconsciousness. The finding of independent bitemporal spike foci in a young adult who has experienced his first convulsion would make it highly improbable that the patient has a localized intracranial lesion such as a neoplasm. A normal interictal EEG does not "exclude" epilepsy, and the report should make this clear. In this manner, prudent and reasonable interpretations can supply the clinician with important information while not misleading him about the specificity or accuracy of the EEG. This discussion proceeds on the assumption that it is directed to the electroencephalographer who sits facing a recording requiring interpretation. Hence, the kinds of EEG abnormality provide the framework for discussion. Since in most laboratories recordings elicit only interictal abnormalities, these receive the majority of the discussion.

RECORDING METHODOLOGY

In order to extract the maximum information from the examination, certain general principles should be borne in mind.

1. Since in some patients with seizures the locus of abnormal discharge is surprisingly small, a sufficient number of electrodes must be routinely used. In our laboratories we use 21 electrodes placed according to the 10–20 system. These include five pairs of parasagittal electrodes, four pairs of temporal electrodes (counting the ear electrodes as temporal electrodes), and three midline electrodes at Fz, Cz, and Pz. Figure 1 illustrates a recording from a child with elementary partial seizures involving the foot. The usual parasagittal recording discloses no abnormality. Unless a vertex electrode (Cz) is used, the spike focus will go undetected.

2. The complex types of abnormality seen in patients with seizures require a sufficient number of channels to delineate the topography of the generators. Sixteen-channel recordings are much superior. Eight channels will often leave unanswered certain important questions about multiple foci, large generators, or unusual generators. A superior technologist can "make do" in recording with eight channels whereas an inexperienced technician may become hopelessly confused.

3. The selection of montages should be flexible and left to the judgement of the technologist. For example, with a spike generator in the temporal region, referential recording can be made using either an average potential reference electrode or the vertex (Cz); however, the ear should *not* be used as a reference electrode (Fig. 2). Given a large parasagittal generator, transverse montages may be necessary to demonstrate a single generator extending across the midline as opposed to two synchronous generators (Fig. 15). With a large single generator, referential recording may be impossible using an average potential reference electrode but feasible with a carefully selected, single reference electrode.

4. If the basal recording shows no significant abnormality, the examination must proceed to activation techniques. Since this cannot be known in advance, sufficient time should be included in the laboratory schedule. Activation procedures include spontaneous or induced sleep, hyperventilation, and photic stimulation.

INTERICTAL ABNORMALITY

Localized Paroxysmal Abnormality

Paroxysmal abnormalities may have several forms. The term *epileptiform* has been applied to any paroxysmal discharge containing spikes or sharp waves, either localized or generalized. In a study of 6,497 unselected, *nonepileptic* patients, spikes and sharp waves

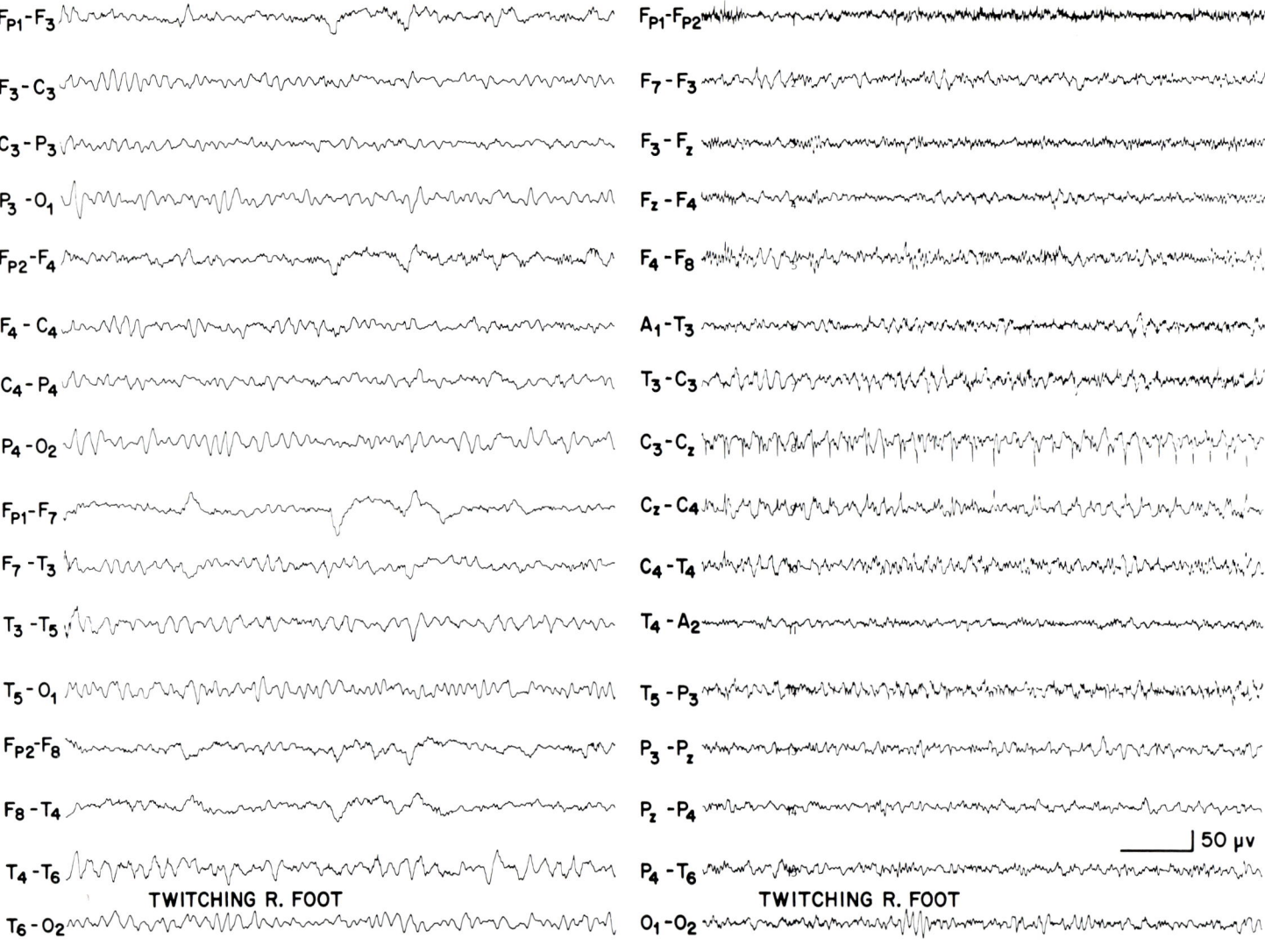

were found in only 2.2% (129). In this subset of patients with paroxysmal discharges, seizures eventually developed in 15%. Zivin and Ajmone-Marsan (129) have concluded that, using appropriately conservative criteria to define spikes, the term "epileptiform" is appropriate.

Spikes and Sharp Waves

Spikes refer to evanescent electrical events lasting, by definition, less than 70 msec (24). As recorded with an inkwriter, they have a biphasic or polyphasic form and are usually surface negative (Fig. 2). They exceed the amplitude of the background rhythms in the region and are usually followed by an aftercoming surface-negative slow wave, which may have a slightly different spatial distribution from the spike generator. Maulsby (93) and Kooi (78) have offered useful guidelines for deciding what constitutes a spike or sharp wave. By definition, sharp waves have durations exceeding 70 msec and occasionally last as long as 200 msec (106). The usual generators of spikes and sharp waves appear equivalent to radially oriented dipoles that are surface negative (Fig. 3). Occasionally a generator appears as a true dipole, tangential to scalp surface, with the positive component lying anteriorly. Curiously, these latter generators seem to occur principally in children (Fig. 4).

The morphology of spikes and sharp waves is uninfluenced by their area of occurrence (46). On the other hand, a correlation exists between the type of seizure and the location of the spike focus. For example, spike foci in the temporal region are commonly associated with complex partial seizures and automatisms (46). In contrast, spike foci in the Sylvian or Rolandic region are commonly associated with tonic or clonic seizures of half the face, oropharyngeal sensations, arrest of speech, and excessive salivation—features compatible with local epileptic discharge in the sensorimotor cortex (82,84).

In the waking state, focal spikes show varying reactivity, for example, being relatively uninfluenced by eye opening or hyperventilation but inhibited by alerting movement or sensory stimulation (113,121). Sleep exerts complex effects on interictal abnormality, effects which are discussed in greater detail in the section on activation [see also ref. 33 for a review]. In 10 to 20% of patients with complex partial seizures, focal spikes appear only during sleep (15,30) whereas in 1 to 7% of patients, temporal spikes disappear during sleep. Blom and Heijbel (15) report the presence of Rolandic spikes only during sleep in 30% of their population of children with "benign Rolandic epilepsy." In slow-wave or nonrapid-eye-movement (NREM) sleep the spike generator often increases in size, and discharges may occur in the homologous area of the opposite hemisphere.

The incidence of spikes varies in different populations. In a study of 1,000 carefully selected normal children, Petersén et al. (109) found focal spikes in 1.5%; Eeg-Olofsson et al. (42) have reported

Fig. 1. Recording of EEG during spontaneous elementary motor seizure involving the right foot. In this and all subsequent illustrations, the 10–20 electrode placement system is used. Horizontal calibration represents 1 sec; vertical calibration indicates microvolts. The patient, a 7-year-old girl, had developed elementary partial motor seizures involving the right foot at age 18 months, followed by a slowly progressive right hemiparesis. At age 6 years radioisotope brain scan, angiogram, and pneumoencephalogram gave normal findings. Chronic encephalitis was suspected but unproven. Both recordings were made during a spontaneous seizure consisting of twitching in the right foot. In the left panel, differential (bipolar) anteroposterior montage is employed. Note that in the top eight channels, recording from the parasagittal areas, no abnormal discharge appears. While the seizure continued the technologist shifted to a transverse montage. Surface negative spikes appeared almost exclusively at Cz (phase reversal between channels 8 and 9). The spikes are extremely short in duration, about 25 msec. After the seizure spikes appeared infrequently, averaging one every 3 to 4 sec.

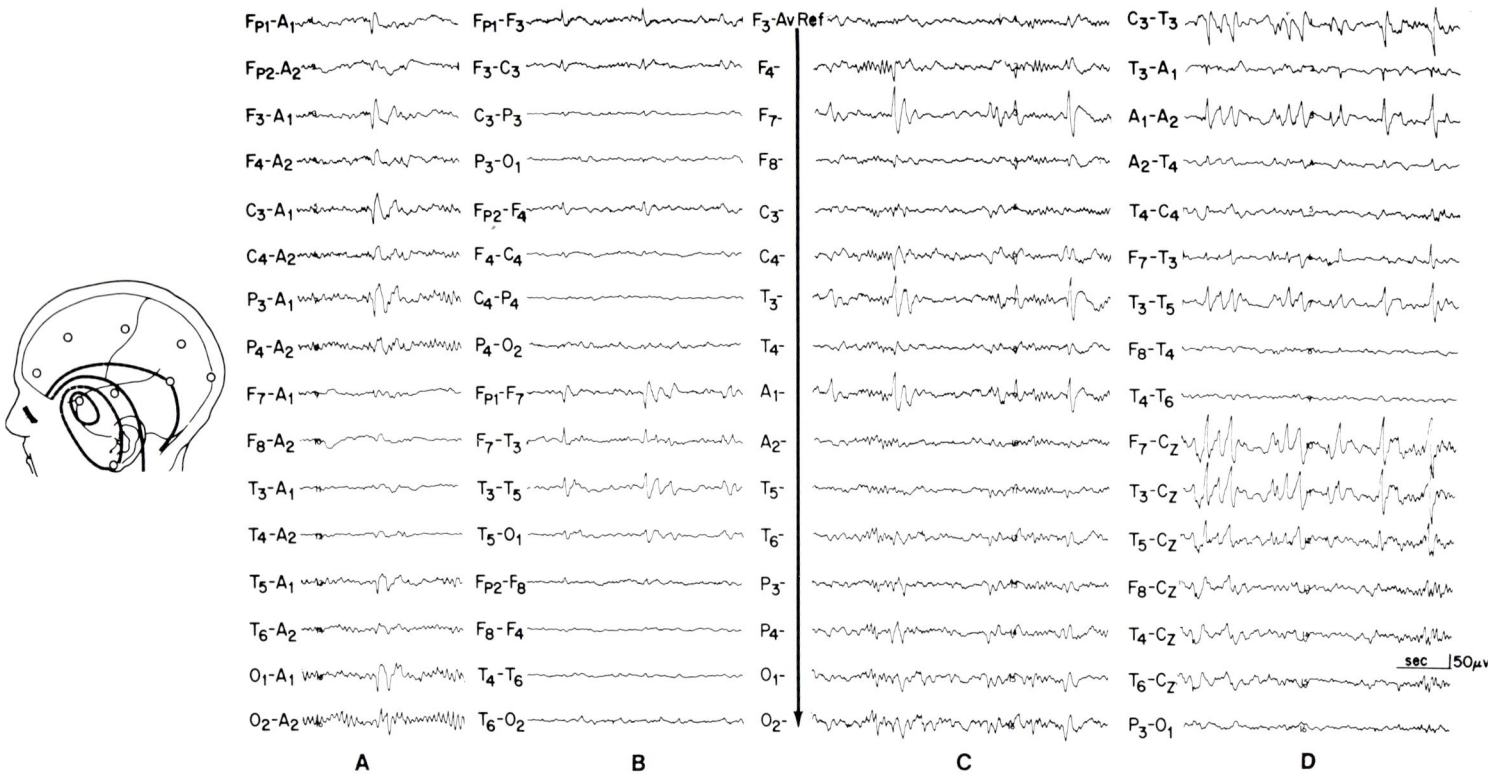

FIG. 2. Radially oriented surface negative spike generator in the temporal region. J. F., a 47-year-old man, was the product of a difficult delivery with postnatal complications. Complex partial seizures appeared at 10 years of age. The seizures began with a "strange [indescribable] feeling," followed by staring, unresponsiveness, flushing, sweating, and flexing of the right hand. Postictally he was aphasic. The diagram shows isovoltage lines at the scalp from the spike generator. Note that F7 is the point of maximal negativity (175 μV) and that the ear electrode (A1) is more negative than the midtemporal electrode T3. **A:** Referential recording using ipsilateral ear electrodes. Note the confusing effect of the reference electrode being located within the generator and hence acting as an active electrode. No apparent discharge occurs in the left temporal region (channels 9 and 11) because of virtual isoelectricity, while what appears to be a surface positive spike occurs widely throughout the remainder of the left hemisphere. **B:** Differential (bipolar) recordings show phase reversal of a surface negative spike at F7 (channels 9 and 10). Upward deflections also occur in channel 11 and 12 since T3 is more negative than T5, which in turn is more negative than O1. **C:** Referential recording using an average potential reference (Goldman-Offner) electrode (24). The spike appears at F7, T3 and A1 but shows maximum negativity (maximum amplitude) at F7. **D:** A montage using both differential and referential derivations. In the top four channels differential recordings in a transverse montage show maximum negativity at A1, phase reversal between channels 2 and 3. Anteroposterior differential derivations indicates maximum negativity at F7 (channel 6). Channels 10 to 15 referential recording using vertex (Cz) reference, maximum negativity is at F7.

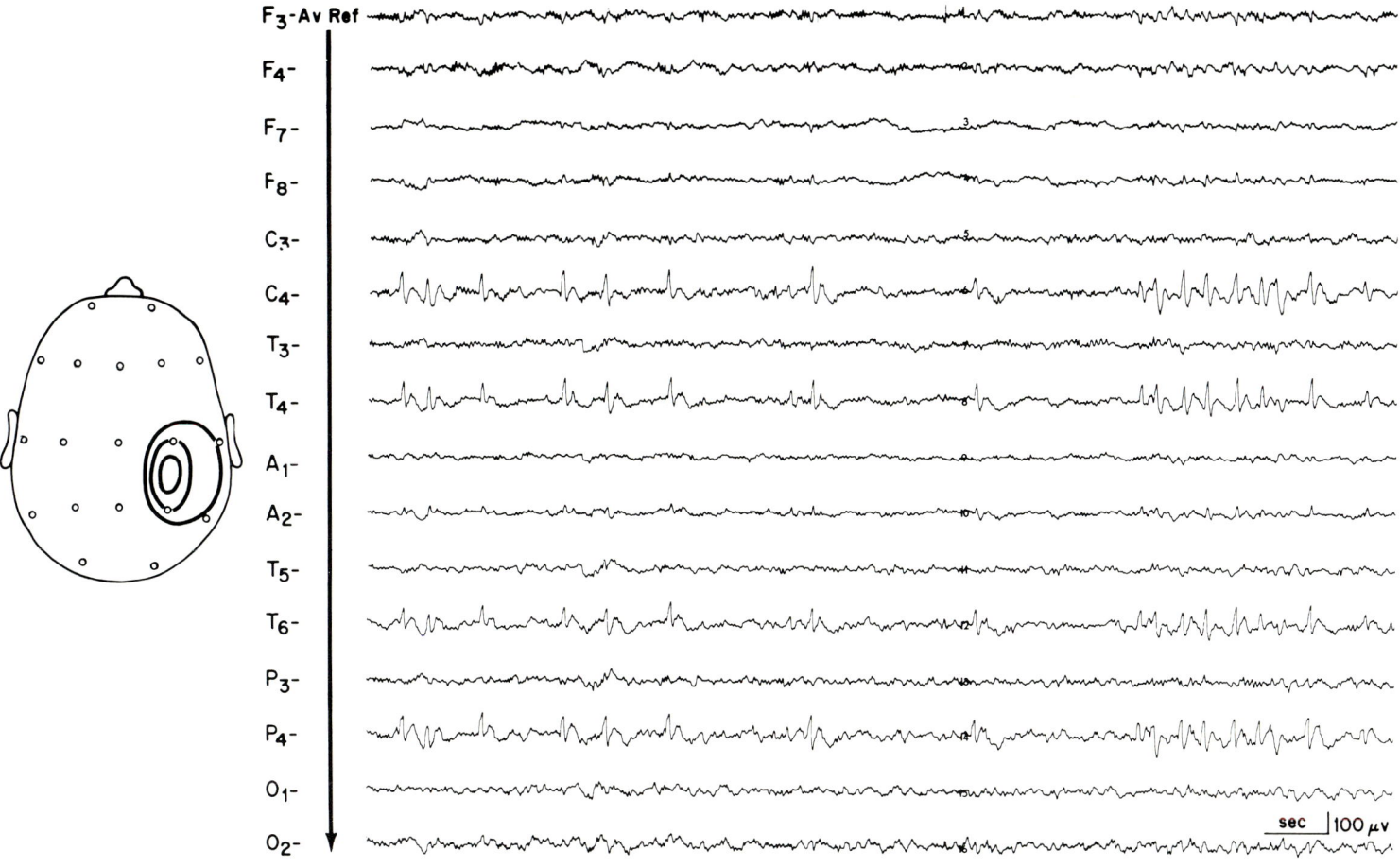

FIG. 3. Surface-negative spike generator. D. F., a 12-year-old boy, developed elementary partial motor seizures involving the left hand and face at age 3 years. The recording uses an average potential reference electrode. The head diagram plots isovoltage lines with maximal negativity at C4-P4. The generator extends inferiorly to the mid (T4) and posterior (T6) temporal electrodes. The generator did not extend to the midline.

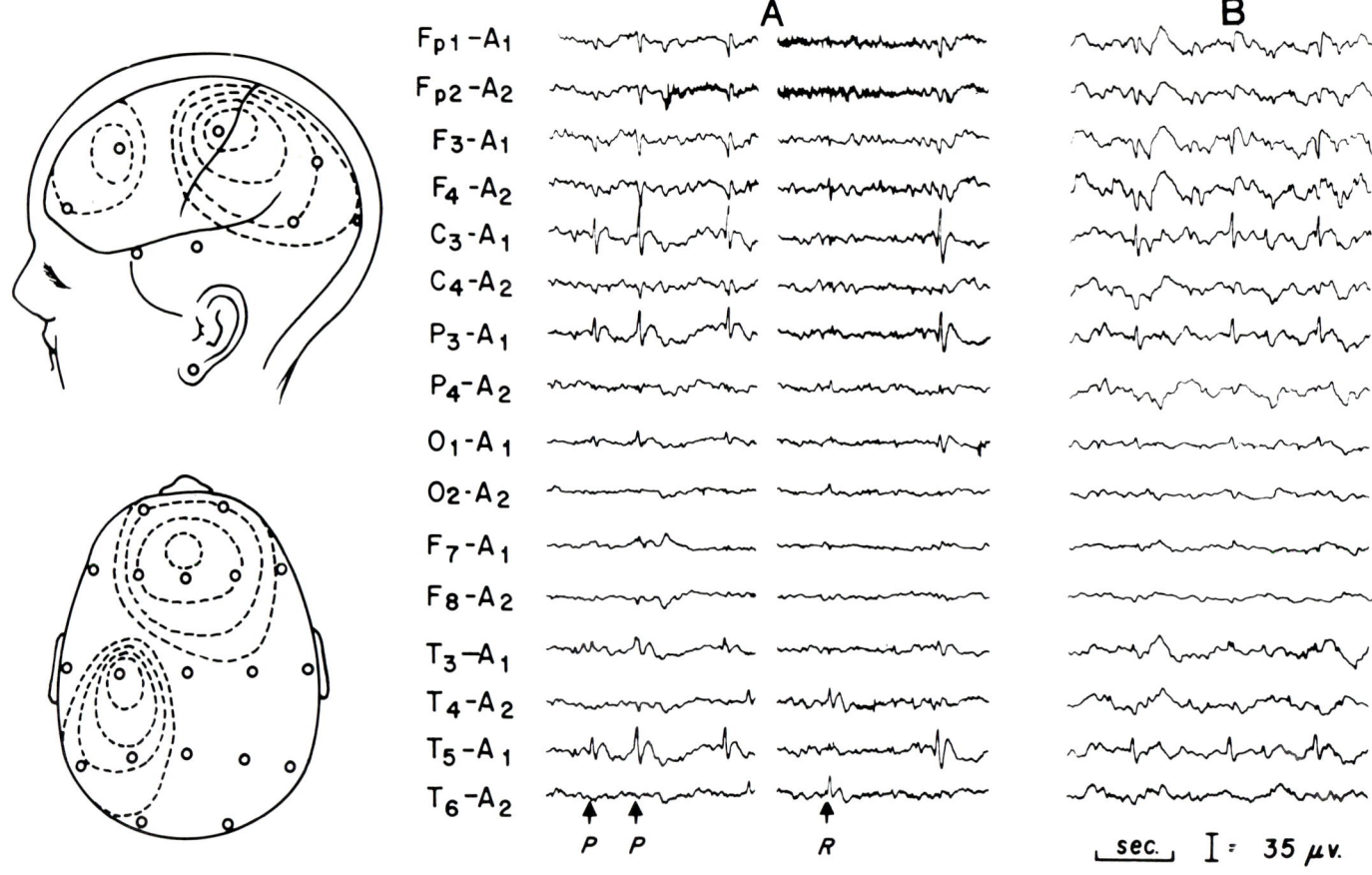

FIG. 4. A: Awake. **B:** Asleep. Parallel or tangential dipole generator of spikes. A. G., a 7-year-old girl, had had a tonic-clonic convulsion during sleep two nights before. Referential recording using the ipsilateral ears was possible since the generator was in the parasagittal region. The discharges occurring from the parallel generator are marked P. Note also, less frequently, the more common type of radially oriented spike generator (R) in the right posterior temporal region. Maximum negativity of the generator appears at C3, indicated by a large upward deflection. Anteriorly, downward deflections appear at FP1, FP2, F3, and F4, indicating positive discharges in these areas synchronous with the negative discharges occurring in the centroparietal region.

similar values (1.9%) in a related population. Trojaborg (123) studied 242 children whose EEG showed spike foci: 82% were epileptic and another 13% without epilepsy had structural disease of the brain, the majority suffering from cerebral palsy. Only 5% were without gross disease, most of these being classified as "behavior disorders" (Fig. 5). Under the age of 2 years, focal spikes occur infrequently but are usually associated with evidence of severe neurological impairment (98,99). These observations may be summarized: (a) focal spikes in children have a high association with clinical evidence of seizures; (b) children without seizures probably have structural disease of the nervous system; and (c) focal spikes rarely occur in normal children. As already mentioned, spikes are equally rare in nonepileptic adults.

Despite the significant association with structural brain disease, with or without seizures, the demonstration of a spike focus on a single examination is not a reliable indicator of underlying focal cortical disease in children. In serial studies of children with spike foci, Trojaborg (123) found that a change in location occurred in 85% of children, and a change from a single focus to two or more foci was observed in two-thirds of children (Fig. 6). Age-related factors appear to operate: in children, temporal foci become increasingly prominent with increasing age and Ajmone-Marsan and Zivin (7) found that focal epileptiform abnormality is most often present in childhood but becomes progressively infrequent after the age of 40.

Careful analysis of patients with spike foci suggests that certain "electroclinical" syndromes exist. The so-called Rolandic or centrotemporal epilepsy of childhood is one instance. In a study of 315 children with Rolandic spikes, Beaussart (12) found seizures in 85%. Seizures were predominantly of the elementary partial type, consisting of tonic or clonic contractions of one side of the face, oral sensations, arrest of speech, tonic contractions of tongue or jaws, and profuse salivation. Convulsions, if they occurred, were secondarily generalized in 82% and happened primarily in sleep. Essentially identical findings have emerged from two independent studies on unrelated populations of patients (16,84). The interictal EEG shows spikes, uninfluenced by hyperventilation and eye opening (12); however, sleep produces a prompt activation (109). The seizures tend to appear between ages 5 and 10 years and, almost without exception, disappear spontaneously by age 15 years (74). A strong genetic factor operates—seizures and Rolandic discharges occurring in 15% of siblings, Rolandic discharges in 19% of asymptomatic siblings, whereas 11% of parents had had seizures in childhood (65). These findings suggest an autosomal dominant gene with age-dependent penetrance, findings strikingly similar to those genetic factors in primary generalized epilepsy with 3-Hz spike-and-slow-wave in the EEG (96).

In studies on slightly older patients, Ajmone-Marsan (6,88) has shown that despite "a much greater complexity and variability (of seizure pattern) than one might expect, a significant correlation exists between the behavioral manifestations of partial seizures and the location of the interictal spike focus." Thus, patients with foci of epileptiform discharge located in the central region show a high incidence of contralateral clonic and tonic motor seizures (Fig. 3) and "somatosensory auras" and an equally significant, low incidence of automatism. In contrast, almost two-thirds of patients with occipital foci described visual sensations as part of their elementary seizures. Automatisms occur most frequently in patients with temporal or frontal foci (60 to 80%), less frequently in patients with occipital foci (40%), and, as mentioned, least frequently in patients with centroparietal foci (25%). In patients with occipital foci, automatisms were almost invariably (87%) preceded by visual sensations, reflecting the selective spread of the ictal process from occipital to temporal regions.

In a large series (666) of patients of all ages selected clinically as having "temporal lobe epilepsy," the EEG showed focal abnormal-

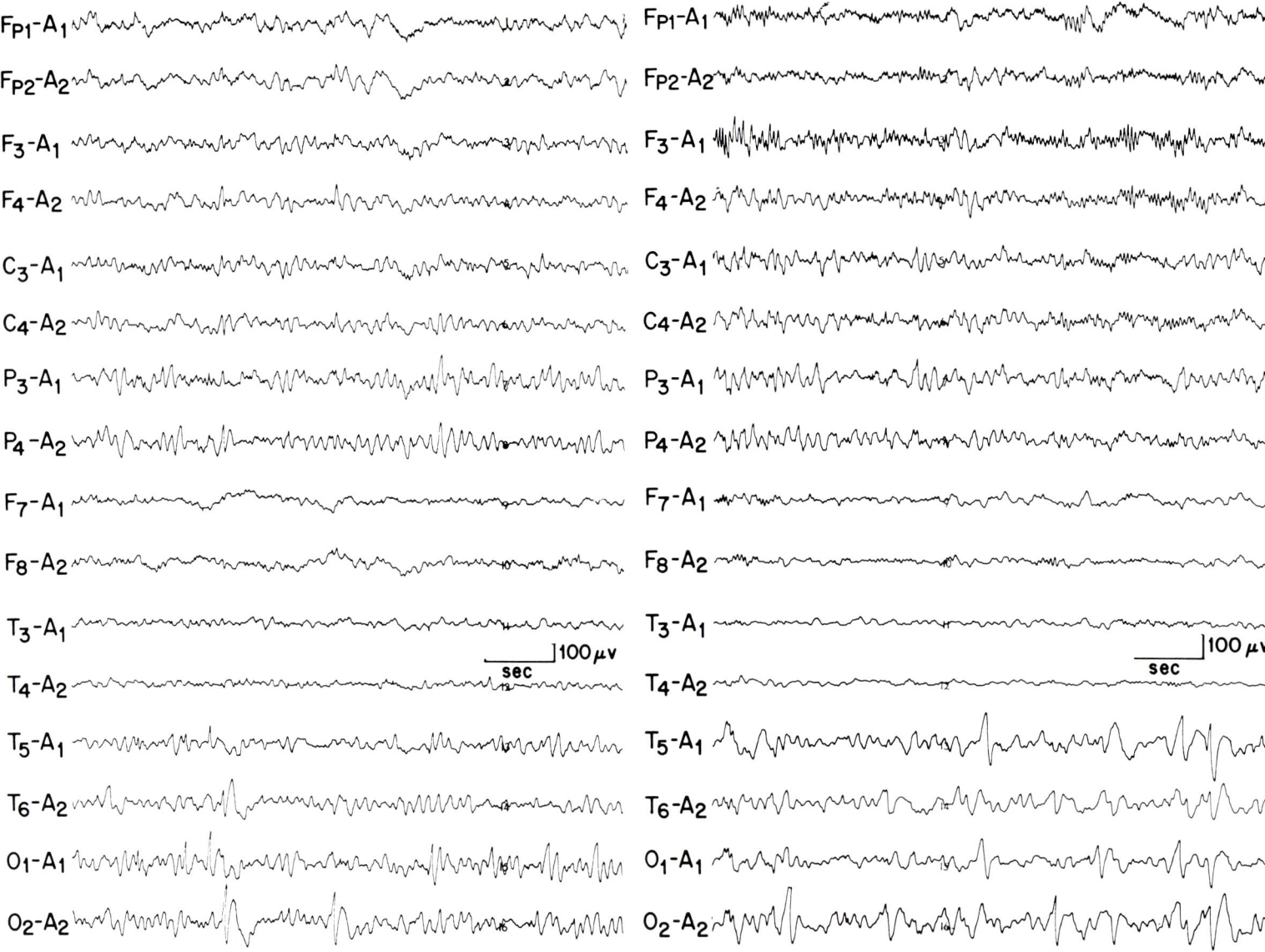

ity in the temporal region in 92% (30); in more than one-half the abnormality consisted of spikes or sharp waves. In patients with complex partial seizures and a stable persistent interictal spike focus in the temporal region, the underlying anatomical abnormality is frequently a static lesion, such as mesial temporal sclerosis due to hypoxia (45), hippocampal herniation (41), or harmartoma (45). If such patients have a homonymous hemianopsia or quadrantanopsia, perinatal occlusion of the posterior cerebral artery may have occurred (112).

Some evidence suggests that, even in the absence of seizures, the location of a spike focus correlates with behavioral defects. Lairy and Harrison (79) have noted a greater incidence of "motor problems" in children with Rolandic foci, as opposed to visual perceptive defects and oculomotor abnormalities in children with occipital foci. In children without seizures who had occipital spike foci, Smith and Kellaway (119) found ocular abnormalities in 27%.

Periodic Discharges

The most frequently seen localized periodic discharge is known under the acronym of PLED, periodic lateralized epileptiform discharge (25), or the less euphonious acronym, PPLD, pseudoperiodic lateralized paroxysmal discharge (91) (Fig. 7). Discharges are biphasic or polyphasic in form, with the initial and predominant components being surface negative. The complexes vary widely in duration, commonly lasting 100 to 200 msec. The average complex has an amplitude of 100 to 200 μV. The complexes usually repeat every 1 or 2 sec. Although they may exhibit relatively constant periodicity over a short time, prolonged observation indicates that fluctuation in the repetition rate invariably occurs. Although the spatial distribution of the electrocardiogram (EKG) differs usually, simultaneous recording of the EKG provides unequivocal differentiation. The discharges appear widely throughout one hemisphere but show maximum negativity in a smaller area. Obtundation frequently limits testing; however, PLEDs seem to show little reactivity, persisting during sleep and after eye opening or noxious stimulation. PLEDs appear out of a background of slow activity in the theta and delta range in both hemispheres. PLEDs may appear independently in each hemisphere (118) or may occur in totally unrelated episodes (91). PLEDs tend to occur only during a limited time of a few days or weeks in the acute stage of an illness and are usually replaced by focal polymorphic delta activity.

PLEDs seem to occur in a fairly stereotyped situation consisting of a depressed state of consciousness (95%), repeated focal seizures (80%), and focal neurological deficits concordant with the seizures (70%). The seizures usually begin abruptly in a patient without a previous history of epilepsy. Patients range in age from children to adults in late life. The prognosis is good with seizures ceasing spontaneously after an interval of 3 to 10 days. A wide variety of pathological disorders precipitates the process, including acute thrombotic or embolic infarction, rapidly growing metastatic tumors or gliomas, and acute necrotizing herpetic encephalitis. Bilateral independent PLEDs are most often seen with herpes encephalitis or multiple vascular lesions due to sickle cell disease. The common pathological

FIG. 5. Independent bioccipital spike foci in children with and without seizures. *Left:* A. C., a 6-year-old boy, had experienced tonic convulsions for 9 months. Surface-negative spikes appear independently at O1 and O2. Both generators extend anteriorly into the parietal and posterior temporal regions. *Right:* J. C., a 6-year-old boy, unrelated to the previous child, had a learning disorder and temper tantrums. Spikes and sharp waves appear independently in both temporooccipital regions. The child was receiving diazepam which may account for the fast activity over anterior head regions.

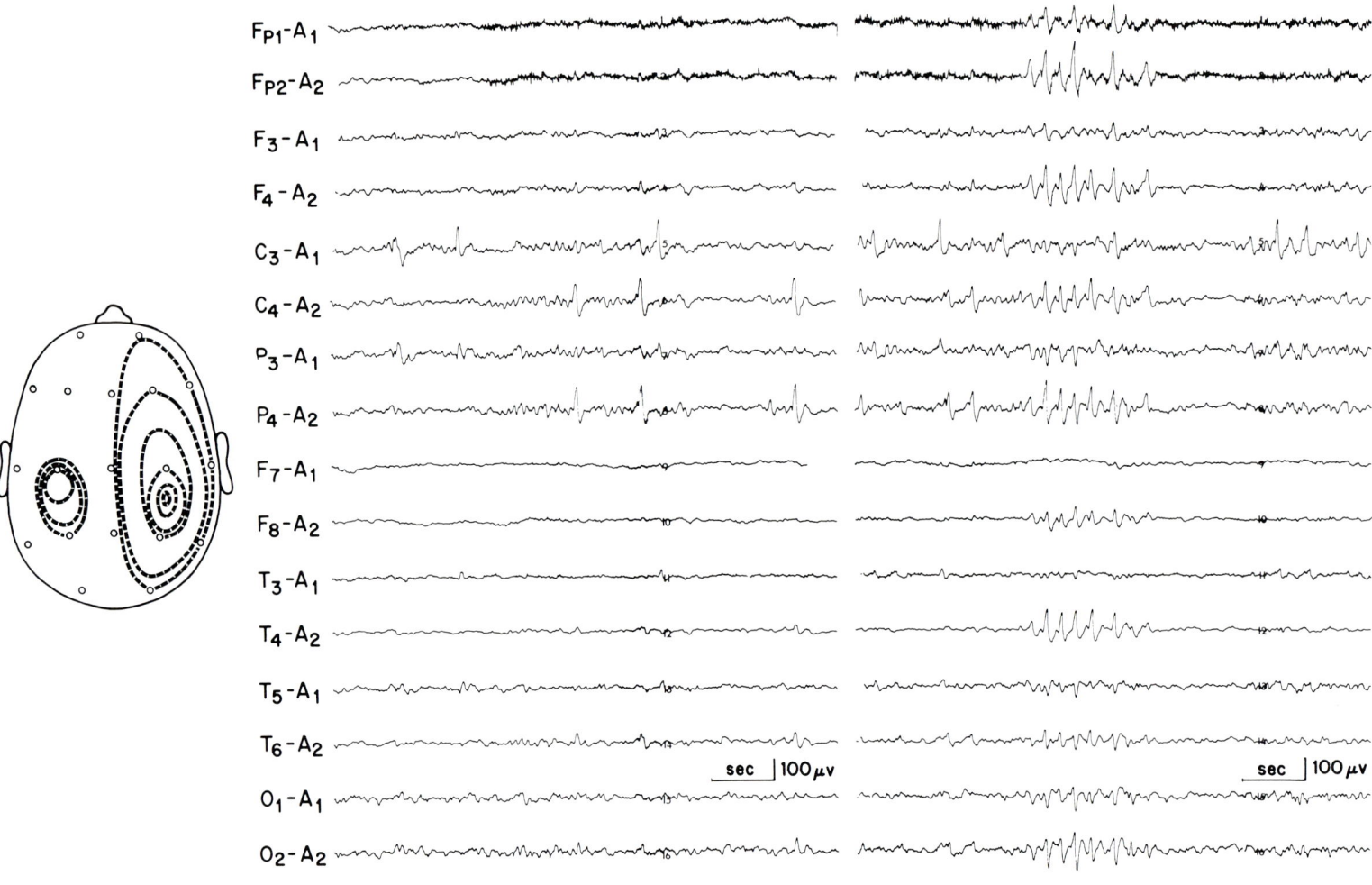

FIG. 6. Independent asymmetric spike foci. R. R., a 14-year-old girl, was the second born twin of a normal pregnancy and uncomplicated delivery. At 6 years of age she developed infrequent tonic-clonic convulsions. Examination revealed dull-normal intelligence (WISC 85) and left exotropia. Two independent spike foci appear in the parasagittal regions. In **A** the left and right foci are of approximately equal size. In **B** the right spike generator is much larger extending throughout the entire hemisphere and across the midline to the left frontal region.

substrate seems to be an acute lesion in white matter undercutting the cortex.

Tharp (122) has reported an unusual form of periodic "sharp slow-waves" occurring in children. The discharges were of relatively long duration (300 msec) and consisted of high voltage (200 μV) monophasic or diphasic surface-negative complexes over one frontal region. The complexes repeated at intervals varying from 0.5 to 2 sec. In the waking state they showed little reactivity; however, NREM sleep enhanced their periodic character. Behavior during the seizures was similar in all children and consisted of initial autonomic signs followed by agitated, frightened, and confused behavior for which the child was amnesic. The agitation was often accompanied by vocalization. Tharp suggested that the seizures arose from the orbital region of the frontal lobe. In a subsequent review of the electrographic changes seen in seizures of orbitofrontal origin, Ludwig et al. (89) have concluded that periodic discharges are uncommon and that the most commonly observed abnormalities consist of paroxysmal unilateral or bilaterally synchronous sharp waves or sharp-and-slow-wave discharges over the anterior head region. Behaviorally the seizures were either complex partial seizures with automatisms or secondarily generalized tonic-clonic convulsions.

Localized Continuous Abnormality

Polymorphic delta activity consists of slow discharges in which the morphology, amplitude, and duration vary for each wave (Fig. 8). Polymorphic delta activity generally shows no reactivity, persisting unchanged during slow-wave and rapid-eye-movement (REM) sleep (32). Localized polymorphic delta activity appears to result from deafferentation of the cortex (35). In a patient presenting with seizures the observation of polymorphic delta activity should, therefore, always raise the question of an underlying structural lesion. The pathological nature of the process cannot be predicted from the EEG. Polymorphic delta activity may occur in conjunction with neoplasms, infarctions, arteriovenous malformations, cerebral contusions, and the like. Admixtures of focal epileptiform discharge and polymorphic delta activity occur in 10% of patients with gliomas, usually slow growing and benign. However, similar abnormalities may appear with metastatic tumors even in the absence of seizures (76).

Multifocal Paroxysmal Abnormality

Multifocal Spikes

Multiple (more than two) sources of spikes appearing during a single examination are to be distinguished from shifting foci observed in serial studies over a long interval. From a study of 238 EEGs on 108 patients, Noriega-Sanchez and Markand (104) have concluded that "independent multifocal spike discharges constitute a distinct electrographic entity with a definable clinical correlation." The patients were primarily children, mean age 6 years with 96% less than 17 years of age. Almost all (94%) had seizures that were frequent, severe (tonic-clonic convulsions in 92%), and resistant to treatment. Most (82%) were retarded, and over one-half showed various neurological deficits. Almost invariably the EEG foci were bilateral and usually located in the temporal regions. In the waking record, background activity was slower than normal. Sleep augmented the spike discharges and often activated new foci. The discharges were largely nonreactive to hyperventilation and photic stimulation. Serial studies in 44 patients showed that the pattern tended to persist. In about one-fourth of patients earlier examination had disclosed hypsarrhythmia or sharp-and-slow-wave complexes (vide infra). The majority

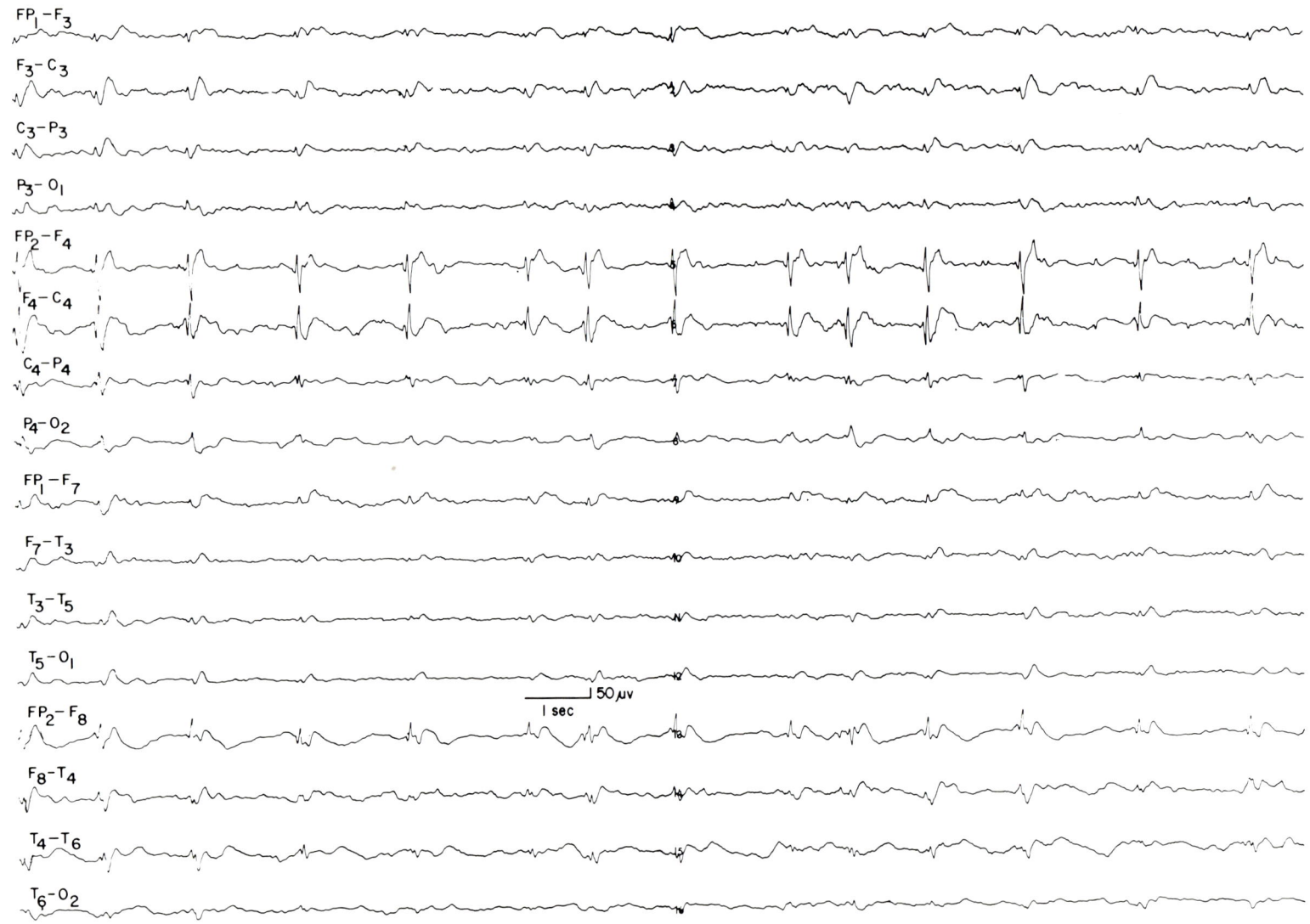

of children were found to have bilateral, multifocal, or diffuse brain disease including hydrocephalus, tuberous sclerosis, perinatal complications of asphyxia and trauma, or postnatal infections of the nervous system.

The so-called mirror focus has provided a fruitful model for experimental studies on epilepsy although its relevance to human epilepsy remains unclear (101,128). In this model, an epileptogenic focus is established in one hemisphere. After an interval of days or weeks spike discharges develop in the homologous area of the opposite hemisphere. Initially these discharges occur synchronously with the discharges at the primary lesion but, as time passes, the discharges in the secondary focus become independent.

Since independent foci of discharge in both temporal regions are commonly found in patients with complex partial seizures, the question regularly arises whether these represent independent foci resulting from multiple lesions, or a primary focus associated with a single lesion that has then led to the development of multiple independent foci by synaptic activation (18). In patients with intractable complex partial seizures the differentiation becomes crucial if the patient is a candidate for surgical intervention to control seizures. The question proves a highly complex one that admits of no simple answer; however, the outlines of an answer appear to be emerging. Engle, Driver, and Falconer (44) have observed that patients with mesial temporal sclerosis have EEGs characterized by a primary spike focus in the medial temporal region, as determined by sphenoidal electrodes, together with independent, contralateral, and extratemporal foci. One-third of these patients also show an ipsilateral decrease in fast activity induced by intravenous administration of barbiturates. Patients with other medial temporal lesions, mostly hamartomas, show similar primary medial temporal foci. In contrast, patients with large scars in the lateral convexity of the temporal lobes demonstrate their foci in scalp electrodes over the lateral convexity and never develop independent secondary foci. Studies using implanted electrodes, electrocorticography, or both, serve to emphasize the disparities between scalp recordings and electrical activity in the depths of the brain (125). Since major questions remain unanswered, the electroencephalographer should use caution in interpreting the significance of bilateral but independent temporal spike foci.

Hypsarrhythmia

In 1952, the Gibbses (56) introduced the term "hypsarrhythmia" to refer to a profoundly disorganized EEG characterized by slow background rhythms with spikes and sharp waves of varying morphology and amplitude occurring in a chaotic fashion from multiple foci in both hemispheres (Fig. 9). Hypsarrhythmia is almost invariably (95%) associated with infantile spasms (70). Infantile spasms are themselves an age-specific type of seizure in response to a wide variety of multifocal or diffuse brain diseases. They appear in two-thirds of cases by 6 months of age and in 90% during the first year of life (23). On the other hand, only about two-thirds of children presenting with infantile spasms show hypsarrhythmia in their initial EEG. The remaining children usually show better organized sharp-and-slow-wave discharges. Depending on the nature of the antecedent

---

FIG. 7. Pseudoperiodic lateralized discharge. A. L., a 65-year-old alcoholic man, was admitted to the hospital after being found in an unresponsive state by his landlady. Examination revealed obtundation and left hemiparesis. Elementary partial motor seizures involving the left upper extremity and left side of the face occurred at intervals of 15 to 60 min. Recording was made approximately 24 hr after admission. Radioisotope brain scan revealed a wedge-shaped area of increased uptake compatible with an acute infarction in the right parietal area. The patient recovered and was asymptomatic on discharge.

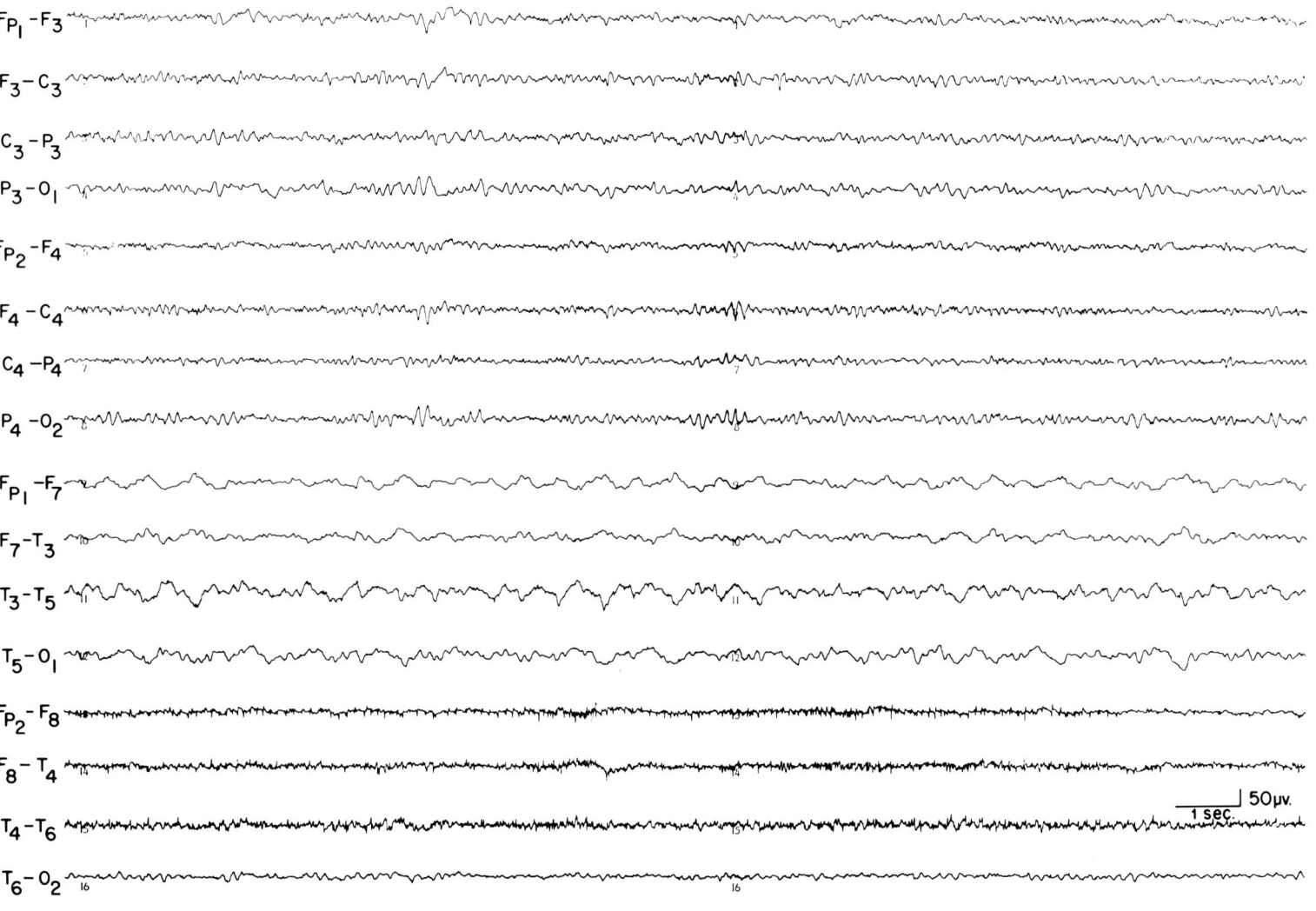

FIG. 8. Focal polymorphic delta activity. D. L., a 46-year-old woman, had experienced complex partial seizures for 8 years. The patient described epigastric "quivering" and a formed visual hallucination of fish swimming in front of her eyes followed by automatism. Examination disclosed interictal aphasia. Operation revealed a glioma in the left temporal lobe. Polymorphic delta appears throughout the left temporal region with irregular slow waves up to 100 μV. Slow waves appear most conspicuously in the anterior to middle temporal region.

insult, hypsarrthymia may evolve from a variety of abnormal EEG patterns in the neonatal and postnatal period—low voltage EEGs, burst-suppression, diffuse slow activity, or multifocal sharp waves (126). Usually by 5 years of age hypsarrhythmia disappears and is replaced either by a normal EEG (55%) or by other types of epileptiform abnormality (36%) (71,104). The association of hypsarrhythmia alternating with periods of flattening, so-called burst-suppression pattern, carries a grave prognosis with high mortality (52%) and little likelihood of normal intelligence (90). A wide variety of neuropathological processes have been reported in these patients including congenital anomalies, perinatal damage, storage diseases, and tuberous sclerosis (73). Huttenlocher (67) has reported a series of patients whose brains appeared grossly and microscopically normal save with heavy metal stains that revealed a decrease in the numbers and branching of dendrites suggesting defective dendritic growth.

Generalized Paroxysmal Abnormality

Three-Hz Spike-and-Slow-Wave ("Classical") Complexes

"Spike-wave bursts" are more often remarked on than carefully described. After studying tracings from 200 patients, Weir (127) has concluded that recognition of only two components in the spike-and-slow-wave complex is an oversimplification. Instead he has observed that the complex usually consists of two surface-negative spikes, a rather long enduring positive transient, and a final surface-negative wave. The initial spike is of low amplitude (25 to 50 μV), short duration (about 10 msec), and appears 5 to 10 msec after the beginning of the positive transient. The second surface-negative spike, the "typical" spike, attains maximum negativity 50 to 60 msec after the first and lasts 40 to 60 msec, occasionally as long as 90 msec. The amplitude, usually maximal in the early part of the burst, may exceed 600 μV. The second spike is most prominent over frontal regions, in contrast to the first spike, which is maximal over the centrotemporal regions. The positive transient attains its maximal voltage within 15 to 20 msec and lasts from 100 to 150 msec, blending into the final, more prominent, surface-negative wave (Figs. 10 and 18; the two spike components are clearly seen in the latter figure). Chatrian et al. (26) have shown that prolonged surface-negative DC potential changes, "paroxysmal negative shifts," invariably accompany bursts of spike-wave discharge. The shifts begin with the onset of the burst and reach a maximal voltage, averaging 350 μV, after 1 to 5 sec. The spatial distribution of the shift parallels that of the slow-wave component of the spike-and-slow-wave discharge and is maximal over the frontal region.

The repetition rate of the complex varies, being highest at the beginning of the burst and gradually slowing as the burst continues. The initial complexes usually repeat at rates between 3 and 4/sec, the majority being between 3 and 3.5/sec (102,117).

The complexes show marked reactivity, being inhibited by eye opening and states of alertness (63). Sleep induces striking changes (Fig. 10). During NREM or slow-wave sleep, marked augmentation occurs with the burst incidence steadily increasing to the deepest levels (stages III to IV) (102,114,117). In contrast, the burst duration becomes increasingly short. Stevens et al. (120) have shown that the burst duration changes from a Gaussian or unimodal distribution during wakefulness to a Poisson distribution, in which extremely short bursts are most frequent, during sleep. As the depth of sleep increases the complexes become increasingly irregular and multiple spikes replace the usual single large spike. The repetition rate of the complexes slows to 1.5 to 2.5/sec, and the bursts tend to recur

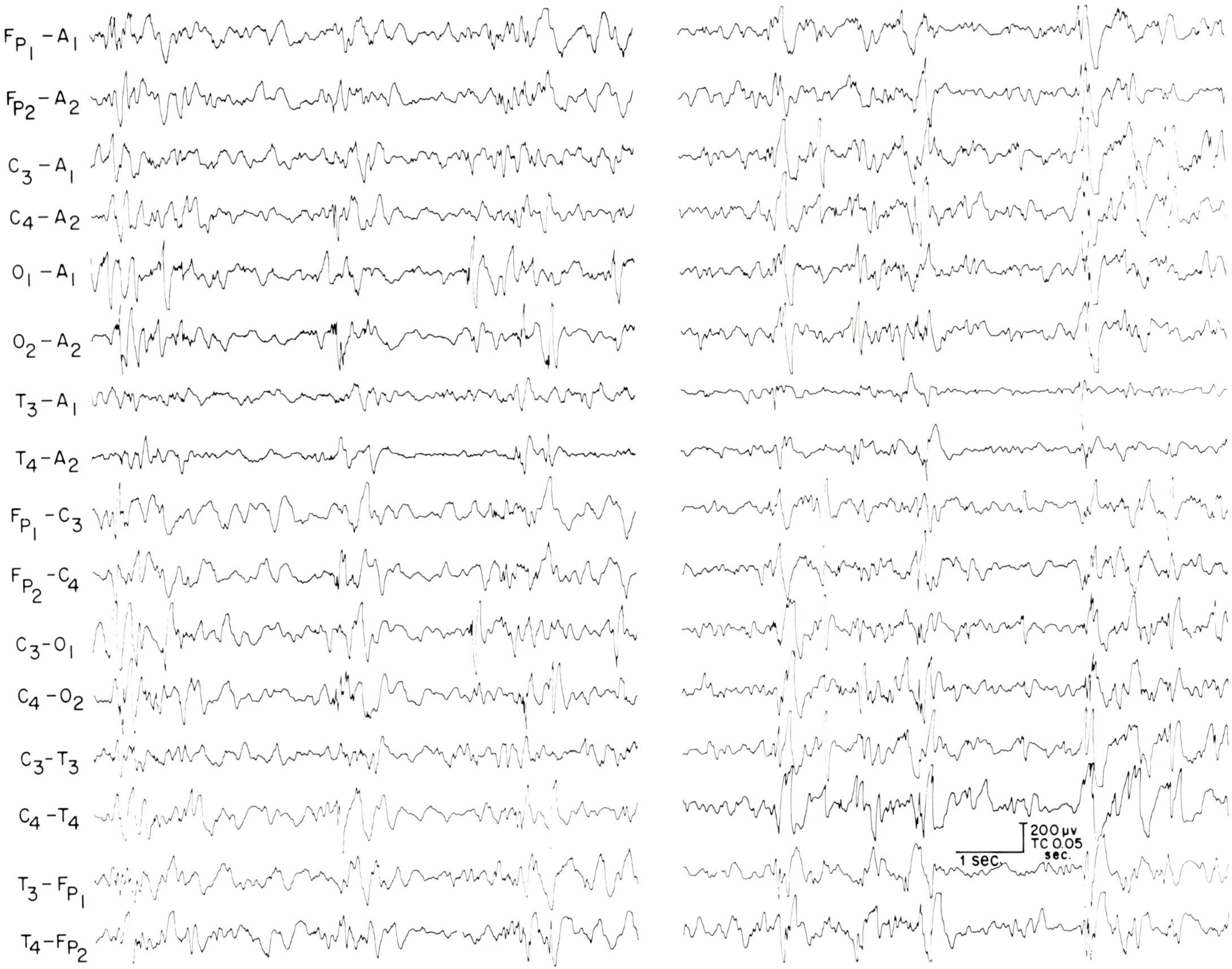

$F_{P_1}-A_1$

$F_{P_2}-A_2$

C_3-A_1

C_4-A_2

O_1-A_1

O_2-A_2

T_3-A_1

T_4-A_2

$F_{P_1}-C_3$

$F_{P_2}-C_4$

C_3-O_1

C_4-O_2

C_3-T_3

C_4-T_4

$T_3-F_{P_1}$

$T_4-F_{P_2}$

200 μV
TC 0.05 sec.
1 sec.

periodically at intervals of 2 or 3 sec. With the onset of REM sleep a dramatic change occurs. The burst incidence falls to slightly below that in the waking state whereas the morphology and duration of the complexes resemble those in waking. Hyperventilation activates the EEG in a high percentage of patients and frequently induces clinical absence (31).

The association of absence seizures with 3-Hz spike-and-slow-wave bursts was one of the early and important contributions to electroencephalography (55). Because of the frequent spontaneous occurrence of absences and their ready induction with hyperventilation, the electroclinical correlations of these seizures have been particularly well studied. Often regarded as the archetype, "simple" absence is in fact a rare form making up less than 10% of absence seizures (108). On the other hand, automatisms, defined as "one or more complex movements," occur in almost two-thirds of absences. Lip-smacking, chewing, and fumbling with the hands are the most common actions (Fig. 18). Impaired responsiveness is the earliest behavioral accompaniment of spike-and-slow-wave bursts. Altered auditory reaction time coincides with the onset of spike-and-slow-wave discharges in 43% of patients, and within 0.5 sec normal reaction times occur in only 20%. Responsiveness returns during the later stages of the paroxysm, and after 4 sec of spike-and-slow-wave discharge, 52% of reaction times are normal (19). In contrast, disruption of more complex behavior, for example, during continuous performance tests, correlates with the duration of the paroxysms and is almost invariably observed in bursts lasting longer than 3 sec (62). Automatisms also relate to burst duration, being seen in almost one-half of seizures lasting more than 6 sec and in 90% of seizures lasting more than 12 sec (108). Clonic twitches occur in about half the patients, almost invariably involving the eyelids and occurring synchronously with the spike component. Clonic twitches occur early in the seizure and usually in attacks of shorter duration (108).

Prolonged periods of spike-wave discharge lasting from ½ hr to 2 days have been referred to as absence status, petit mal status, or spike-wave stupor (8). The impairment of consciousness may range from subjective impairment to deep stupor (Fig. 11). Patients may exhibit confusion, disorientation, inappropriate behavior, variable amnesia, and incontinence. A tonic-clonic convulsion may initiate, interrupt, or terminate absence status. Absence status tends to be a late manifestation of primary generalized epilepsy, and may be the only seizure pattern or occur in patients who also have absences or generalized convulsions.

Terminological confusion has beset attempts to classify the epilepsy associated with 3-Hz spike-and-slow-wave paroxysms. Penfield and Jasper (106) proposed the term "centrencephalic seizures," the "centrencephalon" being defined as a "reticular system" extending from medulla to thalamus but specifically *excluding* cerebral cortex. In contrast, Doose et al. (39) have spoken of "centrencephalic myoclonic-astatic petit mal." The use of this term appears unfortunate since the authors remark that "in most cases dementia develops." Under these circumstances, the neuronal pathology must involve the cerebral cortex as well as any postulated "centrencephalon," clearly an observation inconsistent with the usual course of children with absences. Over the years, an increasing body of evidence (10,

FIG. 9. Hypsarrhythmia. *Left:* T. B., a 6-month-old infant, had developed massive myoclonus 3 weeks previously. Note the generalized slowing of background with paroxysms of high voltage slowing and multifocal spikes. *Right:* B. M., a 6-month-old infant, had developed seizures in the perinatal period and at the time of examination showed severe motor retardation. The EEGs of the two infants are strikingly similar despite the fact that the former had only recently developed seizures.

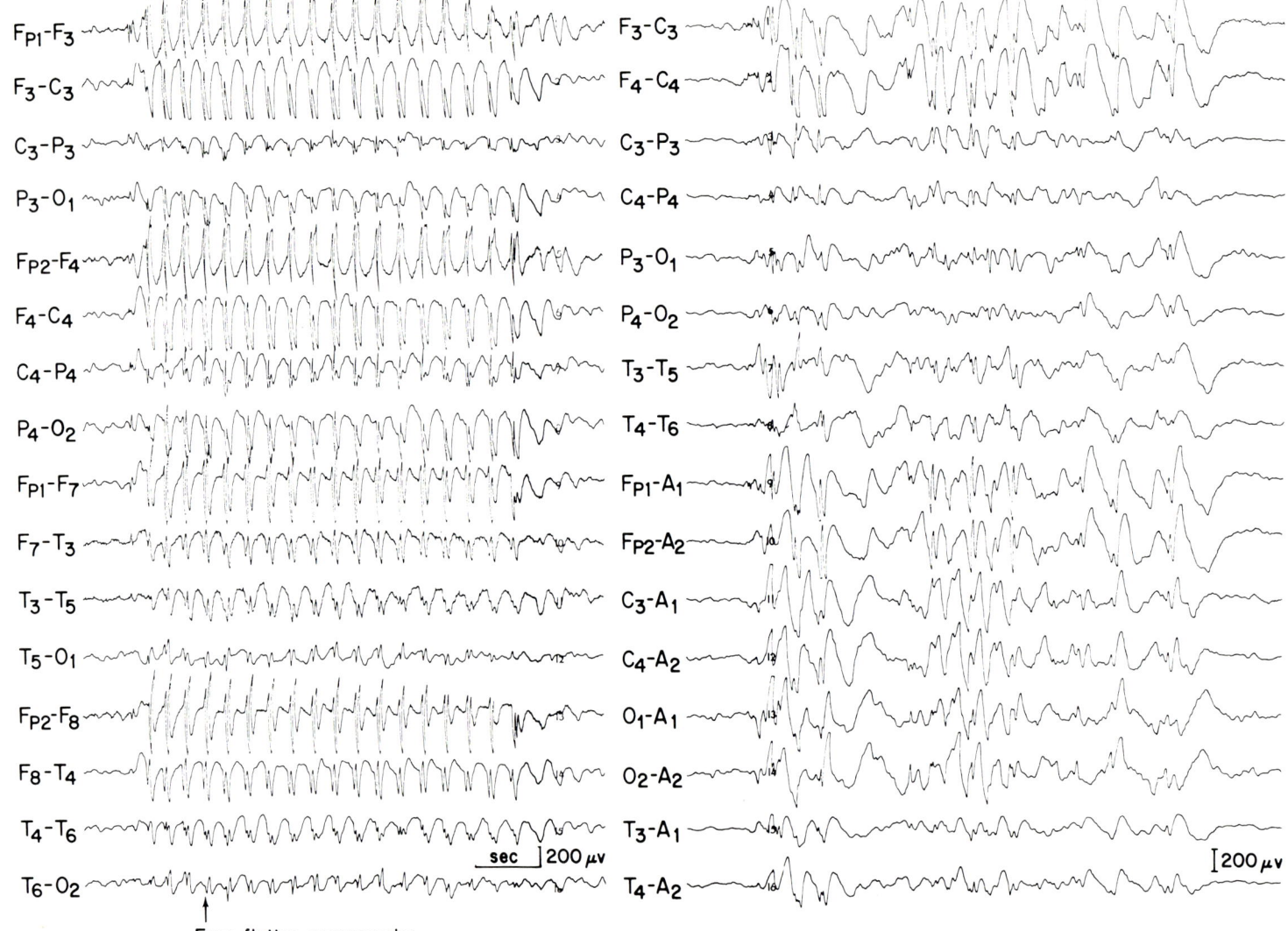

11,57) has indicated that cortical mechanisms do play a major, perhaps sole, role in the physiopathogenesis of these seizures. Gloor (57) has proposed the term "generalized cortico-reticular epilepsies," with one subvariety being the "genetic form" associated with 3-Hz spike-and-slow-wave, whereas Niedermeyer (102) has suggested "common generalized epilepsy." The International Classification adopts the noncommital term "primary generalized epilepsies" (95), which probably represents a better choice in the light of existing gaps in our knowledge.

The role of heredity in patients with absence seizures has long been recognized; however, the advent of EEG permitted recognition of paroxysmal abnormalities in the EEG of asymptomatic relatives. Metrakos and Metrakos (96) have studied kinships in which the proband suffered "generalized cortico-reticular epilepsy" and the EEG showed 3-Hz spike-and-slow-wave complexes. They concluded that the occurrence of such paroxysms reflected a monogenetic factor with age-specific penetrance maximal between 4 and 16 years of age. At such ages, almost one-half of siblings had spike-and-slow-wave bursts although only 12% had clinical seizures (97) (Fig. 12). The EEG of the offspring of probands likewise showed a high (35%) incidence of paroxysms. Because they had passed beyond the age of maximal risk, the parents of probands showed a lower incidence of the electrographic trait. The Metrakoses have concluded that the disorder is transmitted as an autosomal dominant trait with age-specific penetrance. Doose et al. (38) have challenged the concept of single-gene inheritance, arguing "that several genetic factors are responsible, some mutually independent and some either reinforcing or inhibiting the others." It seems likely that this latter study deals with a somewhat different, perhaps nonhomogeneous, population of patients since a subset in their study suffered from a "centrencephalic type of Lennox syndrome . . ." (see following section on sharp-and-slow-wave complexes). Furthermore, this terminology, which consists of mixed eponyms and nominalized postulates, seems more likely to obscure than illuminate the delineation of specific populations. The studies by both groups have been somewhat uncritical in accepting all paroxysmal responses induced by photic stimulation. Reilly and Peters (111) have demonstrated two types of photoparoxysmal responses, only one of which correlates significantly with epilepsy. Studies of children with "simple" febrile convulsions have suggested that a similar or identical genetic factor may be operating. Serial studies of such children over intervals of several years have shown that paroxysmal abnormalities in the EEG appear at 2 to 5 years of age. The most common type is 3-Hz spike-and-slow-waves, which occur in one-third to one-half of patients (80). In this group of children, the paroxysmal discharges tend to appear at an earlier age than in primary generalized epilepsy. Lindsay (81) has suggested that severe febrile convulsions (status) that cause hypoxia may result in selective anoxic damage to the hippocampus (94), mesial temporal sclerosis, and the subsequent development of complex partial seizures. In such instances, a hereditary factor is a necessary but not sufficient link in a more complicated chain of events. These various observations emphasize the incompleteness of our knowledge and the uncertain significance of EEG "signs." Finally, the electroencephalographer should recall that, although these paroxysms may constitute a meaningful "genetic marker," the EEG does not serve as a reliable predictor for the development of seizures.

FIG. 10. Three-Hz spike-and-slow-wave paroxysms. A. C., a 7-year-old girl had had absences for 6 months. The maternal grandmother and a cousin have had convulsions. *Left:* Awake. A spontaneous absence occurs at the point marked by the arrow. The technician noted fluttering of the eyes. The child was unresponsive to a test phase and after the attack was amnesic. *Right:* NREM sleep. The same patient during stage III slow-wave sleep. See text for details.

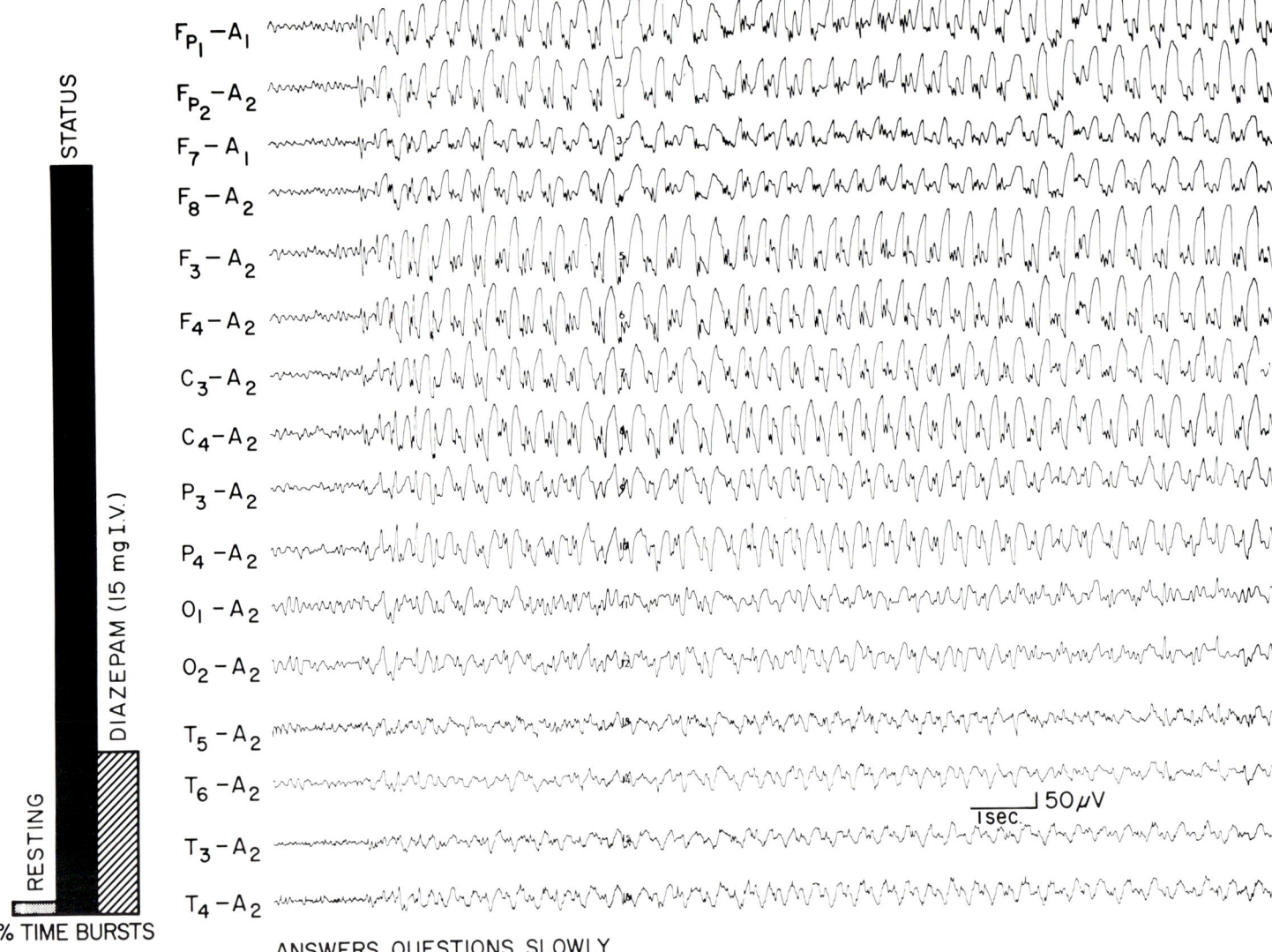

Multiple-Spikes-and-Slow-Wave Complexes

Bursts of multiple spikes followed by a slow-wave repeating at rates of 2 to 3/sec occur interictally and ictally in patients with myoclonic seizures (Fig. 13). The term *myoclonus* has been applied to a variety of movements but is used here to refer to sudden, brief, intense, and involuntary contractions of muscles. The contractions may be symmetric and widespread or limited to an extremity (49). Halliday (64) has proposed that myoclonus results from discharge in the reticular formation of the lower brainstem that "forms part of a generalized non-somatotopic system, subserving the startle response, and . . . is closely integrated with a 'higher level' cortical reflex loop, involving the medial lemniscus, sensorimotor cortex and the corticoreticular fibers." Myoclonic seizures might, thus, be expected to occur in a heterogeneous group of diseases having in common multifocal or diffuse neuronal disease involving both cerebral cortex and brainstem structures. The classification of myoclonic epilepsies has occasioned extensive discussion since some of the diseases are static whereas others are progressive, and some are hereditary whereas others are sporadic (22).

Several recent electroclinical studies have contributed significantly to classification of the myoclonic epilepsies. Loiseau et al. (83) have applied the technique of numerical taxonomy, a statistical method that aims at grouping cases that have in common the greatest number of features. Using this method in the study of 220 patients with myoclonic seizures, they were able to classify 139 patients into three distinct groups. The largest group (100 patients) consisted largely of females who had developed myoclonic seizures after 10 years of age followed almost invariably (87%) a few years later by generalized tonic-clonic convulsions. Both types of seizures characteristically occurred upon awakening. In addition, 22% of the patients had typical absences, and a family history of epilepsy was present in 14%. Intelligence was normal. The interictal EEG showed bursts of multiple-spike-and-slow-waves or brief bursts of "irregular" 3-Hz spike-and-slow-waves. Paroxysms were readily induced by hyperventilation (40%) and intermittent photic stimulation (30%). In a minority of patients (15%), eye closure induced an attack (compare Fig. 18). This group is readily identified with similar groups reported under various names: genetic form of "cortico-reticular epilepsy" (57), "generalized epilepsy of adolescence with myoclonic jerks" (2), "waking epilepsy" of Janz (69), "typical form of common generalized epilepsies" (102), or group II of Aigner and Mulder (3).

The second group comprised 22 patients, predominantly male, whose myoclonic seizures began before the age of 5 years. Seizures tended to be frequent prolonged episodes of generalized myoclonic jerking. Surprisingly, tonic-clonic convulsions occurred in only one-third of patients. Approximately one-half of these patients were mentally retarded. The interictal EEG showed bursts of irregular spike-and-slow-wave complexes of variable duration that were less well organized than the paroxysms of 3-Hz spike-and-slow-waves. Paroxysms with multiple spikes occurred relatively infrequently. The interictal EEG was relatively nonreactive being infrequently activated

---

FIG. 11. Absence status. D. H., a 49-year-old man, since childhood had suffered absence seizures that in adult life had become relatively infrequent. About every 2 months he would experience a day in which he would make many errors at work, appear mildly confused or slow to answer to his wife, and have patchy amnesia. At widely separated intervals he had had three tonic-clonic convulsions. Recording was made on a "bad day." Note prolonged bursts of spike-and-slow-wave discharges, which occupied about 75% of the recording time. Patient answered questions slowly but correctly, usually monosyllabically. In the interictal recordings on "good days" spike-and-slow-wave bursts occurred about 2 to 3% of the time. Intravenous diazepam markedly reduced the percent time of spike-and-slow-wave bursts and was accompanied by a clearing of consciousness.

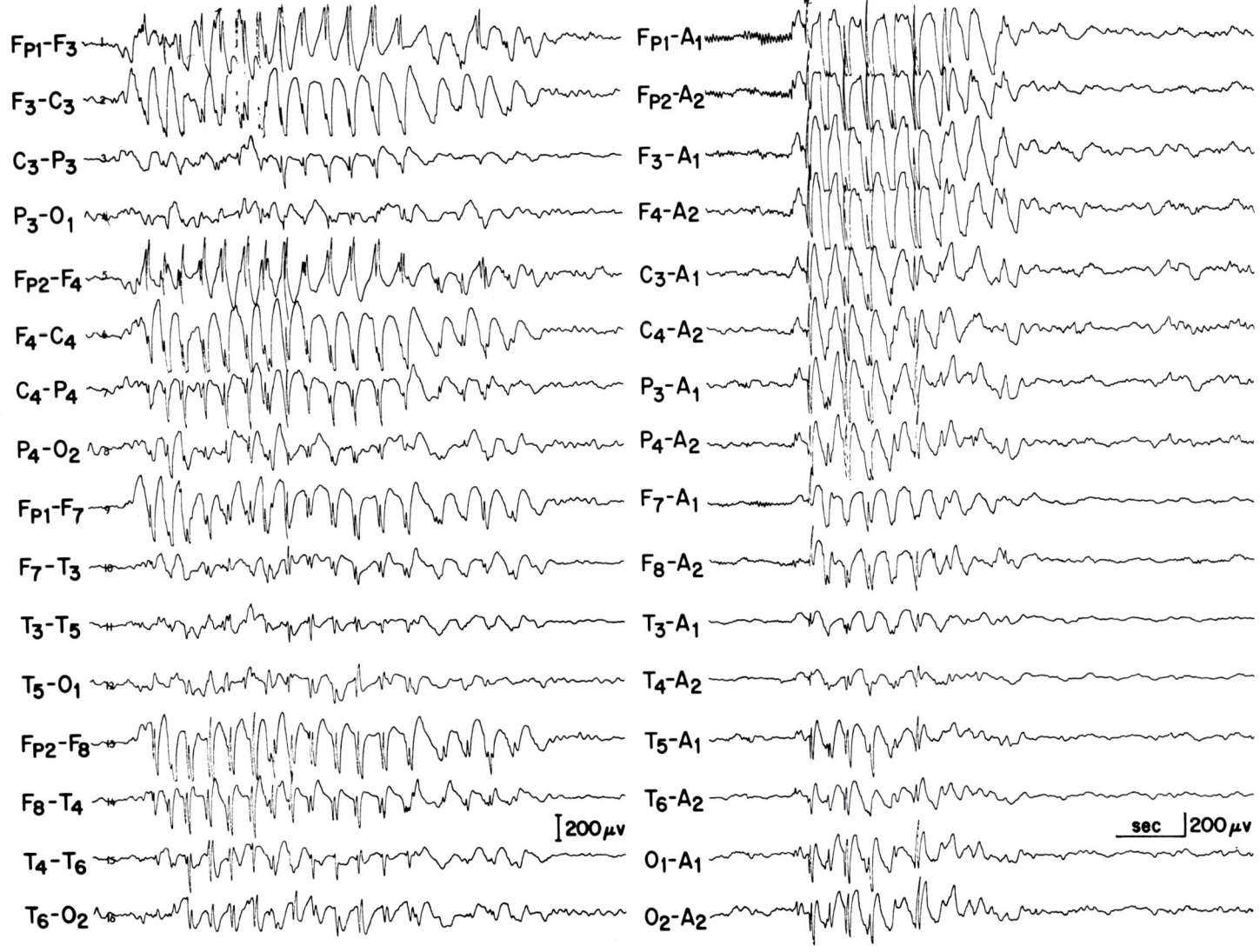

FIG. 12. Three-Hz spike-and-slow-wave bursts in siblings. *Left:* C. L. C., a 12-year-old boy had had absences since 4 years of age. He had never had a convulsion. *Right:* C. R. C., his 9-year-old brother has never had any recognizable absence.

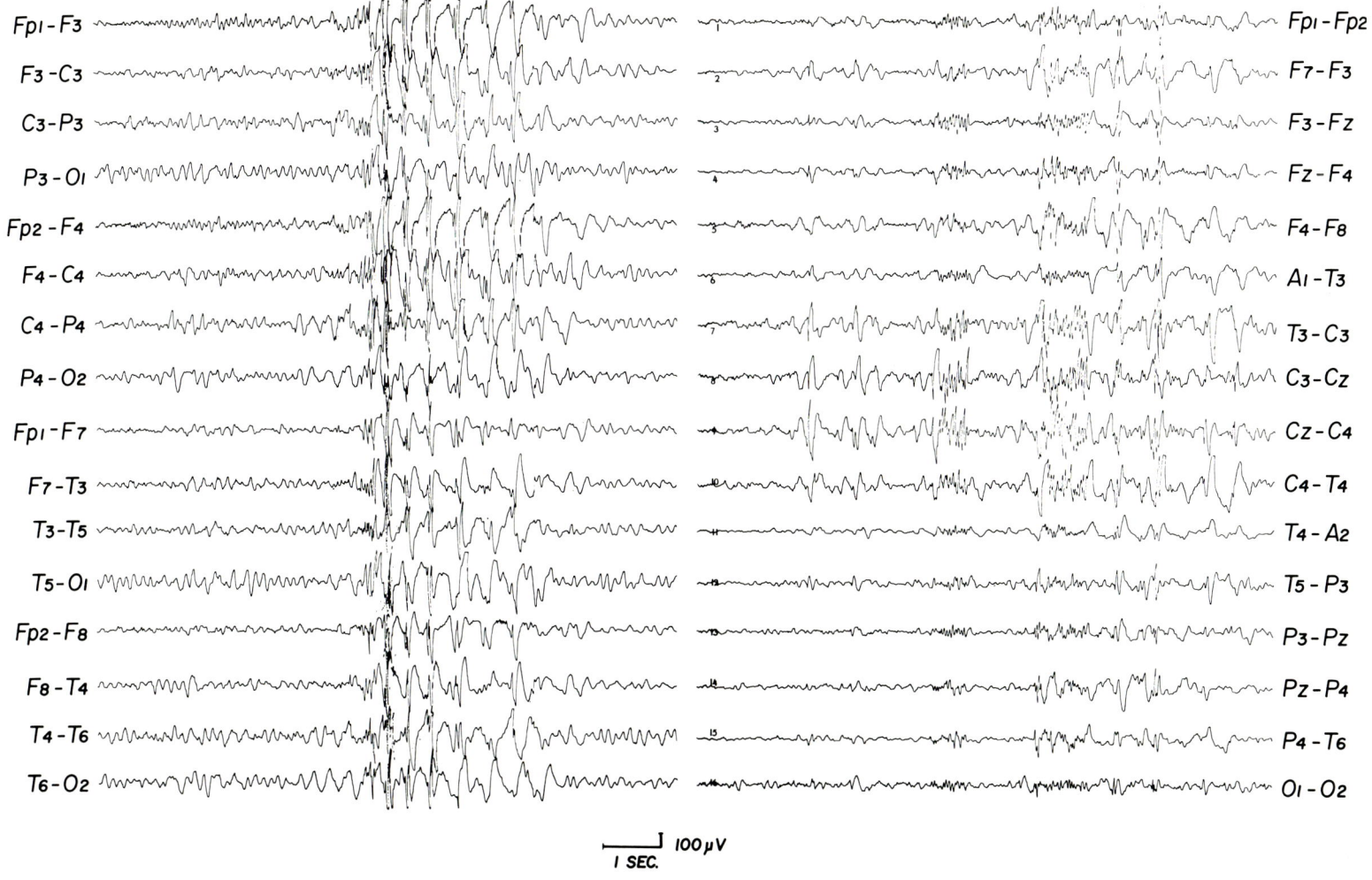

FIG. 13. Multiple spikes and slow waves. H. E., an 8-year-old girl, had developed diurnal myoclonic seizures at age 5 without antecedent illness. No convulsions had occurred, and there was no family history of epilepsy. *Left:* Recording in the waking state. Note bursts of multiple spikes at the onset of the paroxysm followed by slowly repeating complexes of multiple spikes and slow waves. *Right:* Recording during slow-wave sleep using transverse montage. Note bursts of multiple spikes at the vertex in association with vertex waves; Neidermeyer (102) terms this "dyshormia." The more diffuse multiple spikes also appear related to vertex waves.

by sleep or intermittent photic stimulation and responding indifferently to hyperventilation. This category appears to correspond reasonably well with the "myoclonic petit mal" of Aicardi and Chevrie (2) and to relate to some of the patients classified as "centrencephalic myoclonic-astatic petit mal" (39).

The third group of Loiseau et al. (83) consisted largely of girls whose myoclonic seizures began before age 5. Seizures were frequent and usually were single, generalized jerks or jerks limited to the upper extremities, without loss of consciousness. Convulsions occurred rarely. Intelligence was normal, and a family history of epilepsy was reported infrequently. The interictal EEG showed frequent bursts of multiple spikes and slow waves or irregular 3-Hz spike-and-slow-waves. The EEG showed no response to activation procedures. The background activity between the paroxysms tended to be persistently slow. This group has uncertain identity. The patient in Fig. 13 has some of the features of this group; however, the background rhythms are not slow. Loiseau et al. (83) suggest that it resembles the "cryptogenic myoclonic epilepsy of childhood" of Aicardi and Chevrie; however, these latter authors have noted a 75% incidence of retardation in this category and also regarded it as a "nonhomogeneous group" (2).

The 81 unclassifiable cases in this study included *all* 23 cases diagnosed clinically as "Lennox-Gastaut syndrome" (51). The significance of this finding emerges in the following section. "Myoclonus epilepsy with progressive encephalopathy" encompasses a heterogeneous group of diseases including hereditary disorders such as lipidoses, the Ramsay-Hunt syndrome, Lafora body disease, as well as sporadic disorders such as subacute sclerosing panencephalitis (SSPE) and subacute spongiform encephalopathy or Creutzfeldt-Jakob disease (22).

Sharp-and-Slow-Wave Complexes ("Slow Spike-and-Wave")

It was early recognized that complexes composed of sharp waves with a duration of 100 to 200 msec and slow waves of 350 msec that repeat slowly at 1.5 to 2.0 Hz could be distinguished from the more rapid 3-Hz spike-and-slow-wave complexes. Subsequently, Lennox pointed out that these complexes occurred in children who had ictal symptoms differing from those in primary generalized epilepsy and who were often retarded. For this reason the term "petit mal variant" was initially applied to the EEG abnormalities, whereas the clinical syndrome has been described under various names: "Lennox syndrome," "childhood epileptic encephalopathy" (51), and "centrencephalic myoclonic-astatic petit mal" (39). Subsequent studies (17,83) have confirmed that this consists of a heterogeneous group of patients, having in common onset of seizures in the second or third year of life, severe multifocal or diffuse brain disease, and a poor outcome, in terms both of survival rate (88% after 12 years) and of mental retardation (85 to 90%). The incidence of sharp-and-slow-wave complexes is greatest between 2 and 6 years of age and falls off rapidly thereafter, rarely being seen after age 15 (17). The interictal electroencephalographic abnormality (Fig. 14) has been reviewed in detail by Gastaut et al. (51). The background activity between the paroxysms is usually (80%) excessively slow. The paroxysms occur in prolonged bursts and at times may occupy almost

FIG. 14. Sharp-and-slow-wave complexes. A. B., a 5½-year-old full-term dizygotic twin, developed tonic seizures at age 4 months, myoclonic and atonic seizures at age 6 months, and progressive dementia. Etiology was unknown. No behavioral changes were noted during this prolonged burst. Note variability of the sharp-wave component.

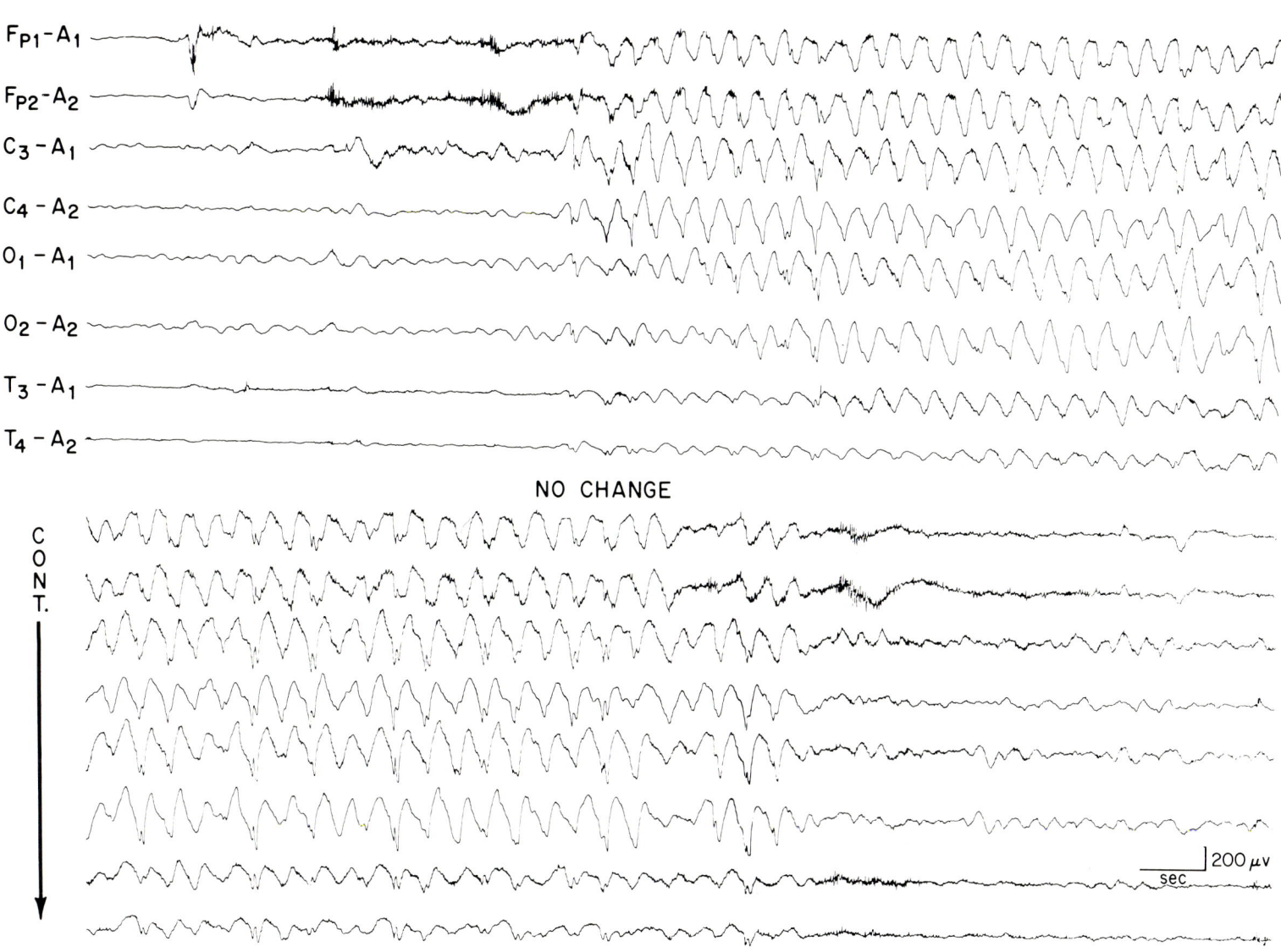

the entire recording. They usually appear diffusely and bisynchronously but at times may be asymmetric. Intermixed with these slow paroxysms may be bursts of fast spike-and-slow-waves (27). Sleep markedly activates the EEG, particularly during NREM sleep (17,51). However, the abnormality is relatively unreactive to hyperventilation and nonreactive to photic stimulation.

Various seizures occur in these children. At younger ages, tonic seizures predominate whereas in older children "atypical absences" (for description see Gastaut and Broughton, ref. 49), myoclonic seizures, and tonic-clonic convulsions replace these (27). In a varying percentage (5 to 25%) of patients, the syndrome develops in children who previously had had infantile spasms with a "hypsarrhythmic" EEG.

In the light of published data, it appears best to regard this syndrome as a nonspecific one related more to the age of the patient and severity of the brain disease than to a specific entity (27).

Secondary Bilateral Synchrony

The concept of secondary bilateral synchrony was introduced by Penfield and Jasper (105) to explain the observation that some patients with unilateral lesions, often on the medial surface of the frontal lobe, exhibited bursts of bilateral discharges in the EEG. The modifier, secondary, signified that the bilateral discharge presumably resulted from secondary excitation of the postulated centrencephalon by unilateral cortical discharge. In a subsequent paper (124) Jasper suggested that the bisynchronous discharges were "often of an irregular spike-and-wave form, with frequencies of 2 to 4 per second." He also noted that differential recordings revealed "a peak voltage at the mid-line or near the mid-line on the side of the lesion." This latter point made by Tükel and Jasper has often been overlooked subsequently. The use of montages employing anteroposterior differential derivations in the parasaggital area can give the false impression of bisynchronous discharge when, in fact, there exists only a single large unilateral generator that extends across the midline. This possibility can be readily resolved by employing transverse montages with midline electrodes (Fig. 15).

In recent years, the intraarterial injection of pentylenetetrazol (Metrazol®) or amobarbital (sodium Amytal®) into the carotid and vertebral arteries has done much to clarify the problem (57,59). In the case of a unilateral lesion, injection of amobarbital into the ipsilateral carotid artery suppresses discharge bilaterally, whereas injection into the contralateral carotid artery has little effect other than reducing the spike component on the side of injection (115). In primary generalized epilepsies, intracarotid injection of pentylenetetrazol on either side induces generalized discharge, whereas injection into the vertebral artery is without effect (57), supporting the

FIG. 15. Apparent bisynchronous paroxysms from single generators. T. S., a 14-year-old girl, had suffered a birth injury with right hemiparesis. At age 6 years complex partial seizures with automatisms developed, followed 2 years later by secondarily generalized tonic-clonic convulsions, initiated with loss of consciousness and turning of the head and eyes to the right. **A:** Montage using referential recording to the ipsilateral ears. Note what appear to be generalized discharges, some of which appear predominantly over frontal regions. A slight amplitude asymmetry exists with higher voltages on the left. **B:** Transverse montage demonstrating two foci that may fire independently or together. The first focus shows phase reversals (maximum negativity) at F3, as indicated by upward and downward pointing arrows. The generator extends across the midline *(first head diagram)* producing the apparent bisynchrony seen in referential recording. A separate generator discharges at the vertex as indicated by the arrows. The generator extends symmetrically to C3 and C4 *(second head diagram)*. **D:** At times, the generators fire synchronously.

Fp1-A1
Fp2-A2
F3-A1
F4-A2
C3-A1
C4-A2
P3-A1
P4-A2
F7-A1
F8-A2
T3-A1
T4-A2
T5-A1
T6-A2
O1-A1
O2-A2
75µv
sec
A
Fp1-Fp2
F7-F3
F3-FZ
FZ-F4
F4-F8
A1-T3
T3-C3
C3-CZ
CZ-C4
C4-T4
T4-A2
T5-P3
P3-PZ
PZ-P4
P4-T6
O1-O2
200µv
B
C
D

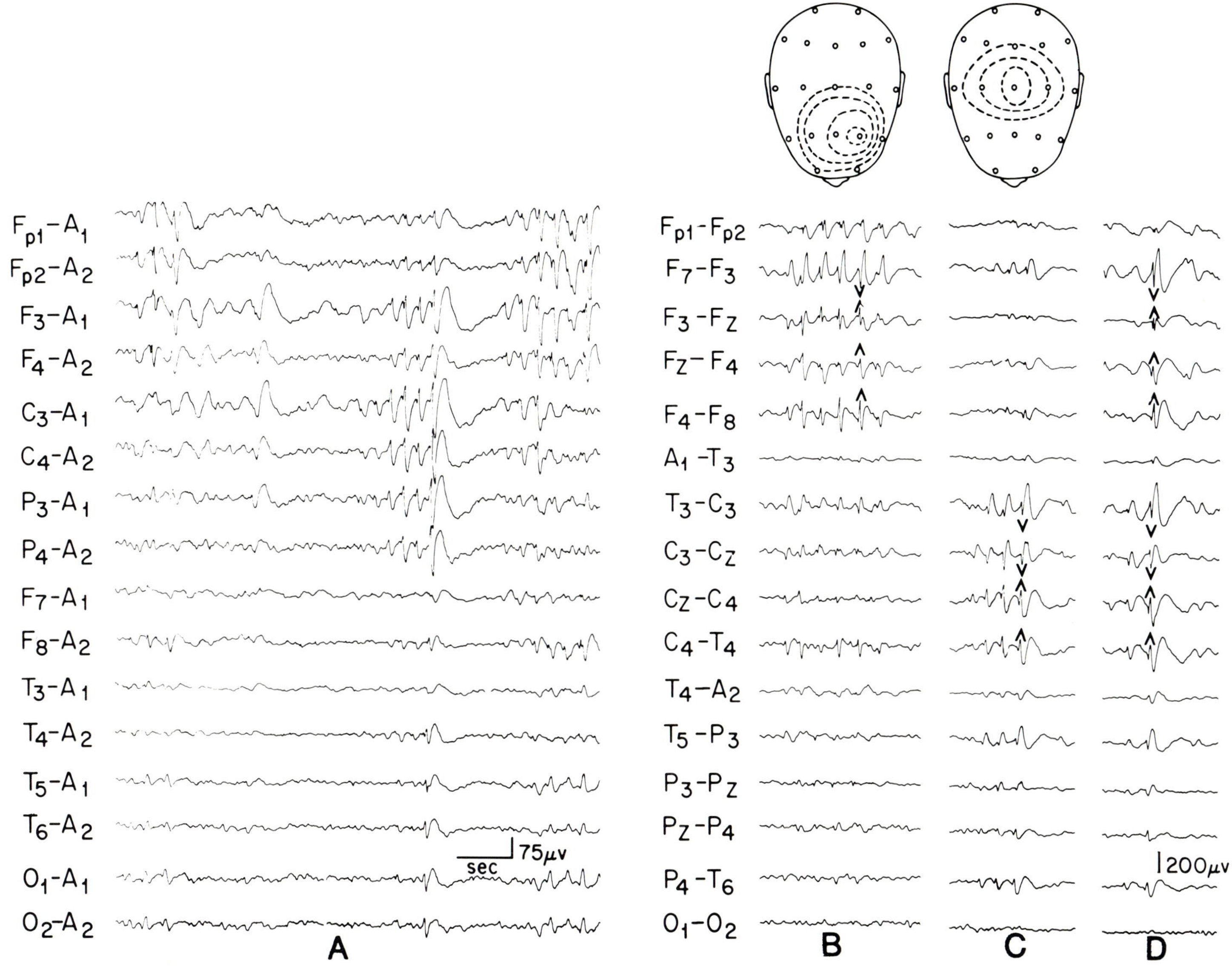

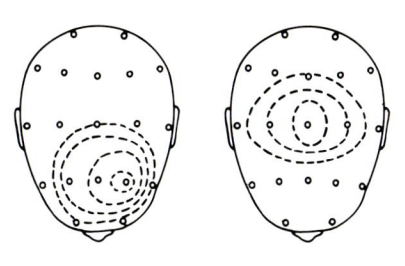

concept that cortical mechanisms predominate in the physiopathogenesis of 3-Hz spike-and-slow wave discharges. Lombroso and Erba (85) have proposed a modification of this test, using repetitive intravenous injections of small doses of thiopental sodium (Pentothal®), that makes it feasible to study young children. Bancaud et al. (11) have reported the initiation of bisynchronous 3-Hz spike and slow waves together with "typical absences" following localized stimulation of the frontal cortex, particularly its mesial aspect. More recently, Gloor et al. (59) have suggested that:

> the classical concept of secondary bilateral synchrony must be revised. This condition probably represents only a particular variety of generalized epilepsy (often caused by widespread brain lesions) in which a localized area of cortex has assumed a dominant pacemaker role in the precipitation of generalized epileptic discharges. There is probably no sharp dividing line between this form of generalized epilepsy with secondary bilateral synchrony and others in which a wide range of asymmetry of the epileptogenic process can be demonstrated.

From these and other studies (89,122), it would appear that no interictal or ictal pattern uniquely signifies an epileptic focus in one frontal lobe. In a study of the coexistence of focal and bilateral diffuse paroxysmal discharges, Gabor and Ajmone-Marsan (46) have concluded "the localizing value of foci in the frontal regions, when associated with bilaterally synchronous discharges, would appear to be questionable . . ." Since most EEG laboratories are not concerned with the intraarterial injections of drugs in the selection of patients for surgical excision, the clinical electroencephalographer is probably well advised to use caution in the interpretation of so-called secondary bisynchrony.

Generalized Periodic Discharges

Although bilaterally synchronous paroxysmal discharges occur in a wide variety of diffuse encephalopathies, periodic discharges have been consistently reported only in two groups: SSPE and subacute spongiform encephalopathy (Creutzfeldt-Jakob disease) (58). However, the characteristics of the periodic complexes differ strikingly in the two diseases.

In Creutzfeldt-Jakob disease, the complex consists of a single wave, usually triphasic in configuration, lasting from 100 to 600 msec (average 360) with an amplitude of about 100 μV. This is usually followed by a burst of rhythmical discharge at 3 to 7 Hz or, alternately, a period of flattening for about 1 sec. The complexes repeat at intervals ranging from 0.5 to 4 sec, but usually average about 1/sec (20). Periodicity develops relatively late in the evolution of the disease and once present is associated with rapid clinical deterioration and death. Myoclonus frequently but not invariably accompanies the discharges; furthermore, the muscular contraction bears no fixed temporal relationship to the complex, sometimes preceding or following the complex. If delivered at slow rates of 1/sec or less, stimuli in different modalities will trigger the complex (103).

In contrast, the periodic discharges of SSPE vary widely in morphology from patient to patient and at different times in the evolution in the illness of any one patient. The idea that "the EEG of (SSPE) passes through a more or less predictable series of changes from normality to complete disintegration before death . . . ," originally proposed by Cobb, has subsequently been rejected by him (28). The complexes last 1 to 3 sec and usually consist of two or more rhythmical slow discharges repeating at about 2 Hz (Fig. 16). Occasionally more rapid components appear, but Cobb has remarked, "Spikes and true sharp waves did not occur." The complexes repeat at relatively slow intervals, ranging from 4 to 14 sec. Celesia (21) has shown that asynchrony characterizes 95% of the complexes that begin in one or the other hemispheres and have a mean latency of 15 msec, approximately the transcallosal transmission time. As with Creutzfeldt-Jakob disease, no constant association exists between the complexes and myoclonus; but, in contrast, the SSPE complexes usually cannot be triggered by sensory stimuli.

Nonspecific Paroxysmal Discharges

Occasionally, bursts of rhythmic bisynchronous slow waves may be the only abnormality observed during a single recording. In such circumstances the electroencephalographer can comment only that paroxysmal slow discharges may be seen in patients without seizures and in normal controls. Based on their frequency, paroxysmal slow bursts may be divided into delta and theta activity.

In the waking record, bursts of monorhythmic delta waves are abnormal at any age; however, the electroencephalographer should be aware that paroxysmal rhythmic delta activity occurs normally during drowsiness in infants and young children. In a study of 100 patients with paroxysmal monorhythmic delta activity in the frontal regions (FIRDA), Cordeau (29) reported "epilepsy" in 25%. However, the most common cause of FIRDA was an intracranial mass lesion. In a subsequent study of a larger and more diverse group of 301 patients with FIRDA, Rowan et al. (116) found tumors were again the most common (30%) cause, with "epilepsy of unknown etiology" the third most frequent (13%) cause after cerebrovascular disease (19%).

Bursts of rhythmic bisynchronous sinusoidal 3-Hz waves in the occipital region have been reported in 40 to 60% of patients with absence whose EEGs show 3-Hz spike-and-slow-waves (4,31). Bursts of rhythmic occipital delta activity also occur commonly in patients with posterior fossa or third ventricle tumors, particularly in patients less than 15 years old (32). Dalby (31) has observed that rhythmical delta activity appears age-dependent, being most common between 6 and 10 years of age. Gerken and Doose (54) have found these rhythms in 6.8% of normal controls, and a slightly higher incidence (10.1%) in the siblings of patients with seizures whose EEGs show this abnormality, suggesting a genetic factor influencing their occurrence. The electroencephalographer must be on the alert to distinguish the so-called alpha variant or "split-alpha," which consists of a second subharmonic of the alpha rhythm and has no significance in relation to seizures (42).

Doose et al. (40) have drawn attention to "monomorphous theta rhythms" that appear predominantly in parietal regions. These occur primarily in 3- to 4-year-old children, usually boys. The authors distinguished these from the theta rhythms normally present at this age and noted them with greater incidence (9.8%) in the siblings of probands whose EEGs exhibit this trait than in normal controls (5.6%). They concluded that these "abnormal" theta rhythms reflect a "genetically determined functional anomaly, which is correlated to an increased seizure susceptibility." Because of the occurrence of theta rhythms in the resting records of normal children and of paroxysmal theta in normal children during drowsiness, the electroencephalographer must be thoroughly familiar with the normal maturational levels of the EEG.

Normal EEG

The finding of a normal interictal EEG in a patient who has unquestioned seizures frequently baffles clinicians. If the patient has epilepsy, how can the EEG be normal? An even more deceptive trap exists

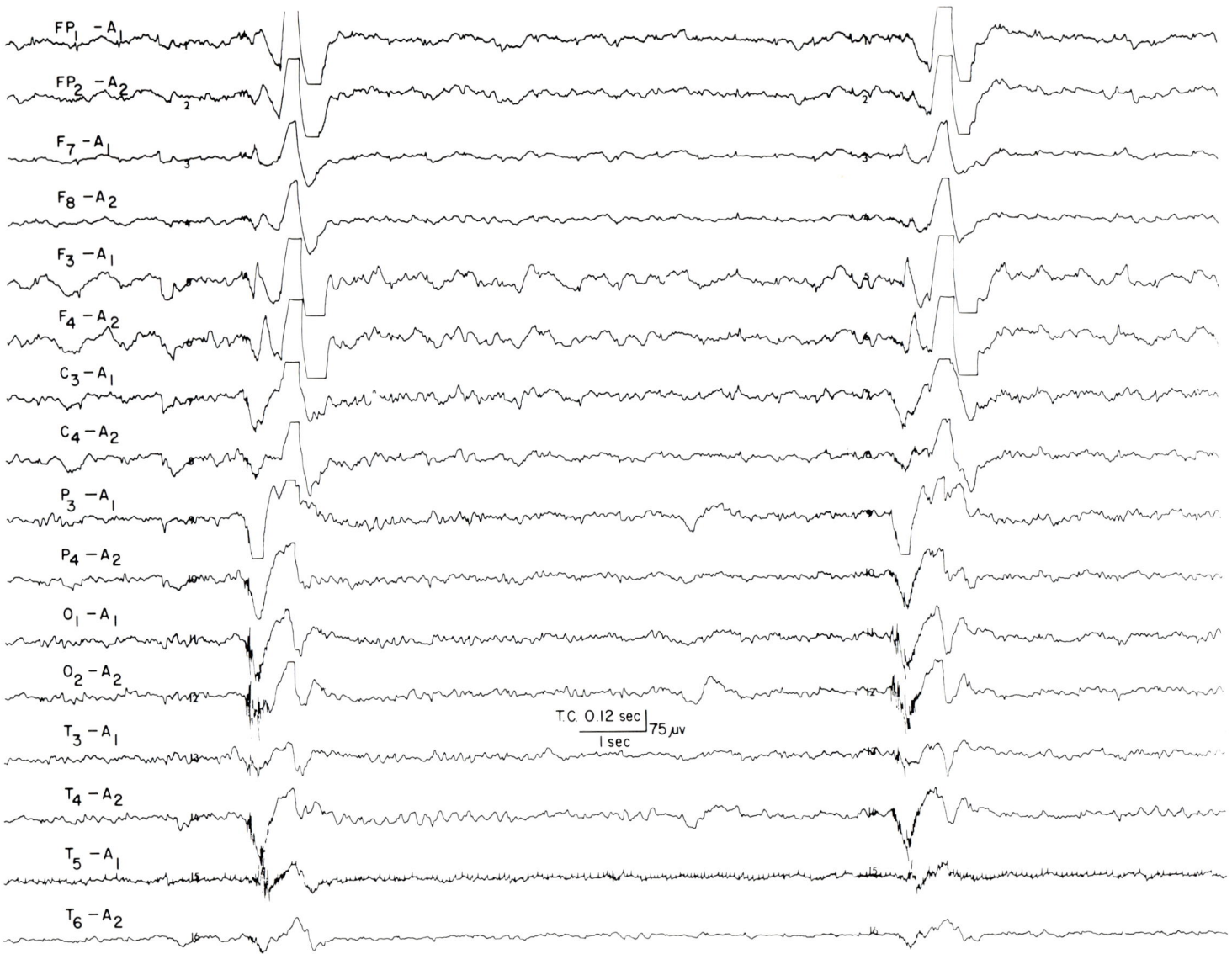

for the clinician who has referred the patient for evaluation of poorly documented episodes. Does the finding of a normal EEG eliminate the possibility of epilepsy? In these situations the electroencephalographer must word his interpretation carefully. Essentially, the finding of a normal EEG does not exclude epilepsy, which, ultimately, must be diagnosed on clinical grounds. After a single examination a significant number of patients with epilepsy are found to have a normal EEG. One or more of several factors may account for this.

As carried out in the EEG laboratory, a routine examination is essentially a sampling procedure. If the recording continues uninterruptedly for an hour, this still consumes less than 5% of the day. Therefore, if interictal abnormality occurs infrequently, the sampling time may be so short that no abnormality appears. Ajmone-Marsan and Zivin (7) have reviewed the factors that appeared to be responsible for the presence or absence of epileptiform activity in 1,824 EEGs made on 308 epileptic patients ranging from less than 1 to 64 years of age. In all patients the EEGs in both waking and sleep states were recorded, as well as EEGs during hyperventilation and photic stimulation. A "positive" record (epileptiform activity present) was obtained on the first examination in 56% of patients. In subsequent recordings an additional 26% of patients had a positive record so that only 18% of patients had consistently "negative" recordings. In contrast, all positive recordings were found in 30% of patients. The authors recognized the semantic questions raised by their approach, which may ignore significant abnormality (for example, persistent focal polymorphic delta activity) if it is not epileptiform. The authors were able to isolate certain factors.

1. *Sampling effect.* This is apparent in the figures above. In a subset of 79 patients followed by repeated examinations over an interval of longer than 1 year, 92% of patients eventually had a positive record, indicating the value of multiple tracings.

2. *Age of the patient.* Age, both at onset of seizures and time of examination, clearly influenced the occurrence of positive tracings. Below the age of 10 years approximately 80% of patients had positive recordings. In subsequent decades there was a continuous decline so that after age 40 only one-third of patients had predominantly positive recordings. By the same token, if seizures developed after the age of 30, all negative recordings were three times as frequent as all positive.

3. *Type of seizure.* Patients with seizures arising in the temporal lobe had a positive EEG at some time in 98%. Inferential evidence suggested that positive EEGs were found in 95% of patients with absences.

4. *Frequency of seizures.* Patients having frequent seizures were more likely to show positive tracings, and a somewhat greater likelihood of obtaining a positive recording existed if the tracing was made within 1 week of a seizure.

5. *Medication effects.* The commonly held view that medication tends to suppress epileptiform activity was *not substantiated*. In fact, the ratio of positive to negative records was lower in patients *off* medication than on.

In a subsequent study, Ludwig and Ajmone-Marsan (87) have reviewed the effects of withdrawal of antiepileptic drugs on 55 patients

FIG. 16. Generalized periodic discharges—subacute sclerosing panencephalitis. S. W., a 12-year-old boy, developed right-sided myoclonic jerks 5 weeks previously. These were rapidly followed by apathy, somnolence, and right hemiparesis. Examination of the spinal fluid revealed 5 lymphocytes/mm^3, protein of 30 mg/100 ml of which 25% was gamma globulin. Recording was made at standard gain to make background activity legible. The periodic complexes show maximal voltage over the anterior head region, and this results in "blocking" (amplifier overload). The complex repeats at 9- 10-sec intervals.

with intractable partial seizures, of whom 76% had focal abnormalities in their EEGs. In 20% the EEG was unchanged after withdrawal, including three of 13 patients whose EEGs consistently showed no focal abnormality. In 25% there was an increase in activity of the focus or activation of a previously inapparent focus, including eight of the 13 patients whose previous EEGs had shown no abnormality. In 29% "complex activation" occurred with an increase in the size of the initial focus or the appearance of independent foci. The most frequent effect was "nonspecific activation," which occurred in 63%. This consisted of various abnormalities including bisynchronous spike-and-slow-wave complexes, sharp-and-slow-wave complexes, or triphasic complexes. The authors suggest this latter effect is "secondary to metabolic derangements resulting from the withdrawal of neurotropic agents and not related to the specific epileptogenic process." Clearly the electroencephalographer must be extremely cautious in interpreting EEGs of patients in whom the clinical diagnosis is uncertain and in whom diffuse or bifrontal epileptiform activity is recorded 1 to 10 days after withdrawal of antiepileptic drugs. In such instances, the examination should be repeated at a more remote interval.

Several points emerge from these observations. If a normal EEG occurs in a patient in whom the clinical evidence of epilepsy is clear, repeating the examination will be more likely to contribute useful information than will stopping medication. The electroencephalographer should make this point clear to the clinician, emphasizing also the possibility of precipitating status epilepticus by withdrawing drugs. If a patient is already on antiepileptic drugs and the diagnosis of epilepsy seems open to serious question, the EEG should be repeated. If the examination consistently yields normal findings, antiepileptic drugs may cautiously be withdrawn and the EEG repeated after a sufficient interval has elapsed to escape the "nonspecific" activation effect of withdrawal. Monitoring of serum levels of antiepileptic drugs prior to and during withdrawal may prove helpful. For example, if the diagnosis of epilepsy is in doubt and the serum levels of the antiepileptic drugs are extremely low, suggesting inadequate dosage or noncompliance, then withdrawal of medication will probably not be clouded by nonspecific activation effects.

Activation Procedures

If the recording in the basal waking state discloses no abnormalities or only nonspecific abnormalities, an attempt must be made to "activate" epileptiform discharge. Over the years numerous techniques have been proposed, many involving the intravenous or intraarterial injection of drugs. This section considers only three noninvasive techniques that can and should be carried out in every EEG laboratory: sleep recording, hyperventilation, and photic stimulation.

Sleep Recording

As is well known, sleep consists of two physiologically distinct states: NREM or slow-wave sleep and REM or "paradoxical sleep." Under ordinary circumstances, such as the diurnal naps recorded in the EEG lab, sleep begins with an interval of NREM lasting approximately 1 hr followed by a phase of REM. In most laboratories routine recording includes only the NREM phase. Night-long polygraphic recordings have shown that different types of interictal abnormalities are selectively influenced by these two phases of sleep.

NREM sleep activates all types of interictal discharge, particularly during stages II and III, stages with spindles and vertex waves (Fig. 17). For a general review see Daly (33) and Klass and Fischer-Williams (77). Paroxysms of generalized 3-Hz spike-and-slow-wave discharges occur during NREM in approximately 90% of patients; Neidermeyer (102) observed paroxysms *only* during sleep (activation)

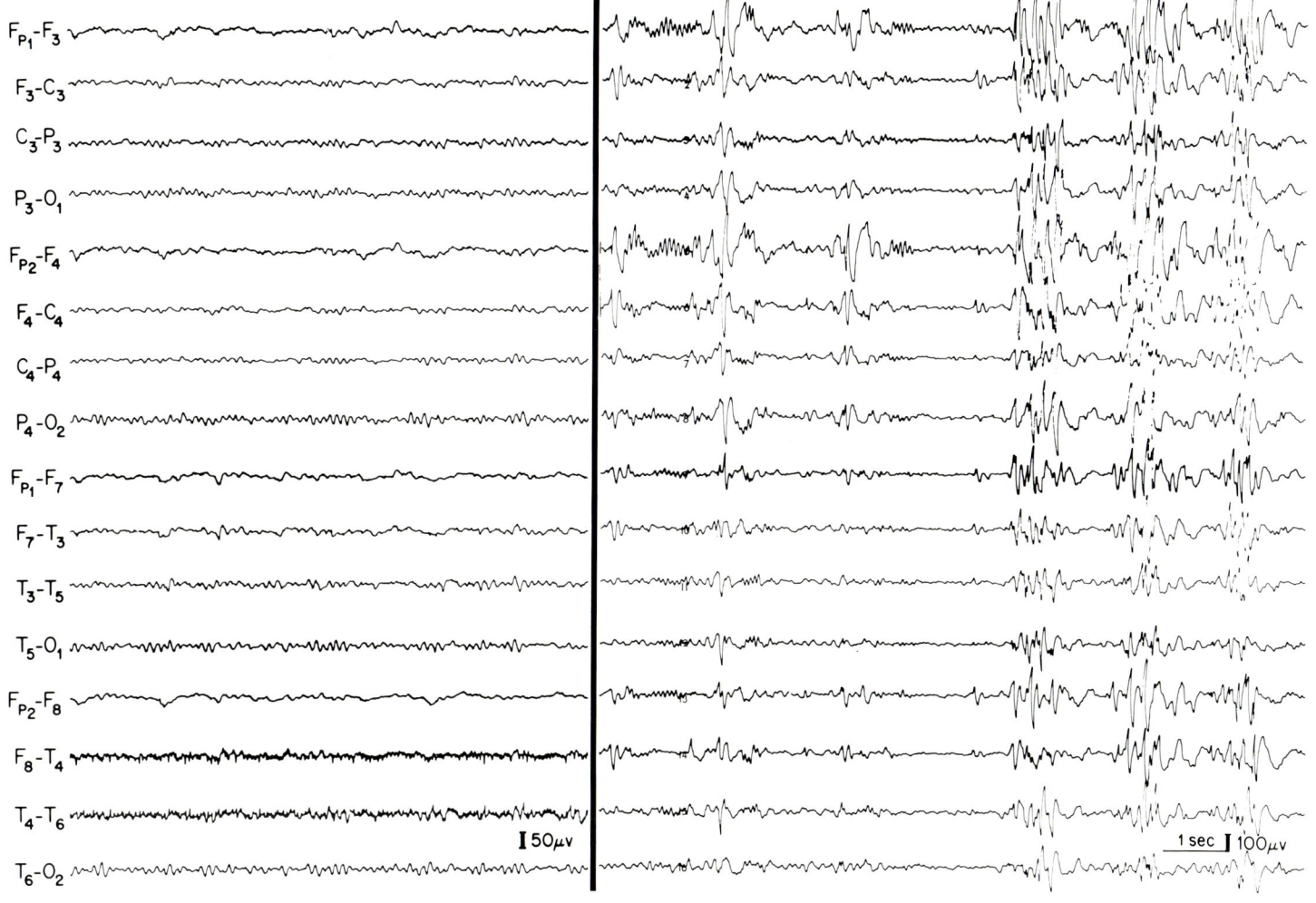

FIG. 17. Sleep activation. C. M., a 16-year-old male, developed nocturnal tonic-clonic convulsions 3 years before. Convulsions always occurred between 3 and 6 A.M. while the patient was sleeping. *Left:* Shows normal waking EEG. *Right:* Recording during NREM (slow-wave) sleep shows bursts of diffuse multiple sharp waves.

in 7% of his patients. Slow-wave sleep activates focal epileptiform discharges also. Rarely temporal spikes may disappear during NREM sleep (Gastaut, cited by Daly, ref. 33). NREM sleep may also modify the morphological features of epileptiform discharges. The bursts of 3-Hz spike-and-slow-waves (Fig. 10) are shortened in duration and replaced by bursts of multiple-spikes-and-slow-waves or single diffuse spikes. The hypsarrhythmic pattern may tend to bisynchrony in place of the multiple independent foci seen in the waking state. The size of discrete spike generators may increase so that the amplitude of the discharge is greater and the area from which it is recorded becomes larger.

During REM sleep generalized discharges disappear entirely or are markedly reduced in incidence. Spike-and-slow-wave bursts become better organized and resume the morphological features seen in the waking state. In contrast, focal spikes tend to persist or may even fire more frequently. The size of spike generators tends to constrict, resembling that seen in the waking state.

Although of theoretical interest, recordings during REM sleep contribute relatively little useful information. Information most useful for clinical purposes usually is found during the first NREM period or during arousal. For these reasons, most laboratories need record only during a diurnal nap. If sleep does not occur spontaneously, the patient may be given a mild sedative such as chloral hydrate.

Lack of sleep has long been recognized as a precipitant of seizures. This led Pratt et al. (110) to use sleep deprivation as an activating procedure. In a study of 114 epileptic patients having normal or borderline interictal EEGs, sleep deprivation for 24 hr resulted in activation of the EEG in 41%. Focal and generalized abnormalities appeared to be activated with equal facility.

Hyperventilation

Three or four minutes of voluntary overbreathing, a universally employed activation procedure, has limitations because of the difficulty in standardizing or quantifying the procedure. Hyperventilation most consistently activates 3-Hz spike-and-slow-wave complexes and often produces a clinical absence (Fig. 18). Dalby (31) noted activation in over 50% of patients with absences with or without convulsions. Activation of spike-and-slow-wave complexes occurs more frequently in those patients whose basal EEGs show rhythmical occipital delta bursts.

Specific data on activation of abnormalities other than spike-and-slow-waves are sparse. When both focal and generalized abnormalities coexist, Gabor and Ajmone-Marsan (46) found that hyperventilation more often activated bisynchronous discharges (29%) whereas in a matched group of patients with only focal discharges hyperventilation caused activation in only 6%. Morgan and Scott (100) have reported observations on 313 patients of whom almost one-half (46%) had supratentorial tumors. They classified EEGs in terms of "localized" abnormality or "paroxysmal" abnormality. The definitions were somewhat blurred since both categories included epileptiform discharges. In both categories of abnormality, hyperventilation was more effective in accentuating or augmenting preexisting abnormality and only marginally effective in activating abnormal discharges not seen

FIG. 18. Absence induced by hyperventilation. J. R., a 7½-year-old girl, developed 10 to 15 daily absences 6 months previously. Absence occurred after 90 sec of overbreathing. One second after onset of the burst *(first arrow)* patient opened eyes and stopped hyperventilating. She failed to respond to, and did not recall, a command. At second arrow, she raised both hands to her face, a *de novo* automatism. Montage combines differential and referential recording; note apparent differences in morphology of complexes that result.

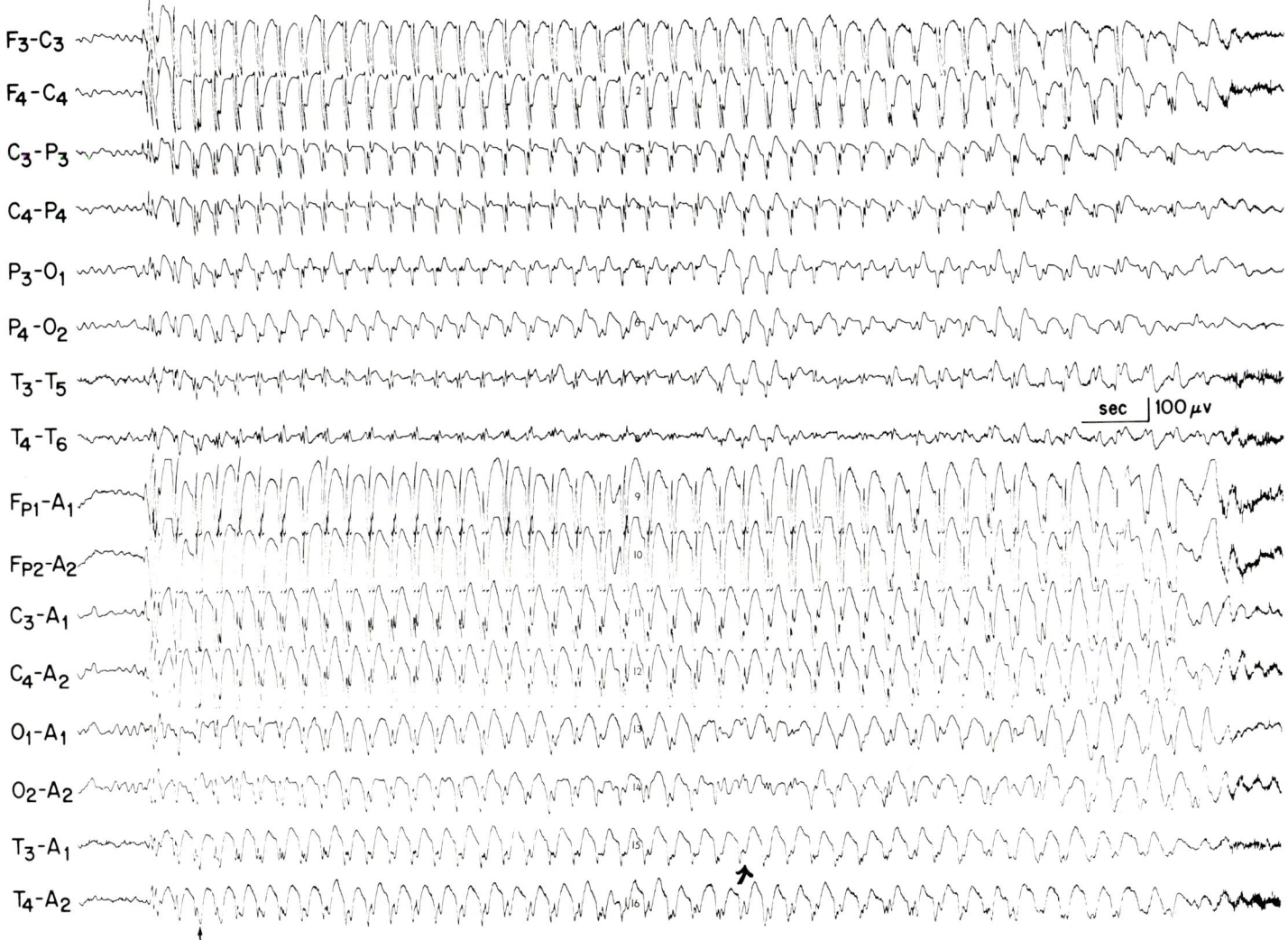

Open eyes, stop HV; unresponsive ↑ raise hands to face

in the basal recording. Although localizing abnormality was more frequent in patients with tumors (73%) than in patients without tumors (27%), hyperventilation activated abnormality in only an additional 4% of patients with tumors as opposed to 9% of patients without tumors. The fact that the group of patients with tumors was somewhat older may have played a role since the efficiency of hyperventilation, as measured by end-tidal carbon dioxide tension, declines with age (14).

Photic Stimulation

The use of photic stimulation to provoke paroxysmal discharges arose out of studies of stimulus-induced seizures or what has traditionally, if inaccurately, been termed "reflex epilepsy." Gastaut and Tassinari (52) and Bickford and Klass (13) provide extended reviews.

Intermittent photic stimulation (IPS) is carried out using a stimulator that permits a wide range of frequencies from less than one to 30 or 40 flashes/sec. Flashes of high intensity and brief duration are produced by a gas-filled flash tube. Stimulation should be carried out systematically over the entire range of frequencies, using stimulation periods of 10 to 15 sec separated by intervals of approximately 30 sec. The patient should be examined with eyes both opened and closed. Certain nonparoxysmal responses occur that are of no clinical significance. If a prominent visual evoked response appears to single flashes, repetitive stimulation will provoke sinusoidal waves over the occipital regions that may also contain harmonic or subharmonic components of the fundamental flash rate. In the photomyoclonic response, brief muscle twitches, usually in the face, occur in a one-to-one relationship with the flash and are due to activation of "microreflexes" (13). These are distinct from stimulus-induced myoclonus seen in certain myoclonic epilepsies.

Paroxysmal responses induced in the EEG by IPS are usually bisynchronous and diffuse (Fig. 19); only rarely can a focal spike be paced or activated by photic stimulation. The morphology of the discharge may vary from well-organized 3-Hz spike-and-slow-wave discharges to irregular spike-and-slow-wave complexes of more variable frequency in which the spike component varies in amplitude from moment to moment. Multiple-spikes-and-slow-waves are often associated with myoclonus. IPS may induce typical absence that at times may progress to a generalized tonic-clonic convulsion. Tonic seizures with an "electrodecremental" pattern may occur. Reilly and Peters (111) have distinguished between "prolonged responses" in which the epileptiform discharge or paroxysmal slow waves continue after cessation of photic stimulation and "self-limited responses" in which the discharge ceases spontaneously while IPS continues, or terminates simultaneously with the cessation of stimulation. In patients showing the prolonged response, 93% had a clinical diagnosis of epilepsy and 80% showed epileptiform discharge in the basal EEG. In contrast, seizures occurred in only 70% of patients with self-limited responses. When compared to an age-matched control group of patients referred to the same laboratory for an EEG, the incidence of epilepsy in the self-limited and control groups was essentially

FIG. 19. Photoparoxysmal response. H. P., a 10-year-old girl, 2 years before had had a tonic-clonic convulsion when a television screen began to flicker. She experienced daily absences with fluttering of the eyelids. Absence was frequently induced by eye closure. **A:** Combined differential and referential recording. A spontaneous brief burst of generalized spike-and-slow-wave discharge. **B:** Brief burst of irregular spike-and-slow-wave discharge with fluttering of the eyelids following eye closure. **C:** Sustained burst of generalized spike-wave discharge induced by photic stimulation at 11 flashes/sec. Bottom channel records output of stimulator. Note persistence of abnormal discharge after cessation of stimulation.

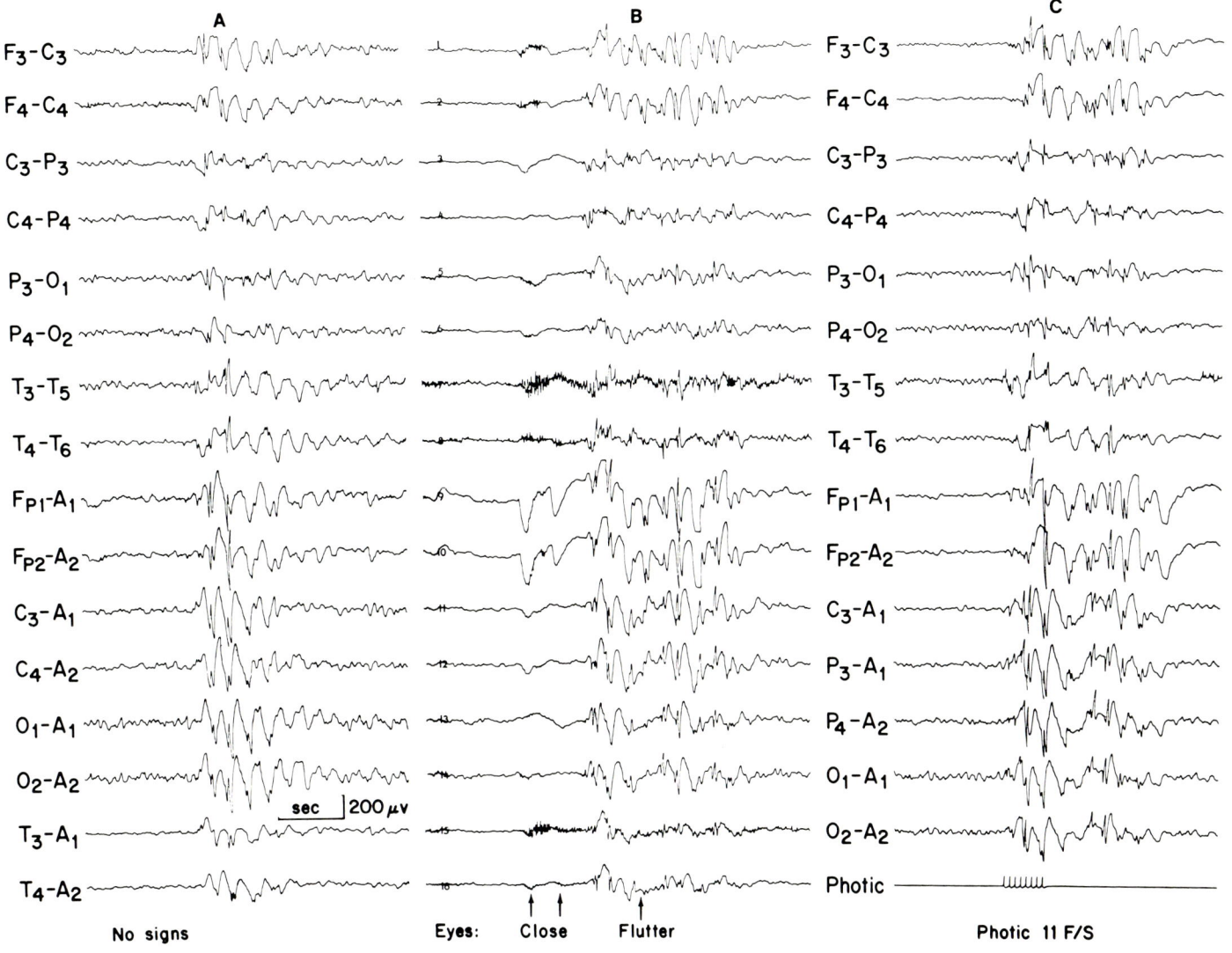

the same. The authors suggest that the classification of "photoconvulsive" response should be qualified by the term "prolonged or self-limited."

As mentioned in the discussion of genetic factors in primary generalized epilepsies, the appearance of spike-and-slow-wave complexes during photic stimulation has been used as evidence for the presence of a genetic "marker." Bearing in mind the caveat of Reilly and Peters, evidence does exist suggesting that photoparoxysmal responses are genetically determined. Doose et al. (38) found evidence of photoparoxysmal responses in approximately 50% of their probands. Photoparoxysmal responses occurred in 12% of the siblings of probands as against 5% of controls. In turn, siblings of photosensitive probands showed a photoparoxysmal response in 15% as opposed to 4% of the siblings of nonphotosensitive probands, a statistically significant difference.

The electroencephalographer must use caution in interpreting the significance of photoparoxysmal responses. However, clinical seizures induced by IPS are abnormal and rarely occur in patients without a history of seizures. More recently, Jeavons et al. (72) have proposed that a grid be fitted over the light to produce a patterned flash, claiming a greater incidence of photoparoxysmal responses. Engle (43) has shown that whereas most patients are sensitive to patterned and diffuse flashes, some will be sensitive only to one or the other. He suggests the routine use of both techniques as a more efficient procedure.

SYNCOPE

Syncope results from cerebral ischemia initiated by one or more extracranial mechanisms. Thus, although syncope occurs paroxysmally, it has no relation to epilepsy. In the intervals between syncope the EEG is normal. Nevertheless, infants and young children are frequently referred for evaluation of "breath-holding spells," and older children and adults because of unwitnessed or ill-described "blackout spells." In recent years several studies (47,61,86) have considerably illuminated the mechanisms operative in breath-holding spells. Lombroso and Lerman (86) have studied syncope in 92 children and found that the majority could be divided into either "pallid syncope" (20%) or "cyanotic syncope" (60%). In 75% of children attacks began between 6 and 18 months of age and terminated spontaneously in 85% by age 5 years. A significant genetic factor operates in that breath-holding spells are reported in 5% of an unselected population whereas, in contrast, 25% of siblings or parents of children with breath-holding spells have suffered similar episodes.

In pallid syncope cerebral ischemia results from profound bradycardia or asystole. Pallid syncope usually follows a minor painful stimulus frequently involving the head. During such an episode, recording the EEG reveals that following asystole generalized slowing appears within a few seconds, succeeded by flattening of the EEG. Generalized clonic jerks may occur in the late phase of slowing and decorticate or decerebrate posturing may appear during the phase

FIG. 20. Syncope. P. M., a 9-year-old girl, for 1 year had had brief attacks of pallor, sweating, and anxiety. She also had had nocturnal episodes of pallor followed by rigidity, jerking, and cyanosis. The episodes had been variously diagnosed as anxiety attacks or epilepsy. An episode occurred during hyperventilation. The recording shows seven channels of referential derivations and one channel of EKG. In the upper panel note the replacement of sinus rhythm by ventricular tachycardia. At this time the child stopped hyperventilating, probably because she felt a change in cardiac rate. The monorhythmic delta activity characteristic of a normal hyperventilation response is replaced by more irregular slow discharges and after about 6 sec by flattening of the EEG. Note electromyographic activity during decorticate posturing. The clonic jerks create movement artifacts that obscure the EEG. Rhythmical slow activity appears 3 sec after resumption of normal cardiac rhythm, and the EEG is almost normal after 10 sec.

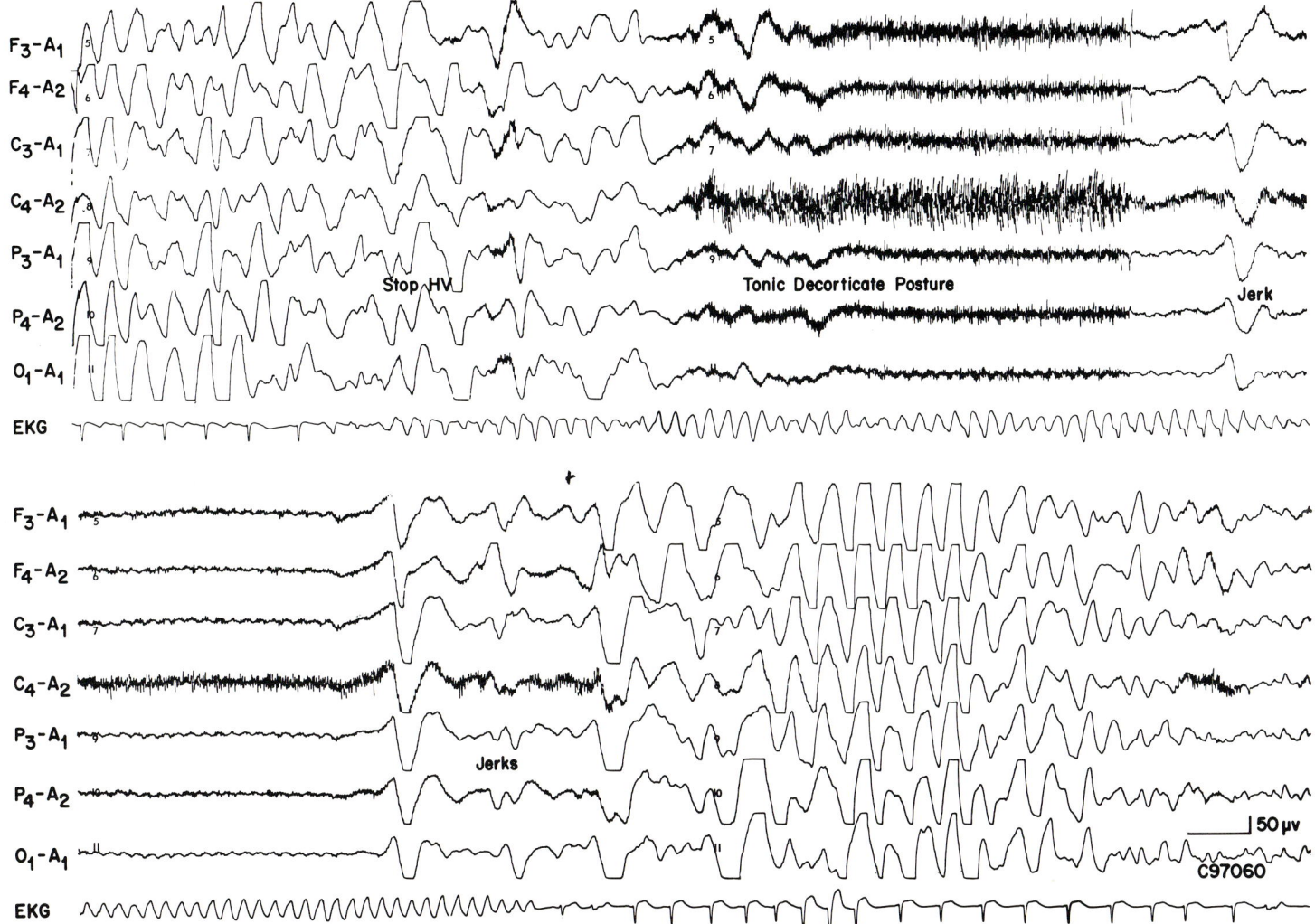

of flattening. With resumption of ventricular contractions, the EEG passes through a phase of generalized slow activity and recovery within 7 to 10 sec. The clonic jerks and decorticate posturing are often misinterpreted as a convulsion. In children with pallid syncope, ocular compression, a painful procedure, will invoke bradycardia or asystole in 60% of children as opposed to 7% of normal children.

Cyanotic syncope arises from the stimultaneous effects of several factors. Its evolution is slower and preceded by an emotional phase induced by frustration or anger associated with crying. Apnea in expiration follows; if prolonged, the child becomes cyanotic, unconscious, and limp. The EEG shows generalized slow activity but usually no flattening. Children with cyanotic syncope show symptomatic oculovagal reflexes in only 10%, although having a generally more hyperactive reflex (24%) than the general population. The precise mechanisms of this type of syncope are less clear cut. It is postulated that crying is associated with hyperventilation, leading to hypocapnia, cerebral vasoconstriction, and ischemia. The apnea is associated with increased intrathoracic pressure, reduction of venous return to the heart (Valsalva maneuver), and lowered cardiac output.

In older children and adults, syncope may result from bradycardia induced by painful stimuli such as venipuncture or from paroxysmal tachycardia (Fig. 20) (see also chapter by Saunders and Westmoreland, *this volume*.)

NARCOLEPSY

Narcolepsy is a disorder of impaired vigilance or wakefulness with repeated progression into episodes of irresistible sleep (37). The disorder is not truly paroxysmal nor does it have any relationship to epilepsy. Occasionally cataplectic attacks or episodes of sleep may be confused with seizures and the patient will be referred for an EEG. The EEG during waking and sleep shows no abnormalities (36). Should a cataplectic attack occur in the laboratory, the EEG shows only a low voltage record without alpha rhythms, resembling that seen when the eyes are open. The contention that REM at the onset of sleep characterizes narcolepsy has been refuted by the studies of Hishikawa et al. (66). In summary, electroencephalography can contribute nothing to establish the diagnosis of narcolepsy, although it may be noted that the patient falls asleep at unusual times such as during hyperventilation or photic stimulation.

REFERENCES*

1. Aicardi, J., and Chevrie, J. J. (1970): Convulsive status epilepticus in infants and children: A study of 239 cases. *Epilepsia,* 11:187–197.
2. Aicardi, J., and Chevrie, J. J. (1971): Myoclonic epilepsies of childhood. *Neuropaediatrie,* 3:177–190.
3. Aigner, B. R., and Mulder, D. W. (1960): Myoclonus. *Arch. Neurol.,* 2:600–615.
4. Aird, R. B., and Gastaut, Y. (1959): Occipital and posterior electroencephalographic rhythms. *Electroencephalogr. Clin. Neurophysiol.,* 11:637–656.
5. Ajmone-Marsan, C. (1965): A newly proposed classification of epileptic seizures: Neurophysiological basis. *Epilepsia,* 6:275–296.
6. Ajmone-Marsan, C., and Goldhammer, L. (1973): Clinical ictal patterns and electrographic data in cases of partial seizures of frontal-central-parietal origin. In: *Epilepsy: Its Phenomena in Man,* edited by M. A. B. Brazier, pp. 236–260. Academic Press, New York.
7. Ajmone-Marsan, C., and Zivin, L. S. (1970): Factors related to the occurrence of typical paroxysmal abnormalities in the EEG records of epileptic patients. *Epilepsia,* 11:361–381.
8. Andermann, F., and Robb, J. P. (1972): Absence status: A reappraisal following review of 38 patients. *Epilepsia,* 13:177–187.
9. Babb, T. L., and Crandall, T. H. (1976): Epileptogenesis of human limbic neurons in psychomotor epileptics. *Electroencephalogr. Clin. Neurophysiol.,* 40:225–243.
10. Bancaud, J. (1972): Mechanisms of cortical discharges in "generalized" epilepsies

---

* On the assumption that citations of articles in English would make the bibliography accessible to the largest number of readers, the bibliography omits all articles in other languages. The omission of numerous informative and important articles is an inevitable, but unfortunate, consequence of this decision.

in man. In: *Synchronisation of EEG Activity in Epilepsies,* edited by H. Petsche and M. Brazier, pp. 368–381. Springer-Verlag, New York.
11. Bancaud, J., Talairach, J., Morel, P., Bresson, M., Bonis, A., Geier, S., Hemon, E., and Buser, P. (1974): "Generalized" epileptic seizures elicited by electrical stimulation of the frontal lobe in man. *Electroencephalogr. Clin. Neurophysiol.,* 37:275–282.
12. Beaussart, M. (1972): Benign epilepsy of children with rolandic (centro-temporal) paroxysmal foci. *Epilepsia,* 13:795–811.
13. Bickford, R. G., and Klass, D. W. (1969): Sensory precipitation and reflex mechanisms. In: *Basic Mechanisms of the Epilepsies,* edited by H. H. Jasper, A. A. Ward, and A. Pope, pp. 543–564. Little, Brown, Boston.
14. Binnie, C. G., Cole, P. A., and Margerison, J. H. (1969): The influence of end-tidal carbon dioxide tension on EEG changes during routine hyperventilation in different age groups. *Electroencephalogr. Clin. Neurophysiol.,* 27:304–306.
15. Blom, S., and Heijbel, J. (1975): Benign epilepsy of children with centro-temporal EEG foci: Discharge rate during sleep. *Epilepsia,* 16:133–140.
16. Blom, S., Heijbel, J., and Bergfors, P. (1972): Benign epilepsy of children with centro-temporal EEG foci. Prevalence and follow-up study of 40 patients. *Epilepsia,* 13:609–619.
17. Blume, W. T., David, R. B., and Gomez, M. R. (1973): Generalized sharp and slow wave complexes. *Brain,* 96:289–306.
18. Brazier, M. A. B. (1973): Electrical seizure discharges within the brain. The problem of spread. In: *Epilepsy: Its Phenomenon in Man,* edited by M. A. B. Brazier, pp. 155–171. Academic Press, New York.
19. Browne, T. R., Penry, J. K., Porter, R. J., and Dreifuss, F. E. (1974): Responsiveness before, during and after spike-wave paroxysms. *Neurology (Minneap.),* 24:659–665.
20. Burger, L. J., Rowan, J., and Goldenshon, E. S. (1972): Creutzfeldt-Jakob disease: An electroencephalographic study. *Arch. Neurol.,* 26:428–433.
21. Celesia, G. G. (1973): Pathophysiology of periodic EEG complexes in subacute sclerosing panencephalitis (SSPE). *Electroencephalogr. Clin. Neurophysiol.,* 35:293–300.
22. Charleton, M. H. (1975): *Myoclonic Seizures,* pp. 167. Excerpta Medica, Amsterdam.
23. Charleton, M. H. (1975): Infantile spasms. In: *Myoclonic Seizures,* edited by M. H. Charleton, pp. 111–120. Excerpta Medica, Amsterdam.
24. Chatrian, G. E., Bergamini, L., Dondey, M., Klass, D. W., Lennox-Buchtal, M., and Petersén, I. (1974): A glossary of terms most commonly used by clinical electroencephalographers. *Electroencephalogr. Clin. Neurophysiol.,* 37:538–548.
25. Chatrian, G. E., Shaw, C. M., and Leffman, H. (1964): The significance of periodic lateralized epileptiform discharges in EEG: An electrographic, clinical and pathological study. *Electroencephalogr. Clin. Neurophysiol.,* 17:177–193.
26. Chatrian, G. E., Somasundaram, M., and Tassinari, C. A. (1968): DC changes recorded transcranially during "typical" three/second spike and wave discharges in man. *Epilepsia,* 9:185–209.
27. Chevrie, J. J., and Aicardi, J. (1972): Childhood epileptic encephalopathy with slow spike-wave: A statistical study of eighty cases. *Epilepsia,* 13:259–271.
28. Cobb, W. (1966): The periodic events of subacute sclerosing leukoencephalitis. *Electroencephalogr. Clin. Neurophysiol.,* 21:278–294.
29. Cordeau, J. P. (1959): Monorhythmic frontal delta activity in the human electroencephalogram. A study of 100 cases. *Electroencephalogr. Clin. Neurophysiol.,* 11:733–746.
30. Currie, S., Heathfield, K. W. G., Henson, R. A., and Scott, D. F. (1971): Clinical course and prognosis of temporal lobe epilepsy. A survey of 666 patients. *Brain,* 94:173–190.
31. Dalby, M. A. (1969): Epilepsy and 3 per second spike and wave rhythms. *Acta Neurol. Scand. [Suppl.],* 40:1–183.
32. Daly, D. D. (1968): The effect of sleep upon the electroencephalogram in patients with brain tumors. *Electroencephalogr. Clin. Neurophysiol.,* 25:521–529.
33. Daly, D. D. (1973): Circadian cycles and seizures. In: *Epilepsy: Its Phenomena in Man,* edited by M. A. B. Brazier, pp. 215–233. Academic Press, New York.
34. Daly, D. D. (1975): Ictal clinical manifestations of complex partial seizures. In: *Complex Partial Seizures and Their Treatment,* edited by J. K. Penry and D. D. Daly, pp. 57–82. Raven Press, New York.
35. Daly, D. D. (1975): Genesis of abnormal activity. In: *Handbook of Electroencephalography and Clinical Neurophysiology,* Vol. 14C, edited by A. Rémond, pp. 5–10. Elsevier, Amsterdam.
36. Daly, D. D., and Yoss, R. E. (1957): The electroencephalogram in narcolepsy. *Electroencephalogr. Clin. Neurophysiol.,* 9:109–120.
37. Daly, D. D., and Yoss, R. E. (1974): Narcolepsy. In: *Handbook of Clinical Neurology, Vol. 15: The Epilepsies,* edited by T. J. Vinken and G. W. Bruyn, pp. 836–852. American Elsevier, New York.
38. Doose, H., Gerkin, H., Horstmann, T., and Völzke, E. (1973): Genetic factors in spike-wave absences. *Epilepsia,* 14:57–75.
39. Doose, H., Gerken, H., Leonhardt, R., Völzke, E., and Völtz, C. (1970): Centrencephalic myoclonic-astatic petit mal. *Neuropaediatrie,* 2:59–78.
40. Doose, H., Gerken, H., and Völzke, E. (1972): On the genetics of EEG-anomalies in childhood. I. Abnormal theta rhythms. *Neuropaediatrie,* 3:386–401.
41. Earle, J. M., Baldwin, M., and Penfield, W. (1953): Incisural sclerosis and temporal lobe seizures produced by hippocampal herniation at birth. *Arch. Neurol. Psychiatr.,* 69:27–42.
42. Eeg-Olofsson, O., Petersen, I., and Selldén, U. (1971): The development of the electroencephalogram in normal children from the age of one through fifteen years. Paroxysmal activity. *Neuropaediatrie,* 4:375–404.

43. Engel, J. (1974): Selective photoconvulsive responses to intermittent diffuse and patterned photic stimulation. *Electroencephalogr. Clin. Neurophysiol.,* 37:283–292.
44. Engel, J., Driver, M. V., and Falconer, M. (1975): Electrophysiological correlates of pathology and surgical results in temporal lobe epilepsy. *Brain,* 98:129–156.
45. Falconer, M. A., and Taylor, D. C. (1968): Surgical treatment of drug resistant epilepsy due to mesial temporal sclerosis. *Arch. Neurol.,* 19:353–361.
46. Gabor, A. J., and Ajmone-Marsan, C. (1969): Co-existence of focal and bilateral diffuse paroxysmal discharges in epileptics: Clinical-electrographic study. *Epilepsia,* 10:453–472.
47. Gastaut, H. (1968): A physiopathogenic study of reflex anoxic cerebral seizures in children (Syncopes, sobbing spasms and breath-holding spells). In: *Clinical Electroencephalography of Children,* edited by P. Kellaway and I. Petersén, pp. 257–276. Grune & Stratton, New York.
48. Gastaut, H. (1970): Clinical and electroencephalographical classification of epileptic seizures. *Epilepsia,* 11:102–113.
49. Gastaut, H., and Broughton, R. (1972): *Epileptic Seizures.* Charles C Thomas, Springfield, Ill.
50. Gastaut, H., Broughton, R., Tassinari, C. A., and Roger, J. (1974): Unilateral epileptic seizures. In: *Handbook of Clinical Neurology, Vol. 15: The Epilepsies,* edited by P. J. Vinken and G. W. Bruyn, pp. 234–245. American Elsevier, New York.
51. Gastaut, H., Rojer, J., Soulayrol, R., Tassinari, C. A., Régis, H., Dravet, C., Bernard, R., Pinsard, N., and Saint-Jean, M. (1966): Childhood epileptic encephalopathy with diffuse slow spike-waves (otherwise known as "petit mal variant") or Lennox syndrome. *Epilepsia,* 7:139–179.
52. Gastaut, H., and Tassinari, C. A. (1966): Triggering mechanisms in epilepsy. *Epilepsia,* 7:85–138.
53. Geier, S., Bancaud, J., Talairach, J., Bonis, A., Szikela, G., and Enjelvien, M. (1975): Clinical note: Clinical and tele-stereo-EEG findings in a patient with psychomotor seizures. *Epilepsia,* 16:119–125.
54. Gerken, H., and Doose, H. (1972): On the genetics of EEG-anomalies in childhood. II. Occipital 2-4/s rhythms. *Neuropaediatrie,* 3:437–454.
55. Gibbs, F. A., Davis, H., and Lennox, W. G. (1935): The electroencephalogram in epilepsy and in conditions of impaired consciousness. *Arch. Neurol. Psychiatr.,* 34:1133–1148.
56. Gibbs, F. A., and Gibbs, E. L. (1952): *Atlas of Electroencephalography, Vol. 2, Epilepsy,* 2nd ed., p. 422. Addison-Wesley, Reading, Mass.
57. Gloor, P. (1968): Generalized cortico-reticular epilepsies: Some considerations on the pathophysiology of generalized bilaterally synchronous spike-and-slow-wave discharge. *Epilepsia,* 9:249–263.
58. Gloor, P., Kalaby, O., and Giard, N. (1968): The electroencephalogram in diffuse encephalopathies: Electroencephalographic correlates of gray and white matter lesions. *Brain,* 91:779–802.
59. Gloor, P., Rasmussen, T., Altuzarra, A., and Garretson, H. (1976): Role of the intracarotid amobarbital-pentylenetetrazol EEG test. The diagnosis and surgical treatment of patients with complex seizure problems. *Epilepsia,* 17:15–31.
60. Gloor, P., Tsai, C., and Haddad, F. (1958): An assessment of the value of sleep-electroencephalography for the diagnosis of temporal lobe epilepsy. *Electroencephalogr. Clin. Neurophysiol.,* 10:632–648.
61. Gomez, M. R., and Klass, D. W. (1972): Seizures and other paroxysmal disorders in infants and children. *Curr. Probl. Pediatr.,* 2:3–37.
62. Goode, D. J., Penry, J. K., and Dreifuss, F. (1970): Effects of paroxysmal spike-wave on continuous visual-motor performance. *Epilepsia,* 11:241–254.
63. Guey, J., Bureau, M., Dravet, C., and Roger, J. (1969): A study of the rhythms of petit mal absences in children in relations to prevailing situations. *Epilepsia,* 10:441–451.
64. Halliday, A. M. (1975): The neurophysiology of myoclonic jerking: A reappraisal. In: *Myoclonic Seizures,* edited by M. H. Charleton. Excerpta Medica, Amsterdam.
65. Heijbel, J., Blom, S., and Rasmussen, M. (1975): Benign epilepsy of childhood with centrotemporal EEG foci: A genetic study. *Epilepsia,* 16:285–294.
66. Hishikawa, Y., Wakamatsu, H., Furuya, E., Sugita, Y., Masaoka, S., Kaneda, H., Sato, M., Nan'no, H., and Kaneko, Z. (1976): Sleep satiation in narcoleptic patients. *Electroencephalogr. Clin. Neurophysiol.,* 41:1–18.
67. Huttenlocher, P. R. (1974): Dendritic development in neocortex of children with mental defect and infantile spasms. *Neurology,* 24:203–210.
68. Ishijima, B., Hori, T., Yoshimasu, N., Fukushima, T., Hirakawa, K., and Sekino, H. (1975): Neuronal activities in human epileptic foci and surrounding areas. *Electroencephalogr. Clin. Neurophysiol.,* 39:643–650.
69. Janz, D. (1974): Epilepsy in the sleep-waking cycle. In: *Handbook of Clinical Neurology, Vol. 15: The Epilepsies,* edited by T. J. Vinken and G. W. Bruyn, pp. 457–490. American Elsevier, New York.
70. Jeavons, P. M., and Bower, B. D. (1974): Infantile spasms. In: *Handbook of Clinical Neurology, Vol. 15: The Epilepsies,* edited by T. J. Vinken and G. W. Bruyn, pp. 219–234. American Elsevier, New York.
71. Jeavons, P. M., Bower, B. W., and Dimitrakoudi, M. (1973): Long term prognosis of 150 cases of "West Syndrome." *Epilepsia,* 14:153–164.
72. Jeavons, P. M., Harding, G. F. A., and Panupopulas, P. C. (1972): The effect of geometric patterns combined with intermittent photic stimulation in photosensitive epilepsy. *Electroencephalogr. Clin. Neurophysiol.,* 33:221–224.
73. Jellinger, K. (1970): Neuropathological aspects of hypsarrhythmia. *Neuropaediatrie,* 1:277–294.
74. Kivity, S., and Lerman, P. (1975): Benign focal epilepsy of childhood: A follow-up study of 100 recovered patients. *Arch. Neurol.,* 32:261–274.

75. Klass, D. W. (1975): Electroencephalographic manifestations of complex partial seizures: In: *Complex Partial Seizures and Their Treatment,* edited by J. K. Penry and D. D. Daly, pp. 113–140. Raven Press, New York.
76. Klass, D. W., and Bickford, R. G. (1958): The electroencephalogram in metastatic tumors of the brain. *Neurology (Minneap.),* 8:333–337.
77. Klass, D. W., and Fischer-Williams, M. (1976): Sensory stimulation, sleep and sleep deprivation. In: *Handbook of Electroencephalography and Clinical Neurophysiology,* Vol. 3D, edited by A. Rédmond, pp. 5–73. Elsevier, Amsterdam.
78. Kooi, K. A. (1966): Voltage-time characteristics of spikes and other rapid electroencephalographic transients: Semantic and morphological considerations. *Neurology (Minneap.),* 16:59–66.
79. Lairy, G. C., and Harrison, A. (1968): Functional aspects of EEG foci in children—clinical data and longitudinal studies. In: *Clinical Electroencephalography of Children,* edited by P. Kellaway and I. Petersén, pp. 197–212. Grune & Stratton, New York.
80. Lennox-Buchthal, M. A. (1973): Febrile convulsions: A reappraisal. *Electroencephalogr. Clin. Neurophysiol.,* (Suppl. 32) 1–138.
81. Lindsay, J. M. N. (1971): Genetics in epilepsy: A model for critical path analysis. *Epilepsia,* 12:47–54.
82. Loiseau, P., and Beaussart, M. (1973): The seizures of benign childhood epilepsy with rolandic paroxysmal discharges. *Epilepsia,* 14:381–389.
83. Loiseau, P., Legroux, M., Grimond, P., dePasquier, P., and Henry, P. (1974): Taxometric classification of myoclonic epilepsies. *Epilepsia,* 15:1–11.
84. Lombroso, C. T. (1967): Sylvian seizures and mid-temporal spike foci in children. *Arch. Neurol.,* 17:52–59.
85. Lombroso, C. T., and Erba, G. (1970): Primary and secondary bilateral synchrony in epilepsy. *Arch. Neurol.,* 22:321–334.
86. Lombroso, C. T., and Lerman, P. (1967): Breath-holding spells. Cyanotic and pallid infantile syncope. *Pediatrics,* 39:563–58.
87. Ludwig, B. I., and Ajmone-Marsan, C. (1975): EEG changes after withdrawal of medication in epileptic patients. *Electroencephalogr. Clin. Neurophysiol.,* 39:173–181.
88. Ludwig, B. I., and Ajmone-Marsan, C. (1975): Clinical ictal patterns in epileptic patients with occipital electroencephalographic foci. *Neurology (Minneap.),* 25:463–471.
89. Ludwig, B., Ajmone-Marsan, C., and Van Buren, J. (1975): Cerebral seizures of probable orbital-frontal origin. *Epilepsia,* 16:141–158.
90. Maheshwari, M. C., and Jeavons, P. M. (1975): The prognostic implications of suppression-burst activity in the EEG in infancy. *Epilepsia,* 16:127–131.
91. Markand, O., and Daly, D. D. (1971): Pseudoperiodic lateralized paroxysmal discharges in electroencephalogram. *Neurology (Minneap.),* 21:975–981.
92. Masland, R. L. (1974): The classification of the epilepsies. A historical review. In: *Handbook of Clinical Neurology,* Vol. 15: *The Epilepsies,* edited by P. J. Vinken and G. W. Bruyn, pp. 1–29. American Elsevier, New York.
93. Maulsby, R. L. (1971): Some guidelines for assessment of spikes and sharp waves in EEG tracing. *Am. J. EEG Technol.,* 11:3–16.
94. Meldrum, B. S. (1972): Neuronal loss and gliosis in the hippocampus following repetitive epileptic seizures induced in adolescent baboons by allylglycine. *Brain Res.,* 48:361–365.
95. Merlis, J. K. (1970): Proposal for an international classification of the epilepsies. *Epilepsia,* 11:114–119.
96. Metrakos, J. D., and Metrakos, K. (1966): Childhood epilepsy of subcortical ("centrencephalic") origin. *Clin. Pediatr.,* 5:536–542.
97. Metrakos, K., and Metrakos, J. H. (1974): Genetics of epilepsy. In: *Handbook of Clinical Neurology,* Vol. 15: *The Epilepsies,* edited by P. J. Vinken and G. W. Bruyn, pp. 429–439. American Elsevier, New York.
98. Monod, N. (1972): Neonatal EEG: Statistical studies and prognosticative value in full-term and pre-term babies. *Electroencephalogr. Clin. Neurophysiol.,* 32:529–544.
99. Monod, N., and Dreyfus-Brisac, C. (1972): Prognostic value of the neonatal EEG in full-term newborns. In: *Handbook of Electroencephalography and Clinical Neurophysiology,* Vol. 15B, edited by A. Rémond, pp. 89–100. Elsevier, Amsterdam.
100. Morgan, M. H., and Scott, D. F. (1970): EEG activation in epilepsies other than petit mal. *Epilepsia,* 11:255–261.
101. Morrell, F. (1969): Physiology and histochemistry of the mirror focus. In: *Basic Mechanisms of the Epilepsies,* edited by H. H. Jasper, A. A. Ward, and A. Pope, pp. 357–370. Little, Brown, Boston.
102. Neidermeyer, E. (1972): *The Generalized Epilepsies,* pp. 247. Charles C Thomas Springfield, Ill.
103. Nelson, J. H., and Leffman, H. (1963): The human diffusely projecting system. *Arch. Neurol.,* 8:544–556.
104. Noriega-Sanchez, A., and Markand, O. N. (1976): Clinical and electroencephalographic correlation of independent multifocal spike discharges. *Neurology (Minneap.),* 26:667–672.
105. Penfield, W., and Jasper, H. (1946): Highest level seizures. *Res. Publ. Assoc. Nerv. Ment. Dis.,* 26:252–271.
106. Penfield, W., and Jasper, H. (1954): *Epilepsy and the Functional Anatomy of the Human Brain.* Little, Brown, Boston.
107. Penry, J. K., and Dreifuss, F. E. (1969): Automatisms association with the absence of "petit mal" epilepsy. *Arch. Neurol.,* 21:142–149.
108. Penry, J. K., Porter, R. J., and Dreifuss, F. E. (1975): Simultaneous recording of absence seizures with video-tape and electroencephalography: A study of 374 seizures in 48 patients. *Brain,* 98:427–440.

109. Petersén, I., Eeg-Olofsson, O., and Selldén, U. (1968): Paroxysmal activity in EEG of normal children. In: *Clinical Electroencephalography of Children,* edited by P. Kellaway and I. Petersén, pp. 167–188. Grune & Stratton, New York.
110. Pratt, K. L., Matteson, R. H., Weikers, N. J., and Williams, R. (1968): EEG activation of epileptics following sleep deprivation. *Electroencephalogr. Clin. Neurophysiol.,* 24:11–15.
111. Reilly, E. W., and Peters, J. F. (1973): Relationship of some varieties of electroencephalographic photosensitivity to clinical convulsive disorders. *Neurology (Minneap.),* 23:1040–1057.
112. Remillard, G. M., Ethier, R., and Andermann, F. (1974): Temporal lobe epilepsy and perinatal occlusion of the posterior cerebral artery. *Neurology (Minneap.),* 24:1001–1009.
113. Ricci, G., Berti, G., and Cherubini, E. (1972): Changes in interictal focal activity and spike-wave paroxysms during motor and mental activity. *Epilepsia,* 13:785–794.
114. Ross, J. J., Johnson, L. C., and Walter, R. (1966): Spike and wave discharges during stages of sleep. *Arch. Neurol.,* 14:399–407.
115. Rovit, R. L., Gloor, P., and Rasmussen, T. (1961): Intracarotid amobarbital in epileptic patients. *Arch. Neurol.,* 5:606–626.
116. Rowan, A. J., Rudolf, N. DeM., and Scott, D. F. (1974): EEG prediction of brain metastases. A controlled study with neuropathological confirmation. *J. Neurol. Neurosurg. Psychiatry,* 37:888–893.
117. Sato, S., Dreifuss, F. E., and Penry, J. K. (1973): The effect of sleep on spike-wave discharges in absence seizures. *Neurology (Minneap.),* 23:1335–1345.
118. Smith, J. B., Westmoreland, B. F., Reagan, T. J., and Sandok, B. A. (1975): A distinctive clinical EEG profile in herpes simplex encephalitis. *Mayo Clin. Proc.,* 50:469–474.
119. Smith, J. M. B., and Kellaway, P. (1964): The natural history and clinical correlates of occipital foci in children. In: *Neurological and Electroencephalographic Correlative Studies in Infancy,* edited by P. Kellaway and I. Petersén, pp. 230–249. Grune & Stratton, New York.
120. Stevens, J. R., Kodama, H., Lonsbury, B. L., and Mills, L. (1971): Ultradian characteristics of spontaneous seizures discharges recorded by radiotelemetry in man. *Electroencephalogr. Clin. Neurophysiol.,* 31:313–325.
121. Tassinari, C. A. (1968): Suppression of focal spikes by somato-sensory stimuli. *Electroencephalogr. Clin. Neurophysiol.,* 25:574–578.
122. Tharp, B. R. (1972): Orbital frontal seizures: An unique electroencephalographic and clinical syndrome. *Epilepsia,* 13:627–642.
123. Trojaborg, W. (1968): Changes in spike foci in children. In: *Clinical Electroencephalography in Children,* edited by P. Kellaway and I. Petersén, pp. 213–226. Grune & Stratton, New York.
124. Tükel, K., and Jasper, H. (1952): The electroencephalogram in parasagittal lesions. *Electroencephalogr. Clin. Neurophysiol.,* 4:481–494.
125. Walter, R. D. (1973): Tactical considerations leading to surgical treatment of limbic epilepsy. In: *Epilepsy: Its Phenomenon in Man,* edited by M. A. B. Brazier, pp. 99–121. Academic Press, New York.
126. Watanabe, K., Iwase, K., and Hara, K. (1973): The evolution of EEG features in infantile spasms. *Dev. Med. Child Neurol.,* 15:584–596.
127. Weir, B. (1965): The morphology of the spike-wave complex. *Electroencephalogr. Clin. Neurophysiol.,* 19:284–290.
128. Wilder, B. J. (1972): Projection phenomena and secondary epilepto-genesis-mirror foci. In: *Experimental Models of Epilepsy,* edited by D. P. Purpura, J. K. Penry, D. B. Tower, D. M. Woodbury, and R. D. Walter, pp. 85–112. Raven Press, New York.
129. Zivin, L., and Ajmone-Marsan, C. (1968): Incidence and prognostic significance of "Epileptiform" activity in the EEG of nonepileptic subjects. *Brain,* 91:751–778.

Chapter 9

Activation Procedures and Special Electrodes

Reginald G. Bickford

EEG Laboratories and Department of Neurosciences, University of California, San Diego, La Jolla, California 92093

Activation Procedures	270
Method of Approach	271
Hyperventilation	272
Interpretation	274
Activation by Sensory Stimulation	276
Photic Stimulation	277
Auditory Activation	284
Somesthetic Triggers	284
Startle-Sensitivity Triggers	285
Hysterical Seizures	285
High-Level Processing Seizures (Internal Triggers)	285
Activation by Sleep	286
Sleep Recording	286
Sleep Deprivation	291

All-Night Sleep Monitoring 291
Pentylenetetrazol Activation 291
Special Electrodes 294
  Nasopharnygeal Electrode 297
  Sphenoidal Electrodes 298
  Electrocorticography 298
  Depth Electrography 300
Conclusions 303
Acknowledgment 304
References 304

ACTIVATION PROCEDURES

Activation has been defined by an international committee (1) as a group of special procedures aimed at "enhancing or eliciting normal or abnormal EEG activity" in the clinical electroencephalogram (EEG) recording. For practical purposes, this definition is too restricted because it should apply importantly to the phenomena of neurologic, behavioral, and mental changes that may (or may not) accompany the alterations in the EEG. Thus, activating methods should be regarded more as clinical EEG procedures than as pure EEG tests. Often, the clinical information gained during the test is more useful in neurologic diagnosis or treatment than the specific EEG changes encountered. When undertaking an activation procedure, the electroencephalographer must be innovative in approach and highly attentive to specific details of the patient's complaint.

Viewed from another standpoint, activation procedures involve an attempt to bias the input or the environment of the brain in ways that we suspect will make it reveal defects in its dynamic function. Thus, we hope to catch this complex and sensitive homeostatic mechanism off balance for a moment, thereby revealing defects that would not otherwise be evident. In exposing the "Achilles heel" of our particular patient, we learn something of far greater significance than the reporting of a normal or abnormal EEG since potentially effective lines of treatment are likely to be revealed. In this sense, activation is dynamic electroencephalography at its best and as such, is a close ally of the neurologist.

Many activation procedures have become part of the routine EEG test, as have stress procedures in the field of electrocardiography. This applies particularly to the techniques of hyperventilation, photic stimulation, and sleep. Even these, however, should be subject to modification after the patient's specific problems have been surveyed. Because of the complexity of neurologic behavior and of EEG data often encountered in seizure-induction tests, the presence of a physician during such a procedure is often mandatory. The physician alone may be able to integrate effectively the diverse information from neurologic, behavioral, and mental changes and the specific EEG discharges that are often encountered in epileptic patients. If a physician cannot be present, a considerable part of this responsibility has to be taken by the senior technician who should be specially trained in this area of clinical-EEG correlation. The documentation and coding of the primary record, indicating the exact timing of convulsive and other phenomena, are very important. For instance, the technician should note the occurrence of such minor happenings as hesitation in the speech of a patient reading aloud who is suspected of a reading epilepsy or slight arm myoclonus in a photosensitive patient viewing a visual pattern. In making such observations, the technician can be aided by a hand-operated switch used to energize an event marker on the EEG record. Vocal comments from the technician or assistants recorded on an audio cassette tape recorder and used in conjunction with the event marker to document the changes during a seizure or other event, are also very helpful. Finally, a simple camera capable of taking multiple pictures (such as the Robot) or a closed-circuit TV camera provide optimum systems for information gathering and for subsequent review by the interpreter or the neurologist.

Table 1 shows a convenient summarized classification of some of the more significant techniques that have been used for activation.

TABLE 1. *Activation procedures*

Chemical	Hyperventilation	
	Pentylenetetrazol	
	Bemegride	
Input modification	*Visual*	Photic
		Pattern
		Reading
	Auditory	Music
		Somesthetic
	Others	Startle
State related	Sleep	
	Sleep deprivation	

Naturally, many other procedures have been used to test specific aspects of a patient's syndrome, and active EEG laboratories make discoveries of new "triggers" that may never reach the literature.

Method of Approach

In the following account, we emphasize techniques that are clinically useful and where possible, illustrate them with patient material. In order to present the data systematically, appropriate comments are made on the following categories of information in the order listed:

1. *General statement.* The applicability of the test, the indications for its use and a summary of the varied techniques that have been employed are discussed.

2. *Recommended procedure.* We summarize the procedure usually employed in our laboratory since results are often dependent on detail about stimulus parameters, etc. Unfortunately, a great diversity of instrumentation and procedures is used in activation techniques in different laboratories leading to variable and discordant statistics in the literature.

3. *Physiology.* When some of the operative mechanisms are adequately understood, the physiology underlying the test is discussed.

4. *Recording and artifact problems.* These are very important for interpretation since specific artifacts are correlated with particular activation techniques and must be thoroughly understood by both technician and interpreter. Montages are suggested for reducing artifact and for enhancing positive aspects of the test when appropriate.

5. *Hazards.* Although some procedures are virtually without hazard, others are associated with some definable risks. The risks must be appreciated and discussed with the patient in order to minimize

medicolegal problems. This section mentions important variables (such as age) that affect the applicability and feasibility of individual activation procedures.

6. *Effects on normal subjects.* All activation procedures have effects on a normal subject's EEG, and these must be understood for correct interpretation of the activation study. Many misdiagnoses result from ignorance of the normal effects of the procedure which can often be dramatic (e.g., drowsiness hypersynchrony in children is often misdiagnosed as an epileptic discharge).

7. *Abnormal pattern.* Activation methods may also evoke highly abnormal discharges in a percentage of normal subjects, e.g., during pentylenetetrazol activation (2).

8. *Seizures.* Some of the activation procedures are capable of precipitating seizures in normal subjects (e.g., photic stimulation and pentylenetetrazol activation). The probabilities of this situation must be taken into account in patients where activation procedures lead to a seizure.

9. *Interpretation.* For all the above reasons, the interpretation of the activation test can be difficult and requires close attention to specific detail of the patient's complaint if pitfalls are to be avoided.

10. *References.* For further information concerning activation procedures to supplement the largely didactic account provided here, excellent articles are available in the *EEG Handbook* (3). References to specific chapters of the *Handbook* are given at the end of each section in this chapter.

Hyperventilation

Hyperventilation competes with sleep activation as the most useful of the commonly employed activation tests. It frequently accentuates questionable discharges seen in the resting record and may precipitate actual seizure discharges with clinical accompaniment. Because it is well tolerated by all but a few patients (such as those with a respiratory difficulty), it is widely employed in virtually all clinical laboratories. Nevertheless, misinterpretation of the results of this test is common among inexperienced electroencephalographers (see also Chapter 5).

The standard test consists of 3 min of vigorous overbreathing (technician monitoring is required to achieve some degree of standardization). The test is usually carried out toward the end of the recording to allow a choice of montage, based on any abnormal or localized findings in the resting record. In patients where an all out effort to produce activation is indicated, the breathing period may be extended to 4 or 5 min. In such a case, some degree of tetany may be produced and because of associated confusion, the patient may continue hyperventilation unless stopped by the technician. The eyes should be closed during hyperventilation so as to observe effects on the alpha and other rhythms, but a short (5-sec) period of eye opening at the end of the test is useful to test the responsivity of any patterns that have been induced.

The activation effects of hyperventilation are thought to result from the cerebral anoxia associated with cerebral vasoconstriction caused by lowering of CO_2 in the arterial blood. This hypothesis is supported by the finding that the anoxia produced by breathing nitrogen often produces identical activation effects (4), e.g., precipitation of spike-wave discharge. The anoxic activating effect of hyperventilation often continues well beyond (30 to 60 sec) the end of overbreathing if the breathing effort has been vigorous because the period of apnea continues until the restoration of normal CO_2 levels. Thus, maximum EEG activation changes may be seen during this period.

Hyperventilation produces artifacts of varied kinds that are often entrained by the breathing rhythm. Muscle and movement artifacts are commonly associated with a vigorous hyperventilation effort.

This may also increase head tremor with the appearance of 4- to 6-Hz muscle spikes in the occipital regions. In sick patients, there may be coughing and swallowing with associated tongue-induced glossokinetic potentials (5) that may mar the record and make it unreliable. Under humid conditions the breathing rhythm may induce slow potential shifts of the psychogalvanic type. Hyperventilation may also produce symptoms of finger paresthesia (possibly related to tetany), feelings of unreality, and mild confusion. Other patients may react with autonomic symptoms, including palpitations, sweating, and syncope. A combination of these symptoms may at times be difficult to distinguish from a seizure, and careful observation and recording by the technician with additional questioning afterward will often be necessary to diagnose correctly any episodes occurring during the test.

However, the problems that cause the most diagnostic difficulties with this activation test are the effects it produces on the EEG of normal subjects. The most frequent misdiagnosis in EEG is probably that of mistaking the normal rhythmic high-voltage 2- to 4-Hz activ-

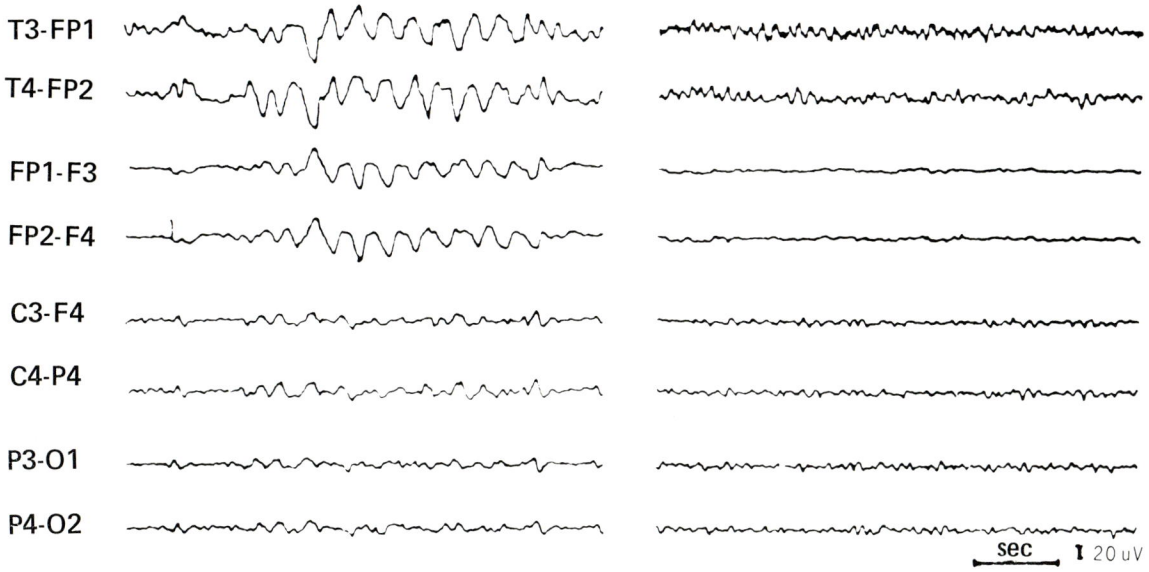

FIG. 1 Effect of blood sugar level on the response to hyperventilation. On the left is shown the typical rhythmic 2- to 3-Hz response to 2½ min. hyperventilation in a normal subject. On the right is demonstrated the effect of an identical period of hyperventilation on the subject following ingestion of 50 g glucose, 15 min before the recording was taken.

ity associated with hyperventilation for an abnormal discharge. This rhythm is often paroxysmal, shows maximal amplitude in the younger age groups (6 to 16 years), and is markedly dependent on the level of blood sugar (Fig. 1). Thus, the hyperventilation "delta" effect is markedly accentuated by lowering of blood sugar and on several occasions has been the first indication of pathologic hypoglycemia (as from islet cell tumor) in a patient referred for an EEG. In younger age groups (2 to 8 years), this rhythm may make its initial appearance in the parietooccipital region (Fig. 2) and spread forward, in contradistinction to older age groups where it appears initially in the frontal regions and spreads backward. This rhythm may produce difficulties in record interpretation because of its fortuitous association with other high-frequency waves, such as beta activity or muscle potentials. The combination of these wave forms can at times give the spurious appearance of a pathologic spike-wave discharge. A careful study of the background activity in relation to the development of the hyperventilation response can usually solve these problems. In normal subjects, hyperventilation commonly increases the amplitude and persistence of the alpha rhythm and may result in the disappearance of minor asymmetries noted in the resting record. If such asymmetries disappear during hyperventilation, they should not be considered to be of any pathologic significance. The normal hyperventilation response has to be distinguished from other rhythmic "projected disturbances," such as frontal intermittent rhythmic delta activity (6) that appears in frontal regions unrelated to hyperventilation. These will be present to some degree in other parts of the record and are often asymmetric. In contrast, the normal hyperventilation response is always symmetric unless rendered unequal by the presence of a lesion. In case of difficulties, giving the patient a glucose drink to produce the suppressive effect on the frontal hyperventilation activity of raising the blood sugar may be helpful (see Fig. 1).

Interpretation

Hyperventilation is frequently of assistance to the interpreter because it may intensify and clarify the wave form of paroxysmal discharges of an uncertain nature that may have appeared in the resting record. It is also an excellent activator of 3-Hz spike-wave discharges such as that seen in Fig. 3. When these are of classic wave form, there is no difficulty in their recognition, although their presence should be documented by behavioral information, which might indicate the occurrence of a petit mal (absence) attack. The occurrence of behavioral changes is of particular significance in deciding whether an atypical paroxysmal discharge of a spike-wave type is to be given epileptic significance. Occasionally, hyperventilation precipitates a focal cortical (partial) seizure which is usually accompanied by localized changes in the EEG. A temporal lobe (complex partial) seizure is occasionally induced by hyperventilation. The induced automatism is usually associated with widespread theta activity which is maximal on the side of origin. Tests of speech function by the technician in the ictal and postictal phases assist in lateralizing the seizure.

In summary, the period of hyperventilation is often the most decisive part of the EEG record for clinical interpretation, but a greal deal of technician skill is needed here so that varied pitfalls mentioned above can be avoided. Further reading on this topic is available in the *EEG Handbook* (7).

FIG. 2. Normal hyperventilation buildup of rhythmic 2- to 3-Hz activity commencing posteriorly in a 6-year-old patient. Note the late involvement of frontal electrodes and the early disappearance of rhythmic activity from this region following cessation of overbreathing.

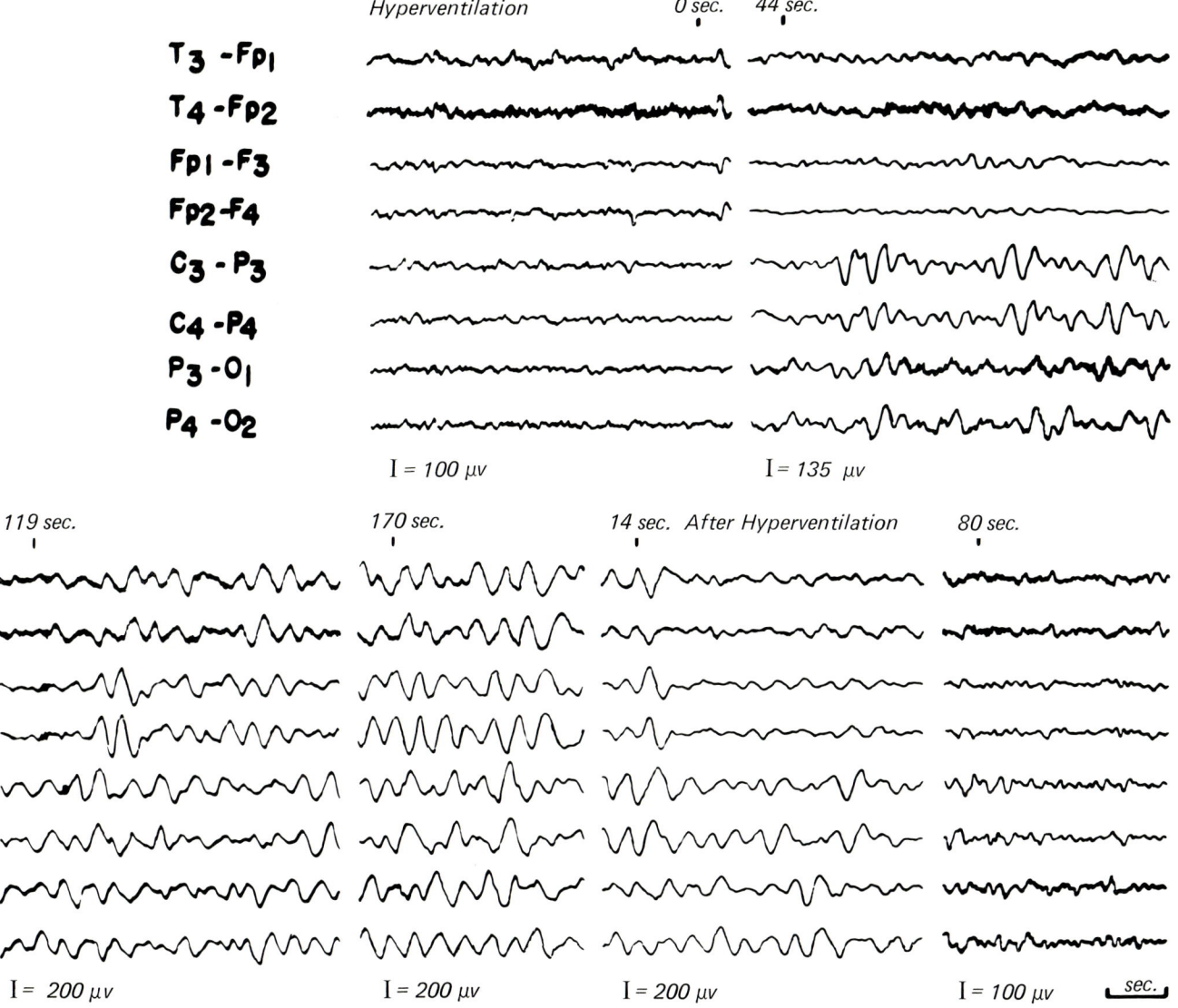

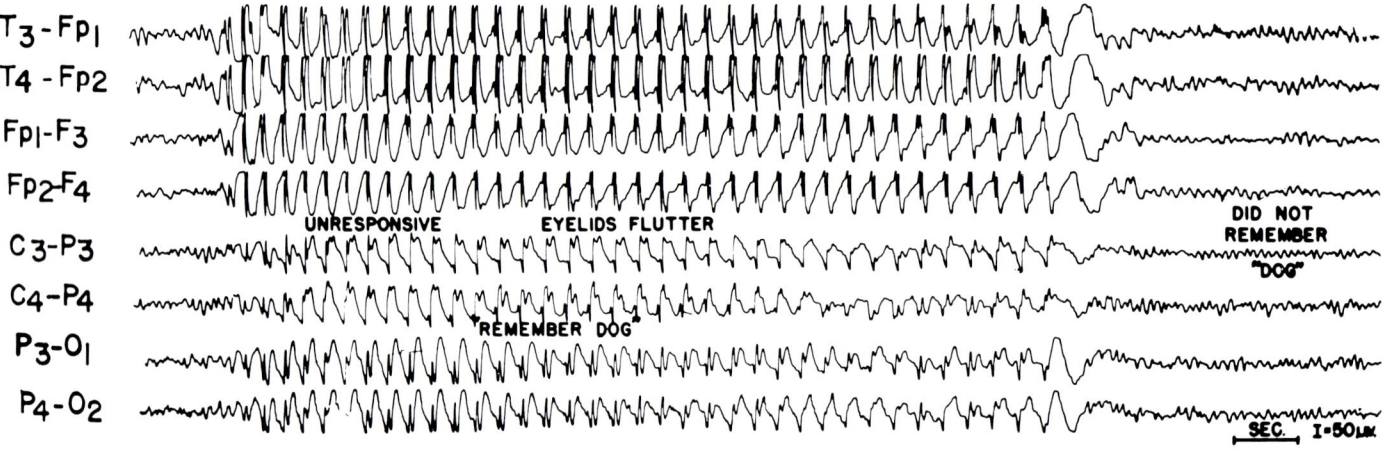

FIG. 3. 3-Hz spike-wave discharge with associated typical absence (petit mal) attack induced by hyperventilation. The discharge occurred 1 min following commencement of overbreathing. Note the marked differences between the pattern of this discharge and that which may be produced normally by hyperventilation (Figs. 1 and 2). Note that tests of responsiveness were carried out and confirmed the paralysis of response during the attack and the absence of memory recording during the discharge ("remember dog").

Activation by Sensory Stimulation

It has been known since antiquity that epileptic seizures in some patients can be precipitated by various types of environmental triggers. The most commonly encountered example of this kind involves visual stimuli, which may give rise to the clinical syndrome known as photogenic epilepsy. However, similar trigger epilepsies have been reported from other sensory input such as auditory and somatesthetic stimuli and others in which the stimulus pattern may be quite complex. Although fully developed trigger epilepsies are not very common (they may account for 5 to 10% of all epileptic patients), environmental stimuli of varied kinds may influence the occurrence of seizures in patients who are not usually considered straightforward trigger epilepsies. The modern urban environment increasingly subjects its population to visual stimulation including flashing neon signs, car headlights, the synchronized music and light of dance floors and discotheques, and the flicker of the TV screen. The investigation of these subliminal triggers may assist the clinician in maintaining seizure control even in cases where medication is the primary factor in suppressing the convulsive disorder. Finally, the clinician who studies the patient's symptoms in detail and the mechanism by which they tend to be accentuated will find that many of the procedures described here provide confirmation by electrophysiologic methods for clinical suspicions that have been generated by the history. The activation methods will be described in the following sequence: (a) photic stimulation, (b) auditory activation, (c) somesthetic triggers, (d) startle-sensitivity triggers, (e) hysterical seizures, and (f) high-level processing seizures.

Photic Stimulation

Although photic stimulation is not as effective for activation as hyperventilation or sleep recording, nevertheless, it produces a variety of electrophysiologic information that often may be usefully integrated in the electroencephalographer's report.

A wide range of techniques have been employed to produce photic stimulation. These include: (a) constant intensity illumination, (b) strobe flashing at varied frequencies, (c) pattern stimulation by viewing pattern materials or by strobing a pattern, (d) solar (sun) stimulation, and (e) self-stimulation techniques. A common test method employed routinely in many laboratories consists of the use of a strobe light (intensities ranging from 500,000 to 2,000,000 foot candles) located at a distance of 12 in from the patient's face. This light is operated at a range of flash frequencies which in our own laboratory include 1,3,6,9,10,11,15,20, and 30 Hz for separate 5-sec runs with the eyes open and with the eyes closed. To test visual pattern response and lambda wave production, a parallel striped black and white or colored pattern is used for the former and a complex picture (8) for the latter. In testing self-stimulation patients (those that induce spike-wave activity and seizures by waving a hand in front of their eyes), a floodlight or the sun may need to be used, but overexposure should be avoided because of the hazard of retinal burn. A referential montage is suitable for recording and should include occipital and parietal leads and at least one frontal lead.

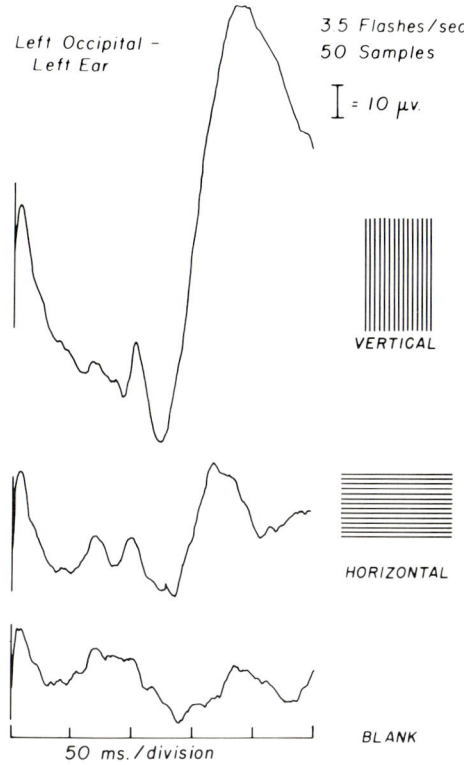

FIG. 4. Abnormal averaged evoked response to pattern stimulus in a pattern-sensitive patient. Patient, a 10-year-old boy, is sensitive to a variety of visual patterns that produce absence attacks. Testing of the patient showed that he had a remarkably specific trigger; viewing horizontal lines was ineffective in producing attacks, whereas viewing of vertical lines was readily effective. This difference is indicated in variation in the later components (150 to 215 msec) of the average evoked response *(upper two tracings).* In these observations, the patterns and a *blank* sheet *(lowermost tracing)* were illuminated by a strobe light flashing at 3.5 Hz, and each tracing represents the summation of 50 responses.

In one channel, the light stimulus should be monitored with photocell or output signal from the stimulator to give an adequate indication of flash timing. The technique of superimposing the photic pulses on the EEG trace is not recommended since it may obscure the relationship between the stimulus and response so necessary for recognizing spurious responses caused by artifact from the photic apparatus. A 5-sec exposure to a particular flash frequency with a 5-sec interval before the next sequence begins is a workable procedure. When searching for low-grade sensitivity, it is sometimes advantageous to have the patient open and close the eyes while the flash rate is continuously varied. Room illumination should be reduced but darkness should be avoided because of the difficulty of observing changes in the patient under these circumstances. Low-level independent illumination avoids the problem of strobing that obscures flash-related myoclonus or other movement.

In spite of extensive investigation, little is known about the mechanism of photic driving or about the manner in which abnormal discharges, such as spike-and-slow-wave complexes, are triggered. There seems to be no simple relationship between the driving response and the development of epileptiform discharge since in most instances one does not lead progressively to the other. Animal experiments (9) have suggested that the occipital cortices are not necessary for the widespread paroxysmal response triggered by photic stimulation, and experimental evidence indicates that this type of response may be mediated by some pathway branching off at the lateral geniculate level. There is no evidence that the normal lambda wave elicited in response to visual pattern relates to the hypersensitive response to pattern present in some photoepileptic patients. In some patients but not all, the average evoked response to photic stimulation may be highly abnormal, as indicated in Fig. 4.

Important instrumental and biologic artifacts occur in association with photic stimulation. These include:

1. *Flash artifact.* A high frequency pickup from the strobe light that occurs simultaneously with the photocell pulse and usually indicates the existence of a high resistance electrode or defective grounding;

2. *The photomyoclonic response.* A muscle reflex appearing maximally around the eyes (Fig. 5).

Photic stimulation carried out with a strobe light is relatively free of hazard to patients since the possibility of retinal burns is eliminated by the shortness of the strobe pulse. However, an appreciable hazard exists with the use of a photoflood bulb or the sun, therefore, exposure to these light sources must be minimized. Photosensitive patients may be driven into a grand mal seizure if minor attacks are repeatedly precipitated.

Photic stimulation produces a variety of rather striking phenomena in the normal subject. These include:

1. *The photic driving response.* A normal phenomenon manifested by symmetric sinusoidal driving of the EEG at the flash frequency and usually maximal in the occipitoparietal regions. In some subjects

FIG. 5. Comparison of photomyoclonic response to photic stimulation **(top)** and photoconvulsive response **(bottom).** Note large muscle contraction spikes *(upper tracing)* associated with palpable muscle jerking in the orbital area. Discharge ceases with light stimulation. This response occurs in the normal population although it may appear in exaggerated form in some patients (drug withdrawal, etc.). The abnormal photoconvulsive response *(lower tracing)* was recorded from a patient who had petit mal (absence) attacks. Note 3-Hz spike-wave discharge, which continues following cessation of photic stimulation (self-sustained discharge) and is associated with behavioral evidence of an absence attack.

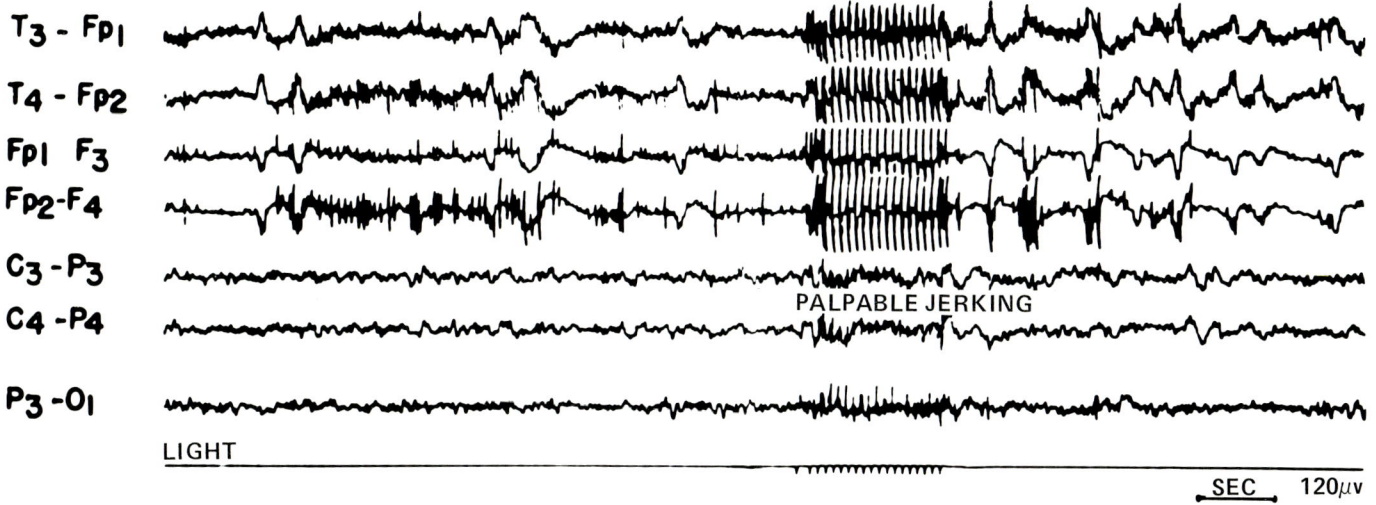
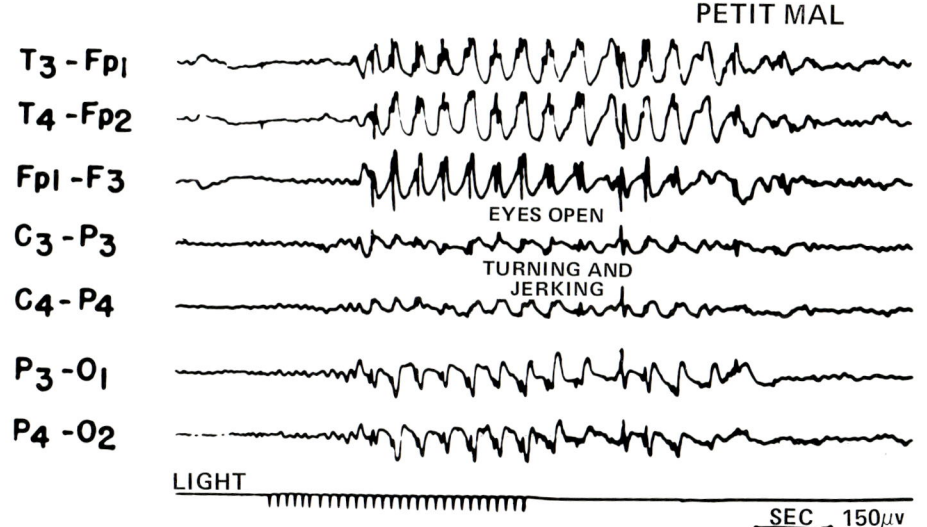

the response may spread widely in both hemispheres. Although this response is usually symmetric on the two sides, it may be asymmetric at some frequencies in the normal subject. Harmonics and subharmonics of the flash frequency may also be generated, but their significance is not understood.

2. *The photomyoclonic response.* Occurs in some 20% of normal subjects and is a muscle reflex maximal in the periorbital muscles. Sometimes it may spread throughout the cranial musculature and even involve the limb musculature. This response appears in the EEG as myogenic "spikes" which follow the photic stimulus with a small delay (about 50 msec). The response often shows recruitment at the beginning of the flash train, is changed by the state of tension of the facial muscles, and ceases abruptly with the last flash (Fig. 5). When present at lower flash rates, it can be mistaken for a spike-wave discharge, particularly when the recording electrode is near the eyes. In these cases the slow wave produced by movement of the eye globe together with the muscle spike may closely simulate a spike-wave discharge of cerebral origin. The technician can verify the existence of photomyoclonus by direct palpation of the facial muscles, since it is often difficult to see the movement because of the strobing effect of the light.

Paroxysmal discharges may be seen in a small percentage of the nonepileptic population (10 to 15%) and consist of complex mixtures of sharp components, spikes, and slow waves that may resemble a photoconvulsive discharge, but they are usually of lower amplitude and there are no clinical accompaniments.

Interpretation

The following aspects of the photic activation record must be considered when a report is made: (a) the amplitude, distribution, and symmetry of the photic driving response, (b) effects of photic stimulation on activity (normal or abnormal) recorded in other parts of the record, and (c) abnormal activity actually precipitated by photic stimulation and not present elsewhere.

Photic driving response. The driving response, when present, can be used as evidence that impressed activity within the visual system is arriving at a cortical level. Thus photic responses in the neonate are reassuring when blindness is in question. The photic driving response may be present in higher cognitive disturbances of visual function and is, for instance, unaffected in hysterical blindness. Not all subjects with normal vision, however, show photic driving. Asymmetry of the driving response can be seen at some frequencies in normal subjects. Cortical lesions of a destructive type may cause unilateral amplitude reduction of the response, whereas irritative lesions, such as those associated with epileptic scars, may produce increased driving on the side of the lesion. For judging significance, the interpreter will want to compare the driving asymmetry with any asymmetry of alpha activity that also may be present. However, many of these problems concerning transmission in the visual system are now solved more definitively by using the average evoked response to flash or to pattern shift and by including information from the electroretinogram (see Chapter 17, Fig. 17).

Effects of photic stimulation on activity recorded in other parts of the record. Photic stimulation sometimes activates and renders more specific paroxysmal discharges seen in other parts of the recording and thus contributes to the final interpretation. Its use (among other evoked sensory measures) has also been recommended in establishing the presence of electrocerebral silence. However, in this instance, there are several problems. The electroretinogram, which is highly resistant to anoxic damage and may be conducted to anterior electrodes, has to be distinguished from cerebral activity. Furthermore,

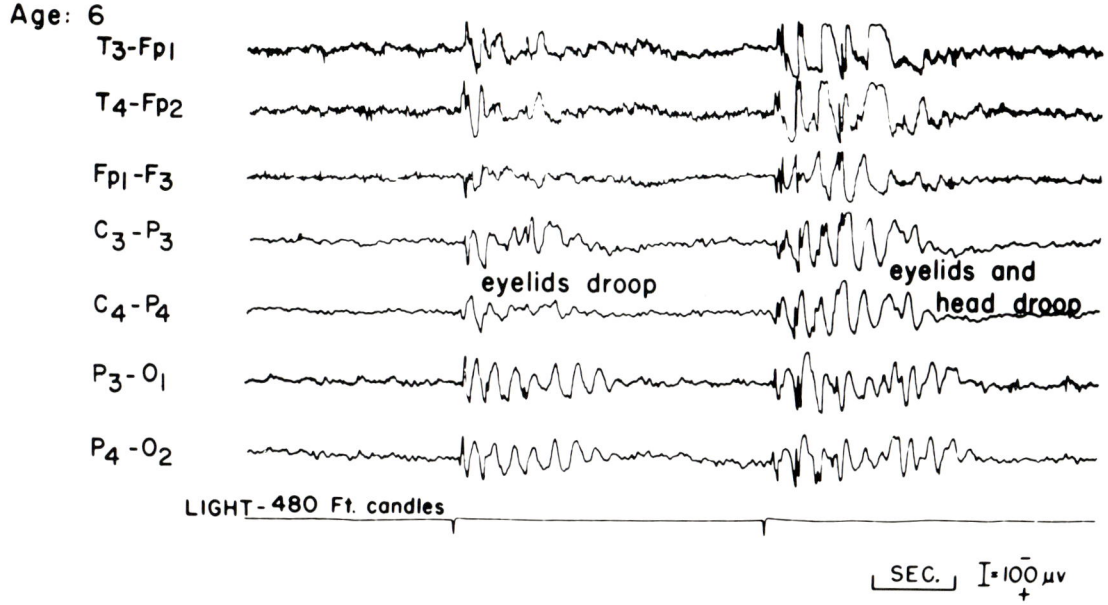

FIG. 6. Spike-wave discharge with associated clinical seizure produced by a single light stimulus. This child was severely retarded and suffered from frequent absence attacks, some of which were self-induced by hand waving while looking at the sun. Note abnormal spike-wave discharges in the EEG produced by the two separate flashes and their association with slightly different absence seizures.

both animal and human observations indicate that at least some kinds of sensory evoked potentials are more resistant to anoxia than spontaneous activity and may be present in the condition of electrocerebral silence (see also Chapter 16).

Abnormal activity precipitated by photic stimulation. Although photic stimulation is not as effective as other activation methods in precipitating abnormal discharges, at times, patients with extreme photosensitivity are encountered (Fig. 6). Some patients show marked variation in response to identical stimuli and in some instances, a periodicity in responsiveness can be demonstrated (10). Such spontaneous fluctuations in responsiveness have to be borne in mind when sensitivity tests (as for dark glasses) are carried out on photoepileptic patients. These photoconvulsive responses, present in some 5 to 15% of epileptic patients, must be distinguished from the photomyoclonic response

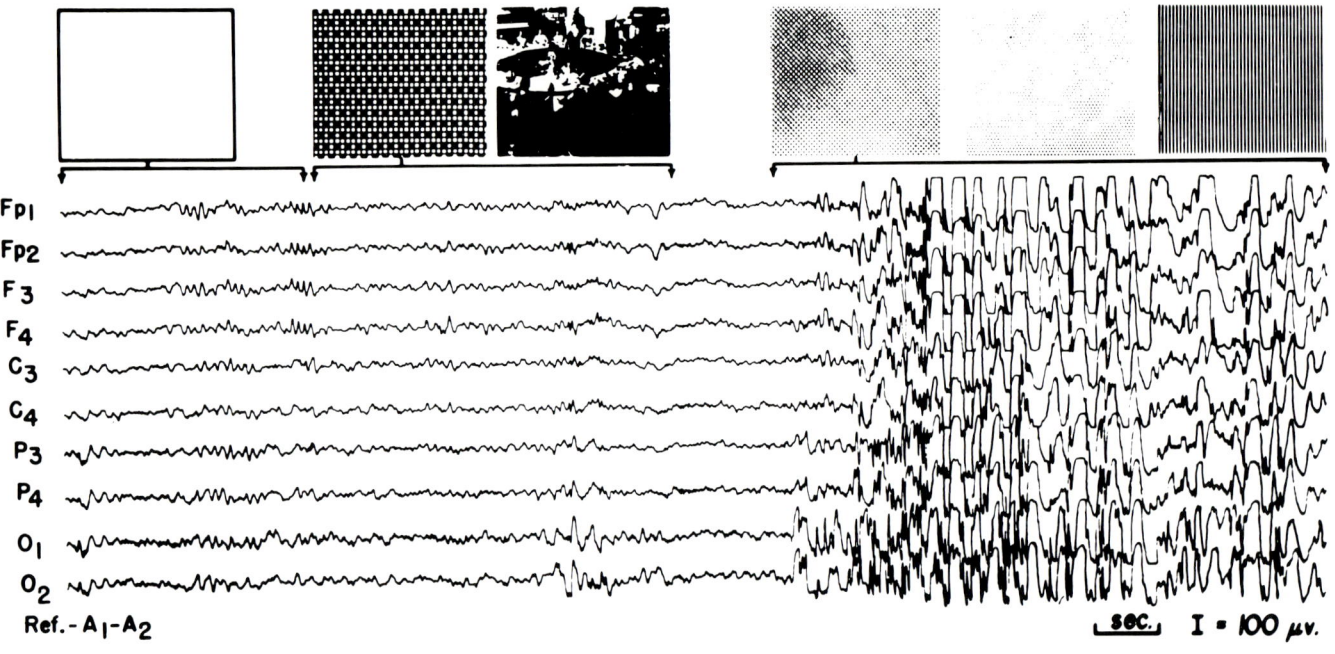

FIG. 7. Response to different stimulus patterns in a child exhibiting visual pattern sensitivity. Patient, age 9, was asked to scan the picture during recording of the EEG. The upper left three patterns (including blank) were ineffective in triggering a seizure. Three fine-grain patterns shown on the right were all effective in inducing a seizure with associated spike-wave discharge, as shown on the right side of the figure. This patient was also sensitive to flash stimuli. In this tracing, A1 serves as a common reference for left-sided leads and A2 serves as a common reference for right-sided leads.

(11). This distinction depends importantly on the fact that the photoconvulsive response is different in wave form and is not synchronized with the stimulus (Fig. 5). Tests of patient responsiveness and observations of behavioral accompaniment also assist in the differentiation since the photomyoclonic response does not affect consciousness.

Patients with seizures who complain of a sensitivity to light indicated by difficulties with snowscapes or with motoring through an avenue of trees in a setting sun should also be tested for the existence of pattern sensitivity. An example of this is shown in Fig. 7.

A small proportion of photosensitive patients acquire the compul-

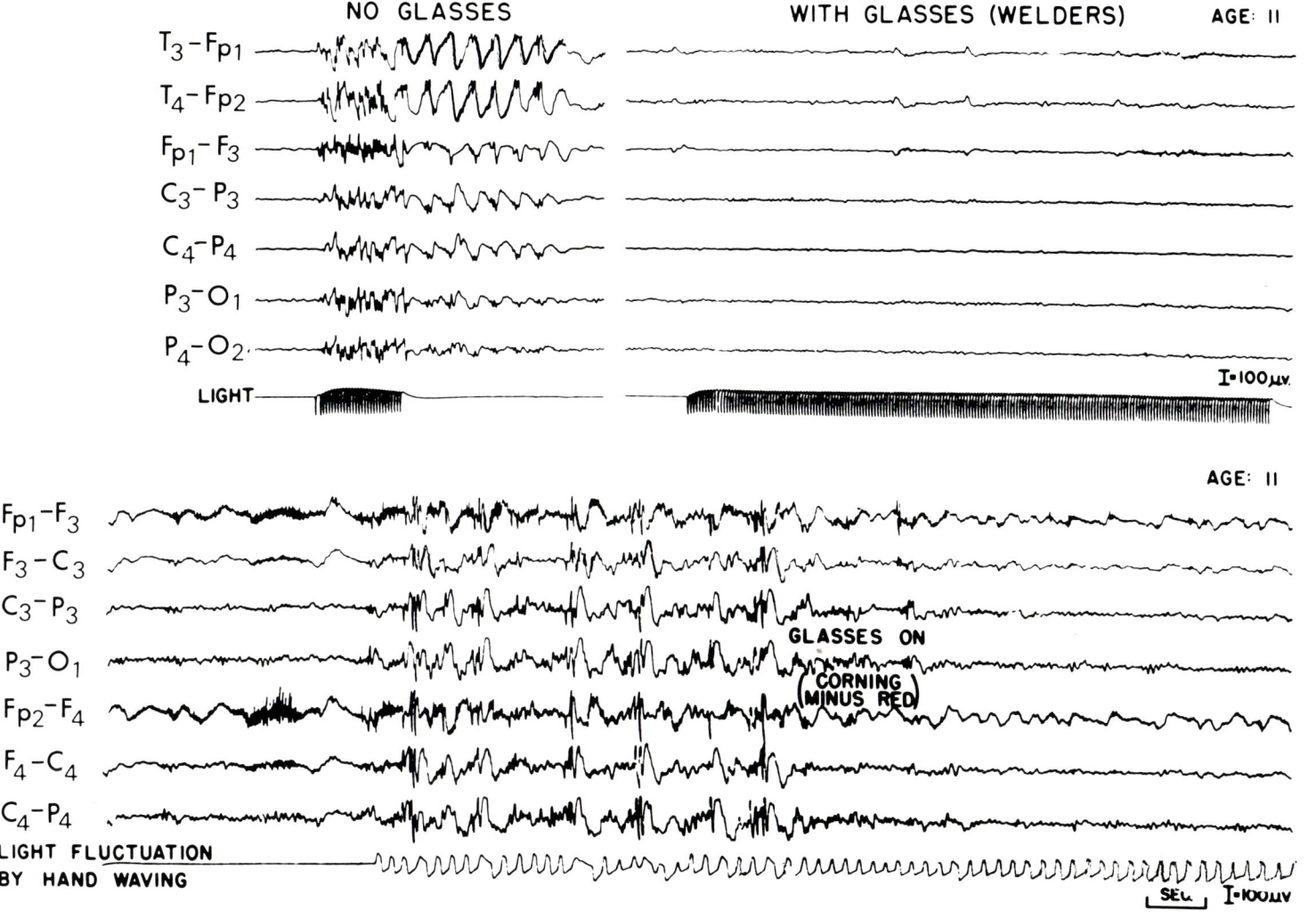

FIG. 8. Protection from convulsive effect of light by dark welder's glasses (top) and by glasses that restrict the red part of the spectrum (bottom). In addition, the patient (bottom) is inducing his attacks by waving his hand between his eyes and a photoflood light. This was a common maneuver the patient employed to induce attacks. A small photocell attached to the face records the hand and finger movements (bottom channel).

sive habit of inducing their own seizures. In these patients, seizure discharges can often be precipitated by having them wave their hands in front of their faces while looking at the sun or a photoflood bulb. Hand movements can be conveniently registered by a small photocell attached to the face below the eye (Fig. 8). Many of these patients can benefit from dark glasses such as welders' glasses (if they tolerate them) as shown in Fig. 8. Also shown is an example of a patient preferentially sensitive to red light who can be protected by excluding this wave length from the spectrum.

The interpretation of the EEG in patients with photosensitivity is usually straightforward when the record shows paroxysmal discharges of the spike-wave type triggered by light and associated with evidence of a petit mal (absence) seizure. However, difficulties may arise when light triggers paroxysmal discharges of a less specific type, since this phenomenon may occur in the nonepileptic population. In this instance, evidence of behavioral accompaniment is valuable since it adds clinical significance to the findings and tends to exclude clinically irrelevant responses that may be encountered in some normal subjects.

Another aspect of growing importance in photosensitivity is its association with drug withdrawal syndromes such as barbiturates (12) and alcohol. A photoconvulsive response may appear in the EEG before the onset of clinical seizures and thus can be usefully employed to monitor patients undergoing a withdrawal regimen. The appearance of a photoconvulsive response indicates the need for anticonvulsant medication during the withdrawal process.

Both the frequency of the basic EEG and the response to photic stimulation can also be employed to monitor electrolyte changes that may lead to convulsions in patients undergoing renal dialysis procedures. The nature of electrolyte changes leading to photosensitivity has been described in both animal and human observations (13).

Auditory Activation

Unlike photic stimulation, rhythmic click or tone stimulation produce little detectable response (except alerting) in the EEG. However, in rare cases the phenomenon of musicogenic epilepsy is observed (14). In these patients, the playing of music gives rise to a seizure (usually temporal lobe in type), and often the type of music that triggers the seizure is very specific (classical, rock, etc.).

These cases do not usually present a diagnostic problem if the clinician is aware of the syndrome and the patient will usually relate the occurrence of the attack (confusion and amnesia, etc.) to the listening to music. The seizure mechanism can be tested by recording the EEG while the offending music is played. A montage covering the temporal lobes bilaterally should be used, and musical stimulation may have to be carried on for a considerable time (1 to 2 hr) before activation is produced. The EEG seizure pattern has to be distinguished from movement and muscle artifacts that may accompany facial mannerisms engendered by the rhythm of rock music or by the seizure itself.

Somesthetic Triggers

In rare instances, skin stimulation is an effective trigger for epileptic seizures. Such cases usually involve a clinical syndrome in which a focal lesion exists on the corresponding somatosensory cortical area. In these cases, the zone of seizure initiation may be quite localized on the patient's body. Testing is usually straightforward and can follow the details of the trigger requirements as supplied by the patient. Some cases initially considered to have a somatosensory trigger on further investigation turn out to have a startle-sensitivity trigger (see below).

Startle-Sensitivity Triggers

A group of cases occur in which startle is the trigger for an epileptic seizure (15). Such patients' seizures begin in reaction to a sudden sound, a light flash, or a touch to the body surface, as long as the element of unexpectedness or startle is present. When testing these patients in the EEG laboratory, it is important that the situation be programmed to supply the requirements of a startle situation (as by the use of a loud unusual sound generated by a gong or other device unknown to the patient). The artifactual components (movement and muscle) generated by the normal startle response may give rise to difficulty in interpretation, but the seizure discharge should outlast the startle response by several seconds.

Hysterical Seizures

Hysterical seizures come in a great variety of forms, and although specific triggers are not usually involved, the environmental situation plays an important part in the initiation mechanism. The diagnostic separation of hysterical attacks from epileptic seizures can sometimes be difficult (16), but the skill of the physician in setting up the appropriate emotional circumstance for precipitating the event is important. Unfortunately, the EEG recording taken during an induced episode is not always helpful because of its likely contamination with muscle and movement artifact. To reduce this problem, an accelerometer should be attached to the head to register movement. A further problem in interpretation is that temporal lobe seizures can occasionally occur with no detectable scalp EEG change. When interpreting the EEG recording of the "event," the EEGer will look for changes in background rhythms and the occurrence of widespread theta activity characteristic of temporal lobe automatism. The observer should also assess any discrepancies between timing of the EEG and behavioral events and should evaluate any neurologic accompaniments, including speech disturbance (as may occur in a temporal lobe lesion effecting the dominant hemisphere).

High-Level Processing Seizures (Internal Triggers)

In rare patients, it has been established that central processing events such as memory recall, calculation, etc., apparently unassociated with sensory input, may precipitate a seizure. Such patients can be tested by recording the EEG during recall procedures, as shown in Fig. 9.

Since the original observation of Bickford and associates (17), it has been known that reading can provide the trigger that induces the jaw myoclonus of primary reading epilepsy. These patients may be tested by having them read (out loud or silently) material that they have noted to be troublesome. Long periods of reading (½ to 1 hr) may be necessary before the syndrome becomes established with the usual complaint of "jaw clicking." This sign, in fact, is myoclonus of the jaw muscles, manifested by the primary reading group, which is usually associated with a relatively inconspicuous paroxysmal discharge maximal in the parietal regions bilaterally (Fig. 10). It is important to establish the relationship of the jaw jerk to the discharge, and because jaw jerking itself can produce movement artifact that may resemble the paroxysm, separate controls should be carried out. In these, patients should be instructed to imitate as closely as possible the kind of jerk they experience in their attack. In general, the seizure discharge is usually found to be different in form and complexity from the simulated movement. Resemblance between the discharge and spontaneously occurring paroxysms unassociated with movement should also be helpful (Fig. 10). Some of these patients have a marked and widespread 3-Hz spike-and-wave discharge appearing diffusely and associated with the jaw myoclonus.

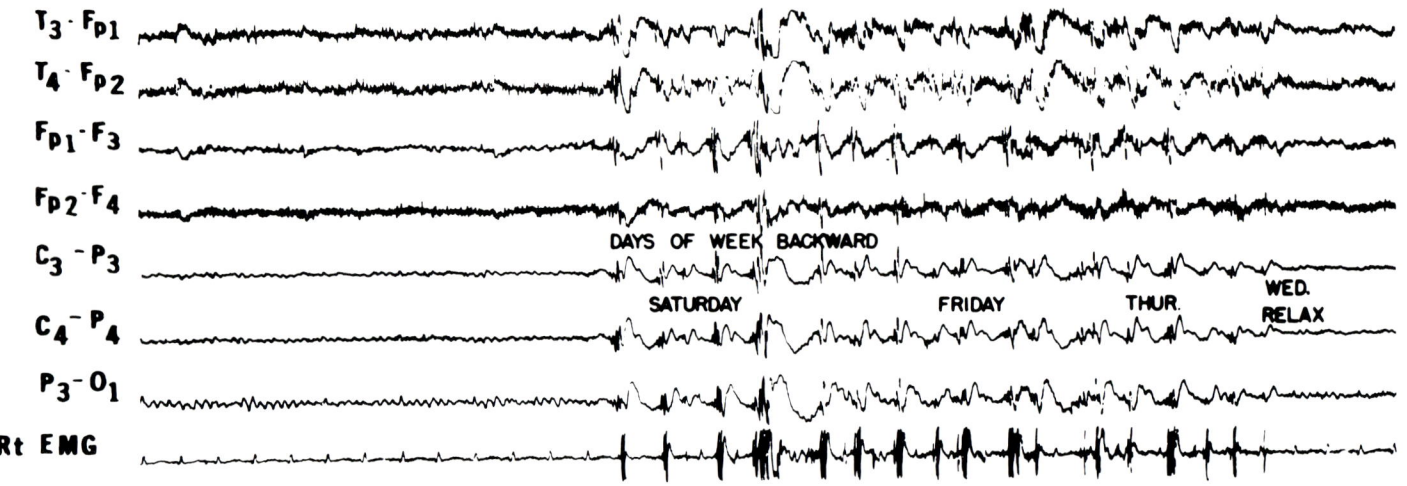

FIG. 9. Seizure discharge with myoclonus related to memory recall. Patient, age 56, had suffered what was probably a stroke a few months previously. Since this incident, she reports jerking of the right arm when she recalls or calculates. EEG is normal until she is asked to name days of the week backwards. Note diffuse spike-wave complexes in the EEG associated with myoclonus (monitored in the bottom channel by surface EMG leads on right forearm).

In these cases, the diagnosis is easily established. The patient should also be tested for pattern sensitivity since a reading text may merely be one of a variety of patterned material that triggers an epileptic seizure (secondary reading epilepsy of Bickford). Once the myoclonus has been established, testing should not be too prolonged; otherwise, the patient may well go into a generalized tonic-clonic seizure.

Activation by Sleep

The sleep state has strong and subtle activating effects on the EEG. In practice the technique is used in three separate approaches: (a) a routine daytime sleep record (with or without sedative medication), (b) a similar recording performed following a period of sleep deprivation, and (c) a recording using the techniques of all-night sleep monitoring.

Sleep Recording

The sleep recording, carried out as part of the routine EEG, is becoming one of the most popular methods of EEG activation and is used routinely in many labs. Furthermore, in some anxious or uncooperative children, it may be the only way to obtain a reliable record. In general, it is a good activation method for both focal

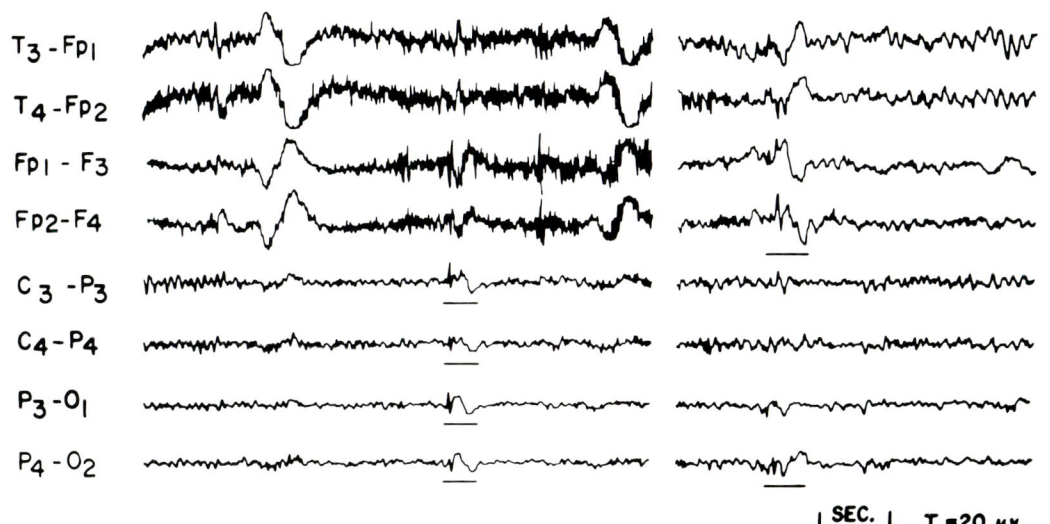

FIG. 10. Case of primary reading epilepsy. Patient, age 29, complains of jaw-jerking following long periods of reading. In the trace on the left, note the occurrence of miniature spike-wave burst (underlined) during a period of reading (eyes open). This was associated with jaw myoclonus. The patient has grand mal attack if he continues reading following the "warning myoclonus." In the trace on the right, a similar spike-wave burst occurs during drowsiness (eyes closed) and is unassociated with movement.

and generalized discharges and should be used in all patients suspected of having a seizure disorder. However, difficulties often arise in the interpretation of sleep recordings. Thus, the clinical significance attached to many of the discharges recorded during sleep remains controversial and undecided. On the other hand, in the important area of neonatal studies, sleep recordings are both important and inevitable, and significant differences exist between the effect of rapid-eye-movement (REM) and nonrapid-eye-movement (NREM) sleep in the assessment of neonatal maturation. Sleep recordings in the neonatal group require additional monitoring of respiration, eye movement (oculogram), and muscle activity for the proper clinical interpretation of the record (18). An example is shown in Fig. 11.

Sleep activation is least complicated in its interpretation when natural sleep is recorded. Thus, after obtaining initial recording in the waking state with eye opening and closing, many laboratories encourage the patient to drift off into sleep. It is commonplace to use ear reference montages preferentially for the sleep part of the record. Because the vertex is an active area in sleep, a vertex reference should not usually be employed and an average reference will have the difficulty of much in-phase activity. If focal discharges are present, their field distribution should be checked using montages with bipolar anteroposterior and coronal derivations.

The physiology of sleep is poorly understood, although a good deal has been learned about the stages of sleep and some of the brainstem control mechanisms (19,20). In the drowsiness or slow-wave phases where most EEG activation occurs, there is evidence of lowering of resistance to synaptic spread of convulsive potentials. Thus, during sleep, many discharges extend widely over the surface

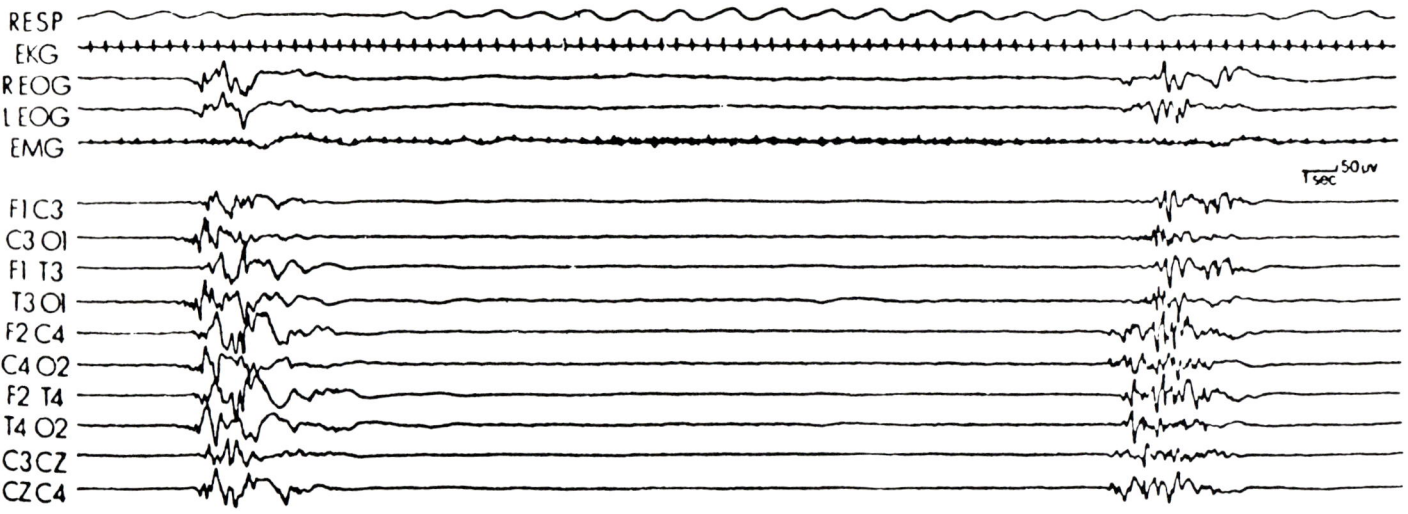

FIG. 11. Recording of newborn infant having apneic attacks. Note utility of extra channels devoted to monitoring (respiration, vertical and horizontal eye movement, and submental muscle) in addition to conventional EEG. This montage is recommended as standard practice for neonatal EEG. Note epileptic discharge leading to cessation of breathing ("convulsive apnea").

of the cortex; discharges that may be confined to deep structures such as the limbic structures tend to fire up to the cortical surface where they can be detected. Such changes in "spike penetrance" related to the onset of sleep have been documented during depth electroencephalographic recordings in man. This tendency for epileptiform discharges to be more widespread during sleep needs to be remembered when interpreting the sleep record. Otherwise such records may be thought to favor the existence of a more extensive lesion than is, in fact, the case. Recordings made during sleep are often relatively free from the kinds of artifacts that appear in the waking record. However, movements can be a problem, particularly if these block the amplifiers and suggest the possibility of widespread paroxysmal discharges. In these cases, technician observations are often helpful.

Sleep recording is probably the safest of all activation. Even when medication is used, it is relatively free from hazard provided the patient is asked about drug allergies and provided that standard doses are not exceeded.

The sleep EEG in the normal subject is a highly complex phenomenon and is quite different in its EEG pattern from one stage to another. Furthermore, normal sleep differs with age (see Chapter 5). In older children and adults, REM stages are not usually encoun-

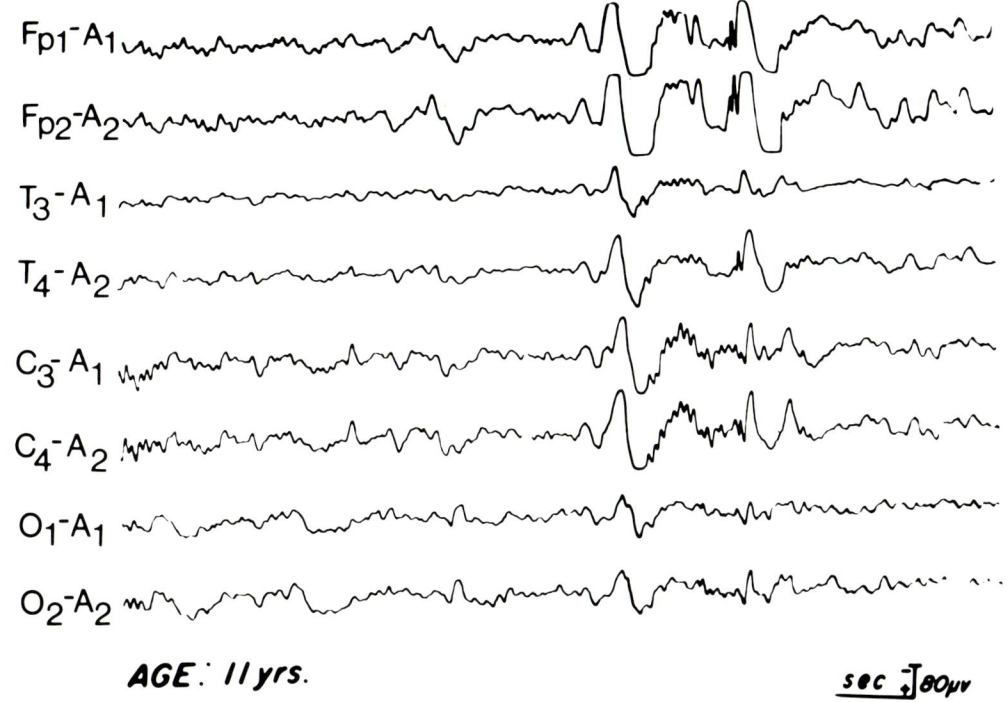

FIG. 12. Difficulties in distinguishing an epileptic spike-wave discharge from a vertex wave of sleep. Patient, age 11, had petit mal (absence) attacks. The first large discharge seen in the tracing is a typical smooth vertex wave followed by spindle activity (K-complex) most evident in the frontocentral region. However, the next discharge to the right has a slightly different distribution and has an added spike component (not due to spindles).

tered in routine daytime sleep recordings, although they are frequently seen in records from the newborn. There are several components of normal sleep that can be mistaken for spikes or sharp waves. Thus, the occipital positive spike-like waves known as positive occipital sharp transients of sleep (POSTS) or "lambdoid waves" are large in some subjects and can be easily mistaken for bioccipital sharp waves. However, the rather constant character of the lambdoid wave and its polarity help to distinguish it from a sharp wave. A more difficult differentiation is that of the vertex wave (V-wave) prominent in stage 2 sleep. In some normal subjects, this transient may have a very sharp contour and may be asymmetric in the two hemispheres. Under these circumstances, it can easily be mistaken for a sharp wave. As shown in Fig. 12, this problem is further complicated by the tendency for many abnormal discharges to appear in the vertex region, where combinations of spindles and V-waves may mimic them. With care, however, the spike-wave discharge can be distinguished. One of the most troublesome problems in the reading of clinical sleep records is the distinction to be made between so-called "small sharp spikes" (SSS) and pathologic focal spike discharges. SSS, which are recorded commonly (about 25%) in the normal population, are regarded by most workers as a normal component of the sleep EEG (see Chapter 14). Further work by Reiher et al. has indicated that amplitude, duration, and other properties of these components of sleep can approach closely the characteristics of more significant spike discharges. However, SSS tend to be distributed more widely over both hemispheres as compared with most focal spikes or sharp waves (21). In spite of the above criteria, these troublesome discharges may be difficult to distinguish from the pathologic spikes.

Because of masking effects of the high-voltage rhythms encountered during sleep, care must be taken to recognize underlying components such as an electrocardiogram (EKG) artifact which may appear intermittently and can simulate a spike or sharp wave. In case of doubt, a monitor EKG trace should solve the problem.

Interpretation

The interpretation of abnormal discharges during sleep is rendered difficult not only for the reasons already discussed, but also because two other commonly occurring patterns, namely, the 14- and 6-Hz positive spike and the 6-Hz spike-wave discharge, remain of uncertain significance (21) (see also Chapter 14). The 14 and 6 positive spike pattern has been regarded as a seizure discharge by Gibbs (22), as indicative of autonomic dysfunction by Kellaway (23), and as related to delinquent behavior. However, early workers did not appreciate its common appearance in the normal population, particularly in the teenage group (24). Thus, at the present time, it appears wise to regard the discharge as having no assignable pathologic significance and records containing this discharge as within normal limits. Similar uncertainty attaches to the significance of the 6-Hz spike-and-wave discharge occurring during drowsiness and light sleep (25). Some believe it is related to the 6-Hz component of the 14 and 6 phenomenon, but it is more likely to be entirely separate. Some evidence indicates that this discharge is seen more commonly in patients with convulsive disorder, but the statistics are not very convincing. Again, it is wise to regard this phenomenon as being within normal limits.

The utility of sleep recordings is indicated by the fact that approximately 65% of the records from epileptic patients undergo some form of activation during sleep. The significance of this activation is, however, greater in the case of focal discharges because other methods (hyperventilation and photic stimulation) are relatively less effective in this situation.

Sleep tends to modify discharges that are observed in the waking EEG. Thus: (a) the continuous pattern of hypsarrhythmia in the waking state may become fragmented and less specific during sleep, (b) spike discharges often become more widespread during sleep, and (c) myoclonus associated with a spike discharge in the waking state often disappears during sleep.

In considering sleep activation, a comment concerning the adequacy of sleep recording alone seems appropriate since there are laboratories in which this is a standard practice. The majority opinion on this question is that the waking record is a highly important and necessary part of any EEG study (see Appendix) since it includes observation of important background rhythms such as the alpha rhythm, and of diagnostically significant procedures such as eye opening, hyperventilation, and photic stimulation. Furthermore, the widespread slow activity of a sleep recording often makes it more difficult to recognize focal slow-wave abnormality. The suggestion, attributable originally to Silverman (26), that sleep recording assists in the estimation of the depth of a mass lesion, has not turned out to be very useful from a practical standpoint. It is evident that the full weight of diagnostic acumen in electroencephalography can be best brought to bear when there is detailed comparison of phenomena seen in the waking state with those seen or activated in the sleeping state. Thus, sleep recordings alone should only be acceptable under exceptional circumstances, namely, inadequate cooperation on the part of the patient for a waking record. In these situations, the waking record may be unreliable for interpretation.

Sleep Deprivation

Many routine sleep recordings are associated with some degree of sleep deprivation since the patient is commonly instructed to limit sleep the night before the test in order to increase the likelihood of obtaining a satisfactory sleep record. However, there is now much evidence in the literature indicating that sleep deprivation per se provides an additional degree of activation compared with sleep unrelated to deprivation. The extensive studies of Mattson et al. (27) on epileptic patients indicate that an additional 34% activated significantly following sleep deprivation than activated with sleep alone. In view of these results, it seems appropriate to prepare the patient coming to the EEG lab with some degree of sleep deprivation when this is feasible.

All-Night Sleep Monitoring

In a small percentage of epileptic patients (approximately 5%) seizures occur only or preferentially during sleep. Although abnormalities may be present in the waking record of such patients, it is more satisfactory to monitor the EEG during all-night sleep since the appropriate stage may not be encountered in routine daytime sleep activation studies. Furthermore, in patients who do not describe a sleep relationship for their seizures, the specific discharges (spikes or spikes-and-slow-waves) are sometimes confined to a specific sleep stage. In these instances, a standard recording (preferably at 1.5 cm/sec paper speed) can be carried out during the night in the EEG laboratory. However, more specific information will be obtained if eye movement and muscle (submental) monitors are employed as recommended in the sleep recording manual (19). This additional information assists in determining the sleep stage at which the discharge is more prevalent.

Because the bulk of such recordings makes them inconvenient and costly, attempts have been made to compress the data generated into a computer-derived sleep summary known as the somnogram (see Chapter 17) (28). In this three-page all-night spectral sleep display, the epileptic pattern (such as spike-and-wave discharge) can be distinguished from sleep rhythms (29). A very useful section on sleep recording and its clinical application is available in the *EEG Handbook* (30).

Pentylenetetrazol Activation

Pentylenetetrazol (Metrazol) is a convulsant drug originally used to produce convulsions in schizophrenic patients. The pentylenetetrazol test for activation of epileptic discharges in the EEG has been used in various ways by different investigators. Some have sought to activate the EEG only, thereby precipitating focal or generalized EEG discharges. The pentylenetetrazol test is best employed, however, as a clinical-EEG procedure in which precipitation of the seizure is often the most important part of the test.

The procedure used in my laboratory and in a number of others is to inject pentylenetetrazol intravenously at the rate of 50 mg/min up to 500 mg and at 100 mg/min thereafter. This schedule is

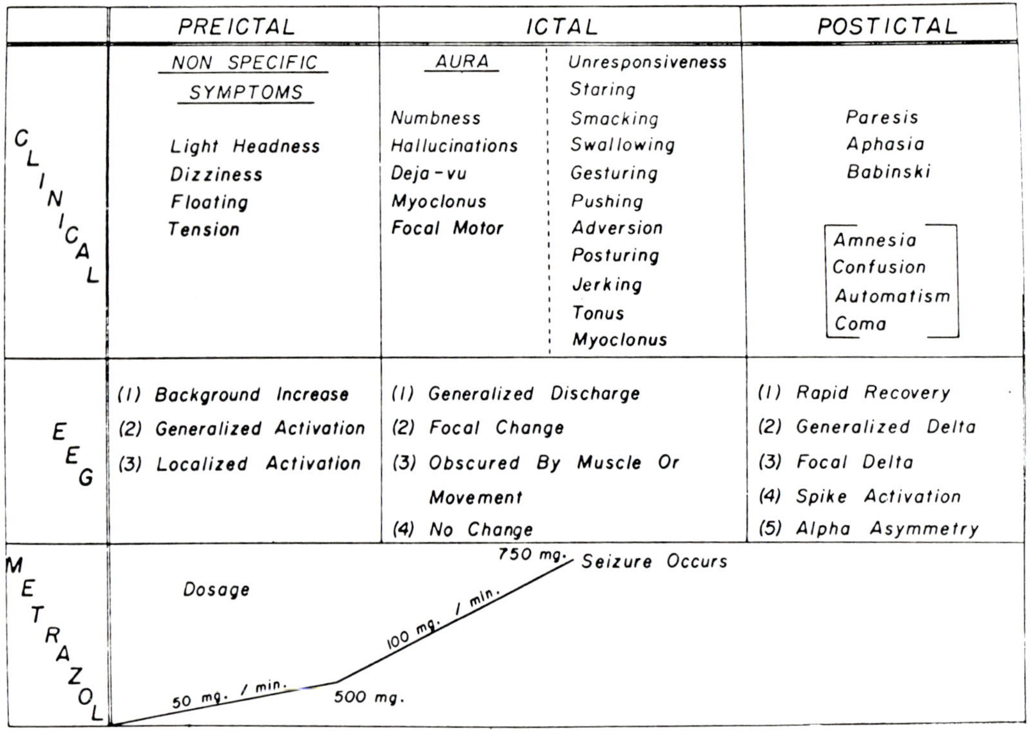

	PREICTAL	ICTAL		POSTICTAL
C L I N I C A L	NON SPECIFIC SYMPTOMS Light Headness Dizziness Floating Tension	AURA Numbness Hallucinations Deja-vu Myoclonus Focal Motor	Unresponsiveness Staring Smacking Swallowing Gesturing Pushing Adversion Posturing Jerking Tonus Myoclonus	Paresis Aphasia Babinski Amnesia Confusion Automatism Coma
E E G	(1) Background Increase (2) Generalized Activation (3) Localized Activation	(1) Generalized Discharge (2) Focal Change (3) Obscured By Muscle Or Movement (4) No Change		(1) Rapid Recovery (2) Generalized Delta (3) Focal Delta (4) Spike Activation (5) Alpha Asymmetry
M E T R A Z O L	Dosage — 50 mg./min. — 500 mg. — 100 mg./min. — 750 mg. Seizure Occurs			

FIG. 13. Diagram of the pentylenetetrazol test. The diagram shows the relationships of changes in the EEG to the clinical accompaniments that may be seen in the preictal, ictal, and postictal stages of the test. Below is a hypothetical pentylenetetrazol dosage schedule such as might be encountered in an average case. Notice the emphasis placed on interpretation of clinical and behavioral signs. Note that the postictal phase may be the most important part of the test. Thus, both EEG and clinical testing should be extended into this period.

shown in the lower part of Fig. 13. The maximal dosage employed is 2,000 mg. As the drug is given, the patient is almost continuously interrogated for changes in sensation or consciousness with particular emphasis on the recognition of features relating to the particular aura of which the patient complains. When an aura is established, administration of the drug is terminated since the seizure usually develops its full complement without further injection. Termination of the test may also be dictated by a number of complications, including a complaint from the patient of undue tension, dizziness, or nausea. However, minor degrees of these sensations are common in the pentylenetetrazol test, and the patient should be reassured. In addition, a metallic taste in the mouth normally accompanies each injection of the drug (usually most prominently after the first injection) and should be disregarded. This taste can usually be separated from gustatory hallucinations often part of a temporal lobe seizure process by its relation to the injection and its difference from the patient's usual sensation. It is important to terminate the test if increasing tendency to generalized myoclonus appears, since this is usually the precursor of a generalized tonic-clonic seizure (so-called "Metrazol seizure"). Diazepam or sodium amytal can be used to counteract these undesirable effects of pentylenetetrazol.

The physiology underlying the action of pentylenetetrazol as a convulsant is poorly understood, although it is often stated that it acts at a cortical level. However, recent work has shown that both unit discharges and fast activity appear early in the brainstem reticular activating system, indicating that pentylenetetrazol, in fact, acts at many levels in the central nervous system.

A number of recording artifacts are often encountered during pentylenetetrazol activation attributable to anxiety and proneness to myoclonus. Thus, myoclonus occurring around the eyes may give rise to a spurious discharge resembling spike-and-wave that disappears when the eyelids are held closed. The montage employed should be designed to give adequate coverage for the suspected area of focal disturbance (such as the temporal lobe), but with adequate coverage of homologous areas of both hemispheres and a "thin" coverage of other regions, such as frontal, occipital, and central, etc. As indicated in Fig. 13, different EEG changes may be seen in the preictal and postictal phases. Of course special problems do occur during the seizure that need careful observation and documentation, and skilled handling of the patient as the seizure occurs is necessary in order to prevent injury.

In the pentylenetetrazol test, it is always possible that a generalized seizure will eventuate, even though the administration of the drug is carefully controlled and is terminated when signs, such as frequent myoclonus, appear. Thus, the test should not be given to patients with orthopedic or cardiac problems in whom a generalized seizure might be injurious. Surprisingly, children often tolerate pentylenetetrazol far better than adults since they appear to suffer less from symptoms such as tension, anxiety, and vertigo.

A well-known effect of pentylenetetrazol is the production of diffuse spike-wave discharges in a portion of the normal population (2). Although such discharges might not be associated with clinical accompaniments, in contrast to petit mal (absence) seizures, this test is clearly not a satisfactory method for spike-wave activation per se. The concept that a threshold level of pentylenetetrazol for EEG activation distinguishes the epileptic from the nonepileptic is no longer tenable.

Pentylenetetrazol activation is rarely carried out purely for its EEG effects of local or generalized spike or spike-and-wave activation, since such discharges can be more easily provoked with less hazardous methods of activation, such as sleep or hyperventilation. Thus, the method is most useful in patients who have a well-specified and repetitious event in their history which may or may not represent a partial seizure. Its second important use is in centers that specialize in epileptic surgery, since these procedures demand careful study of the patient's seizure before proceeding to such special methods as electrocorticography, depth electrography, or actual cortical excision. Even so, the use of this test in North American laboratories has greatly decreased in recent years. It should be emphasized that to be carried out successfully, the pentylenetetrazol test requires a good deal of experience and expertise and should not be attempted in laboratories that have not had previous experience in its administration or that are not adequately equipped to take advantage of recording all features of the seizures (visual, auditory, and electrographic) when it occurs. An example of a successful pentylenetetrazol test is shown in Fig. 14. Pentylenetetrazol activation may be combined with other activating procedures, such as reading, listening to music, etc. It has also proved to be useful during electrocorticography (see

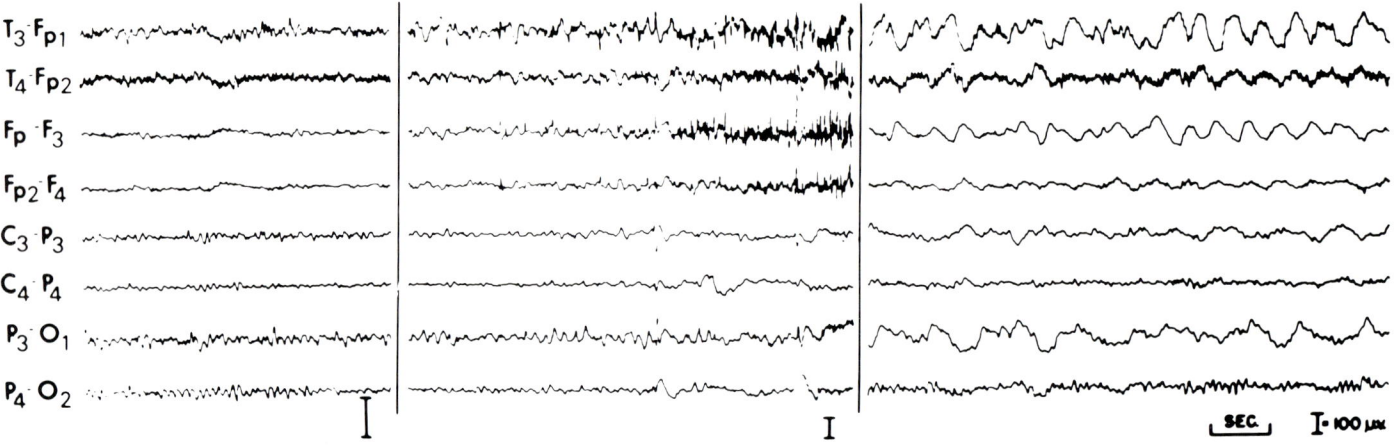

FIG. 14. Pentylenetetrazol activation. The EEG of a patient with the normal EEG before pentylenetetrazol **(left)**, who develops focal spike discharges (left temporal-parietal) during pentylenetetrazol administration **(middle segment)**. The EEG was obscured during the later ictal phase, but postictal recordings showed a clear left temporal-parietal delta focus **(right)**. The right-sided Todd's paralysis confirms the left-sided involvement.

Fig. 15) and depth electrography (see Fig. 16) in patients with infrequent spontaneous seizures.

Further information concerning this activation method is available in the *EEG Handbook* (31).

SPECIAL ELECTRODES

Clinical EEG diagnosis using special electrodes parallels the activation procedure in that with both, we are trying to record significant abnormalities when the usual EEG test has given normal or equivocal results. The need for additional approaches to the recording of brain activity is evident when we consider that the area of the brain available to conventional scalp leads probably represents considerably less than half of its cortical surface. Much inaccessible cortex is located on the mesial surface of the two hemispheres and on the under surface of the frontal, occipital, and temporal lobes. Also, large nuclear masses that are situated deeply, such as the thalamus and caudate nucleus and much deeply enfolded cortex, are anatomically quite distant from scalp electrodes. As partial solutions to these problems, a variety of procedures have become available, some of which are relatively simple, without hazard, and noninvasive (such as the nasopharyngeal electrode), and others of which may require the insertion of depth probes through holes drilled in the skull. The technique of electrocorticography requires a craniotomy and exposes considerable areas of the brain in order to apply the recording electrodes.

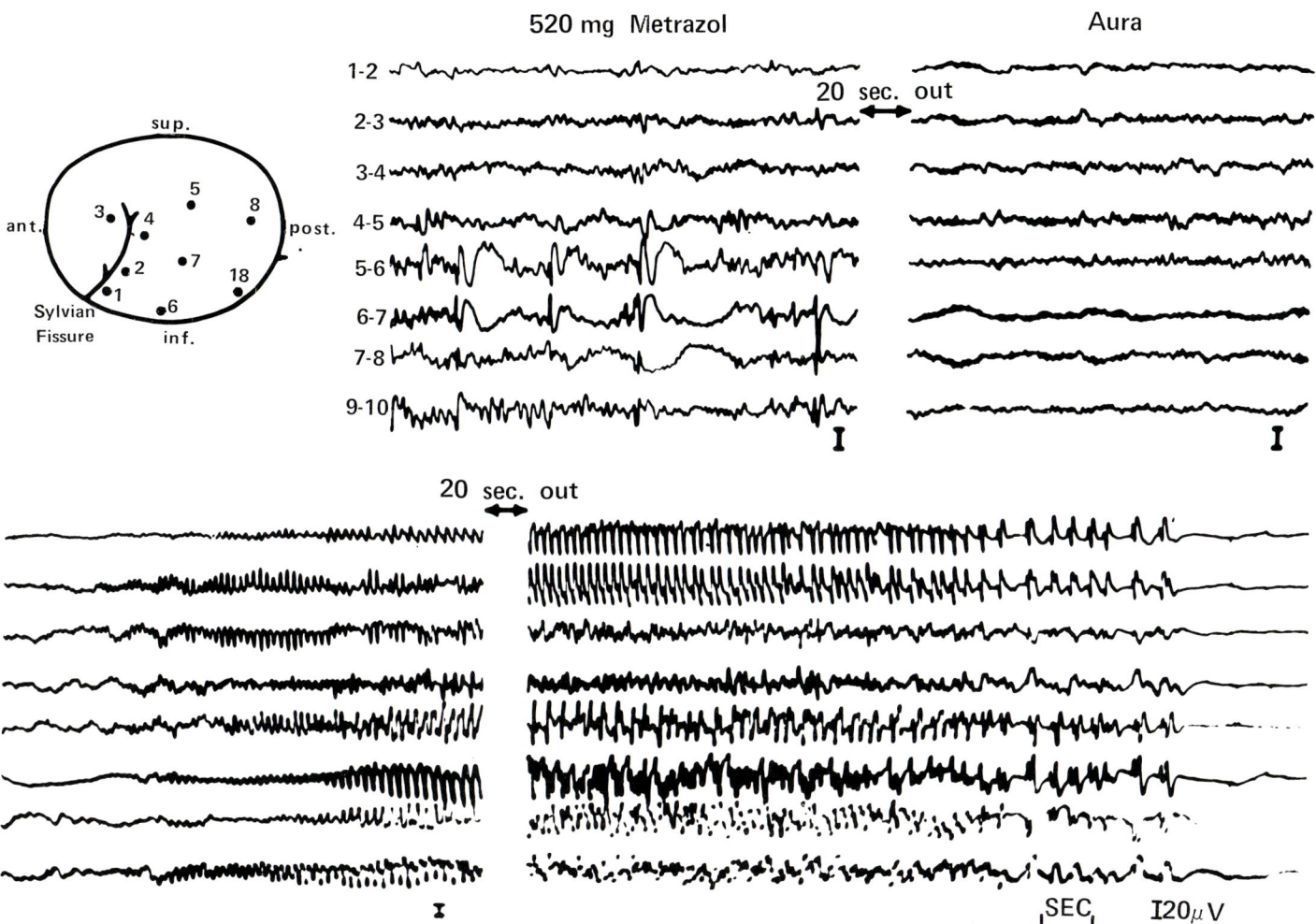

FIG. 15. Recording taken in the operating room from exposed cortex (electrocorticogram). Focal spike discharge was induced in electrode 6 at a total dose of 520 mg pentylenetetrazol **(upper left)**, followed by a seizure discharge and clinical seizure that appears to begin in electrode 3 and spreads rapidly to the other leads **(bottom traces)**. Note absence of visible discharge during aura **(upper right)**. Patient, age 41, had temporal lobe seizures.

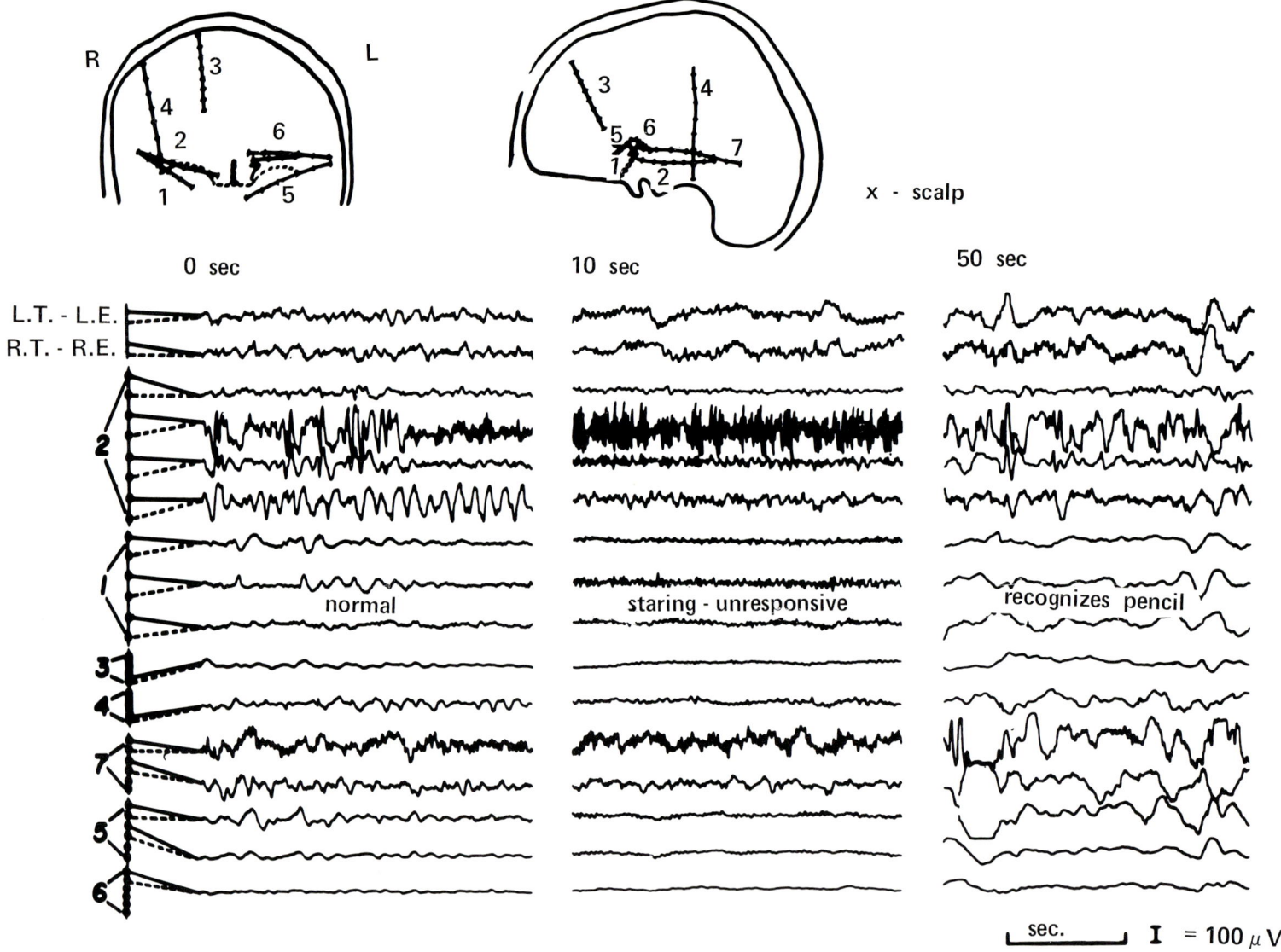

Because they require neurosurgery, because the objective is to determine the feasibility of surgical therapy, and because they are complex procedures, both electrocorticography and depth electrography are carried out largely in specialized centers. This fact, however, should not lead the average electroencephalographer to ignore important data gleaned by these techniques. By studying the findings yielded by these special procedures, he or she will come to realize both the strengths and limitations of the more commonly employed conventional scalp recording methods.

Nasopharnygeal Electrode

This technique, which involves recording from a special malleable electrode (or pair of electrodes) inserted through the nares to rest in the nasopharynx under the base of the skull, has been employed with varying degrees of success in clinical laboratories. There are some who feel strongly that it should be used in all cases where a lesion of the inferior parts of the hemispheres and particularly of the temporal lobes is suspected. However, opinions about its use are divided (see Discussion of Chapters 8 to 14).

The flexible type of nasopharnygeal lead is relatively easy to insert and can be positioned by a physician or a specially trained technician without use of local anesthesia. Some patients, however, do not tolerate the leads well, and a nasal spray of topical anesthetic may be required. Nasopharyngeal leads are usually employed bilaterally and are positioned so that there is maximal separation at the tips. Skill is needed in placing them so that artifacts from respiratory movement and vascular pulsation are minimized. A coronal montage is useful since it tends to reduce eye movement artifact and gives important correlative information from the surface of the temporal lobe.

Evidence indicates that the nasopharyngeal leads, when properly positioned, record from the undersurface of the mesial temporal lobe at least. As far as local discharges are concerned, recordings from these leads resemble those obtained from sphenoidal electrodes, indicating that the discharges are probably conducted through nearby skull foramina (foramen ovale).

Unfortunately, nasopharyngeal electrodes are prone to artifacts that seriously reduce their utility. The most troublesome of these are the spike-like discharges produced by contractions of the nasopharyngeal muscles. The contour of these myogenic potentials can be difficult to distinguish from epileptiform spikes. However, these problems can be considerably reduced if the discharges occurring in the nasopharyngeal lead are compared with the relatively artifact-free records that should be obtainable from adjacent temporal regions of the scalp with a coronal montage. If there are reflections of the discharge in these other leads, even to a minimal degree, the validity of the nasopharyngeal spike can be accepted. Recently a specially constructed nasopharyngeal lead has been introduced in which the ball electrode contains a movement transducer (R. G. Bickford and J. Casler, *unpublished data*). In the use of this electrode a separate EEG channel is employed to register fine movement (such as naso-

---

FIG. 16. Depth electrogram with automatism. Example of depth recording illustrating electrographic changes arising from right temporal lobe during an automatism. Note spike discharge from depth electrode 2 (right temporal lobe) before seizure **(left)**. During seizure associated with staring and unresponsiveness, there is fast discharge (25 to 35 Hz) in the midregions of electrode 2 **(left and middle).** This discharge and the associated automatism occurred at a total dose of 150 mg pentylenetetrazol. Fifty seconds later, the seizure is over **(right),** the patient has some postictal confusion, and the spike discharge is reestablished. The scalp electrodes **(upper two channels of each segment)** did not reflect these complex changes related to the seizure.

pharyngeal muscle contractions, pulse, and respiration artifact) and thereby to assist the EEGer in the clinical interpretation of these records. Preliminary results indicate that it can be quite helpful. Because of the difficulties encountered with the nasopharyngeal lead, some laboratories with a special interest in temporal lobe recordings have preferred to use the relatively artifact-free sphenoidal lead described below.

Those requiring further information on the use of the nasopharyngeal lead should consult the *EEG Handbook* (32).

Sphenoidal Electrodes

A more satisfactory approach to recording from the inferior aspect of the temporal lobe (a region which is often epileptogenic) is the use of a sphenoidal electrode. This lead requires the skill of a trained physician or surgeon for insertion since the tip has to be located in the region of the foramen ovale. The insertion procedure is quite similar to that employed for anesthetization of the Gasserian ganglion, and detailed instructions are available in neurosurgical textbooks. Some electroencephalographers favor the technique of inserting a fine wire that is insulated except at the tip. It is introduced within a needle that is subsequently removed, leaving the wire in place (33).

Sphenoidal lead recordings are highly satisfactory from a technical standpoint since they do not have nearly as much of the extraneous artifactual activity that occurs so frequently in recordings with nasopharyngeal leads. However, the difficulty of positioning them in the proper location and the need for a surgical procedure to insert them has resulted in their use only in a few specialized clinics. Their EEG recording zone appears to be roughly similar to that of the nasopharyngeal leads. Thus, in practice, their use is likely to be confined to cases where there is a question about whether more complex procedures such as electrocorticography or depth electrography should be undertaken in patients with temporal lobe seizures who are candidates for surgical therapy.

A more comprehensive discussion of the use of sphenoidal electrodes can be found in the *EEG Handbook* (34).

Electrocorticography

This technique is highly specialized and is used only in the neurosurgical operating room for the purpose of locating epileptic discharges from abnormal cortical tissue that subsequently may be subject to surgical excision. The technique varies considerably in different neurosurgical centers. In the method originally employed by Penfield (35) in Montreal, the operation is performed under local anesthesia so that communication with the patient can continue during the varied testing procedures. This approach facilitates the observation of the clinical phenomena associated with an induced seizure. After adequate exposure of the cortical surface, an electrode holder is attached to the bone edge. This holder can be U-shaped or rectangular and holds up to 18 mobile electrodes that can be placed on the cortex after they have been moistened with saline. The actual placement of electrodes is often dictated by visible abnormalities of the cortical surface, such as a scar or cyst. Naturally, the edges of such pathologic lesions are given preferential coverage since it is here that epileptogenic activity and seizure discharges are commonly encountered. EEG abnormalities also influence the electrode placement, since the objective is to delineate the limits of an area giving rise to paroxysmal discharges.

Ideally the natural physiologic state of the cortex is maintained as far as possible, and for this reason general anesthetics are avoided. However, some surgeons prefer to perform the operation with general anesthesia and muscle relaxants, and in very young patients and those who are temperamentally unsuited to the rigors of an operation under local anesthesia, a general anesthetic such as halothane may be essential. In this case, unless the anesthetic level is lightened prior to recording, there may be some reduction in spike discharges, and the surgeon is robbed of clinical information such as effects on speech, etc., if a seizure occurs.

Many artifacts are associated with electrocorticography, including 60-cycle pickup related to a ground loop or inadequate grounding of neurosurgical instruments and interference from the electrocautery equipment. Pulsation artifacts can also be troublesome but are usually eliminated by slight shifts of the electrode. Positions of electrodes should be marked by a number system and a photograph taken of the exposed cortex, for subsequent reference in relation to the EEG recording electrodes.

A bipolar montage connection of the cortical electrodes is commonly employed although not mandatory. Experience with electrocorticography and depth electrography has indicated that the origin of a sharp wave or spike discharge often involves multiple foci and does not necessarily indicate the point of origin of the patient's seizure. For this reason, many neurosurgeons like to record the patient's seizure while the cortex is exposed. Unless a spontaneous seizure is encountered, pentylenetetrazol activation may be required in the operating room (Fig. 15). If the cortical recordings indicate that the focus may lie deeply as, for instance, in the amygdala or uncus, it is sometimes useful to use a multicontact depth probe for recording to see if a subcortical spike focus or seizure discharge can be located by this means.

Another technique available in electrocorticography is electrical stimulation of the brain. During electrocorticography this is carried out for two reasons:

1. To locate functional regions of the brain that are not always closely related to observable landmarks on the cortical surface. Thus, the motor cortex is often outlined early in the procedure and checked by observing the contralateral movement induced during passage of the current. Furthermore, in operations on the dominant hemisphere the possibility of producing speech disturbance is usually investigated, particularly in an area likely to be chosen for subsequent excision.

2. To delineate the cortical focus where the patient's seizure is originating. Thus, successful induction of the patient's seizure or of sustained electrographic seizure discharge from a localized area of cortex suggests that this region is the epileptogenic lesion. However, it has to be borne in mind that it is possible to produce seizures at a distance by conduction along fiber tracts or even as a result of volume conduction of the stimulus itself.

If it is decided to carry out a cortical excision, the electroencephalographer is usually asked to make further recordings after the excision has been completed. If spiking is still detected the neurosurgeon may wish to extend the area of excision, if this is feasible, to eliminate the focus more effectively.

In summary, electrocorticography is a specialized procedure employed almost exclusively in cases where surgical excision of a spiking focus or epileptogenic area is contemplated. In other situations, where a patient has a mass lesion such as a tumor that has been associated with epilepsy, some surgeons use electrocorticography as a guide to the degree of excision necessary to prevent postoperative seizures, which can be a problem in this group.

For further information on this topic, the comprehensive account by Ajmone-Marsan and O'Connor should be consulted (36).

Depth Electrography

Depth electrography is a highly complex procedure only carried out in special clinics where surgical treatment of epilepsy is undertaken. It is unique in allowing the investigator to sample from virtually any part of the cortex or subcortex by means of fine probe electrodes that are introduced surgically and usually under stereotactic control. In addition, it allows the electroencephalographer to stimulate electrically, through the implanted electrodes, various parts of the cortex and subcortex with a view to investigating their function (memory, speech, movement, etc.) before a decision is made about the surgical removal of epileptogenic areas. In addition, by using special techniques, single unit studies of the human cortex and subcortex can be carried out, although at present, these have not been shown to have any special diagnostic value.

The procedures used and the type of electrode implanted vary widely, depending on laboratory experience and preference. Our philosophy has been that the epileptic process tends to vary considerably among different individuals and to involve areas in the temporal lobe or other parts of the brain without consistent limitation to particular nuclear cell masses. Therefore, depth electrodes are implanted over a wide area to delineate the extent of the epileptic process. This wide coverage facilitates the investigation of functional localization (speech, memory, movement) within an area that may subsequently need to be excised surgically. Other laboratories believe that the epileptic process is largely concentrated in specific structures in the temporal lobe such as the hippocampus, uncus, or amygdala, and therefore tends to restrict the electrode targets to these structures.

In choosing suitable patients for these procedures, rigid criteria have to be met, although they vary somewhat in different laboratories. They usually include: (a) a patient having a long history of focal epilepsy with poor control from adequate and varied anticonvulsant medication and with surveillance of anticonvulsant drug levels, (b) evidence of severe and long-term functional incapacity, evidenced by work record, etc., (c) clinical and electrographic evidence suggesting a localized epileptic focus (since attempts to improve generalized seizure disorders by localized lesions have not yet been proven successful), and (d) the existence of adequate clinical function demonstrable in other areas of the brain and the demonstration that the proposed region for excision has little importance in major functions such as speech and memory.

There are some differing philosophies concerning the use of specific diagnostic techniques such as electrocorticography and depth electrography for evaluating the feasibility of surgical excision in the epileptic patient. If the problem is relatively straightforward and there is no question of bilateral brain involvement, the surgeon may proceed from the initial EEG investigations (including seizure induction) directly to electrocorticography. In more complex cases involving the possibility of bilateral disease, uncertainty about the primary location of the epileptogenic area, or uncertainty about dispensibility of function in the area likely to be excised, a period of depth electrographic investigation lasting some 2 to 3 weeks is usually desirable in order to obtain the best therapeutic result.

Although this account has dealt summarily with the very extensive topic of depth electrography and its many technical aspects, examples of actual patient investigations have so much relevance to clinical EEG and the general topic of montage strategies that they are worth presenting for their didactic value. Thus, some lessons learned from implanted depth lead procedures carried out on 76 epileptic patients (at Mayo Clinic and University of California, San Diego) could be summarized as follows:

1. In most patients, spike foci tend to be far more complex and multiple in their origin than is apparent when the scalp recording

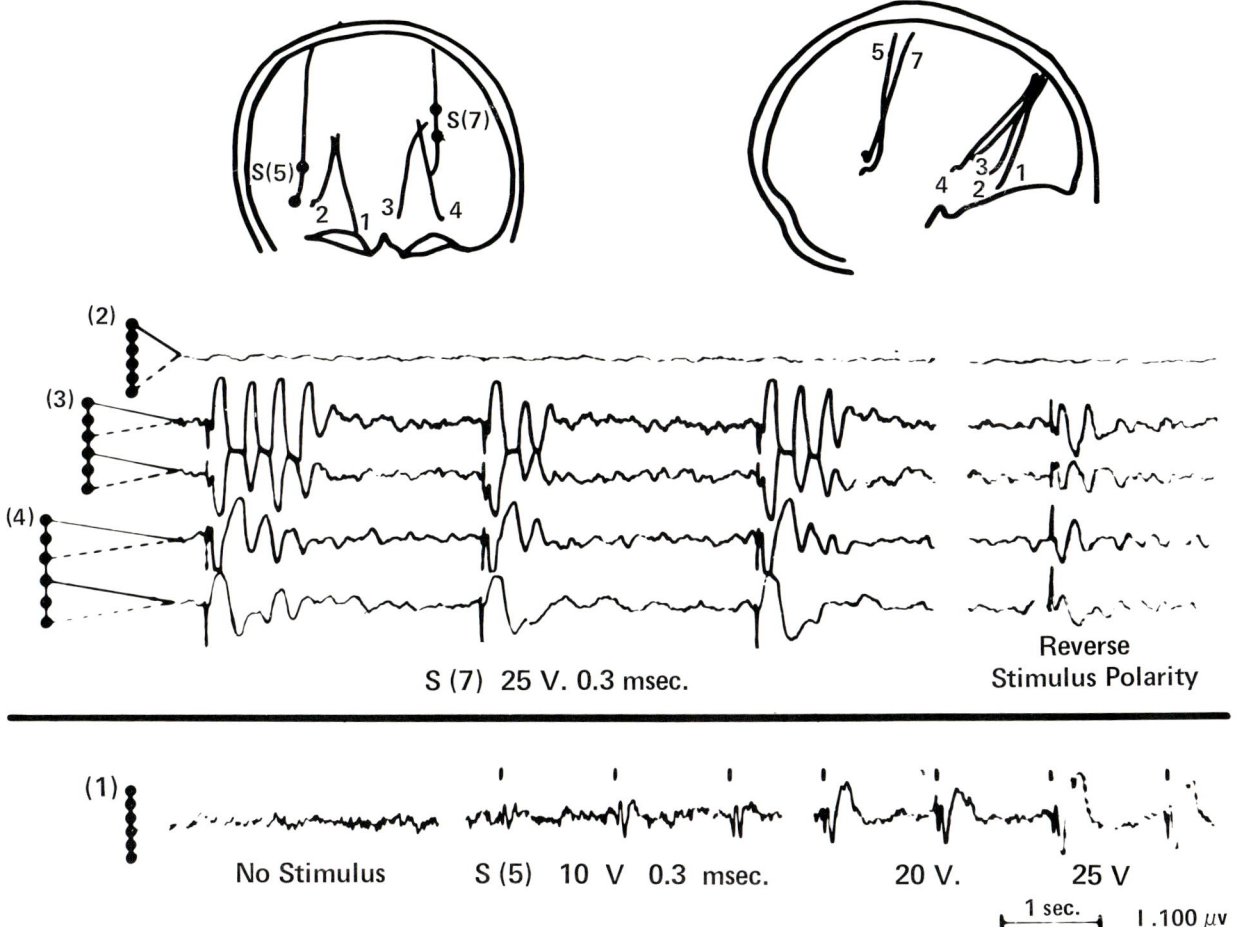

FIG. 17. Depth electrogram. Widespread rhythmic discharges induced by electrical stimulation through depth leads in the parietal region transmitted widely to frontal leads. Stimulation of S (7) elicits responses in electrodes 3 and 4 *(above horizontal line)* and stimulation of S (5) elicits responses in electrode 1 *(below horizontal line)*. This is an example of a widely transmitted response to single pulse depth stimulation which, in spite of high amplitude (several hundred μV), did not produce any detectable clinical accompaniment.

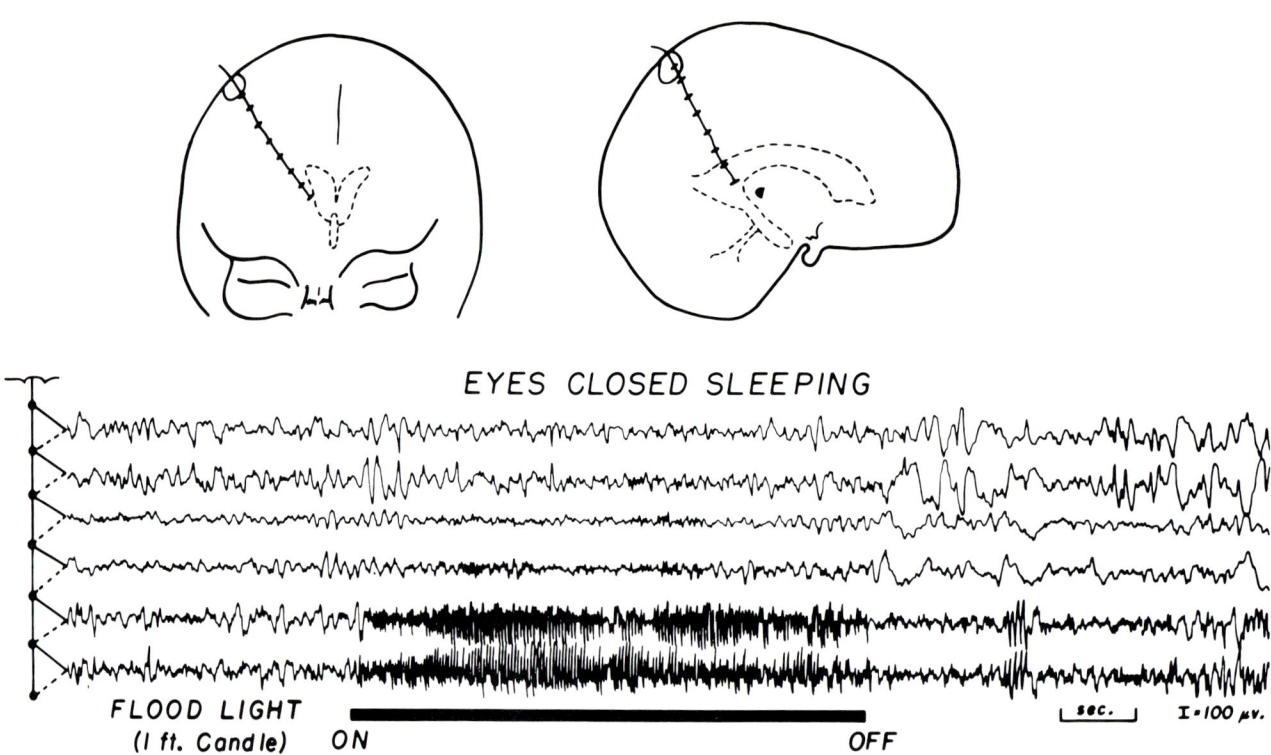

FIG. 18. Depth electrogram with light stimulation. Example of fast response to constant light stimulation appearing in patient with epilepsy from an implanted depth lead in the calcarine region. This is an example of what is regarded as a physiologic rhythm recorded in man and not yet duplicated in animals (37).

is considered alone, even when additional electrode strategies have been employed.

2. Spike discharges are often far more active in the depth of the brain than on the cortical surface when the patient is awake.

3. The existence of independent spike foci often well outside the primary target (such as the temporal lobe) tends to reduce the EEG-er's confidence in these interictal discharges as necessarily reliable indicators of the origin of the patient's seizures. Thus, it is apparent

that recordings of the patient's EEG during a seizure are a far more valuable indicator of localized epileptogenicity than are recordings of sporadic spikes or sharp waves.

4. High amplitude and conspicuous electrographic events (spontaneous or induced) can occur in various parts of the cortex and subcortex without being detectable by the patient or producing any behavioral or mental effects (Fig. 17). Although it can be argued that more sensitive tests might detect the occurrence of these widespread spontaneous and induced electrographic events, a more likely explanation seems to be that they occur in neuronal systems separate from those involved directly in cerebral processing.

5. Many physiologic processes have been revealed by depth electrography that have not yet found a precise equivalent in animal work. An example is the fast activity evoked by continuous light stimulation (37) shown in Fig. 18.

6. Temporal lobe seizures are highly complex disturbances of temporal lobe function which, in spite of rather similar clinical manifestations (staring, unresponsiveness, and the motor features of an automatism), may have completely different electropathic discharge mechanisms. Thus, in different patients showing a roughly similar automatism, recordings from deep temporal lobe structures have yielded at least three separable electrographic changes: (a) repetitive spike discharge, (b) fast rhythmic activity (Fig. 16), and (c) background flattening without evident discharge.

7. Simple concepts of spike generation taken from animal models do not appear to fit the reality of synchronized spike distribution as it occurs in depth recordings.

Thus, synchronous spiking often appears to extend without evident interruption over considerable distances (2 to 4 cm), which, anatomic studies indicate, must cross several enfolded cortical and white matter barriers. Thus, the cortical penicillin spike with its localized field spread seems to be an inadequate model of spike mechanisms as they are encountered in the cortex and subcortex of the epileptic patient.

The risks of electrocorticography and depth electrography are minimal now that optimal electrodes have been developed and the risk of infection minimized. In fact, these risks should be weighed against the very beneficial therapeutic effects obtained when patients are carefully selected and the complex diagnostic procedures are handled in clinics with extensive background and experience.

CONCLUSIONS

The use of activation methods and of special techniques for recording in the depth of the brain has taught us some important lessons concerning epilepsy that are perhaps worthy of mention in concluding this section. For instance, it is evident that the expression of a particular epileptic discharge, such as a spike, sharp wave, or spike-wave paroxysm, can be greatly altered during an activation procedure. Thus, in pentylenetetrazol activation, a spike-and-wave discharge may produce no detectible effect on a patient's response before the drug is given and yet one of the same general duration and electrographic contour may result in a complete "absence" attack after a moderate dosage of the drug is administered. Similar changes in what might be called "expressivity" are noted; sharp-wave discharges arising from the motor cortex, in the waking state, may be associated with a myoclonus, but, during sleep, the same or indeed a larger discharge may not have any detectable myogenic accompaniment. These observations and much other evidence have suggested to us (38) that the proper understanding of the relationship between electrographic discharges and the clinical response requires the interposition of a third concept for which we have suggested the name, "gating mechanism." This is a conceptual rather than an anatomically precise formulation that may operate at several levels in the nervous system and clearly implies a number of inhibitory mechanisms. The operation of a gating mechanism may explain why many discharges of a potentially epileptogenic type recorded in depth do not in fact have any clinical accompaniment.

Finally, depth techniques point up the variable reliability of the electrographic spike from a diagnostic standpoint and challenge us as electroencephalographers to search for other concomitant changes when this phenomenon is encountered. Additional tests should surely include coherence analysis, shown by Brazier (39) to be a potent tool in deciding which of many dispersed electrographic discharges is actually responsible for initiating a seizure.

Additional information relating to depth electrography and the surgical treatment of epilepsy can be obtained from the following sources: (35,40,41).

ACKNOWLEDGMENT

This work has been supported by USPHS grant N.S. 08962–09.

REFERENCES

1. Chatrian, G. E. (1974): The report of the committee on terminology. *Electroencephalogr. Clin. Neurophysiol.,* 37:529.
2. Baker, R. N., and Klass, D. W. (1965): The metrazol activation of the normal brain. *Bulletin LA Neurol. Soc.,* 30:201–209.
3. Remond, A. (editor) (1976): *Handbook of Electroencephalography and Clinical Neurophysiology,* Vol. 1–16. Elsevier, Amsterdam.
4. Gastaut, H., Bostem, F., Naquet, R., and Fernandez-Guardiola, A. (1959): L'activation hypoxique de l'E.E.G. par inhalation d'azote. 1. Premiers resultats obtenus dans les épilepsies généralisées. *Rev. Neurol.,* 100:501–515.
5. Klass, D. W., and Bickford, R. G. (1960): Glossokinetic potentials appearing in the electroencephalogram. *Electroencephalogr. Clin. Neurophysiol.,* 12:235.
6. Cordeau, J. P. (1959): Monorhythmic frontal delta. *Electroencephalogr. Clin. Neurophysiol.,* 11:733–746.
7. Bostem, F. (1976): Section II. Hyperventilation. In: *Handbook of Electroencephalography and Clinical Neurophysiology,* Vol. 3D, edited by A. Remond, pp. 74–88. Elsevier, Amsterdam.
8. Scott, D. F., Groethuysen, U. C., and Bickford, R. G. (1967): Lambda responses in the human electroencephalogram. *Neurology (Minneap.),* 17:8:770–778.
9. Hunter, J., and Ingvar, D. H. (1955): Pathways mediating metrazol induced irradiation of visual impulses. *Electroencephalogr. Clin. Neurophysiol.,* 7:39–60.
10. Bickford, R. G., and Klass, D. W. (1969): Sensory precipitation and reflex mechanisms. In: *Basic Mechanisms of the Epilepsies,* edited by H. H. Jasper, A. A. Ward, and A. Pope, pp. 543–564. Little, Brown, Boston.
11. Bickford, R. G., Sem-Jacobsen, C. W., White, P. T., and Daly, D. (1952): Some observations of the mechanism of photic and photo-metrazol activation. *Electroencephalogr. Clin. Neurophysiol.,* 4:275–282.
12. Wulff, M. H. (1959): The barbituate withdrawal syndrome: A clinical and electroencephalographic study. *Electroencephalogr. Clin. Neurophysiol.,* Suppl. 14.
13. Klass, D. W., Wakim, K. G., and Johnson, W. J. (1970): Paroxysmal electroencephalographic abnormalities experimentally induced by electrolyte alterations. *Electroencephalogr. Clin. Neurophysiol.,* 28:93.
14. Poskanzer, D. C., Brown, A. E., and Miller, H. (1962): Musicogenic epilepsy caused only by a discrete frequency band of church bells. *Brain,* 85:77–92.
15. Alajouanine, T., and Gastaut, H. (1955): La syncinésie-sursaut et l'épilepsie-sursaut à déclanchement sensoriel ou sensitif inopiné. I. Les faits anatomicocliniques (15 observations). *Rev. Neurol.,* 93:29–41.
16. Rodin, E. A., Mulder, D. W., Faucett, R. L., and Bickford, R. G. (1955): Psychologic factors in convulsive disorders of focal origin. *AMA Arch. Neurol. Psychiatry,* 74:365–374.
17. Bickford, R. G., Whelan, J. L., Klass, D. W., and Corbin, K. B. (1956): Reading epilepsy: Clinical and electroencephalographic studies of a new syndrome. *Trans. Am. Neurol. Assoc.,* 81:100–102.
18. Werner, S. S., Stockard, J. E., and Bickford, R. G. (editors) (1977): *Atlas of Neonatal Electroencephalography.* Raven Press, N.Y.
19. Rechtschaffen, A., and Kales, A. (editors) (1968): *A Manual of Standardized Terminology, Techniques and Scoring System for Sleep Stages of Human Subjects.* NIH Publication No. 204. U.S. Govt. Printing Office, Washington, D.C.
20. Hobson, J. A. (1974): The cellular basis of sleep cycle control. In: *Advances in Sleep Research,* Vol. 1, edited by E. D. Weitzman, pp. 217–248. Spectrum Publications, N.Y.
21. Reiher, J., and Klass, D. W. (1968): Two common EEG patterns of doubtful clinical significance. *Med. Clin. North Am.,* 52:933–940.

22. Gibbs, F. A., and Gibbs, E. L. (1952): *Atlas of Electroencephalography, Vol. 2, Epilepsy,* 2nd ed., p. 422. Addison-Wesley, Reading, Mass.
23. Kellaway, P., Drawley, J. W., and Kagawa, N. (1960): Paroxysmal pain and autonomic disturbances of cerebral origin: A specific electro-clinical syndrome. *Epilepsia,* 1:466–483.
24. Wiener, J. M., Delano, J. G., and Klass, D. W. (1966): An EEG study of delinquent and nondelinquent adolescents. *Arch. Gen. Psychiatry,* 15:144–150.
25. Thomas, J. E., and Klass, D. W. (1968): Six-per-second spike-and-wave pattern in the electroencephalogram: A reappraisal of its clinical significance. *Neurology (Minneap.),* 18:587–593.
26. Silverman, D., and Groff, R. A. (1957): Brain tumor depth determination by electrographic recording during sleep. *Arch. Neurol. Psychiatry,* 78:15–28.
27. Mattson, R. H., Pratt, K. L., and Calverley, J. R. (1965): Electroencephalograms of epileptics following sleep deprivation. *Arch. Neurol.,* 13:310–315.
28. Hanson, K. R., Stockard, J. J., Kalichman, M. W., and Bickford, R. G. (1974): Compressed spectral somnogram—a multiparameter spectral sleep display. *Proc. San Diego Biomed. Symp.,* 13:545–548.
29. Burchiel, K. J., Myers, R. R., and Bickford, R. G. (1976): Visual and auditory evoked responses during penicillin-induced generalized spike-and-wave activity in cats. *Epilepsia,* 17:293–311.
30. Klass, D. W., and Fischer-Williams, M. (1976): Section IB. Sleep and sleep deprivation. In: *Handbook of Electroencephalography and Clinical Neurophysiology,* Vol. 3D, edited by A. Remond, pp. 48–73. Elsevier, Amsterdam.
31. Bancaud, J. (1976): Section IV. EEG activation by metrazol and magimide in the diagnosis of epilepsy. In: *Handbook of Electroencephalography and Clinical Neurophysiology,* Vol. 3D, edited by A. Remond, pp. 105–120. Elsevier, Amsterdam.
32. Binnie, C. D., MacGillivray, B. B., and Osselton, J. W. (1976): Section I4a. Electrodes and their use. In: *Handbook of Electroencephalography and Clinical Neurophysiology,* Vol. 3C, edited by A. Remond, pp. 17–19. Elsevier, Amsterdam.
33. Townsend, H. R. A. (1968): An introducer for sphenoidal wire electrodes. *Proc. Electrophysiol. Technol. Assoc.,* 15:67–72.
34. Binnie, C. D., MacGillivray, B. B., and Osselton, J. W. (1976): Section I4b. Electrodes and their use. In: *Handbook of Electroencephalography and Clinical Neurophysiology,* Vol. 3C, edited by A. Remond, pp. 19–20. Elsevier, Amsterdam.
35. Penfield, W., and Jasper, H. (1954): Electrocorticography. In: *Epilepsy and the Functional Anatomy of the Human Brain,* chapter 17, pp. 692–736. Little, Brown, Boston.
36. Ajmone-Marsan, C. (1976): Volume 10-C. Electrocorticography. In: *Handbook of Electroencephalography and Clinical Neurophysiology,* edited by A. Remond, pp. 1–49. Elsevier, Amsterdam.
37. Chatrian, G. E., Bickford, R. G., and Uihlein, A. (1960): Depth electrographic study of a fast rhythm evoked from the human calcarine region by steady illumination. *Electroencephalogr. Clin. Neurophysiol.,* 12:167–176.
38. Bickford, R. G. (1975): The concept of a seizure gating mechanism in epilepsy. *Electroencephalogr. Clin. Neurophysiol.,* 38:551–552.
39. Brazier, M. A. B. (1973): Electrical seizure discharges within the human brain: The problem of spread. In: *Epilepsy: Its Phenomena in Man,* edited by M. A. B. Brazier, pp. 153–167. Academic Press, New York.
40. Crandall, Paul H. (1973): Developments in direct recordings from epileptogenic regions in the surgical treatment of partial epilepsies. In: *Epilepsy: Its Phenomena in Man,* edited by M. A. B. Brazier. Academic Press, New York.
41. Ajmone-Marsan, C. (1976): Volume 10-B. In: *Handbook of Electroencephalography and Clinical Neurophysiology,* edited by A. Remond, pp. 1–65. Elsevier, Amsterdam.

Chapter 10

Use of the EEG for Evaluation of Focal Intracranial Lesions

Eli S. Goldensohn

Department of Neurology, College of Physicians and Surgeons, Columbia University, New York, New York 10032

Continuous PDA	308
Intermittent Rhythmic Delta Activity	310
Local Depression or Absence of Background Rhythmic Activity	311
Epileptiform Discharges	311
Nonspecific Changes	312
Characteristics of Tumors	312
Deep-Seated and Infratentorial Tumors	312
Lesions Involving Hemispheric White Matter	316
Lesions of White Matter and Cortical and Subcortical Gray Matter	321
Lesions Involving Subcortical Gray Matter Structures	326
Extra-axial Lesions	330
Serial EEG Studies	331
EEG and CTT in Focal Structural Lesions	331
References	340

Berger, the founder of human electroencephalography, indicated in 1929 that intracranial tumors affect the electroencephalogram (EEG) (18), and subsequently Walter (42) demonstrated the usefulness of the EEG in the diagnosis of brain tumor in man. Surgeons and electroencephalographers, recording directly from the brain, soon demonstrated that tumor masses themselves do not produce EEG waves, but that brain tissue affected directly and indirectly by neoplasms generate the electrical abnormalities seen at the cortex and the scalp (39). By 1957 Drift (15) was able to report that the EEG could localize or lateralize supratentorial tumors approximately 80% of the time, and that over 90% of EEGs in hemispheric tumors showed electrical characteristics outside the limits of normality. These figures remain essentially accurate today (25).

As might be expected from the fact that the neoplasm itself does not produce EEG waves, focal abnormalities not infrequently fail to coincide with the major portion of a lesion, and sometimes the EEG focus is remote from the lesion. Although absence of electrical activity at some mass lesions can be found in the electrocorticogram, localized complete absence of all activity is seldom found in the EEG at the scalp. The reasons for this and for other discrepancies between what is present at the surface of the cortex and what is seen at the scalp (EEG) are discussed by Abraham and Ajmone-Marsan (1), Hirsch et al. (26), and Goldensohn and colleagues (21). Some factors which affect the degree of attenuation of electrical activity between the cortical surface and the scalp are discussed in Chapter 15 and include: (a) variations in the size of cortical areas involved in generating the in-phase synaptic potentials responsible for the EEG waves; (b) the larger area of the cortex surveyed by the relatively distant scalp electrode compared to an electrode placed directly on the cortex; and (c) variations in distances between the cortical surfaces and the scalp electrodes over different lobes of the brain. Awareness of attenuations and distortions that occur between electrical activity generated at the cortex and its appearance in the scalp recording is helpful when extracting clinically useful information from the EEG for evaluating focal intracranial lesions.

The discussion which follows is oriented toward the avoidance of false localizations and toward maximizing the ability to localize lesions by distinguishing between EEG signs of local injury and signs indicating effects from distant structures. Further, it is directed toward identifying features in the EEG record that give clues about the nature of the destructive agent and supply information concerning prognosis, including threatened decompensation of brain function.

EEG features characteristic of focal intracranial lesions include: (a) continuous focal delta waves that are irregular in wave form [polymorphic delta activity (PDA)]; (b) intermittent delta waves that are regular in wave form [intermittent rhythmic delta activity (IRDA): focal, generalized, or both]; (c) depression or absence of usual background activity in the vicinity of the local slowing; and (d) paroxysmal or epileptiform discharges in the form of spikes, sharp waves, or spike and wave complexes that remain or begin as local discharges. The most reliable of these signs for localizing destructive lesions is continuous focal PDA and focal depression or absence of usual background activity in the vicinity of the focal slowing (3).

CONTINUOUS PDA

In 1953 Jasper and VanBuren made the important observations that polymorphic delta waves were usually associated with lesions involving the white matter and that bilateral synchronous rhythmic slow waves in the delta range were usually found in deeply located tumors near the floor of the third ventricle and aqueduct of sylvius (28). Gloor and colleagues, in a study of the EEG in diffuse encephalopathies, pointed out similar correlations (20). Bilaterally synchronous rhythmic EEG discharges were shown to be characteristic of diffuse cortical and subcortical gray matter disease. In contrast, the EEGs in diffuse encephalopathies that involved primarily white matter were characterized by continuous nonparoxysmal irregular discharges (PDA waves) and a virtual absence of rhythmic bilaterally synchronous discharges. A combination of prominent bilaterally synchronous paroxysmal discharges and continuous nonparoxysmal PDA occurred in diffuse encephalopathies that involved both gray and white matter. Rhee et al. (38) conducted a further study of such relationships in focal intracranial lesions, and many of the illustrations in this chapter come from that work, which has not yet been published in full. Their findings, which correlated the EEG with the nature and locations of brain lesions measured at autopsy in relation to their calculated distances from electrodes on the scalp (International 10–20 System), confirmed and extended the earlier studies. PDA characteristically consists of irregularly formed arrhythmic delta waves (0.5 to 2.5 Hz) and usually shows little or no reactivity to visual or arousal stimuli and little or no change with sleep. PDA arises from altered synaptic activity of neurons lying within or peripheral to the tumor, but the mechanisms by which the EEG changes occur is conjectural. Among the factors possibly responsible for PDA are edema, cerebral blood flow reduction, change in metabolism, and disruption of axons going between the deep gray matter nuclei and the cortex. Daly (12) suggested that deafferentation of the cortex by the disruption of these fibers is the cause of PDA. This mechanism was also suggested by Gloor et al. (19) to explain the PDA they created by making destructive lesions of the white matter in cats.

Although it is not an infallible sign, in most instances continuous focal PDA indicates a destructive lesion in cerebral white matter. Among the causes of focal destructive lesions in man, those most frequently encountered are tumors, abscesses, infarcts, hematomas, and contusions. A not uncommon exception is focal PDA after a migraine attack (27). The localizing significance of the polymorphic delta focus increases with the degree of slowness of the waves and with their irregularity and amplitude. The amplitude of PDA, however, is not necessarily maximum over the area of structural damage. A region of maximal destruction may show low-voltage PDA with depressed superimposed faster frequencies, and it may be surrounded by larger-amplitude delta waves.

Tumors in the frontal temporal and occipital areas are more likely to produce PDA than similar lesions in central and parietal areas near the vertex. There is a tendency for PDA to localize excessively in the temporal regions in adults and the temporo-occipital areas in children. Correct localization of the tumor by PDA is possible most often with frontal and temporal lobe tumors, whereas with tumors in other locations PDA tends to be at higher voltage and more abundant in adjacent temporal areas (24). It is therefore important to bear in mind that temporal delta foci may signify tumors in adjacent lobes. If both background rhythm depression and PDA are present in the temporal region, the likelihood of a tumor having a temporal location is very high.

Parasagittal frontal and parietal tumors often do not demonstrate PDA. Other EEG characteristics often seen in parasagittal and parietal lobe tumors are attenuation of alpha and beta rhythms, and slight slowing of basic frequencies and theta waves. Theta wave foci have been reported to be twice as commonly associated with parietal tumors (30%) than with other sites (33). Theta foci are also seen in relatively slow-growing lesions (e.g., tuberculomas and oligodendrogliomas), but this is not consistent and delta activity is often prominent.

INTERMITTENT RHYTHMIC DELTA ACTIVITY

In 1945 Cobb (7) drew attention to the significance of rhythmic sinusoidal slow waves that occur in bursts or runs, whose characteristics were later further described by others (10,12,28). This intermittent rhythmic delta activity (IRDA) is composed of runs of sinusoidal or sawtooth waves with more rapid ascending than descending phases at frequencies around 2.5 Hz. The waves are consistent in form and frequency, and occur in bursts. Unlike PDA, which is relatively unmodified by stimuli, IRDA is markedly reactive. It is augmented by eye closure and hyperventilation, and attenuated by alerting stimuli (e.g., eye opening and mental activity). It usually increases during drowsiness, ceases during deeper levels of slow wave sleep, and reappears during rapid eye movement (REM) sleep (41).

IRDA has two characteristic distributions. Frontally localized IRDA (FIRDA) shows maximal amplitude over the frontal or anterior head regions, and occipital IRDA (OIRDA) is most prominent over the occipital or occipitotemporal areas. These two types of rhythmic delta activity in large part are age-related. FIRDA is usually seen in adult patients, whereas OIRDA is found mainly in children.

The two distributions of the activity do not signify either different locations for cerebral lesions or different pathologies. When either occurs in bilaterally synchronous fashion, it is considered to indicate that cortically generated EEG activity has been modified by interaction with midline structures, e.g., the thalamus and reticular core of the midbrain. Although probably indicative of altered function in those structures, IRDA does not necessarily indicate that the major pathology is in that region. OIRDA and FIRDA were found in 53% of 145 children with posterior fossa tumors (36). In supratentorial tumors the incidence of FIRDA varies from 33% (33) to as high as 56% (24). It has little value in localizing cerebral hemispheric lesions except in deep frontal lobe tumors where FIRDA may be the only abnormality in the record. The rhythmic delta in those instances is usually quite slow (1.5 to 2.0 Hz) and may be accentuated on the side of the tumor (25). Although generally useless for localization to a single lobe, FIRDA has lateralizing value in hemispheric tumors. A strong accentuation of FIRDA to one side is highly suggestive of an ipsilateral supratentorial lesion, although contralateral accentuation of theta has been encountered in some supratentorial lesions (16). In infratentorial lesions IRDA is usually bilaterally symmetrical or shows shifting asymmetries. It is important to keep in mind that IRDA is nonspecific and is seen in many non-space-occupying conditions, including systemic metabolic disorders affecting the brain, aqueductal stenosis, encephalitis, and cerebral trauma (see also Chapter 11).

The basic mechanisms for the production of IRDA are only partly understood. IRDA most likely represents a dysfunction of the interaction between subcortical gray matter structures and cortical neurons (12). The activity cannot be produced by simply raising intracranial pressure artificially in man, and IRDA is characteristically absent in patients with benign increased intracranial pressure (4a). In patients with posterior fossa tumors, the appearance of IRDA correlates best with acute or subacute dilation of the third ventricle (36). This may explain its presence in patients with aqueductal occlusion and its prompt disappearance following shunting or relief of the blockage (see Figs. 17 and 18 below). In such patients it is postulated that disturbed thalamic function consequent to third ventricle dilation may be responsible for the appearance of the IRDA.

LOCAL DEPRESSION OR ABSENCE OF BACKGROUND RHYTHMIC ACTIVITY

A solid indication of brain dysfunction is unilateral absence or depression of background activity. Since tumors are electrically inactive and also destroy neurons, areas of absence of electrical activity are found in the corticogram (39). It is rare, however, to observe complete absence of electrical activity in the scalp EEG overlying a tumor, as was explained by field studies (21). When complete local silence does occur, it is associated with very large superficial necrotic lesions (see Fig. 15, below). Incomplete depression of background activity, however, is common. Unilateral local depression of frontal beta, central rhythms, alpha, or sleep spindles in association with PDA (even if the PDA is not at highest voltage at that area) reliably localizes the area under those electrodes as overlying the destructive lesion (see Fig. 3, below). The combination of depression of superimposed faster frequencies and PDA was referred to as "flat polymorphic delta" by Arfel and Fischgold (3), who emphasized its reliability for localization.

EPILEPTIFORM DISCHARGES

Focal spikes and sharp waves are seen in the EEG of 20% or 30% of cerebral tumors (30,33) and are much more frequently encountered in tumors than in subacute or chronic lesions caused by vascular accidents. The association of spikes and sharp waves correlates well with a tendency toward seizures; but of the approximately 40% of hemispheric brain tumor patients who have seizures, many show no evidence of epileptiform discharges, and many patients with brain tumor and no seizures demonstrate paroxysmal activity. Periodic lateralized epileptiform discharges (PLEDS), which commonly occur immediately after and up to 2 weeks following acute vascular accidents, are occasionally seen in brain tumors (5).

The presence of a spike focus may be the only abnormality in the early stages of a cerebral tumor, but usually there is also some focal polymorphic slowing. Epileptogenic foci, which are common with hemispheric tumors, occur in only 5% of diencephalic and infratentorial tumors (25).

In hemispheric tumors spike discharges are found more commonly in the temporal regions than in the frontal and rolandic areas. Most authors (3,25) emphasize the limitations of using an interictal spike focus for tumor localization as the spikes may be found at the margin of the lesion or in homologous areas of the opposite hemisphere and, on rare occasions, only on the opposite side. One should therefore be cautious when localizing a tumor to a given area if focal spiking is the only abnormality seen. In general, slow-growing tumors such as astrocytomas or oligodendrogliomas produce more epileptiform discharges than do rapidly growing tumors such as metastases and glioblastoma (29). Epileptiform activity is commonly seen following surgical removal of tumors, particularly meningiomas. This is partly related to the cortical irritation from damage by the tumor and its removal. Also the spike discharges are more easily seen after surgery as there is less attenuation of the discharges owing to the skull defect.

Parasagittal and frontal tumors can produce bilaterally synchronous spike and wave discharges. They are usually easy to distinguish from the primary bilateral synchronies found in epilepsies of unknown etiology in that they are atypical in form. Focal PDA, which persists postictally for more than 5 min after a seizure, is strongly suggestive of a structural lesion in that area. Focal discharges during an ictus have better localizing value than interictal spikes (25).

NONSPECIFIC CHANGES

Generally distributed mild to moderate slowing with mainly theta rhythms and some delta activity indicates diffuse cerebral dysfunction resulting from medication, metabolic derangement, changes secondary to increased intracranial pressure, or other causes. Such changes do not usually interfere with the detection of EEG signs of focal intracranial lesions. If a moderate degree of slowing is present without a distinct focus, and a local lesion is present, it is likely to be deeply located.

Severe generalized abnormalities consisting mainly of diffusely distributed delta range activity with superimposed theta activity is seen in brain tumors that have caused elevated intracranial pressure and displacement of diencephalic and brainstem structures leading to alterations in level of consciousness. Focal signs of hemispheric tumors under such circumstances may be obscured so that the absence of focal signs in a severely diffusely slow EEG cannot be considered evidence against a hemispheric lesion. Generalized slowing immediately after a seizure may also obscure a focus, but such postictal effects are usually of short duration. Nonspecific generally distributed abnormalities are more commonly seen in infratentorial tumors (25) where they may be the major or even the only changes encountered. It should be recalled that a small percentage of healthy adults have mild degrees of slowing in the form of scattered excess theta activity that is classified as abnormal (see also Kellaway, *this volume*). Such mild nonspecific changes are of no diagnostic value for brain tumor.

CHARACTERISTICS OF TUMORS

Deep-Seated and Infratentorial Tumors

Intraventricular tumors, thalamic tumors, and tumors of the basal ganglia are difficult to diagnose by means of the EEG. Tumors of the thalamus and basal ganglia may produce FIRDA that is bilaterally synchronous and symmetrical or has some lateralization to the side of the tumor. Thalamic tumors more commonly result in ipsilateral widespread PDA with alpha depression. Intraventricular meningiomas in the region of the trigone and the temporal horn usually cause focal slowing in the temporal region (9).

The EEG is of limited diagnostic help in infratentorial tumors because most records are either normal or contain nonspecific generalized abnormalities. If there is no clinical evidence of increased intracranial pressure, normal EEGS are seen in about 50% of adults with infratentorial tumors, including brainstem gliomas and cerebellar pontine angle tumors. Considering infratentorial tumors of all types, and including children (in whom the majority of brain tumors are located below the tentorium), roughly one-fourth to one-third of all patients have normal EEGs with infratentorial tumors (14,-24,36). According to Hess (25), normal EEGs occur with 4% of hemispheric tumors, whereas the incidence for infratentorial tumors is 31%. When a patient shows clinical evidence of increased intracranial pressure and has a normal EEG, a posterior fossa tumor is a much more likely possibility than a hemispheric tumor.

In some series more than half of infratentorial tumors are associated with intermittent rhythmic slowing (14,36). The discharges are waves in the delta range (IRDA) or in the theta range. The intermittent slowing usually appears as bisynchronous rhythmic activity in generalized bilateral distribution or, particularly in children, in the posterior electrodes only (OIRDA) (36). Rhythmic slow activity is sometimes seen mainly frontally (FIRDA), and this occurs more often in adults. The distribution of the rhythmic activity is not related to the location of the tumor within the posterior fossa.

Bilateral PDA also occurs with infratentorial tumors, particularly in children, and was reported by Martinius et al. in half their patients (36). It occurs more often in rapidly growing tumors and is usually

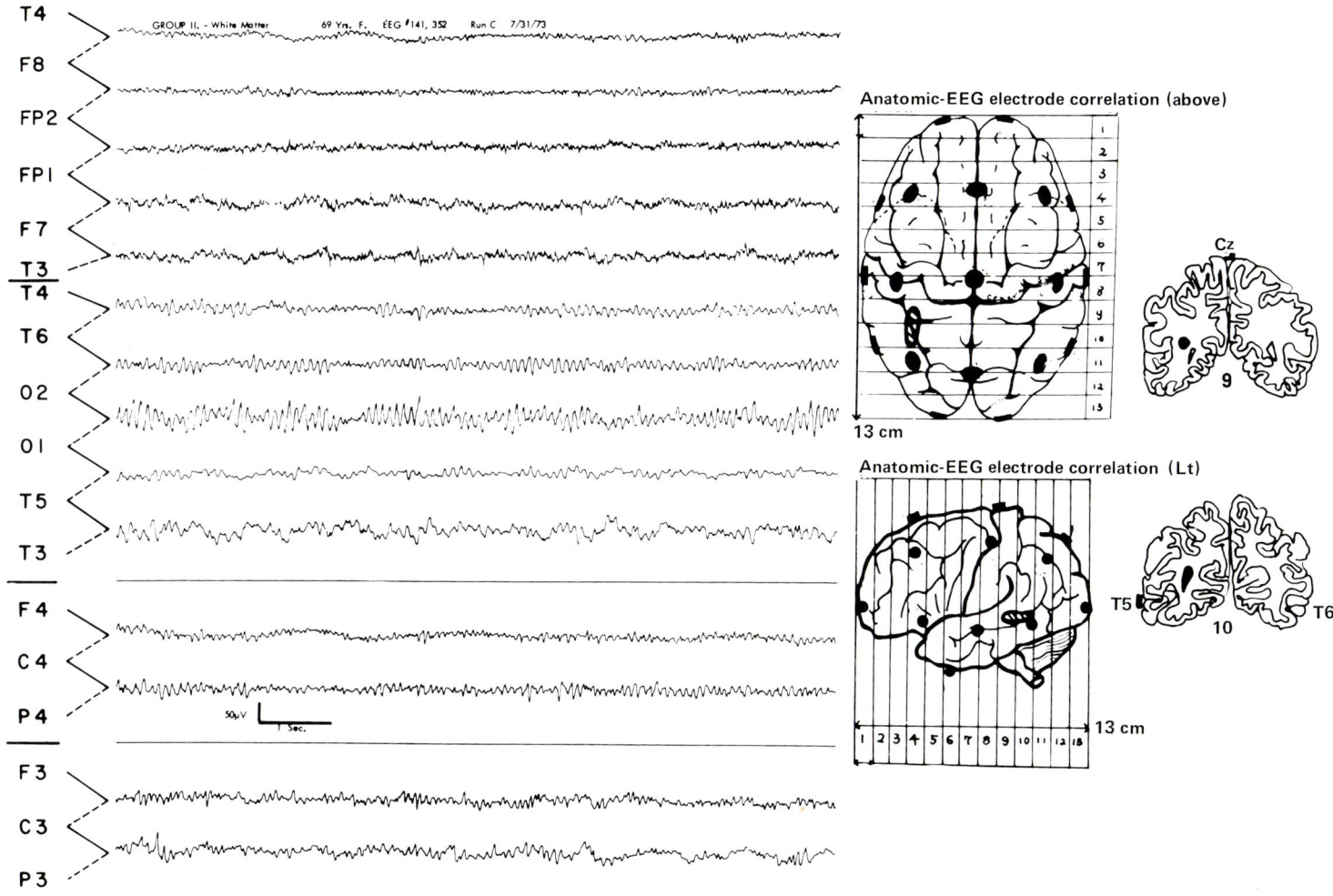

FIG. 1. PDA focus at highest voltage at electrodes T3 and P3. There is depression of alpha activity at T5 and T3. The location of the lesion is in the white matter of the left temporal-parietal area, as shown in the accompanying diagrams.

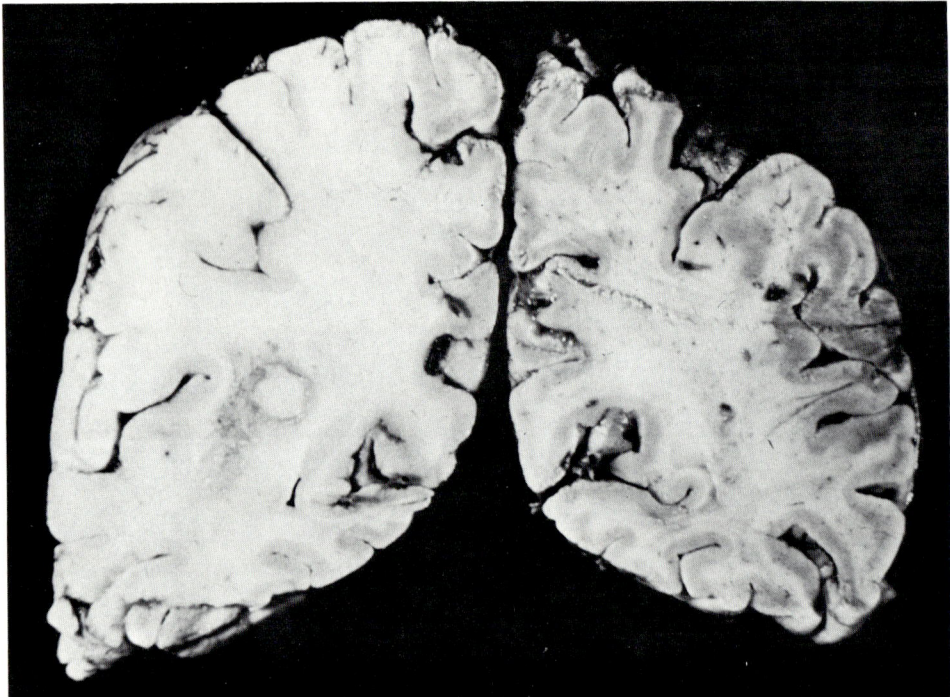

FIG. 2. Specimen obtained 4 weeks after the EEG in Fig. 1 was done. The lesion is a glioblastoma limited to the white matter of the left temporal-parietal area.

bilateral, occurring predominantly in the posterior areas; it may show shifting asymmetry but no consistent focal accentuation.

As was previously mentioned, bilaterally synchronous IRDA in the EEG of posterior fossa tumors correlates with dilation of the third ventricle (14,36). The relationship is not a simple one, however, and the rate of ventricular dilation and other factors influence the appearance of OIRDA in posterior fossa tumors. It has been suggested that PDA seen in posterior fossa lesions may be the result of pressure directly on the occipital lobes by the neoplasm or by its interference with the posterior circulation (36).

FIG. 3. The first of a series of tracings taken over a 6-year period (January 1971 to December 1976) in a patient with a right frontal lobe astrocytoma. The tumor was subtotally removed 12 weeks before this tracing was obtained. Continuous PDA is seen at electrodes FP2 and F8. Beta activity is at higher amplitude at electrode FP2 than at FP1 owing to the skull defect.

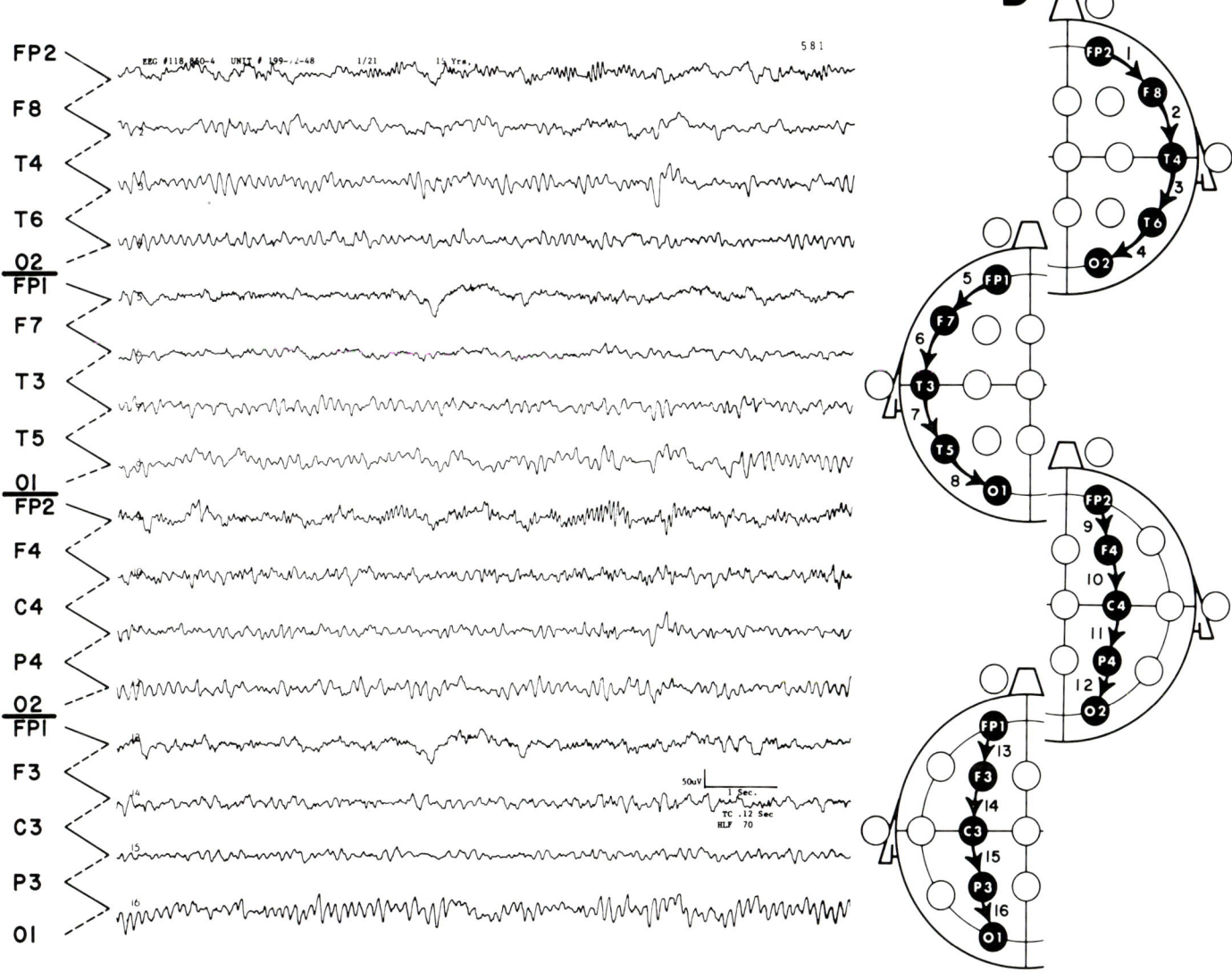

Lesions Involving Hemispheric White Matter

Continuous PDA usually indicates a destructive lesion in the underlying white matter. Figures 1 and 2 illustrate a white matter lesion in the left temporoparietal area. The pathology is glioblastoma, and the EEG shows widespread PDA that involves electrodes T3, P3, T5, and F7, with maximum slowing at T3 (Fig. 1). There is a depression of alpha in the vicinity of T5. In this case the voltage depression localized the lesion that was closest to electrode T5 more accurately than did the highest voltage of the PDA. The gross aspects of the lesion are shown in Fig. 2.

Although continuous irregular PDA of focal distribution is usually indicative of a destructive lesion in the white matter, the likelihood of such a lesion becomes even greater when there is also continuous depression or absence of superimposed background activity in the area of irregular slowing. Exceptions exist, however, and both focal background activity depression and focal PDA can be seen for many days following a migraine attack (27).

There is usually worsening of the EEG as a brain tumor progresses, but such a course can be markedly altered by surgical intervention, x-ray treatment, and particularly by the administration of steroids to reduce pressure. Steroids (e.g., dexamethasone) can profoundly improve the EEG records of patients with extensive tumors. Such EEG changes correlate well with improvement in the patient's state of awareness and to a degree with improvement of focal neurological deficits. Often there is very little or no associated change in the computerized transaxial tomogram (CTT). Figures 3 through 8 show a sequence of changes over a period of years in a progressive lesion involving the white matter. It illustrates interactions of surgical treatment, radiation, and the administration of steroids on the basic progressive nature of the lesion. The patient was initially referred because of uncontrolled short absences lasting a few seconds each. An initial EEG showed bilaterally synchronous 2- to 3-Hz generalized spike and wave complexes with bifrontal accentuation, greater on the right side, and PDA at the right frontopolar electrode (FP2). The first record (Fig. 3) was taken in January 1971, 12 weeks after a grade II astrocytoma of the right frontal lobe was removed subtotally because part of the lesion extended deeply and was surgically inaccessible. Radiotherapy followed. The record shows a focus of PDA at FP2 which also involves F8 to a lesser degree. Beta activity is at higher voltage in the frontal area on the right side (Electrode FP2) compared to the left side. This is attributable to decreased attenuation of underlying cortical activity by defects in the skull and other coverings consequent to the operation.

Over the next 2.5 years the patient's condition remained stable and his seizures were completely controlled. In June 1973 the delta focus was less extensive and a few sharp waves had appeared at the anterior frontal area (Fig. 4). However, by November 1975, 4 years after subtotal removal of the tumor, focal PDA in the right anterior frontal area had markedly increased and runs of FIRDA also appeared in that area (Fig. 5). The patient at that time was noted to have mild weakness in his left upper extremity and a recurrence of mild subjective seizures without recognizable abscences. In spite of radiotherapy, the seizures and neurological deficits in-

FIG. 4. Two and one-half years later (June 1973) the delta focus is confined to FP2 and is less prominent than in the earlier record. Part of the slowing in the previous record, which has receded, could be attributed to the surgical procedure; some of the improvement in this tracing may be related to the effect of radiotherapy on the tumor. A few sharp waves have appeared in the frontal area.

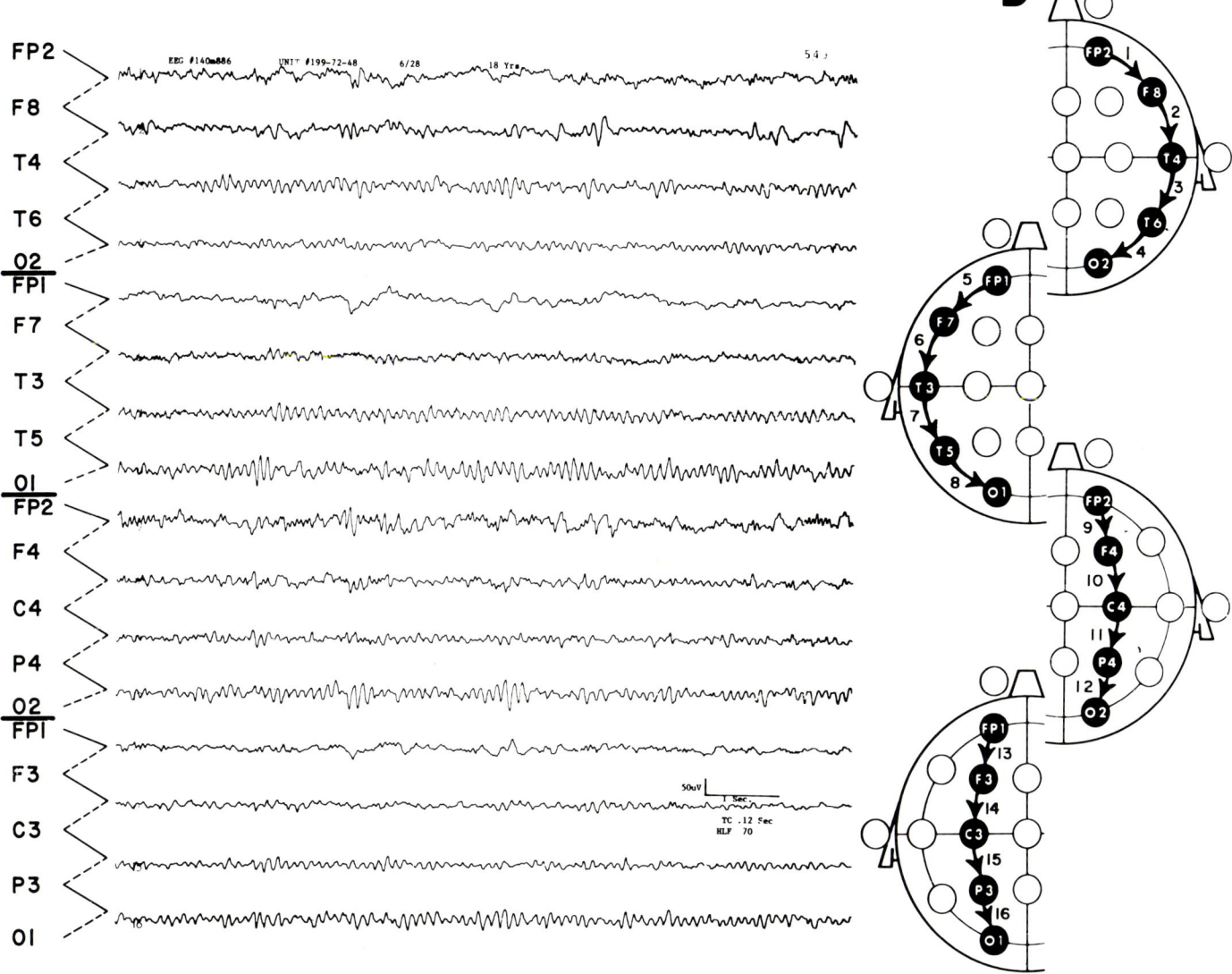

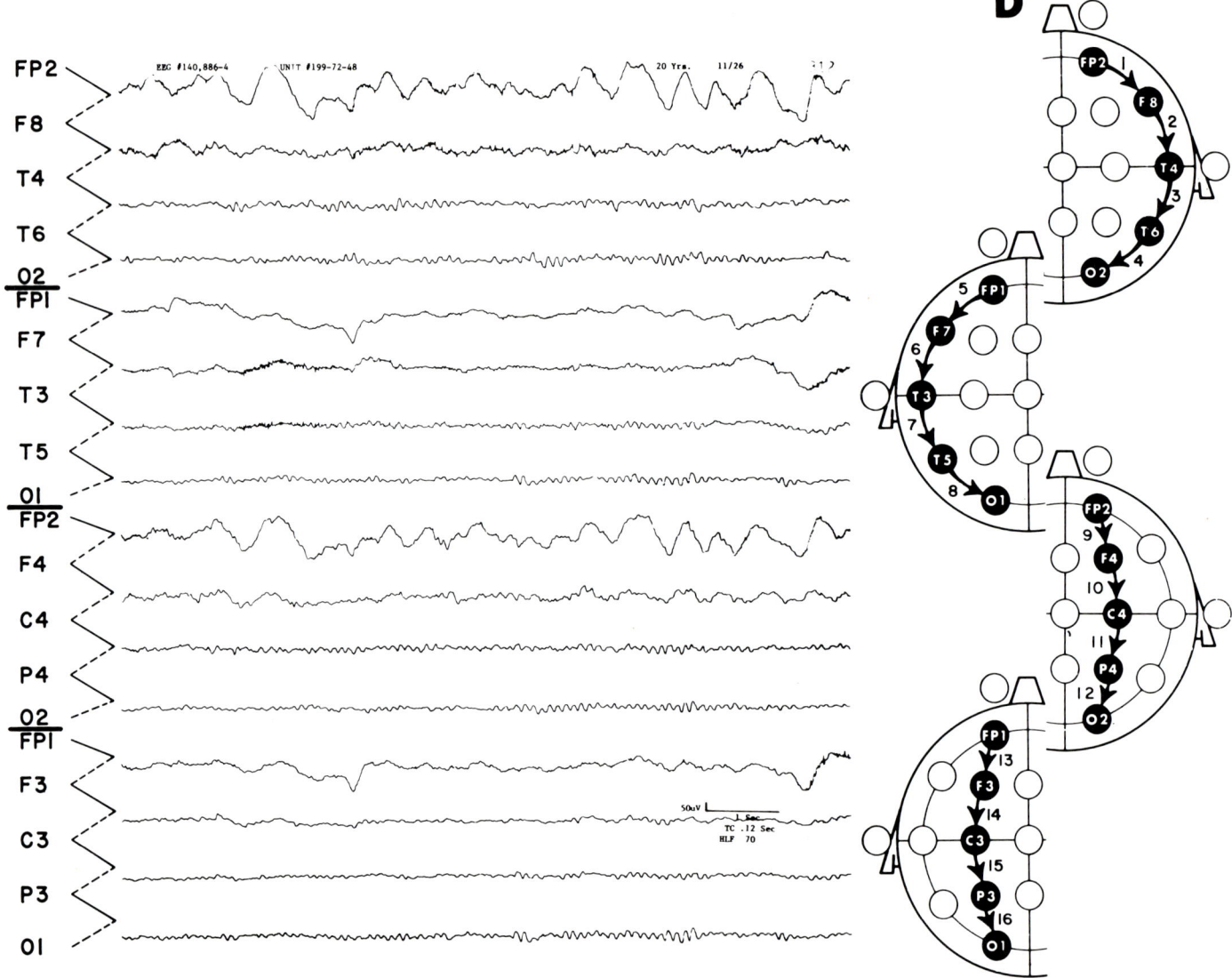

creased. By March 1976 the maximal voltage of the PDA had moved posteriorly into electrode F4, and PDA extended over a wider area, including the temporal and central regions (Fig. 6). In addition, background activity was depressed and slowed to a considerable extent over the entire right hemisphere and to a lesser extent on the left side. The record was considered consistent with progression of the clinical signs, which now included lethargy. Figure 7 shows the CTT scans, demonstrating an increase in the size of the lesion during the interval. Following this, dexamethasone was prescribed orally. An improvement in the state of awareness of the patient occurred, and the background records of both hemispheres markedly improved (Fig. 8). Later the general downhill course of the patient and his EEG resumed until his death in 1977.

Solitary metastatic lesions are indistinguishable by EEG from gliomas or other focal intracerebral destructive lesions involving mainly the white matter (17). A focus of PDA with associated depression of local background activity often overlies the sites of metastatic lesions, and as with primary brain tumors epileptogenic discharges are often seen (31). Common metastatic tumors to the brain are those secondary to carcinomas of the lung, kidney, and breast, as well as from melanomas and chorionic carcinomas. Periodic lateralized epileptiform discharges, which are often seen in acute vascular accidents, may occur early in metastatic tumors, particularly in rapidly growing ones. Sporadic focal spikes may be seen in metastatic as well as in more slowly growing tumors. It is possible only rarely to demonstrate multiple foci in patients with multiple metastatic lesions. The EEG in such cases shows either a single PDA focus or more widespread unilateral or bilateral PDA without definite foci.

Brain abscesses are most often located in the cerebellum and the frontal and temporal lobes. Using rapid and serial EEGs, it is possible to demonstrate almost daily the progression of clinical and EEG changes relative to other expanding lesions. The electrical changes are similar to those of other progressive destructive lesions, but focal PDA tends to be exceptionally slow, irregular, and of higher amplitude and wider distribution. The slowing frequently involves the entire hemisphere, so the lesion cannot be located accurately. At times the PDA is so generalized and bilaterally equal there is no EEG evidence of a focal process. Ziegler and Hoefer (44) correctly localized only half of the abscesses in their patients and were unable to lateralize in 20%. As an abscess becomes encapsulated, the generalized slowing may recede, with focal PDA becoming more recognizable. Flattening of the background activity overlying the cerebral abscess in the frontal or occipital areas is sometimes seen (37). An extensive and rapidly growing lesion involving primarily white matter is shown in Figs. 9 and 10. The abscess is in the right frontal lobe. The abnormality consists of continuous PDA activity at FP2 and F3 with maximal slowing at FP2, which is closest to the lesion. FIRDA is seen in the homologous region in the opposite side. Suppression of frontal background activity can be seen at electrode FP2, and alpha activity is absent bilaterally. Random sharp waves are present rarely. The postmortem specimen (Fig. 10) was obtained 1 week after the EEG was taken. Multiple hemispheric abscesses only rarely produce recognizable multiple slow-wave foci. They usually cause either widespread lateralized delta activity or, more often, diffuse bilateral delta. Epileptiform discharges occur with cerebral abscesses (34).

FIG. 5. Four years and 10 months after subtotal removal of the tumor (November 1975). Focal PDA in the right frontal area has markedly increased, and IRDA is prominent at electrode FP2. PDA is apparent at F8 and F4. At the time of this recording, weakness of the left upper extremity was noted and mild subjective seizures had reappeared. A CTT scan showed extension of the tumor.

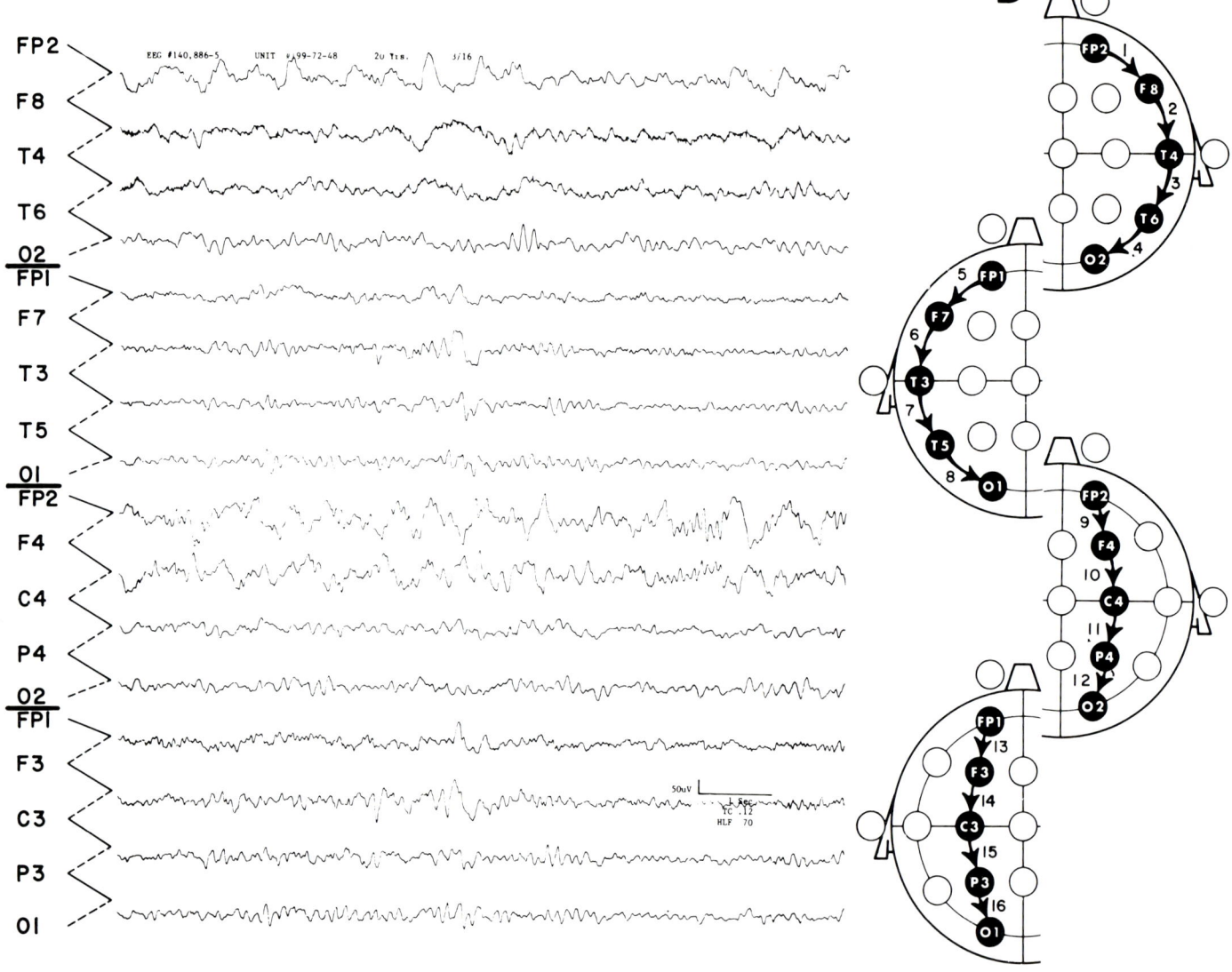

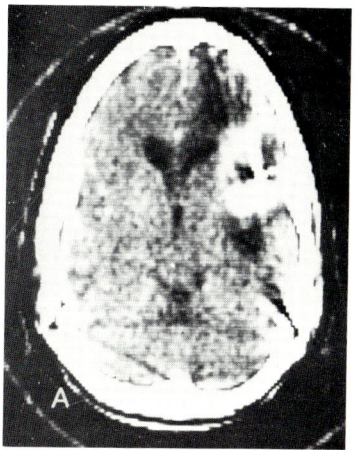 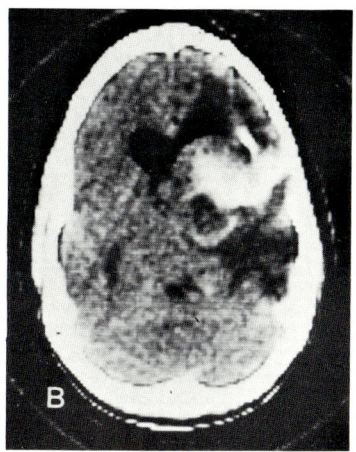

FIG. 7. CTT scans between **(A)** December 15, 1975 before dexamethasone and **(B)** March 1976 demonstrate an actual increase in the size of the lesion during an interval when the EEG showed improvement, coincident with dexamethasone administration.

In cerebellar abscesses the EEG usually shows IRDA or generally distributed PDA. Rarely, but more often than for hemispheric abscesses, the EEG is normal. Following successful combined medical and surgical treatment, the EEG rapidly improves, but some focal theta and delta activity may persist indefinitely. Within a few days to a year, epileptiform discharges appear in a large number of patients. The incidence of clinical epilepsy resulting from brain abscess is usually cited at about 50%, but after several years the incidence may rise to as high as 72% (35). Although the onset of epilepsy usually occurs earlier, a considerable number of patients develop seizures 3 or 4 years after operation. Epileptogenic activity (e.g., spikes, sharp waves, and spike and wave discharges) are common in patients who develop clinical seizures but are not necessarily predictive of clinical seizures as they are often seen in patients who do not develop clinical epilepsy.

Lesions of White Matter and Cortical and Subcortical Gray Matter

Large, rapidly growing lesions involving white matter and extending deeply into the midline structures may result in diffuse PDA, a reduction or absence in background activity, and IRDA. The patient whose record is shown in Fig. 11 was deeply stuporous. There is diffuse PDA with a degree of asymmetry, a loss of background rhythms, and some intermittent runs of superimposed theta waves. The CTT scan (Fig. 12) shows a large midline frontal mass obliterating the right frontal horn, involving the corpus callosum and extending deeply. Autopsy revealed a large glioblastoma in the septum pellucidum extending into the septal area and the right caudate and left lenticular nuclei.

Figures 13 and 14 demonstrate the presence of a lesion that is mainly in the thalamic gray matter without involving the centrum ovale but with some extension into the adjacent ventricular white matter, more on the right side. The record is characterized by bilateral and diffusely distributed 5- to 7-Hz activity. In addition, PDA is

FIG. 6. Five years and 3 months after subtotal removal of the tumor (March 1976). PDA has extended over a wider area than that seen in the previous record and now includes the temporal and central regions (T4, T6, and C4). Highest voltage slowing has moved posteriorly into electrode F4. In addition, background activity has become slower over the entire right hemisphere and to a lesser degree on the opposite side. Dexamethasone was given in large doses following this recording and a second course of radiotherapy begun.

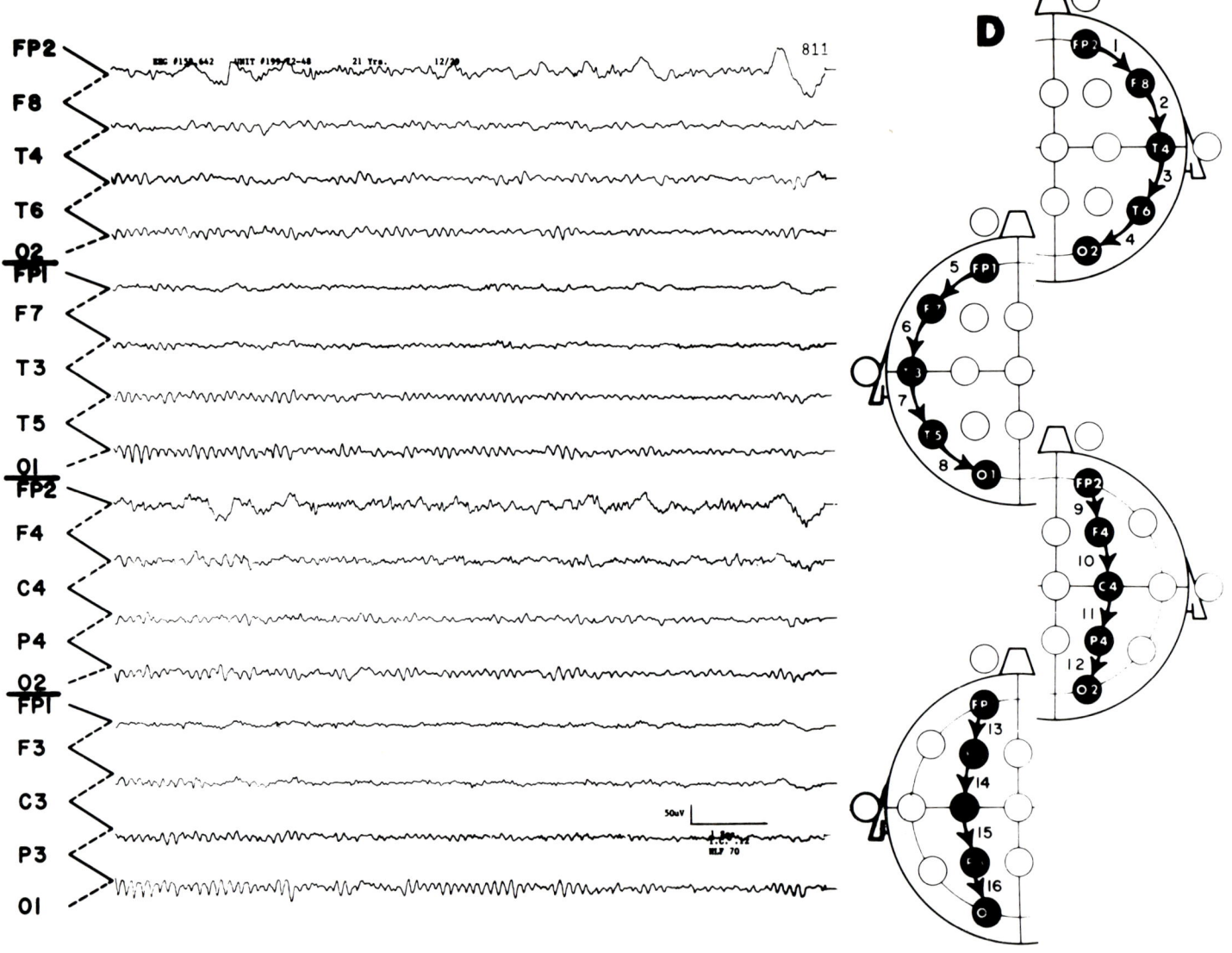

FIG. 8. Eight months after the previous EEG (December 1976). Although the CTT scan showed further extension of the tumor, dexamethasone has markedly improved the EEG. The patient improved clinically, particularly by becoming more alert for several months, but he then reverted to his downhill course.

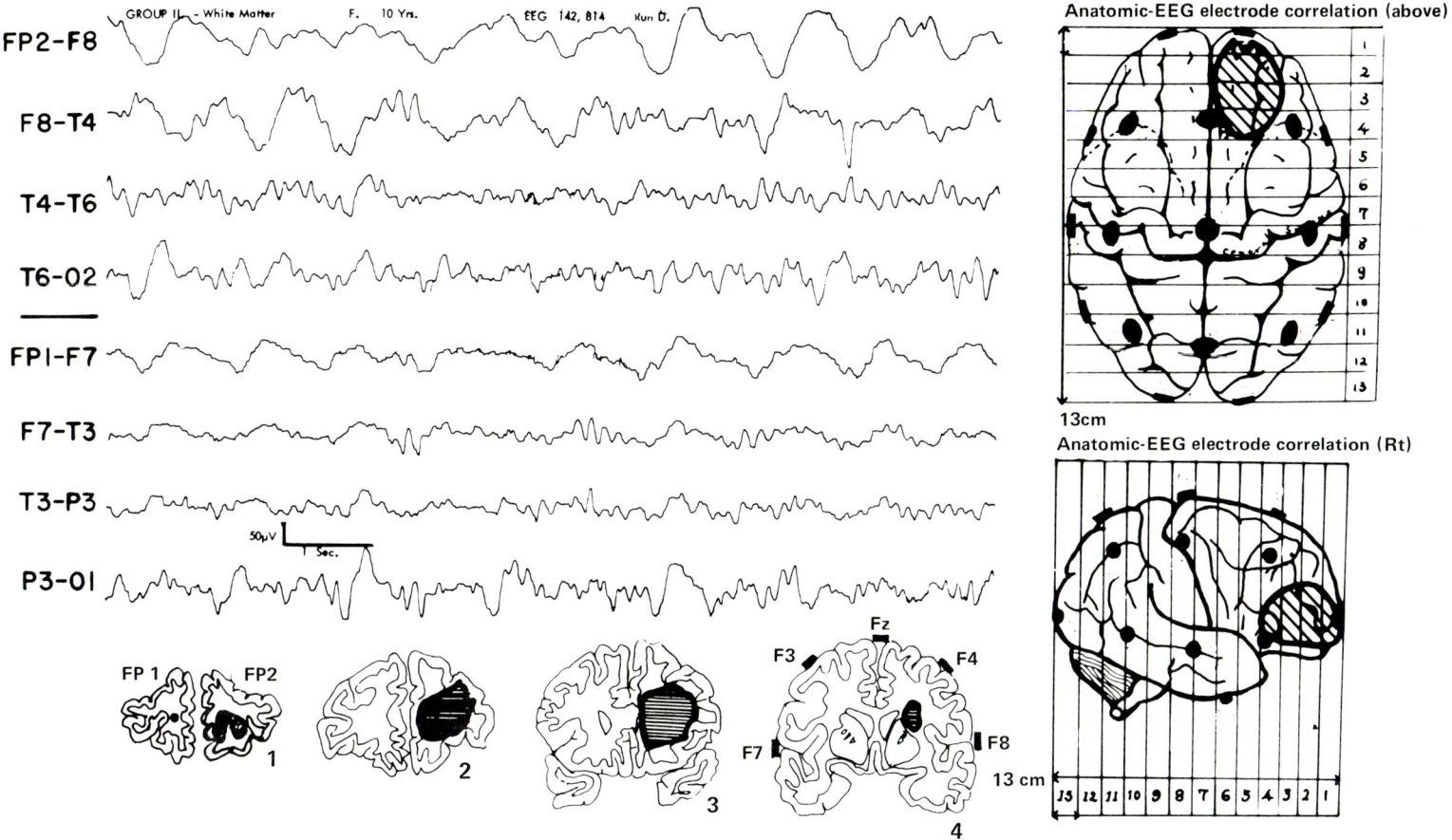

FIG. 9. EEG taken 1 week prior to death in a patient with a large abscess involving primarily white matter of the right frontal lobe. The record shows continuous focal PDA at FP2, F8, and FP1, and generalized rhythmic slowing at about 7 Hz. Background activity is depressed at electrodes FP2 and F8, and FIRDA can be seen at FP2 and FP1 during the last 4 sec of the tracing. The diagrams show the proximity of the electrodes to the lesion.

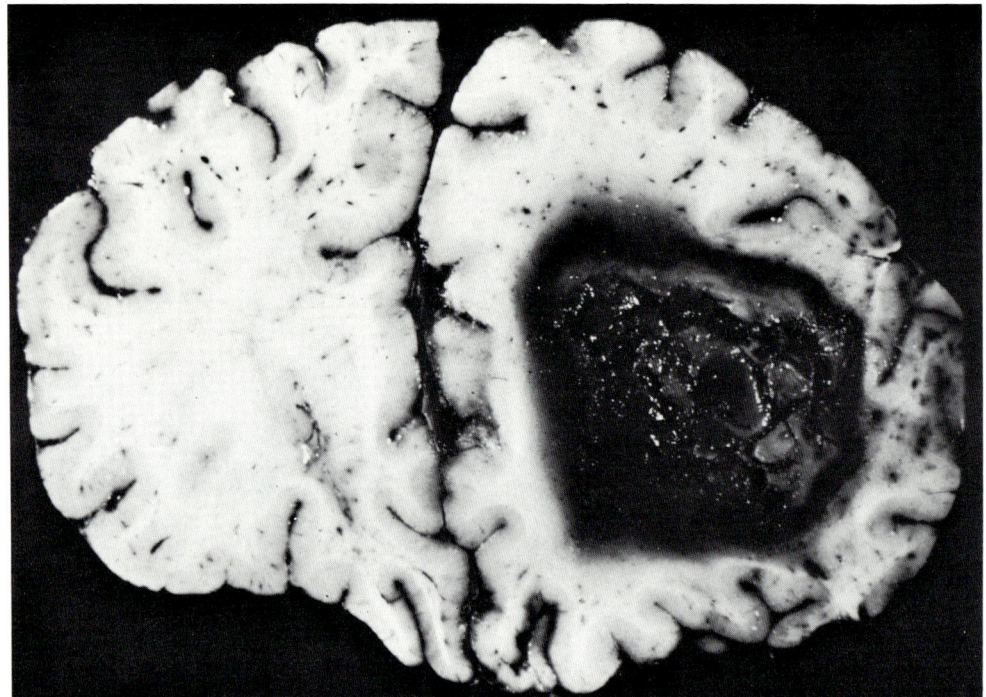

FIG. 10. This specimen was obtained 1 week after the EEG in Fig. 9. A large abscess is present in the white matter of the right frontal lobe.

noted on the right side. PDA is less prominent than in previous examples that had more extensive lesions of the white matter. Nevertheless, recognizable continuous PDA is seen in this case on the right side, where the tumor has invaded the white matter.

When the cerebral cortex and underlying white matter are severely damaged over an extensive portion of the hemisphere, nearly complete electrical silence can occur. This is demonstrated in Figs. 15 and 16, where an infarction of most of the right hemisphere occurred

FIG. 11. PDA in generalized distribution appears more on the right, with reduction in background activity and intermittent runs of theta waves. The patient is deeply stuporous. The lesion involves the white matter and extends deeply into the midline structures. The relationship of the lesion to the recording electrodes is shown in the diagrams. The CTT scan is shown in Fig. 12.

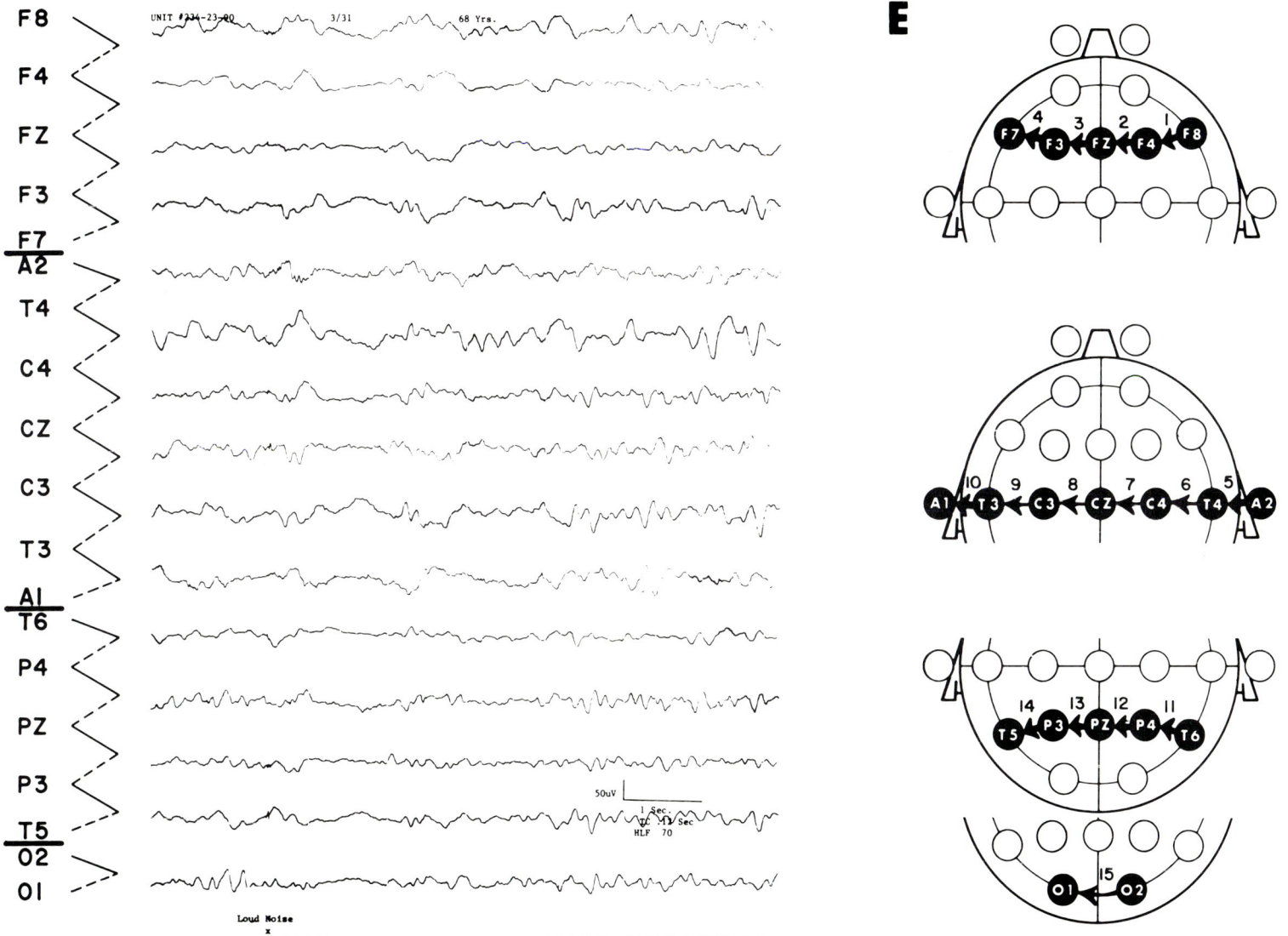

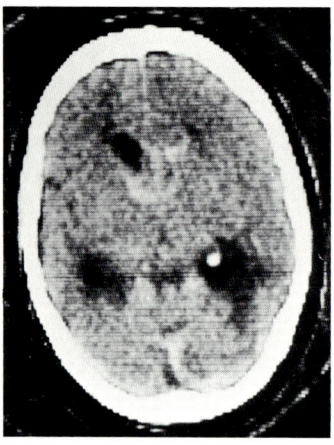

FIG. 12. CTT scan indicates a large midline frontal mass that involves the corpus callosum, obliterates the right frontal horn, and extends deeply. Autopsy revealed a large glioblastoma in the septum pellucidum extending into the septal area and the right caudate and left lenticular nuclei. The adjacent periventricular white matter on the right side was involved, but the centrum ovale was spared.

consequent to complete occlusion of the right middle and anterior cerebral arteries. The EEG in this case shows an almost complete absence of activity on the right side. On the left side, PDA and IRDA are seen in general distribution, and background alpha activity is absent. The left-sided abnormalities seen in Fig. 15 are the result of secondary effects on the diencephalon, upper brainstem, and right hemisphere. Most gliomas and other invasive tumors, even though they may extend widely into the white matter and subcortical gray masses, do not cause almost complete suppression of cortical activity such as can be seen in cases of complete major vascular infarctions. This is because the major infarctions cause death of nearly all cortical neurons in the area of ischemia, in contrast to most tumors, which directly involve relatively small amounts of cortical tissue. Because of this it may be said generally that large cerebral hemispheric tumors produce more high-voltage PDA and less depression of background than do large infarcts (23). It should be clearly understood, however, that the EEG cannot reliably differentiate between tumors and vascular accidents (16). Although focal spikes and sharp waves are encountered more commonly in brain tumors than in vascular accidents (22), repetitive paroxysmal discharges of sharp waves referred to as periodic lateralized epileptiform discharges (PLEDS), although not shown in the case illustrated, are frequently encountered during the first few days following an acute cerebral vascular accident, as mentioned earlier. PLEDS are encountered less frequently in progressive lesions (5).

Up to this point all the focal destructive lesions illustrated have included at least some damage to the hemispheric white matter. The PDA that is characteristic of such lesions may be related to deafferentation or isolation of the cortex from afferent influences. It has been hypothesized that the modified synaptic potentials that generate polymorphic slow waves may result from loss of cholinergic influences on postsynaptic membranes following cortical deafferentation by the destruction of axons ascending through the white matter (19). It appears that edema of the white matter per se does not produce PDA (40).

Lesions Involving Subcortical Gray Matter Structures

Lesions involving deep midline gray matter structures characteristically result in IRDA. Intermittent delta rhythm, like all EEG activity, is generated by neurons in the cortex but reflects influences projected from dysfunctioning diencephalic or upper brainstem gray matter. The IRDA usually occurs in relatively brief bursts. As men-

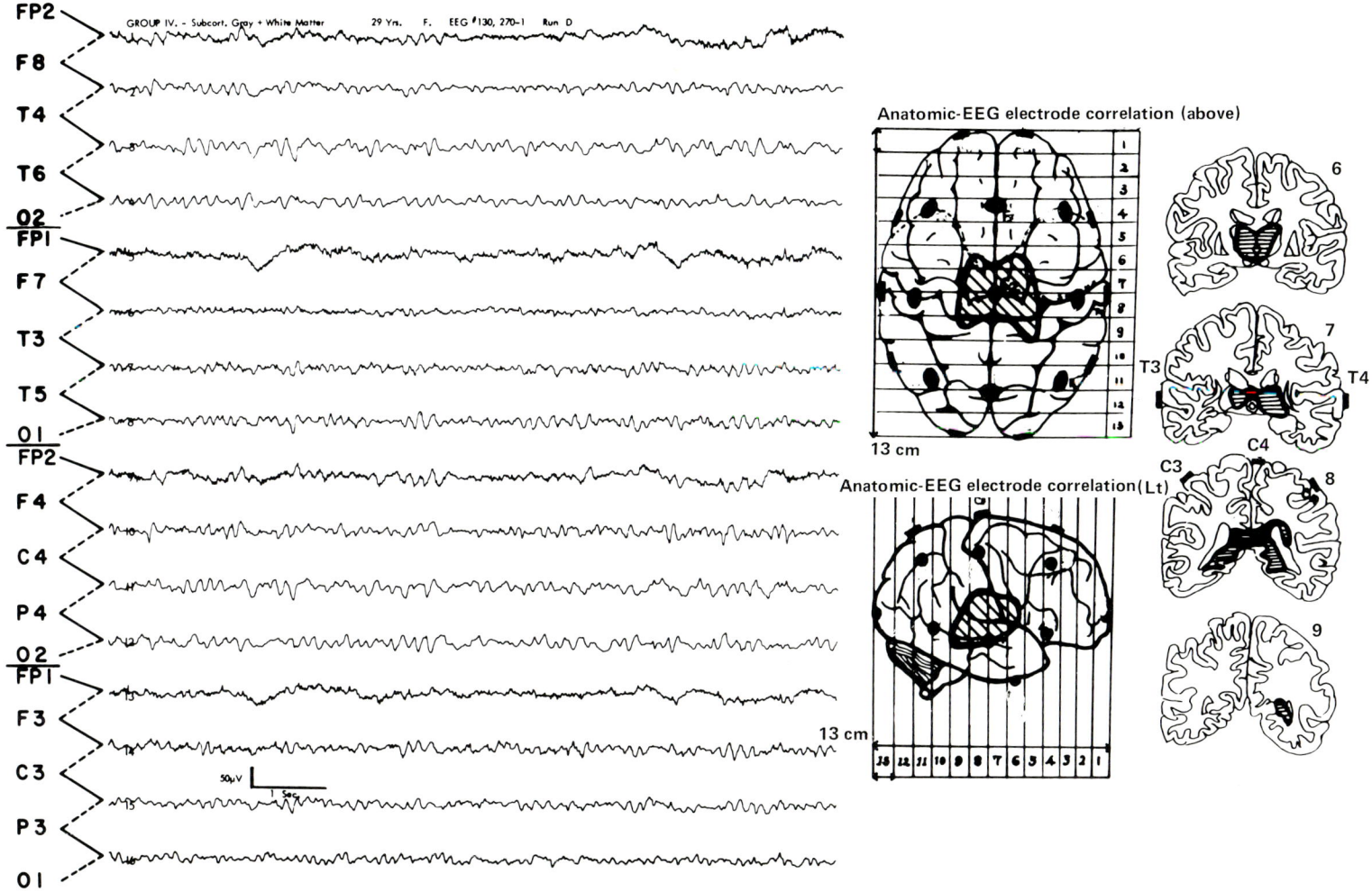

FIG. 13. A tumor is present, mainly in the thalamic gray matter with some extension into the white matter, more on the right side, as indicated in the diagrams. The record has generally distributed rhythmic activity at 5 to 7 Hz. PDA is present on the right side, mainly in the right posterior temporal-parietal area.

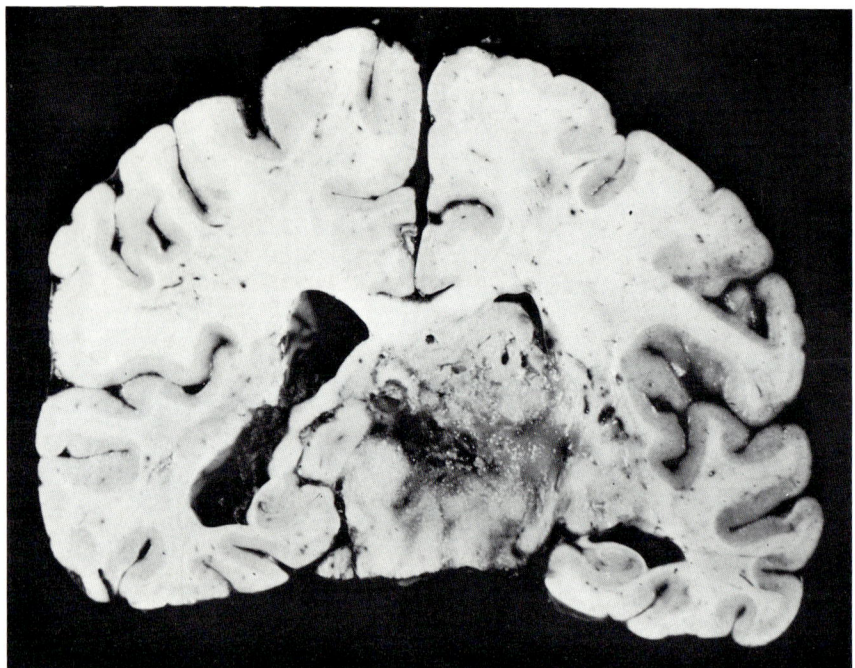

FIG. 14. Specimen shows a glioblastoma in the thalamus, extending into the white matter of the right parietal lobe.

tioned earlier, in adults the intermittent delta is at highest voltage frontally and is referred to as FIRDA. In young children it is usually more prominent in the occipital areas and is referred to as OIRDA (11). IRDA can be differentiated from PDA by form and by the fact that PDA usually persists during attention, eye opening, and sleep, whereas IRDA becomes attenuated or disappears with attention, eye opening, and during the slow-wave stages of continuous sleep. However, IRDA persists during drowsiness and is present during REM sleep. In destructive lesions IRDA, which alternates with normal background rhythms, occurs as the result of direct or indirect effects from those lesions on the gray matter, mainly the thalamus. The development of intermittent delta rhythms and their disappearance in a patient with a pinealoma is shown in Fig. 17. The disappearance followed radiotherapy, which resulted in shrinkage of the tumor and alleviation of the obstructive hydrocephalus that caused dilation of the third ventricle, distorting the thalamus. Figure 18 shows the changes in the tumor and ventricular size before and after radiotherapy.

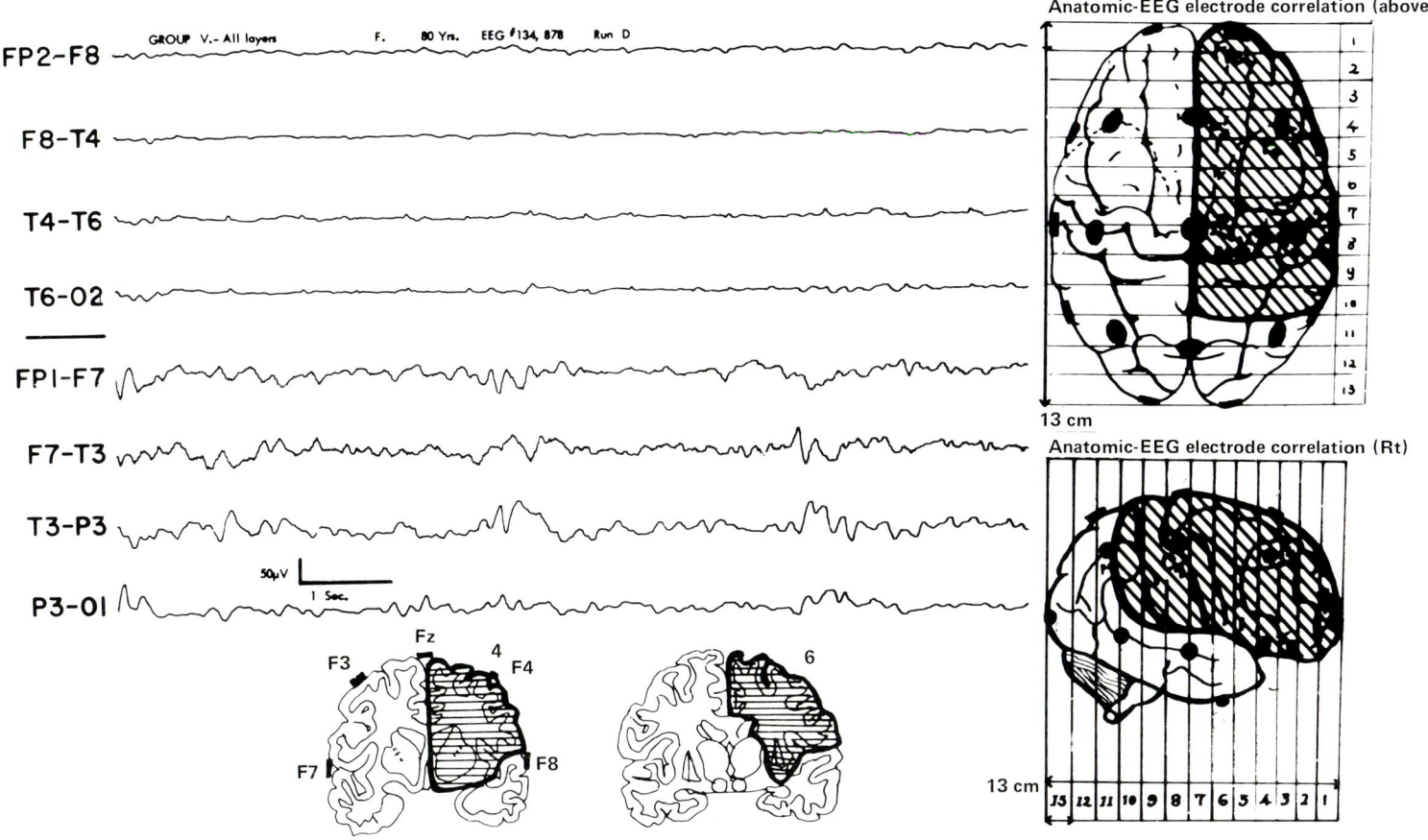

FIG. 15. The record shows almost complete absence of activity on the right side. On the left side PDA and some rhythmic waves mainly in the theta range are widely distributed. There is no alpha activity. The diagrams indicate the extent of the lesion at postmortem examination.

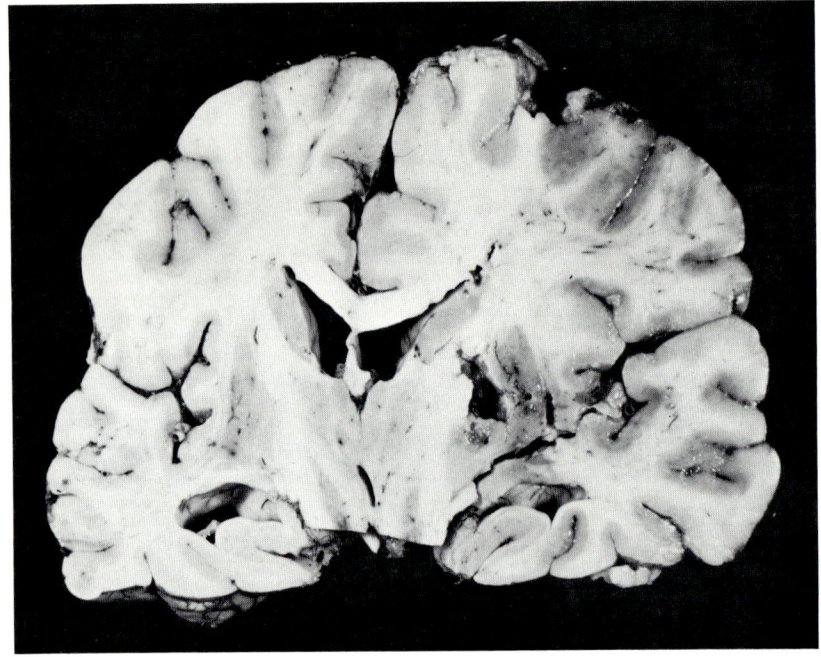

FIG. 16. Specimen obtained 1 week after the EEG in Fig. 15. There is an extensive cerebral infarct consequent to complete occlusion on the right middle and anterior cerebral arteries. Swelling of the entire right hemisphere distorts the left hemisphere, diencephalon, and brainstem.

Lesions which directly destroy major portions of the reticular formation of the midbrain may result in generalized disorganization of EEG background activity, an absence of alpha rhythm, and generalized PDA associated with depression of consciousness. This is shown in Figs. 19 and 20.

Lesions in reticular formation that do not ascend as high as the upper part of the midbrain (e.g., those that occur in pontine hemorrhage) may have either the normal characteristics demonstrated here (Fig. 21) or contain central rhythm in the alpha frequency range which may be mistaken for alpha but is not responsive to eye opening (6). Persistent alpha activity, which may be responsive to eye opening and noxious stimuli, occurs in the locked-in syndrome in which the patient is conscious but unresponsive because of quadriplegia (Figs. 21 and 22) (43).

Extra-axial Lesions

Slow-growing extra-axial lesions, which do not significantly disrupt or only slowly compress the white matter, usually cause mild changes;

these take the form of either local spikes from cortical irritation or local theta activity. An example of this is shown in Fig. 23 in which a rather large meningioma gives rise to relatively mild slowing. Clinical neurological deficits are also usually mild in such cases, as was true in this example. More rapidly developing and larger extra-axial lesions (e.g., subdural hematoma) produce focal background depression and focal PDA.

SERIAL EEG STUDIES

An initial record with a focus of continuous PDA is indicative of an underlying structural lesion, and unless the patient is known to have recently had a severe typical migraine attack, a structural lesion should be strongly suspected. Serial EEGs can confirm the presence of an expanding lesion (e.g., a tumor or abscess) when progressive deterioration in the record is detected (13,32). After a previously normal study, the appearance of a focus of PDA or focal paroxsymal activity for the first time in a patient with seizures should raise the suspicion of a progressive lesion. Patients with epilepsy may harbor slowly infiltrating gliomas which interdigitate among the fibers of the white matter of the brain without destroying tissue until late in the course, and repeated EEGs may show no significant changes for years. Conversely, in malignant tumors EEG deterioration is often recognizable within weeks. Ventricular obstruction and cerebral herniation consequent to a space-occupying lesion can result in bilateral generalized IRDA and/or PDA within a matter of hours.

The widespread use of steroids, particularly dexamethasone, has greatly modified the use of the EEG for assessing progressive lesions. Striking improvement in the EEG may occur in patients with space-occupying lesions following the administration of corticosteroids (Fig. 8). Such changes with steroids usually correlate with physiological improvement. If steroids are not used, serial studies are helpful in the management of patients after surgical removal of tumors and often provide evidence of recurrence. During the immediate postoperative period, deterioration of the EEG is not uncommon, with severe generalized slowing and prominent focal PDA following the surgical procedure (which includes some degree of trauma, subarachnoid bleeding, and marginal edema). EEGs usually stabilize within 2 months after surgery, and IRDA and generalized PDA usually disappear. Focal PDA frequently persists but is improved, having a more restricted area with lower voltage and less continuous activity. Often epileptiform discharges are seen for the first time after surgery over the region of excision in successfully treated cases. They are regarded to be the result of diminished attenuation of discharges related to the craniotomy defect, and if the field of the spike is very restricted they may have no clinical significance. However, if spiking becomes pronounced or focal PDA increases or IRDA reappears, recurrence of the tumor is likely.

EEG AND CTT IN FOCAL STRUCTURAL LESIONS

Computerized transaxial tomography (CTT) shares with electroencephalography the advantage of being noninvasive. It does, however, expose the patient to radiation varying from relatively insignificant to appreciable amounts, depending on the methods used. The CTT has many obvious advantages over other less-sensitive and invasive procedures used in the detection and evaluation of brain lesions. The comparatively recent introduction and limited availability of CTT does not yet permit evaluation of its full impact on the uses of electroencephalography in the management of intracranial disease. It is recognized, however, that CTT has already revolutionized the diagnosis of focal intracranial lesions. Also, as CTT methodology

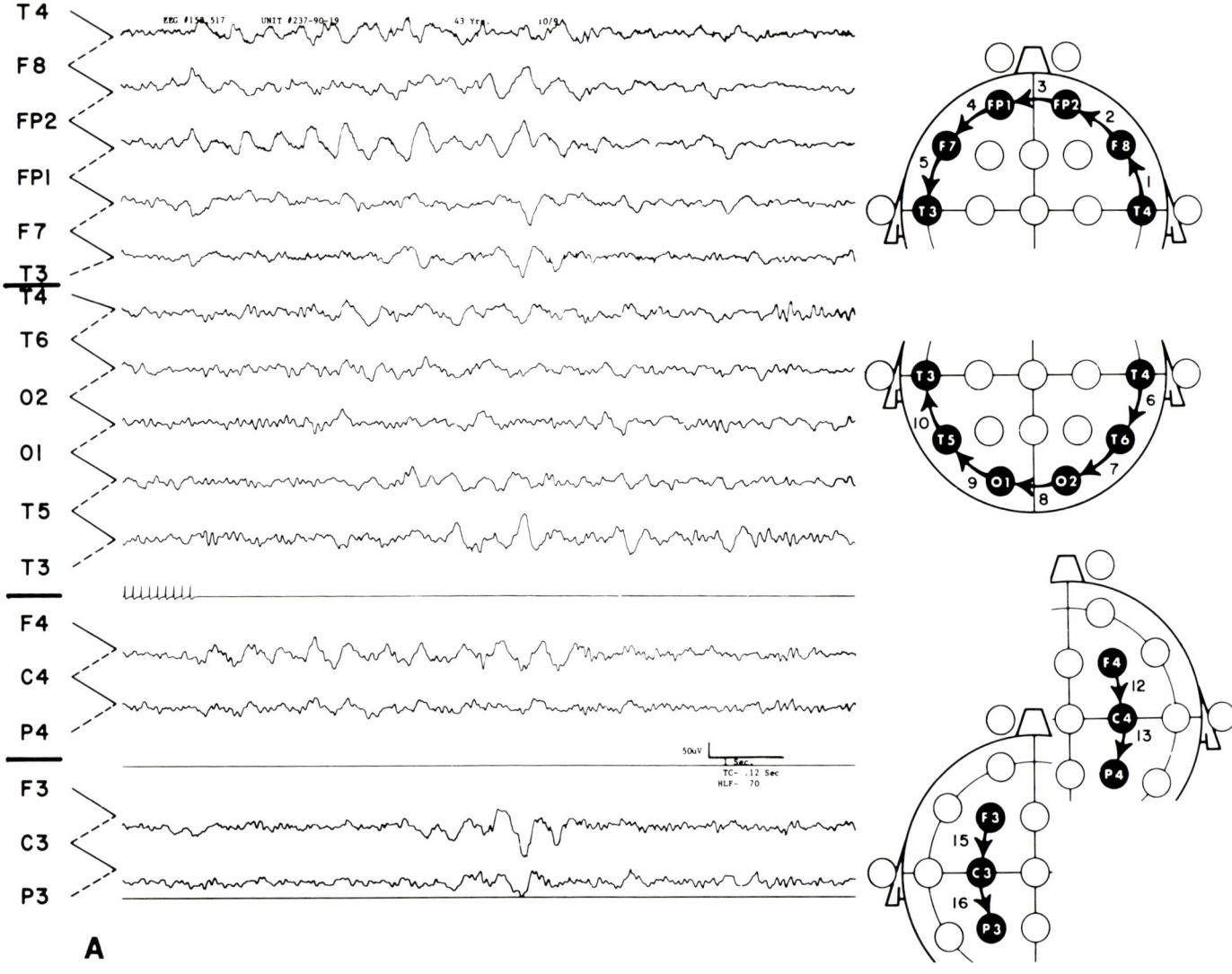

FIG. 17. A: FIRDA is seen best in FP2 and F4 leads but is also present bilaterally and in generalized distribution in a lethargic patient with a pinealoma obstructing the third ventricle. **B:** Note the disappearance of FIRDA and resumption of alert characteristics of the record following alleviation of the obstructive hydrocephalus *(facing page)*.

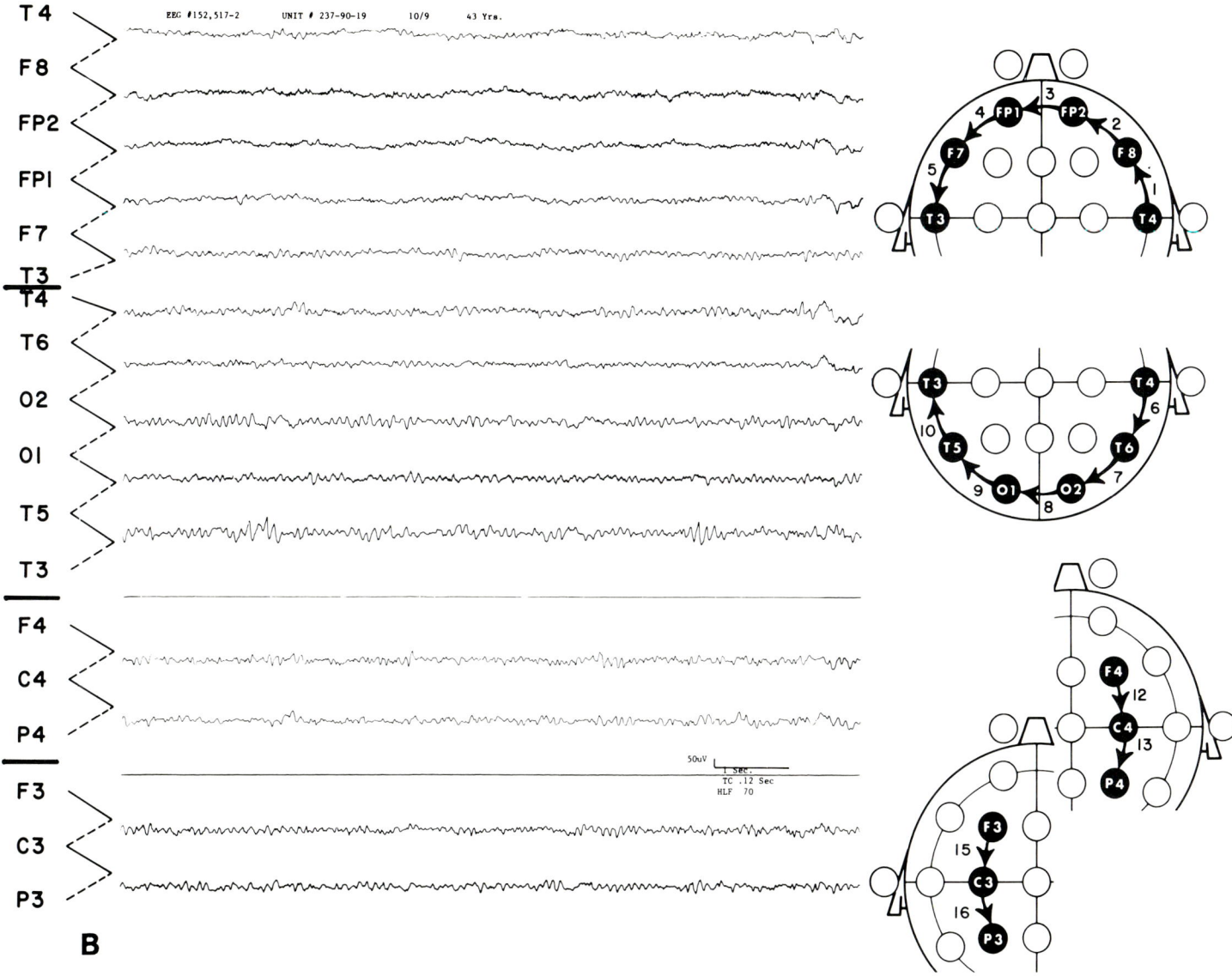

FIG. 17. B.: (See legend facing page.)

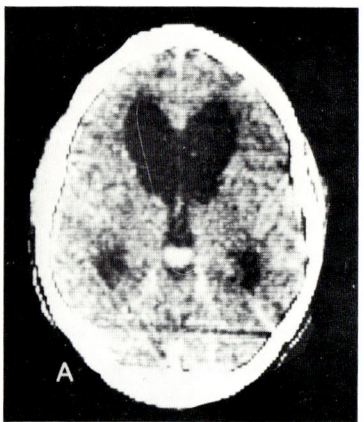 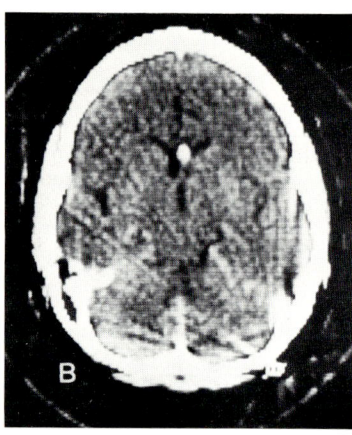

FIG. 18. A: CTT scan done on the same day as the EEG in Fig. 17A. The scan shows a large midline pinealoma with dilation of the third and lateral ventricles. **B:** CTT scan after radiotherapy resulted in reduction of tumor size and disappearance of ventricular dilation.

improves, allowing more precise definition, its effects on the comparative usefulness of the EEG in the identification, characterization, and management of structural lesions of the brain will be fully felt. It seems likely that, in the future, in highly suspected structural lesions the EEG will often be bypassed in favor of the CTT scan. Up to this time, however, at the Neurological Institute of New York and at the Mayo Clinic there has been no significant change in the number of EEGs in spite of a prompt precipitous decrease in the use of pneumoencephalography, radioactive brain scanning, and arteriography (4). Although some 90% of brain tumors in the cerebral hemispheres result in EEG abnormalities, localization is accurate in only 68% compared to 96% accuracy with CTT (2). Nevertheless, because the EEG reflects functional changes (local and distant) that structural examinations cannot reveal, the EEG will continue to have a unique role in the clinical diagnosis, management, and prognosis of focal intracranial lesions.

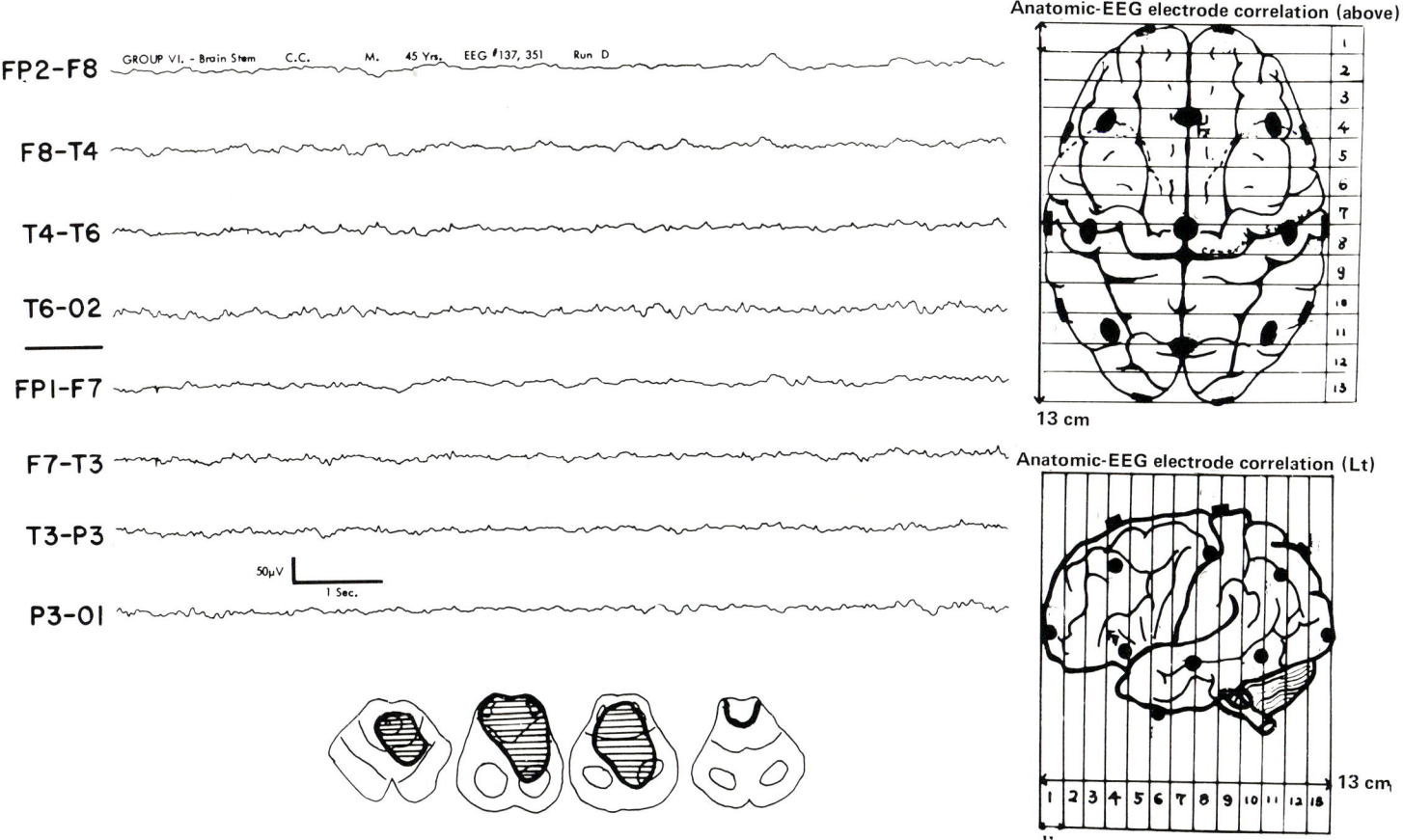

FIG. 19. Comatose patient with pontine hemorrhage extending into the midbrain. The record is generally disorganized, with mainly bilaterally distributed PDA and theta waves and some low-voltage activity resembling sleep spindles.

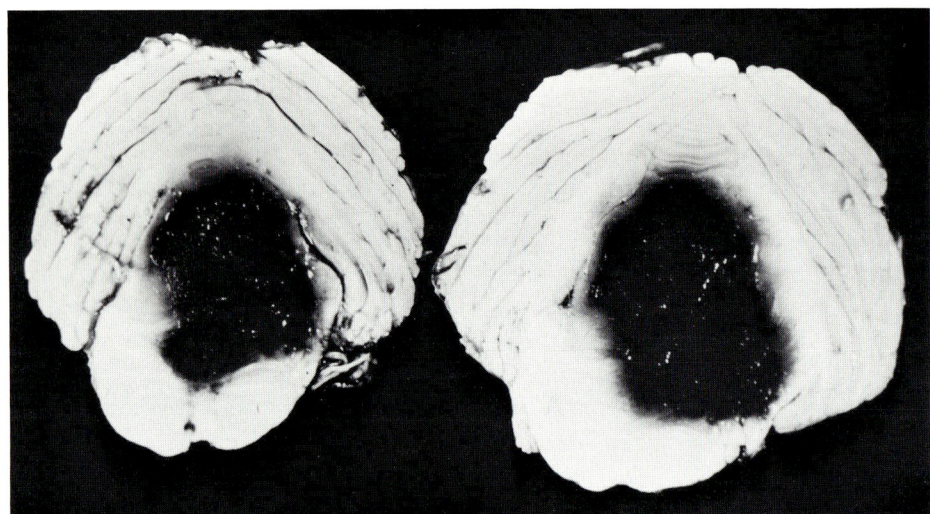

FIG. 20. This specimen was obtained 1 week after the EEG in Fig. 19 was taken. There is extensive hemorrhage into the midbrain reticular formation.

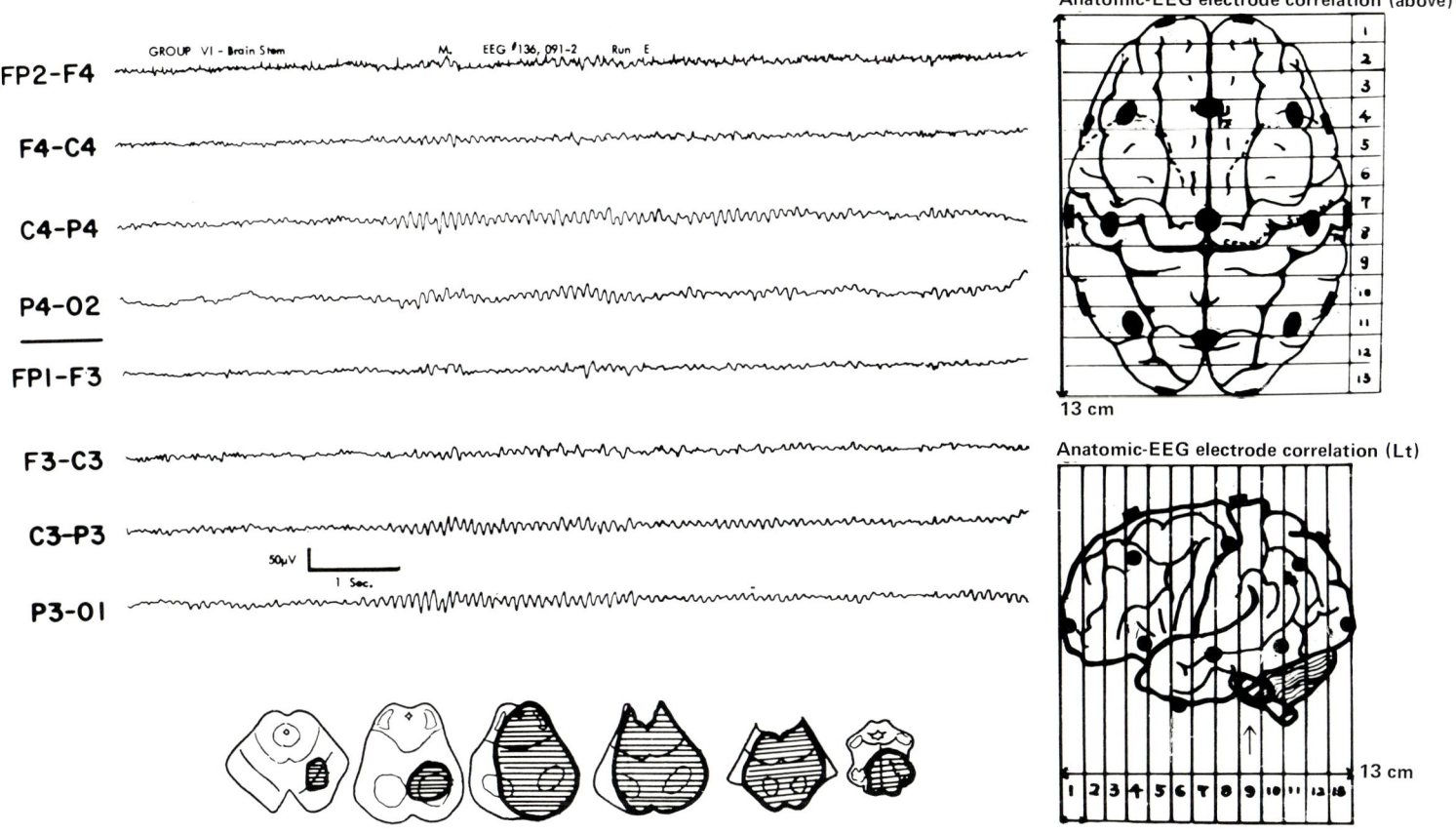

FIG. 21. EEG with reactive alpha activity in a patient who is mute and quadriplegic but conscious. Diagrams indicate extent of lesion in the brainstem.

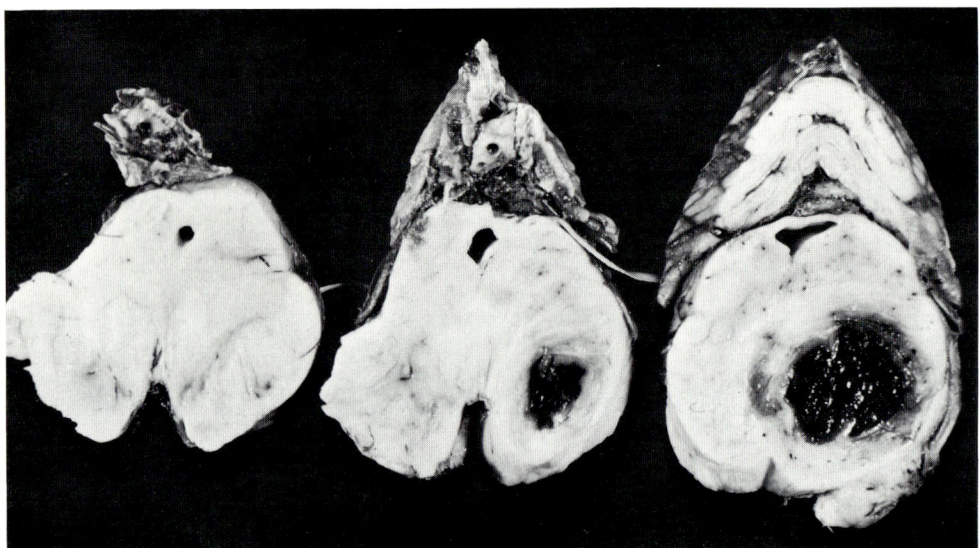

FIG. 22. Specimen shows a hemorrhage within, located in the pons and medulla, which is an astrocytoma. It fails to involve the midbrain periaqueductal gray matter, such as is seen in Fig. 20.

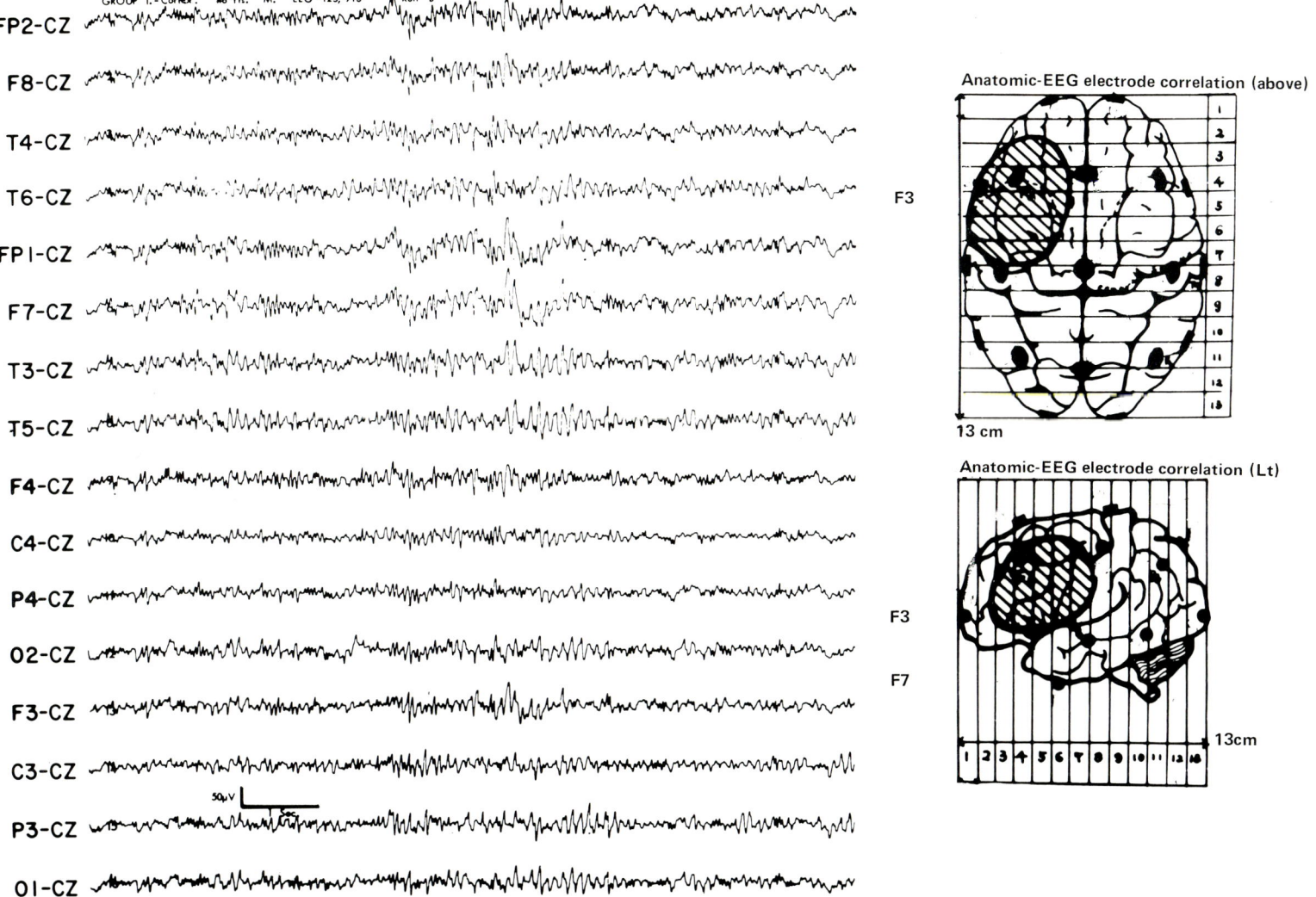

FIG. 23. Record shows rhythmic theta activity and sharp waves from the left hemisphere without significant amounts of delta in a patient with a convexity meningioma.

REFERENCES

1. Abraham, K., and Ajmone-Marsan, C. (1958): Patterns of cortical discharges and their relation to routine scalp electroencephalography. *Electroencephalogr. Clin. Neurophysiol.,* 10:447–461.
2. Ambrose, J., Gooding, M. R., and Richardson, A. E. (1975): An assessment of the accuracy of computerized transverse axial scanning (EMI scanner) in the diagnosis of intracranial tumours: A review of 366 patients. *Brain,* 98:569–582.
3. Arfel, G., and Fischgold, H. (1961): EEG-signs in tumours of the brain. *Electroencephalogr. Clin. Neurophysiol. (Suppl),* 19:36–50.
4. Baker, H. L. (1976): Computed tomography and neuroradiology: A fortunate primary union. *Am. J. Roentgenol.,* 127:101–110.
4a. Boddie, H. G., Banna, M., and Bradley, W. G. (1974): "Benign" intracranial hypertension. *Brain,* 97:313–326.
5. Chatrian, G. E., Shaw, C. M., and Leffman, H. (1964): The significance of periodic lateralized epileptiform discharges in EEG: An electrographic, clinical and pathological study. *Electroencephalogr. Clin. Neurophysiol.,* 17:177–193.
6. Chatrian, G. E., White, L. E., Jr., and Shaw, C-M. (1974): EEG pattern resembling wakefulness in unresponsive decerebrate state following traumatic brain-stem infarct. *Electroencephalogr. Clin. Neurophysiol.,* 16:285–289.
7. Cobb, W. A. (1945): Rhythmic slow discharges in the electroencephalogram. *J. Neurol. Neurosurg. Psychiatry,* 8:65.
8. Cobb, W. A. (1950): Intracranial tumours. In: *Electroencephalography,* edited by D. Hill and G. Parr, pp. 273–301. Macdonald, London.
9. Cobb, W. A., and Gassel, M. M. (1961): The EEG with lateral ventricle meningiomas. *Electroencephalogr. Clin. Neurophysiol. (Suppl),* 19:111–124.
10. Cordeau, J. P. (1959): Monorhythmic frontal delta activity in the human electroencephalogram: A study of 100 cases. *Electroencephalogr. Clin. Neurophysiol.,* 11:733–746.
11. Daly, D. D. (1968): The effect of sleep upon the electroencephalogram in patients with brain tumors. *Electroencephalogr. Clin. Neurophysiol.,* 25:521–529.
12. Daly, D. D. (1975): Brain tumors and other space occupying processes. In: *Handbook of Electroencephalography and Clinical Neurophysiology, Vol. 14: Clinical EEG,* pp. 5–10. Elsevier, Amsterdam.
13. Daly, D. D., and Thomas, J. E. (1958): Sequential alterations in the electroencephalograms of patients with brain tumors. *Electroencephalogr. Clin. Neurophysiol.,* 10:395–404.
14. Daly, D., Whelan, J. L., Bickford, R. G., and McCarthy, C. S. (1953): The electroencephalogram in cases of tumors of the posterior fossa and third ventricle. *Electroencephalogr. Clin. Neurophysiol.,* 5:203–216.
15. Drift, J. H. A. van der (1957): *The Significance of Electroencephalography for the Diagnosis and Localisation of Cerebral Tumours.* H. E. Stenfert Kroese, Leiden.
16. Drift, J. H. A. van der, and Magnus, O. (1961): The value of the EEG in the differential diagnosis of cases with cerebral lesions. *Electroencephalogr. Clin. Neurophysiol. (Suppl),* 19:183–196.
17. Drift, J. H. A. van der, and Magnus, O. (1961): Cerebral metastases. *Electroencephalogr. Clin. Neurophysiol. (Suppl),* 19:138–140.
18. Gloor, R. (1969): Hans Berger and the discovery of the electroencephalogram. *Electroencephalogr. Clin. Neurophysiol. (Suppl),* 28:1–36.
19. Gloor, P., Ball, G., and Schaul, N. (1977): Brain lesions that produce delta waves in the EEG. *Neurology (Minneap),* 27:326–333.
20. Gloor, R., Kalabay, O., and Giard, N. (1968): The electroencephalogram in diffuse encephalopathies: Electroencephalographic correlates of grey and white matter lesions. *Brain,* 91:779–802.
21. Goldensohn, E. S., Zablow, L., and Salazar, A. (1977): The penicillin focus. I. Distribution of potential at the cortical surface. *Electroencephalogr. Clin. Neurophysiol.,* 42:480–492.
22. Grunnet, G. L., and Goldensohn, E. S. (1967): Some differences in the EEG of brain tumors and cerebral vascular accidents. *Electroencephalogr. Clin. Neurophysiol.,* 23:491–494.
23. Hass, K. W., and Goldensohn, E. S. (1959): Clinical and electroencephalographic considerations in the diagnosis of carotid artery occlusion. *Neurology (Minneap),* 9:575–589.
24. Hess, R. (1958): *Elektroencephalographische studien bei Hirntumoren,* p. 106. Thieme, Stuttgart.
25. Hess, R., editor (1975): Brain tumors and other space occupying processes. In: *Handbook of Electroencephalography and Clinical Neurology, Vol. 14: Clinical EEG.* Elsevier, Amsterdam.
26. Hirsch, J. C., Buisson-Ferey, J., Sachs, M., Hirsch, J. C., and Scherrer, J. (1966): Electrocorticogramme et activities unifaires lors de processus expansif chez l'homme. *Electroencephalogr. Clin. Neurophysiol.,* 21:417–428.
27. Hockaday, J. M., and Whitty, C. W. (1969): Factors determining the electroencephalogram in migraine: A study of 560 patients, according to clinical type of migraine. *Brain,* 92:769–788.
28. Jasper, H., and Van Buren, J. (1953): Interrelationship between cortex and subcortical structures: Clinical electroencephalographic studies. *Electroencephalogr. Clin. Neurophysiol. (Suppl),* 4:168–188.
29. Kershmann, J., Conde, A., and Gibson, W. C. (1949): Electroencephalography in differential diagnosis of supratentorial tumors. *Arch. Neurol. Psychiatry,* 62:255–268.
30. Kirstein, L. (1953): The occurrence of sharp waves, spikes and fast activity in supratentorial tumours. *Electroencephalogr. Clin. Neurophysiol.,* 5:33–40.
31. Klass, D. W., and Bickford, R. G. (1958): The EEG in metastatic tumors of the brain. *Neurology (Minneap),* 8:333.

32. Klass, D. W., and Daly, D. D. (1960): Electroencephalography in patients with brain tumor. *Med. Clin. North Am.*, 44:1041–1051.
33. Krenkel, W. (1974): The electroencephalogram in tumours of the brain. In: *Handbook of Clinical Neurology*, Vol. 16. Elsevier, Amsterdam.
34. Le Beau, J., and Dondey, M. (1959): Importance diagnostique de certaines activités électroencéphalographies latéralisées, périodiques ou a tendance périodique au cours des abcès du cerveau *Electroencephalogr. Clin. Neurophysiol.*, 11:43.
35. Legg, N. J., Gupta, P. C., and Scott, D. F. (1973): Epilepsy following cerebral abscess: A clinical and EEG study of 70 patients. *Brain*, 96:259–268.
36. Martinius, J., Matthes, A., and Lombroso, C. T. (1968): Electroencephalographic features in posterior fossa tumors in children. *Electroencephalogr. Clin. Neurophysiol.*, 25:128–139.
37. Pine, J., Atoynatan, T. H., and Margolis, G. (1952): The EEG findings in eighteen patients with brain abscess: Case reports and a review of the literature. *Electroencephalogr. Clin. Neurophysiol.*, 4:165–179.
38. Rhee, R. S., Goldensohn, E. S., and Kim, R. C. (1975): EEG characteristics of solitary intracranial lesions in relationship to anatomic location. *Electroencephalogr. Clin. Neurophysiol.*, 38:553 (abstract).
39. Scarff, J. E., and Rahm, W. E., Jr. (1941): Human electrocorticogram: Report of spontaneous electrical potentials obtained from exposed human brain. *J. Neurophysiol.*, 4:418–426.
40. Schaul, N., Ball, G., Gloor, P., and Pappius, H. M. (1976): The EEG in cerebral edema. In: *Dynamics of Brain Edema*, edited by H. M. Papius and W. Fendel, pp. 144–149. Springer-Verlag, Berlin.
41. Scollo-Lavizzari, A. (1970): The effect of sleep on EEG abnormalities at a distance from the lesion: All night study of 30 cases. *Eur. Neurol.*, 3:65–87.
42. Walter, W. G. (1936): Location of cerebral tumours by electroencephalography. *Lancet*, 2:305–308.
43. Westmoreland, B. F., Klass, D. W., Sharbrough, F. W., and Reagan, T. J. (1975): Alpha-coma: Electroencephalographic, clinical, pathologic and etiologic correlations. *Arch. Neurol.*, 32:713–718.
44. Ziegler, D. K., and Hoefer, P. F. (1952): EEG and clinical findings in 28 verified cases of brain abscess. *Electroencephalogr. Clin. Neurophysiol.*, 2:41–44.

Current Practice of Clinical Electroencephalography,
edited by D. W. Klass and D. D. Daly.
Raven Press, New York © 1979.

Chapter 11

The EEG in Evaluation of Disorders Affecting the Brain Diffusely

*Michael G. Saunders and **Barbara F. Westmoreland

*Formerly Section of Electroencephalography; Computer Department and Department of Physiology, Faculty of Medicine, University of Manitoba, Winnipeg, Canada; and **Mayo Clinic and Mayo Foundation, Rochester, Minnesota 55901*

Metabolic Conditions	345
Glucose Metabolism	347
Hypoglycemia	347
Hyperglycemia	349
Hypoxia	349
Hepatic Disease	352
Renal Disease	357
Calcium Metabolism	357
Hypocalcemia	357
Hypercalcemia	358

* Deceased April 4, 1975.

Electrolyte and Water Disturbances... 359
Toxic States... 359
   Drug Toxicity... 359
   EEG Changes with Therapeutic and Toxic Levels of Medication 359
   Drug Overdosage... 359
   Withdrawal from Drugs 361
   Alcohol Withdrawal... 362
Degenerative Conditions... 364
Inflammatory Diseases... 370
Head Injury 371
Summary.. 377
References.. 378

The value of the electroencephalogram (EEG) in the epilepsies and in focal cerebral disease has tended to overshadow its use in various other conditions directly or indirectly disturbing cerebral function. These conditions include the various metabolic, toxic, degenerative, inflammatory, and posttraumatic disorders that diffusely affect cerebral functioning and cause acute, subacute, or chronic changes. They may affect the brain directly, by primary involvement or damage to the nerve cells, or indirectly, by altering systemic, metabolic, or electrolyte factors secondarily affecting brain function.

The symptoms or signs leading the physician to request an EEG vary widely, but frequently the EEG is requested because of a change in mentation or an alteration in consciousness. Usually no localizing neurologic signs are present. The EEG, however, often is a good indicator of a disturbance of cerebral functioning and usually serves as a measurement of the severity of the disease process.

In general, the EEG often shows rather nonspecific changes, that is, changes that are frequently encountered and are common to most of the conditions to be described herein. Usually, the most consistent change is diffuse slowing of varying degrees of severity, ranging from a slowing of the alpha rhythm to generalized delta slowing. The slower the frequency, the more severe the abnormality. Thus, theta slowing usually reflects a mild-to-moderate abnormality, while slowing in the delta frequency range indicates a more significant abnormality in the EEG.

Two main types of slow wave abnormalities are seen in the EEG. Polymorphic and arrhythmic delta slowing, which persists throughout the tracing and shows little or no reactivity to afferent stimuli, usually indicates a disturbance of cerebral functioning (Fig. 1). Generalized slowing reflects a diffuse disturbance of cerebral functioning; focal slowing indicates a localized disturbance of cerebral functioning.

Intermittent, rhythmic, and bilaterally synchronous slow wave activity, which attenuates with eye opening or following an alerting stimulus, is indicative of a distant rhythm (Fig. 2). This type of abnormality reflects a disturbance arising at a distance from the

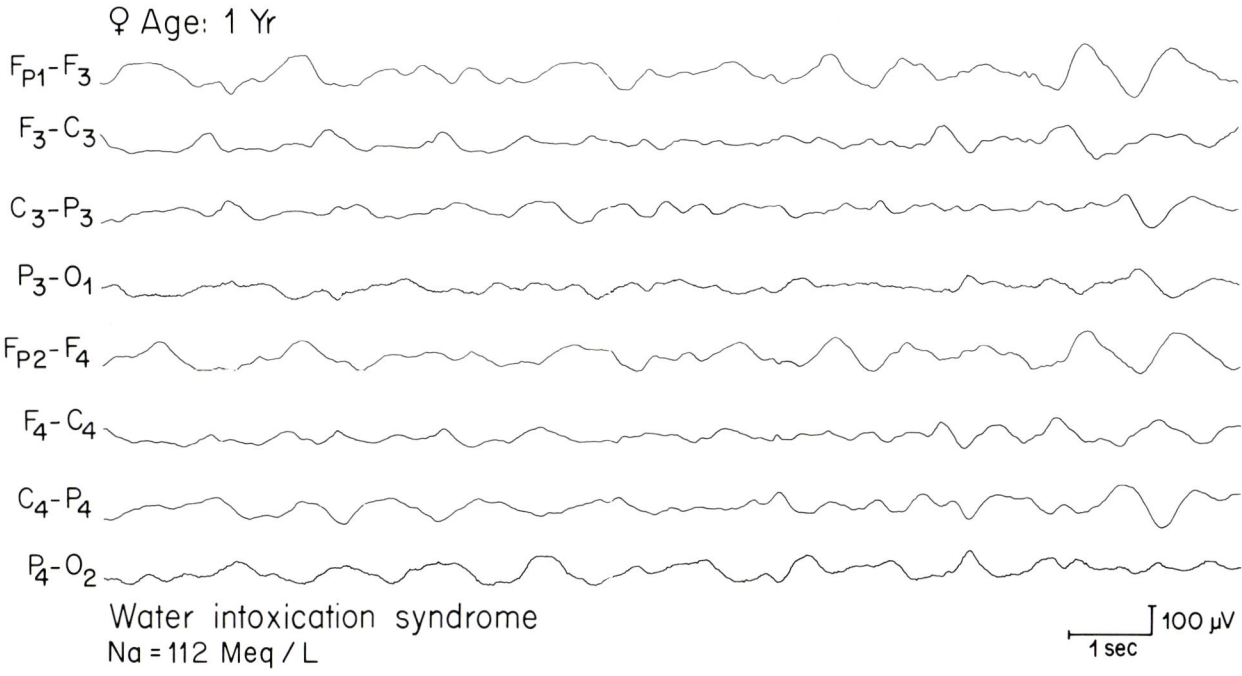

FIG. 1. Diffuse and persistent polymorphic delta activity in a 1-year-old child with water intoxication.

recording electrodes, probably from more deep-seated midline structures, particularly the diencephalon and periventricular structures, and projecting to the surface. The "projected" rhythm can occur however as a result of a primary lesion affecting the midline structures, as a result of increased intraventricular pressure, as a secondary effect of a shift or distortion of the midline structures from a supratentorial mass lesion, or as the result of a metabolic or toxic disturbance.

METABOLIC CONDITIONS

Many metabolic conditions can diffusely affect cerebral functioning and cause changes in the EEG. The earliest changes in the EEG that occur with many of the toxic or metabolic disturbances are a decrease in frequency of background rhythms and the appearance of diffuse theta activity. These changes, when minimal, may mimic

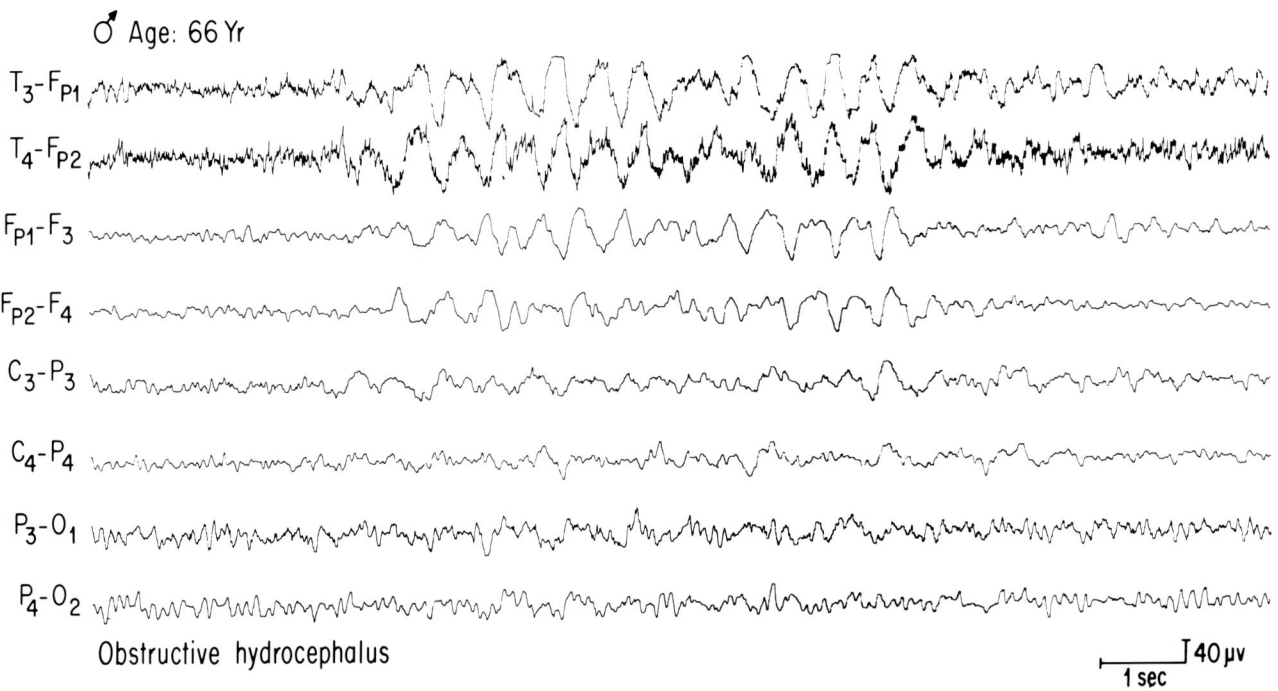

FIG. 2. Projected type of abnormality in a 66-year-old patient with obstructive hydrocephalus. Note intermittent bilaterally synchronous slow waves occurring maximally over the anterior regions.

drowsiness, and a decision as to whether or not abnormal amounts of theta activity are present can be very subjective. They have been reported with such varied descriptions as "excessive diffuse slow activity," "nonspecific activity," or "borderline normal activity." Such reports may not be specific, yet the EEG patterns are warnings that some organic change is present. Figure 3 shows an example of this nonspecific pattern. Note the diffuseness of the slow activity and its tendency to appear for short periods, and then disappear.

With more severe disturbances of cerebral functioning, slower frequencies prevail. Slowing, either in the theta or delta range, that is intermittent and blocks when a stimulus is given, implies less severe involvement than does persistent slowing without blocking. This lat-

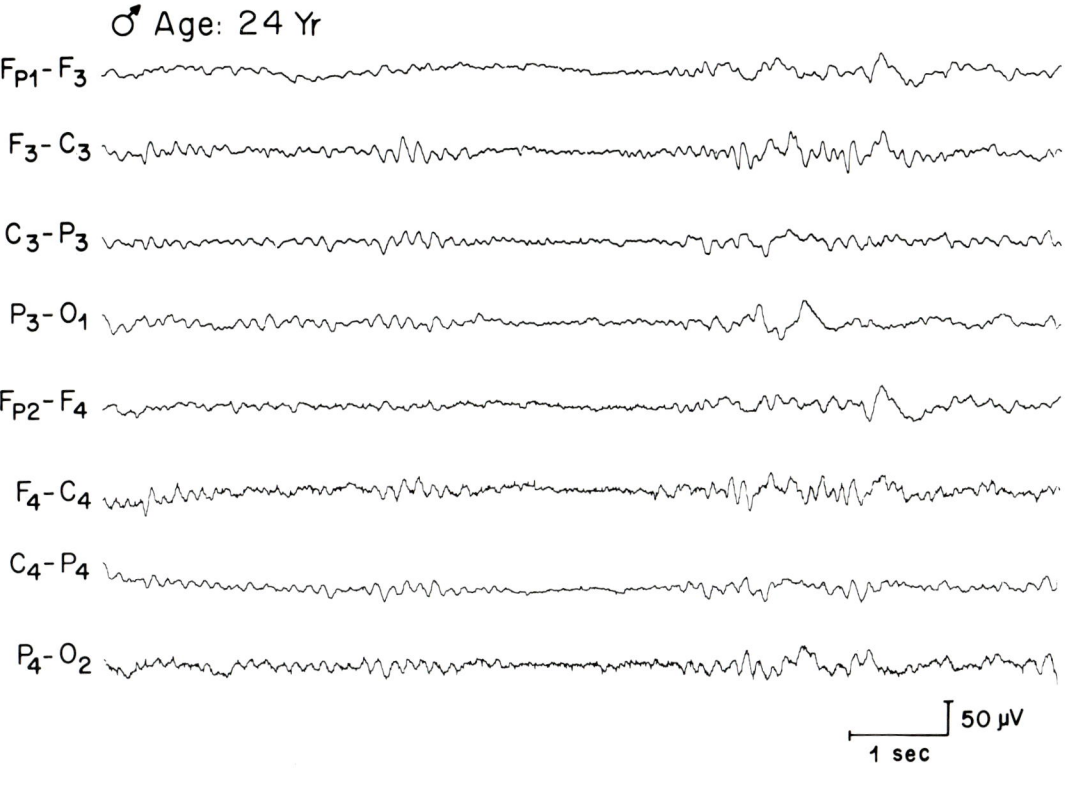

FIG. 3. Nonspecific slowing of background activity with intermittent abnormal slow waves in a 24-year-old patient with uremia.

ter level of suppression of the arousal effect is rare in metabolic or toxic disorders except with very severe changes or with coma.

The most common metabolic disorders that may produce changes in the EEG are those associated with glucose metabolism, hypoxia, hepatic disease, renal disease, and electrolyte disturbances.

Glucose Metabolism

Hypoglycemia

Changes in the EEG that may be associated with hypoglycemia include an exaggerated response to hyperventilation, generalized

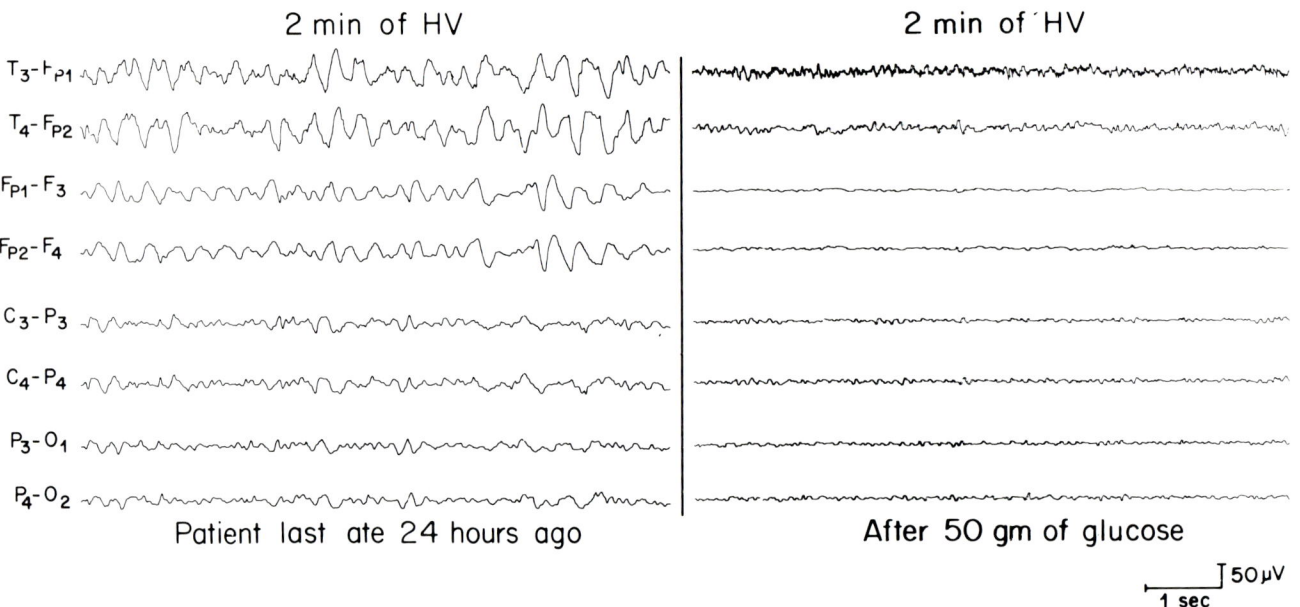

FIG. 4. Effect of glucose on EEG response to hyperventilation in a 42-year-old man. The segment on the left shows rhythmic slow wave activity occurring bilaterally over the anterior regions of the head during hyperventilation when the patient was in a fasting state. The segment on the right was recorded after glucose had been given and shows no slowing.

slowing of the EEG, and accentuation of preexisting epileptiform abnormalities.

One of the earliest EEG changes in response to hypoglycemia is an increased or exaggerated response to hyperventilation in which bilaterally synchronous slow waves may appear earlier and to a greater degree than if the individual had a normal blood sugar (1). This type of response can be seen in normal persons in a fasting state (Fig. 4).

Mild changes may become apparent in the resting record when the blood sugar ranges between 50 and 80 mg/dl (2). These changes consist of a slowing of the alpha rhythm, together with diffusely intermingled theta components. As the blood sugar level decreases, the EEG shows more prominent slowing together with intermittent bursts of bisynchronous slow waves (projected rhythm).

With further lowering of the blood sugar and as the patient becomes comatose, generalized delta slowing occurs. In most cases the EEG abnormalities disappear rapidly when the blood sugar is restored to normal (Fig. 5). After deep or prolonged hypoglycemic coma, however, it may be several days before the abnormalities disappear (1). Occasionally, a focal abnormality persists, implying the possible existence of a focal vascular compromise in association with the hypoglycemia.

With regard to epileptiform abnormalities, hypoglycemia may enhance the presence of 3-Hz spike-and-wave discharges (3), and sometimes relative hypoglycemia is used to help precipitate petit mal seizures and the 3-Hz spike-and-wave pattern. Other generalized spike-and-wave patterns are less sensitive to blood sugar levels. Activation of focal epileptiform abnormalities by lowering blood sugar levels, such as with the tolbutamide test (4), is variable.

Infants usually can tolerate a lower blood sugar level than adults. However, one of the most common causes of neonatal seizures is hypoglycemia, and the EEG may show multifocal epileptiform abnormalities in association with this condition.

Hyperglycemia

The EEG is usually normal or shows only mild nonspecific irregularities in uncomplicated diabetes mellitus, and the tracing may be relatively normal with blood sugar levels as high as 300 mg/dl (5). In diabetic acidosis, however, if the patient has clouding of consciousness, the EEG often shows generalized slowing, the degree of which usually reflects the degree of obtundation of the patient. As a rule, seizures are not common in ketoacidosis because the ketoacidosis may act as a protective mechanism against convulsions.

In nonketotic hyperglycemia, however, recurrent focal seizures and epilepsia partialis continua may occur in association with focal EEG abnormalities. This condition usually is related to an underlying focal cortical lesion, most often vascular in nature, which is "activated" by hyperglycemia, hyperosmolality, and dehydration (6).

Hypoxia

The main effects of progressive hypoxia on the EEG are reduction and slowing of alpha activity, increased theta activity, generalized delta slowing, and finally, suppression of activity (1,5).

During a syncopal episode, the EEG may show slowing within 7 to 13 sec after the arrest of circulation (7). Initially, there may be a decrease in the frequency and an increase in the amplitude of alpha activity and then slowing in the theta range. Often this is followed by the rather abrupt onset of high amplitude and bilaterally synchronous semirhythmic delta waves, which often have a maximal emphasis over the anterior region of the head. If the arrest of circulation is prolonged, attenuation of activity and flattening of the EEG occur, and the patient may have generalized myoclonic jerks or generalized tonic spasms. If recovery occurs shortly after this, then the reverse sequence takes place (7) (Fig. 6).

With a more prolonged period of anoxia, severe damage to the brain occurs and a wide variety of patterns can be recorded (1,8). The type of EEG pattern that is present, particularly if sequential recordings are obtained, may be of prognostic value in determining the patient's potential for recovery. An EEG showing spontaneous cyclic variability, a polymorphic sleep pattern, and a return of more normal rhythms associated with reactivity to external stimuli, indicates a potential for improvement. On the other hand, patterns that indicate a poor prognosis include a burst suppression pattern, periodic discharges associated with myoclonus, an invariant monorhythmic pattern such as the "alpha coma" pattern, and electrocerebral silence.

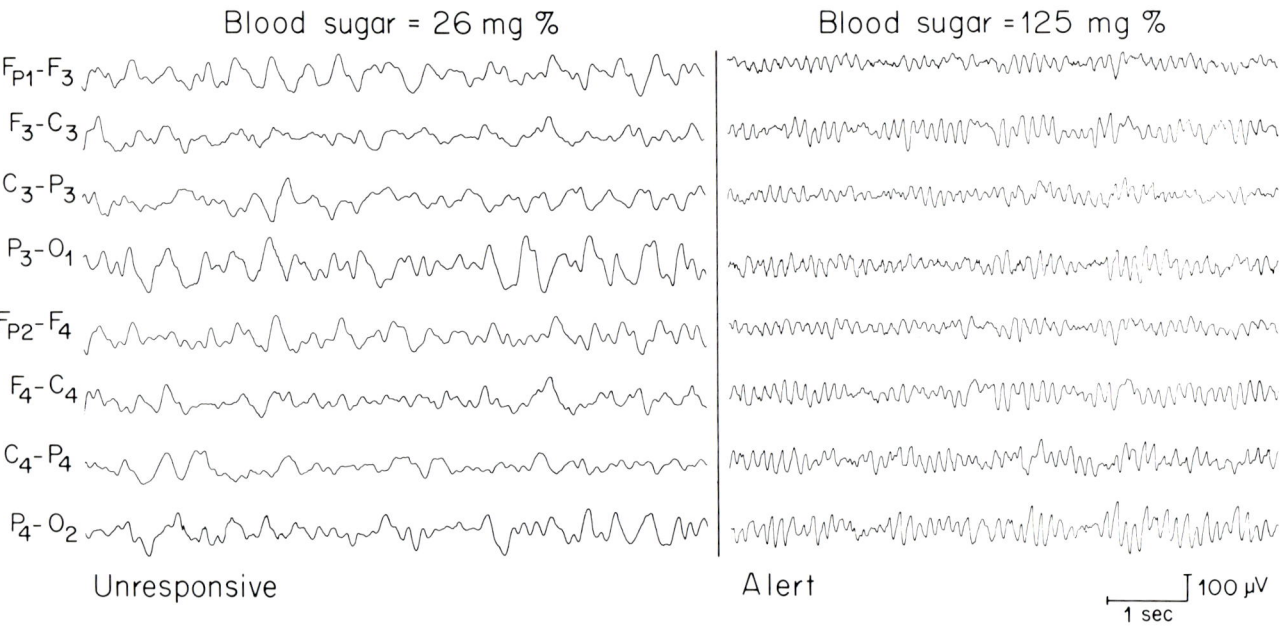

FIG. 5. EEG during a hypoglycemic episode in a 10-year-old boy. The segment on the left shows generalized slow wave activity when the patient was unresponsive. The segment on the right shows the return to a normal EEG when the blood sugar level was increased.

The burst suppression pattern consists of periodic bursts of activity of mixed frequencies with intervening periods of electrocerebral inactivity (Fig. 7). Often the bursts are accompanied by myoclonic jerks of the body. This pattern indicates a severe disturbance of cerebral function, which may occur with any severe insult to the central nervous system (CNS). However, it can also be seen during deep anesthesia and after a drug overdosage, which are potentially reversible conditions.

Another unfavorable pattern is the occurrence of periodic generalized epileptiform discharges with isoelectric intervals. The discharges may consist of spike-and-slow-wave, multiple-spike-and-slow-wave, or sharp wave discharges, usually recurring every 1 to 2 sec and often accompanied by myoclonic jerks of the body (Fig. 8).

On occasion, a comatose patient may show an EEG pattern containing alpha activity comparable to that of a normal awake pattern. This paradoxical "alpha coma" pattern has been seen in comatose patients with brainstem infarcts and as a transient phenomenon in comatose patients after cardiac or respiratory arrest (Fig. 9). The

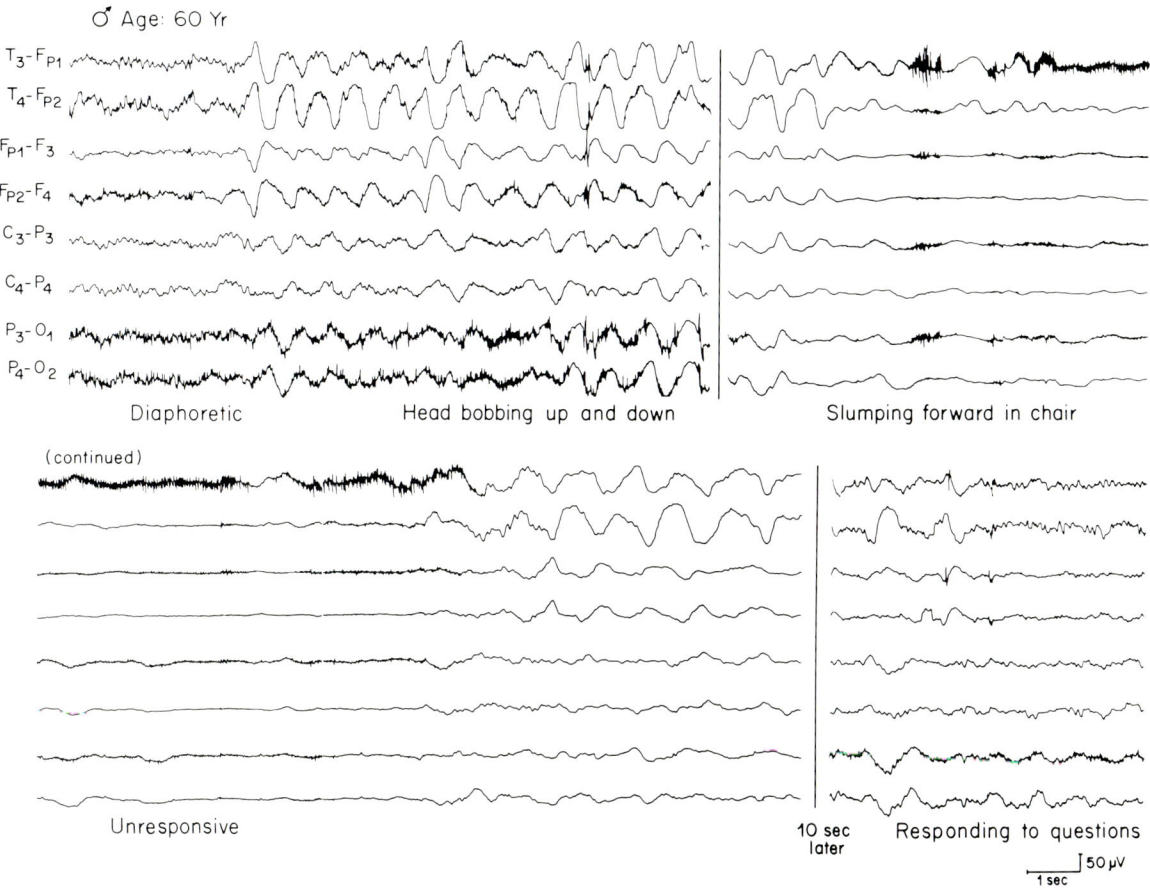

FIG. 6. Recording showing the sequence of changes during a syncopal episode with the EEG initially showing high amplitude bisynchronous slowing *(upper left)* followed by generalized attenuation of activity *(upper right)* and then a return of background rhythms with first slower wave components *(lower left)* and then faster frequencies *(lower right)*.

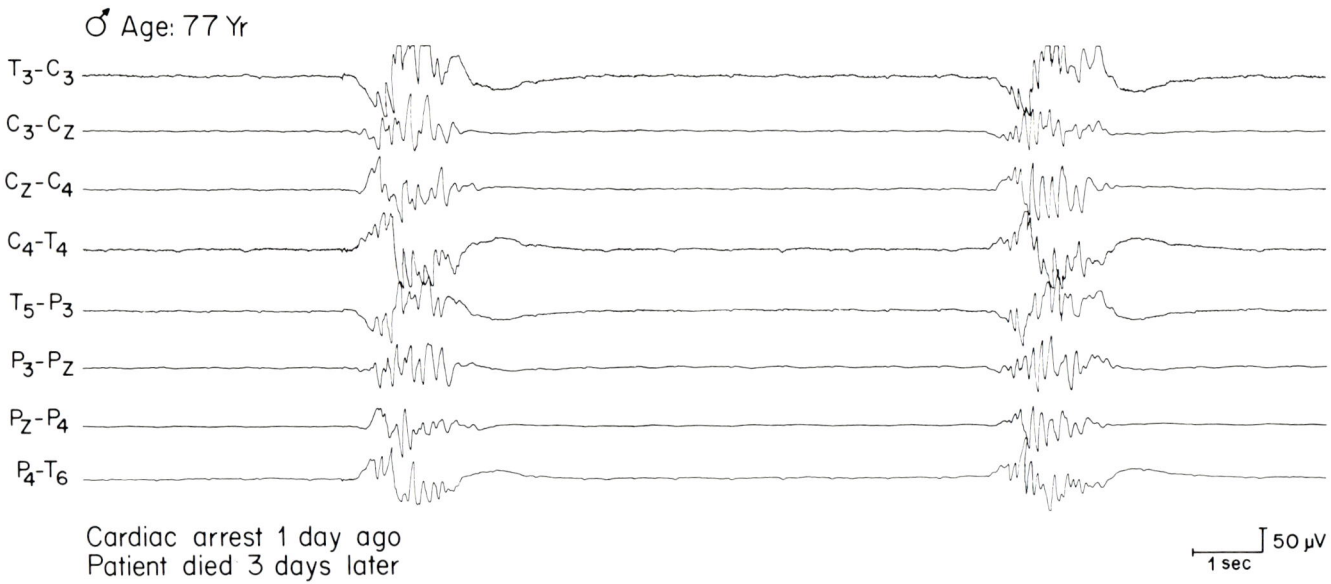

FIG. 7. Burst suppression pattern, consisting of intermittent bursts of high amplitude activity with suppression of background between bursts.

alpha activity in this latter type of EEG, in contrast to the normal alpha rhythm, shows a more diffuse distribution, is often maximal over the anterior head regions, and shows little or no reactivity to external stimuli (9). The presence of this pattern in a comatose patient usually indicates a poor prognosis for clinical recovery.

The terminal phase is electrocerebral inactivity (Fig. 10). Determination of electrocerebral inactivity may not be simple (10). The requirements for recording EEGs in suspected cerebral death are different from those for recording routine EEGs, and the minimal technical requirements for recording cerebral death are included in Chapter 7 and the Appendix.

Hepatic Disease

The EEGs of patients with liver disease often show some type of abnormality by the time hepatic dysfunction is severe enough to cause an alteration in consciousness. In the early stages of hepatic encephalopathy, the EEG shows progressive slowing of the alpha

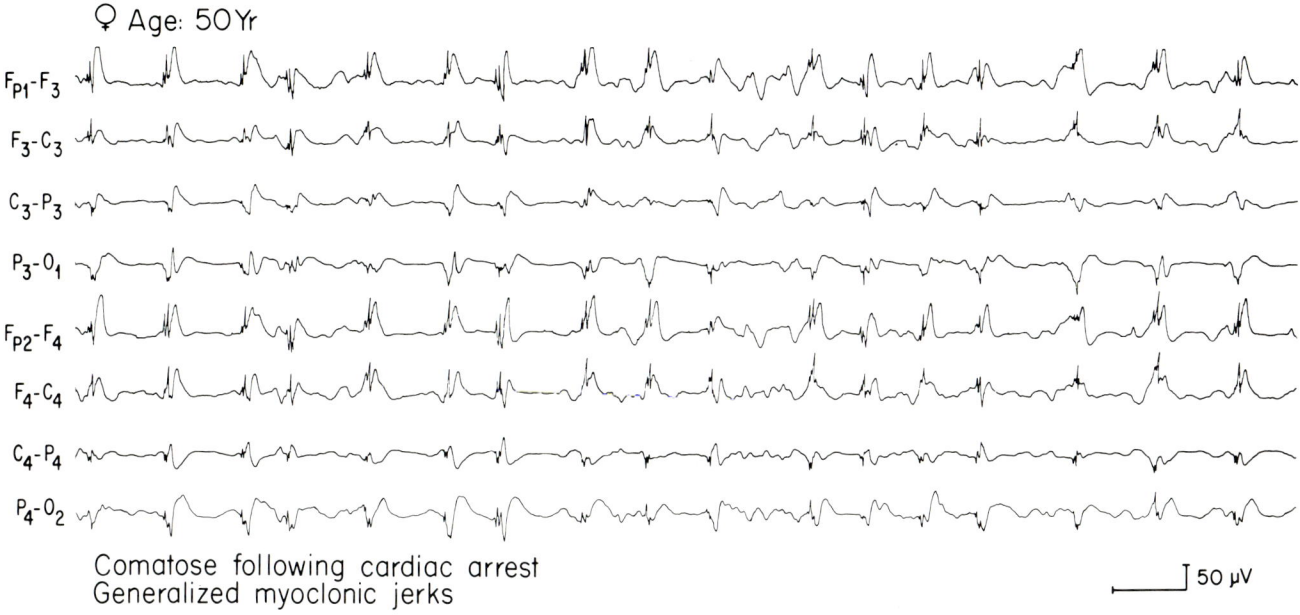

FIG. 8. EEG of a 50-year-old woman showing periodic spike-and-slow-wave discharges associated with myoclonic jerks after cardiac arrest.

rhythm, with diffusely intermingled theta activity (1). With further clouding of consciousness, slower delta frequencies occur. As the patient becomes progressively more comatose, alpha activity disappears and the triphasic wave pattern, a distinctive pattern associated with hepatic coma, may occur. However, patients in hepatic coma do not always show this pattern. It is a transient and ephemeral pattern that is present during certain stages of hepatic coma, usually when the patient is stuporous but still responsive to painful stimuli.

The characteristic EEG features of the typical triphasic wave pattern of hepatic coma consist of medium to high amplitude, broad triphasic waves, occurring rhythmically or in serial trains at a rate of 1.5 to 2.5 Hz in a bilaterally synchronous and symmetric fashion over both hemispheres and having a fronto-occipital or occipitofrontal time lag (11). These wave forms often have a frontal predominance, and care should be taken not to mistake this for an eye-blink artifact (8). Figure 11 shows the typical triphasic wave pattern in a patient with hepatic coma.

With regard to the specific association of triphasic waves with

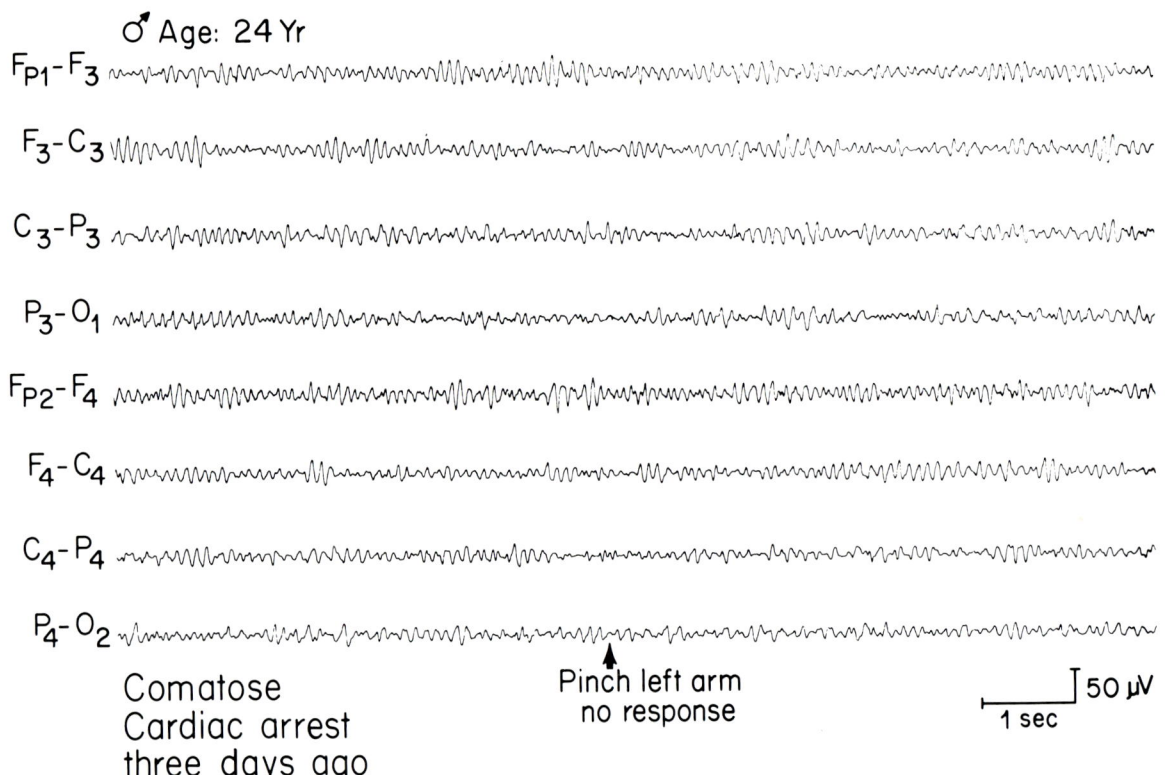

FIG. 9. "Alpha coma" pattern in a patient who had had cardiac arrest 3 days before the tracing. The EEG showed continuous and widespread 10-Hz activity throughout the recording, which showed no reactivity to afferent stimuli.

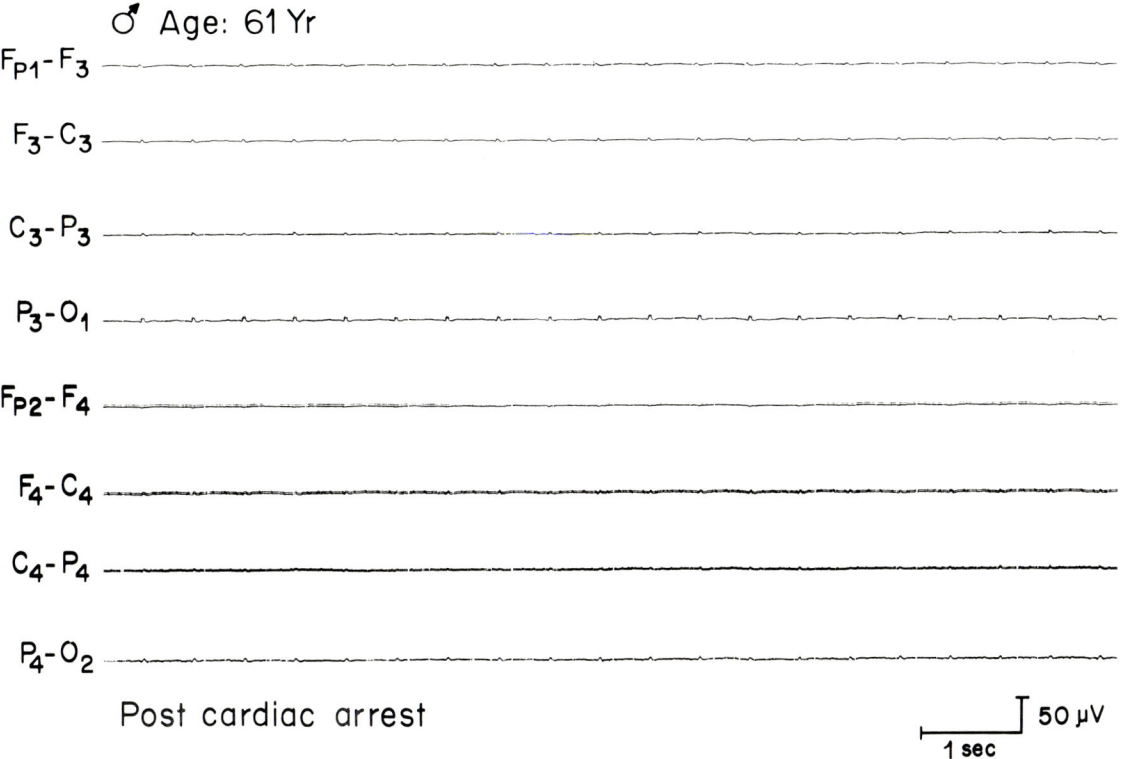

FIG. 10. Electrocerebral inactivity in a patient who had had a cardiac arrest 2 days earlier. (The periodic deflections represent ECG artifact.)

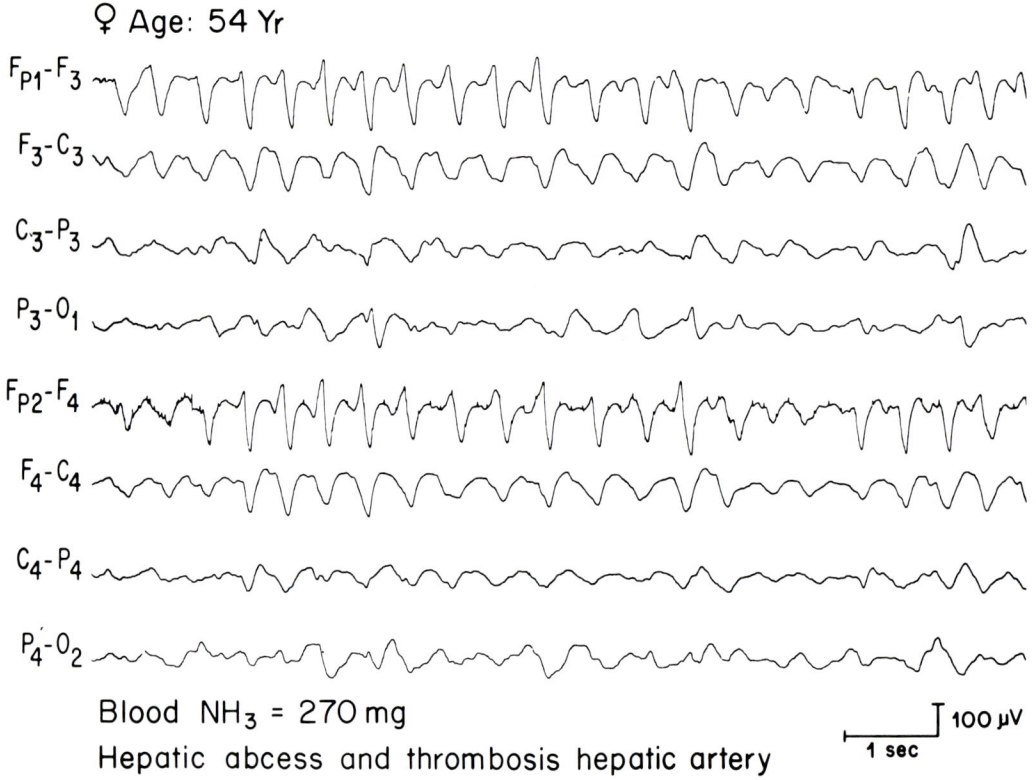

FIG. 11. Typical triphasic waves in a 54-year-old patient with hepatic coma.

hepatic coma, if all of the foregoing EEG criteria are met, there is a high correlation with the presence of hepatic disease (11). On the other hand, triphasic waves that do not meet all of these criteria, i.e., atypical triphasic wave forms, are a more nonspecific finding which can be present in a variety of conditions, including other types of metabolic derangements, electrolyte disturbances, toxic states, degenerative processes, or following an anoxic episode or head trauma.

The nature of the specific metabolic derangement responsible for the electrographic alterations and, in particular, the triphasic wave pattern, is still unknown. Blood ammonia levels correspond in part to the clinical picture and EEG pattern; however, a one-to-one correlation does not always exist and other metabolic products also may be involved (1,5).

Renal Disease

In uremia, as in other encephalopathies, there is a correlation between the EEG changes and an alteration in consciousness (1). As the patient becomes more obtunded, disorganization and slowing of the background occur with replacement by theta and delta frequencies (Fig. 12). There may be paroxysmal and intermittent bursts of semirhythmic slow waves (projected rhythm); and an abnormal or exaggerated arousal response to afferent stimuli may be present, with bursts of slow waves occurring in response to noise or other stimuli. Photic stimulation may elicit a photoparoxysmal or photomyogenic response, and paroxysmal epileptiform abnormalities may sometimes be present in the absence of clinical symptoms or just prior to the onset of convulsions (12).

In renal disease, only a loose correlation exists between the EEG and the blood urea levels; instead, the EEG relates more to levels of obtundity and to the acuteness of decompensation. Other complex factors, including electrolyte and calcium imbalance, acidosis, other toxic metabolites, edema, and hypertension also may play a role in producing the EEG abnormalities (1,12).

During hemodialysis, marked EEG changes may occur during or immediately after dialysis (12), particularly if the patient exhibits a dialysis disequilibrium syndrome (Fig. 13). These changes may consist of increased slow wave activity, paroxysmal abnormalities, increased photosensitivity, and exaggerated visual evoked responses. The findings are related, in part, to the osmotic disequilibrium; however, rapid changes in electrolytes, particularly sodium, with resultant hyponatremia, may be a more critical factor (13).

Another syndrome that has recently been recognized in patients maintained on chronic hemodialysis is the dialysis dementia syndrome (14). This is a progressively fatal disorder that is characterized by a slowly progressive dementia, speech disturbances, involuntary movements, myoclonus, and convulsions. Patients with this syndrome have significantly abnormal EEGs consisting of diffuse slowing of the background with superimposed bursts of high amplitude slow waves, triphasic contoured waves, sharp waves, or spike-and-slow-wave complexes (Fig. 14). EEGs recorded shortly after dialysis often show more prominent abnormalities than do predialysis tracings. The EEG abnormalities may be present before the onset of the clinical signs and may be of help in predicting the occurrence of this syndrome (14).

Calcium Metabolism

Hypocalcemia

In hypocalcemia there may be diffuse slowing of the background frequencies, an accentuation of slowing during hyperventilation (1,5), and an exaggerated response to photic stimulation. In some cases, there also may be an accentuation of paroxysmal epileptiform activity with severe hypocalcemia.

In infants, hypocalcemia is one of the most common causes of neonatal seizures (15) and often the EEG shows focal epileptiform abnormalities consisting of spikes, sharp waves, or electrographic seizure discharges (Fig. 15). Sometimes the discharges occur predominantly in one region, giving the false impression of a focal cortical abnormality. On other occasions multifocal independent or shifting epileptiform abnormalities are present, which may not necessarily correlate with the location of the clinical seizures.

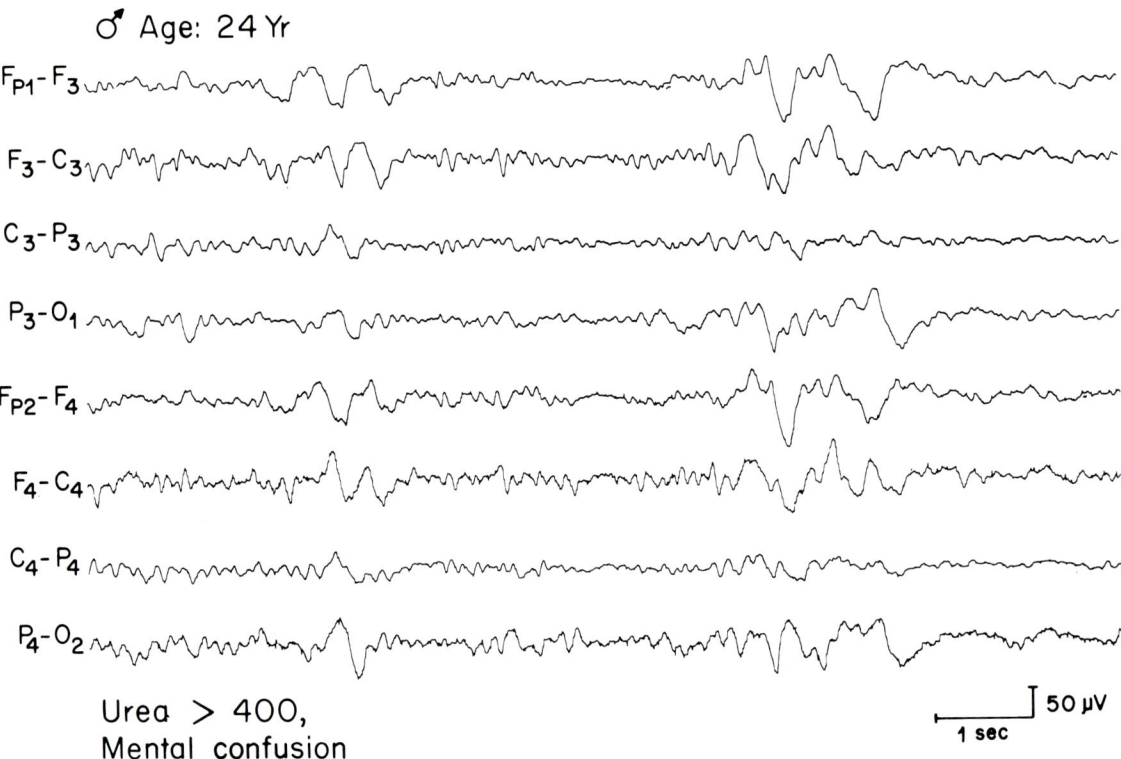

FIG. 12. Diffuse rhythmic theta activity and intermittent bursts of high amplitude delta waves in a 24-year-old patient with renal disease.

Hypercalcemia

In hypercalcemia, the EEG may show diffuse slowing of the background, an excess of theta and delta frequencies, occasional intermittent and semirhythmic slowing enhanced by hyperventilation, and prominent lambda and photic responses (16). Some authors, however, think that most of these changes are not related to the hypercalcemia *per se* but to the associated electrolyte changes, renal derangement, and other complicating factors associated with the hypercalcemia (17).

Electrolyte and Water Disturbances

Water intoxication or severe hyponatremia may give rise to a diffuse encephalopathy with the EEG showing generalized delta slowing (Fig. 1) or intermittent bursts of bisynchronous slow wave activity superimposed on an abnormally slow background. Dehydration, hypernatremia, hypokalemia, and hyperkalemia, contrarily, usually are associated with little or only mild nonspecific changes in the EEG (1,5).

TOXIC STATES

Drug Toxicity

The most common cause of a toxic effect on the EEG is that caused by drugs or medications. Since patients with drug toxicity can present with changes in mentation and behavior or signs suggestive of an organic disease process, the EEG may be helpful in suggesting the presence of a toxic medication effect. Changes in the EEG can occur at therapeutic levels of drugs, and diffuse abnormalities can be seen with excessive drug levels, with a drug overdosage, or after an abrupt withdrawal of medications.

EEG Changes with Therapeutic and Toxic Levels of Medication

One of the earliest signs of medication effect on the EEG is the presence of excessive beta activity. The most common drugs producing this effect are the barbiturates, the sedative drugs such as diazepam (Valium), chlordiazepoxide (Librium), meprobamate, glutethimide (Doriden), and the anticonvulsants—phenobarbital, primidone (Mysoline), and mephenytoin (Mesantoin). With increasing drug levels, progressive slowing of the background results with diffusely intermingled theta activity. With higher drug levels, the EEG may show generalized theta and delta slowing, as well as intermittent paroxysmal slow wave activity suggestive of a projected rhythm.

Phenytoin (Dilantin) can cause significant changes in an EEG, and this can range from mild slowing of the background frequencies at therapeutic levels to marked delta activity and paroxysmal slow wave abnormalities at toxic levels (18). Also, on occasion, the changes due to phenytoin may be asymmetrical if there is focal brain disease or a skull defect (Fig. 16).

Carbamazepine (Tegretol) may also cause diffuse slowing of the EEG as well as an increase in paroxysmal epileptiform abnormalities; it should be noted, however, that the latter does not necessarily correlate with the incidence of clinical seizures.

Phenobarbital, primidone, and mephenytoin, in addition to inducing an excessive amount of fast activity, can also cause diffuse slowing of the background. Ethosuximide (Zarontin) and trimethadione (Tridione) on the other hand usually have little effect on the resting background frequencies of the EEG.

The effects of other drugs on the EEG and, in particular, the psychotherapeutic drugs, are discussed more fully in Chapter 13 by Low.

Drug Overdosage

A characteristic EEG pattern may be present in patients who are comatose as a result of taking an overdosage of a drug, usually as a suicide attempt, and the recognition of this pattern is important

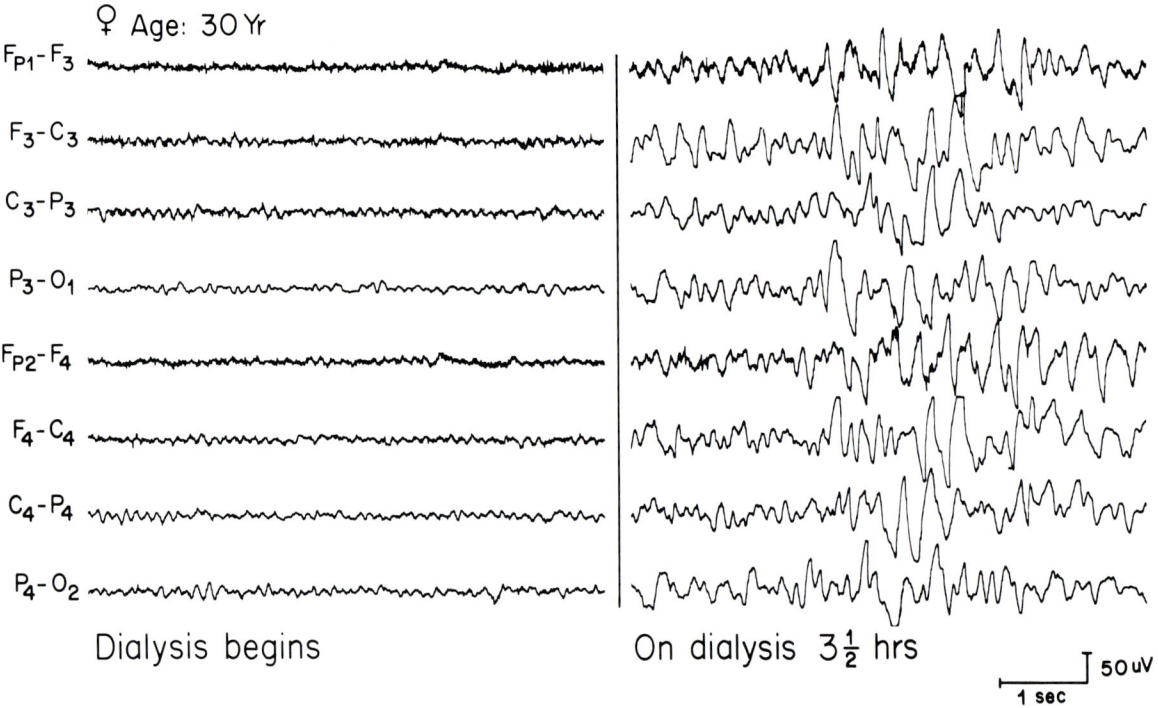

FIG. 13. EEG changes during dialysis. The segment on the left was recorded before dialysis and showed only minimal slowing of the background. The segment on the right was recorded 3½ hr after dialysis had begun and showed paroxysmal bursts of high amplitude mixed frequency activity.

in making the prompt diagnosis of a potentially treatable condition. If one sees an EEG showing moderate-to-high amplitude generalized abnormal fast activity in the range of 10 to 16 Hz having a maximum over the anterior head regions and superimposed on underlying delta slowing, then one should consider drug overdosage. This type of pattern, which has some features similar to an anesthetic pattern, is most commonly seen after an overdosage of barbiturates, benzodiazepines, or other sedative drugs that produce beta activity in the EEG (Fig. 17). With even higher drug levels, a burst suppression pattern or generalized suppression of the EEG may occur.

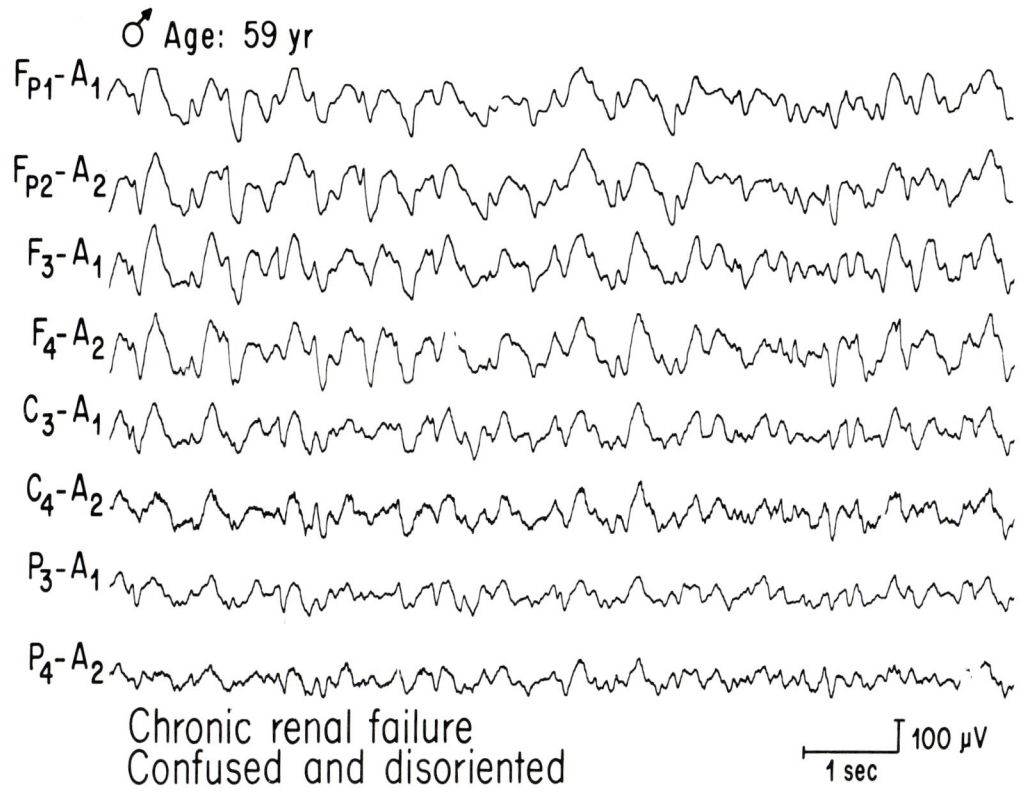

FIG. 14. EEG showing serial trains of slow waves and triphasic contoured waves in a 59-year-old man with dialysis dementia syndrome.

Withdrawal from Drugs

Paroxysmal abnormalities can occur in the EEG after a sudden withdrawal from certain drugs, in particular, the sedative drugs such as the short-acting barbiturates and the benzodiazepines. They are manifested most often as some degree of light sensitivity, either a photomyogenic or photoparoxysmal response.

The photomyogenic (or photomyoclonic) response (19) is a noncerebral response characterized by the presence of brief repetitive muscle spikes over the anterior regions of the head. This may often

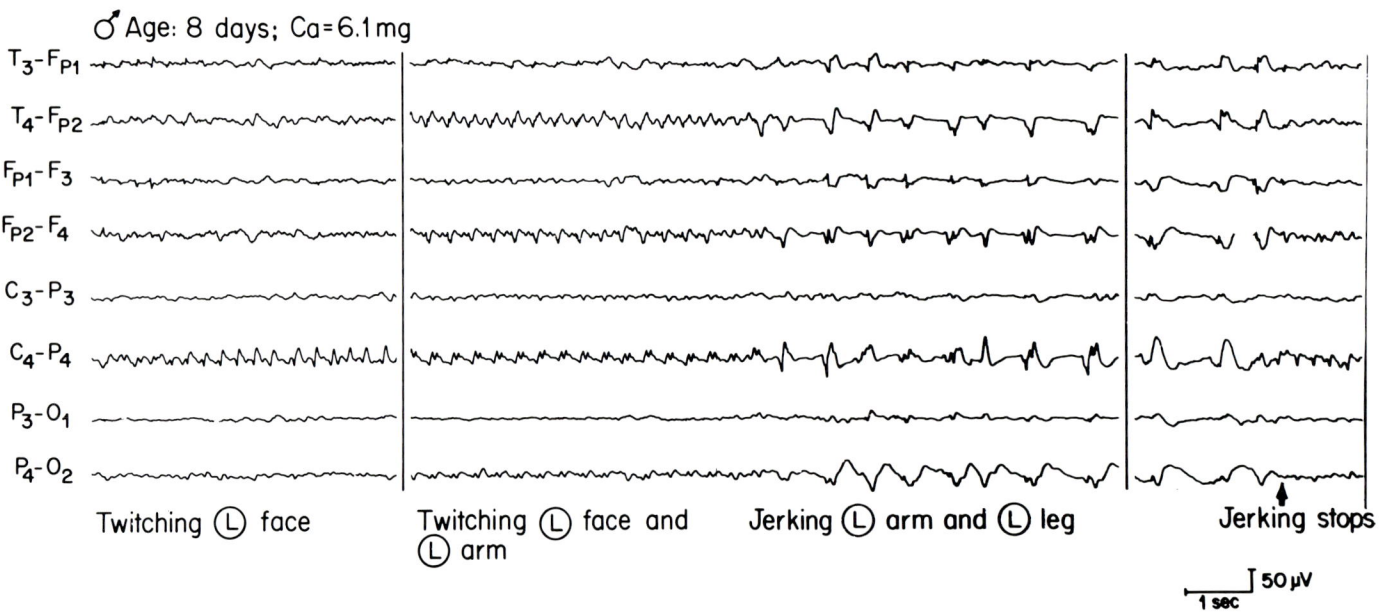

FIG. 15. Recorded focal motor seizure in an 8-day-old infant with hypocalcemia consisting of the onset of focal discharges in the right central region followed by spread to the right frontal and parietal regions.

be associated with eye flutter and myoclonic twitchings of the forehead and eyelids (Fig. 18).

The photoparoxysmal (photoconvulsive) response (19) is an abnormal cerebral response to intermittent photic stimulation characterized by the appearance of generalized spike-wave or multiple-spike-and-slow-wave discharges that may outlast the stimulus (Fig. 19).

These changes are usually transient in nature and most often occur within the first few days after withdrawal from the drug. On occasion, however, the paroxysmal abnormalities may persist for 3 to 4 weeks following withdrawal from the drug (20).

Alcohol Withdrawal

Similar changes may be seen with sudden withdrawal from alcohol, particularly after a heavy drinking spree. During this time the EEG may show generalized paroxysmal abnormalities with or without a photomyogenic or photoparoxysmal response to light stimuli. Usually these abnormalities occur within the first 2 days after cessation of ethanol intake, a time when seizures may occur. It has been suggested that the paroxysmal abnormalities may be related to hypomagnesemia and alkalosis (21).

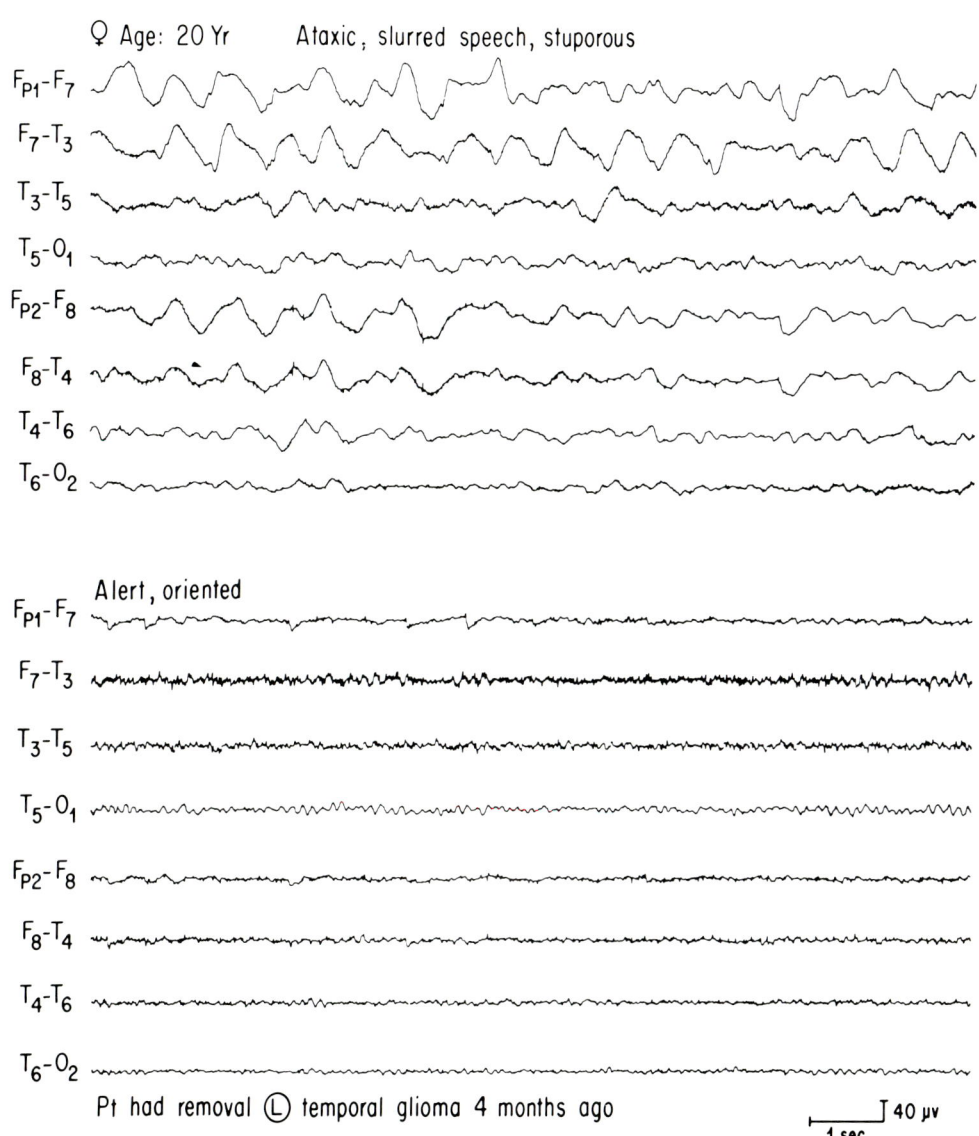

FIG. 16. Effect of phenytoin (Dilantin) on EEG. The upper tracing was recorded when the patient was on toxic doses of phenytoin and shows generalized slowing, maximal over the left temporal region where the patient had a left temporal glioma removed 4 months before the recording. The bottom segment was recorded after the dosage of phenytoin had been reduced to a therapeutic range and shows a marked improvement.

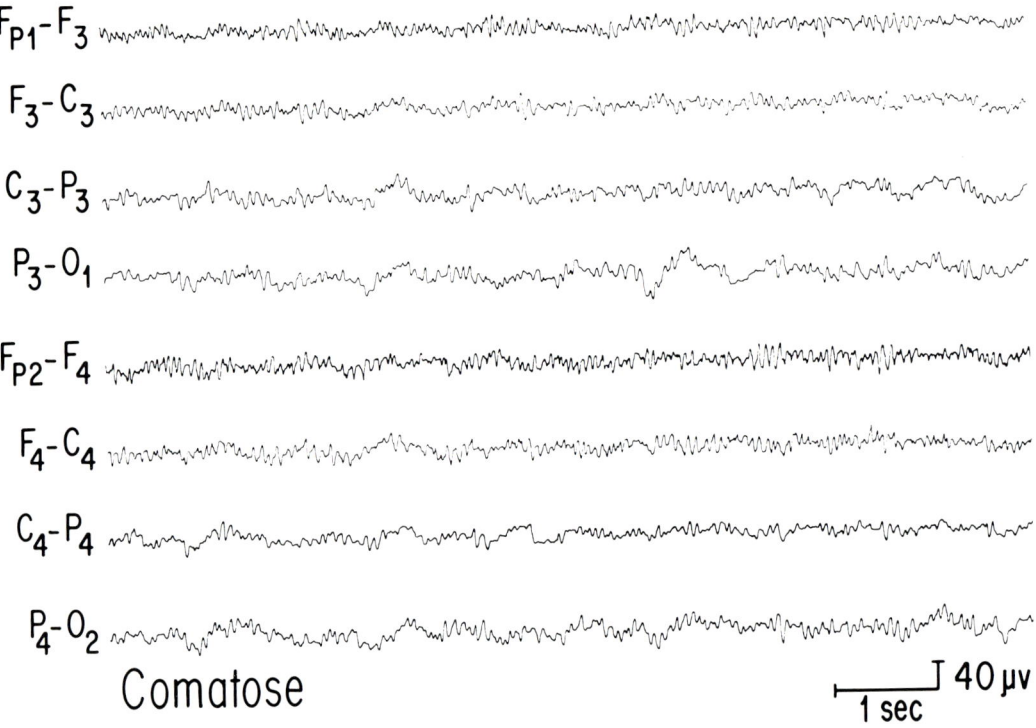

FIG. 17. Drug-induced pattern in a 16-year-old girl who was brought to the emergency room in a comatose state after taking an overdose of a barbiturate.

DEGENERATIVE CONDITIONS

Numerous degenerative disorders diffusely affect cerebral function and cause generalized changes in the EEG. The EEG abnormality usually consists of diffuse slowing, and the degree of the abnormality is often related to the rapidity of progression of the disease process and the severity of involvement.

Cerebrovascular insufficiency is one of the most common causes of cerebral degeneration in the adult, and the EEG may show diffuse or focal changes depending on the area(s) involved. The clinical

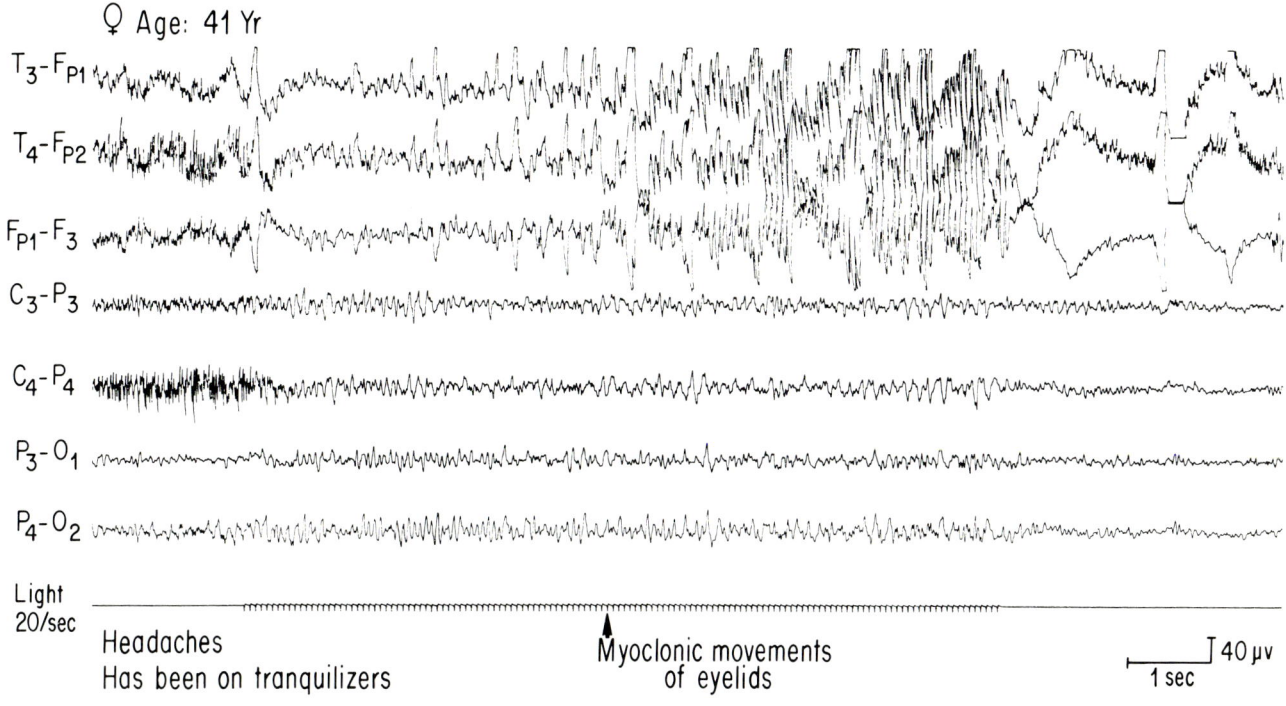

FIG. 18. Photomyogenic response recorded from the frontal regions (upper 3 channels) associated with drug withdrawal.

manifestations of generalized cerebral vascular disease are often those of presenile or senile changes and the EEG may show diffuse slow wave abnormalities. These changes are nonspecific in nature and are similar to those seen with toxic and metabolic disturbances and other degenerative processes. The similarity of the EEG changes in cerebrovascular diseases to those caused by toxic or metabolic states is unfortunate. A regrettable tendency is to assume that these rather nonspecific changes in the geriatric age group are caused by cerebrovascular degeneration and to neglect adequate investigation of the patient for other possible etiologic factors. The EEG can help, however, particularly if sequential recordings are obtained, in differentiating a transient metabolic derangement from a more chronic process. The EEG is also of value in distinguishing a static or resolving vascular process from a progressive neoplastic lesion and in differ-

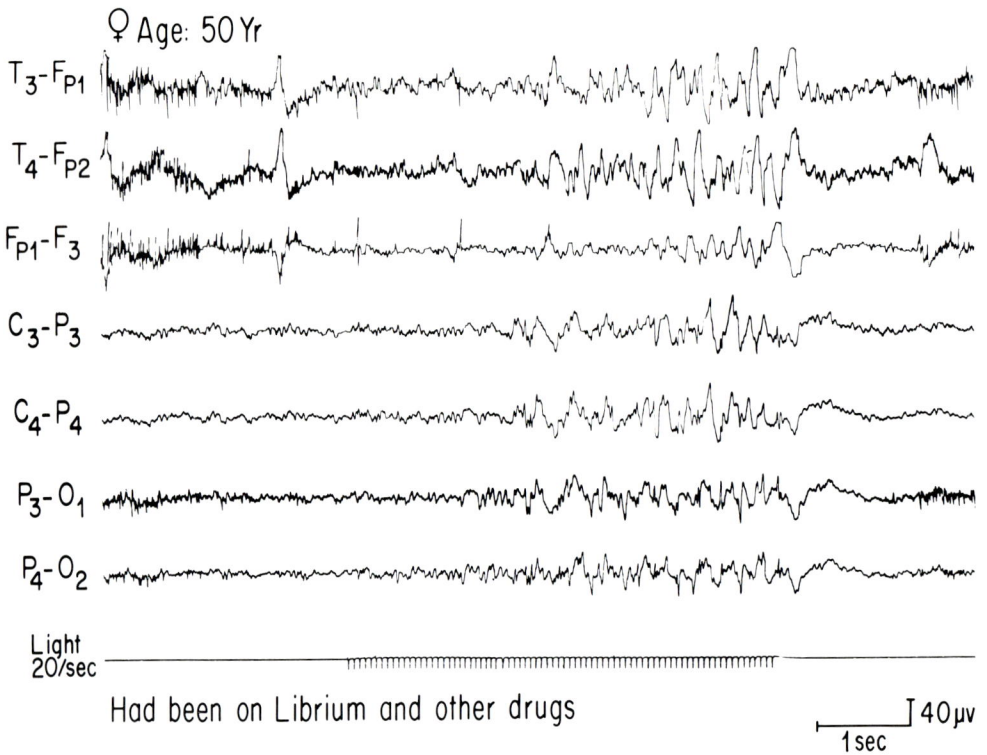

FIG. 19. Photoparoxysmal response after abrupt drug withdrawal.

entiating transient ischemic attacks or syncopal episodes from seizures.

Other degenerative diseases such as Alzheimer's disease, Pick's disease, Parkinson's disease, and Huntington's chorea may also produce diffuse changes in the EEG. Alzheimer's disease is associated with a high incidence of abnormal EEGs, usually consisting of diffuse theta and delta slowing (22) and which may be accompanied by superimposed bursts of intermittent rhythmic slow waves. In Pick's disease and senile dementia, the EEG may show a slowing of the alpha rhythms or diffuse theta and delta waves, but the slowing is often less severe than that seen with Alzheimer's disease (22). Patients with severe Parkinson's disease may also have EEGs showing generalized theta and delta slowing with intermittent rhythmic slow wave abnormalities. In advanced stages of Huntington's chorea, the EEG

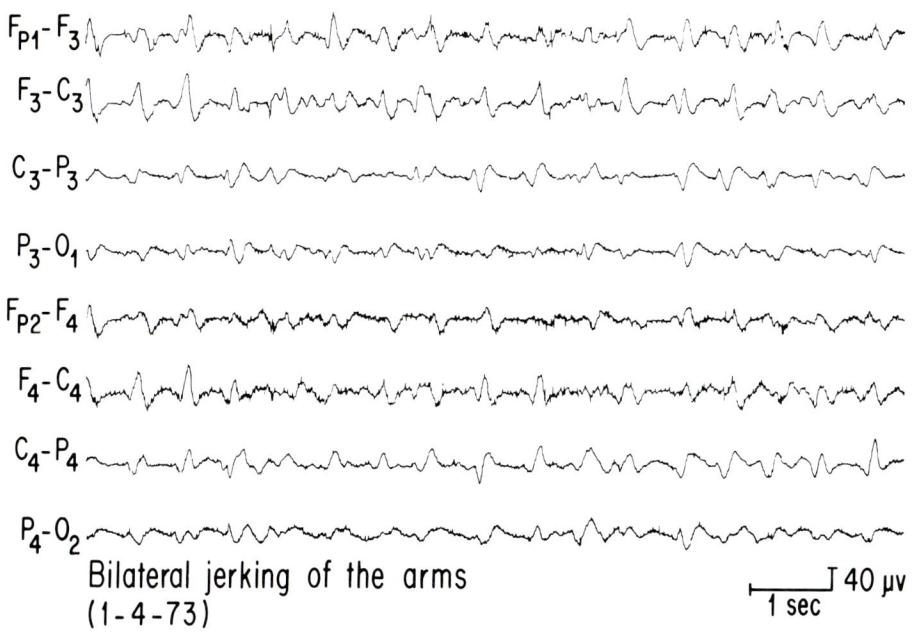

FIG. 20. Repetitive and bilaterally synchronous periodic sharp waves, often accompanied by myoclonic jerks of the arms, in a 48-year-old man with Jakob-Creutzfeldt disease.

is often abnormal, consisting of a low amplitude background, a poorly developed alpha rhythm, and random, low-to-medium amplitude slow wave abnormalities (23).

Most of these conditions are associated with nonspecific slow wave abnormalities in the EEG. A more distinctive EEG pattern, however, may be present in certain degenerative conditions that are thought to be caused by a slow viral infection. Jakob-Creutzfeldt disease, which occurs in middle-aged adults, may be associated with a distinctive EEG pattern (5) consisting of generalized, repetitive, and stereotyped, bilaterally synchronous sharp waves, usually occurring at a frequency of 1 to 2 Hz and often associated with myoclonic jerks (Fig. 20). Subacute sclerosing panencephalitis (SSPE), which occurs in children and adolescents, often shows a characteristic EEG pattern of periodic bursts of stereotyped slow and sharp wave complexes occurring at intervals of 3 to 10 sec. This pattern, when present, is usually diagnostic for the disease process (24) (Fig. 21). The periodic complexes are often associated with jerks or movements that may cause artifacts in the EEG, and at times they may cause one to overlook the underlying abnormality. It may be helpful to record the EEG during sleep in these patients since the movements then disappear but the EEG abnormalities remain.

Infants with cerebral lipoidosis may show a characteristic EEG

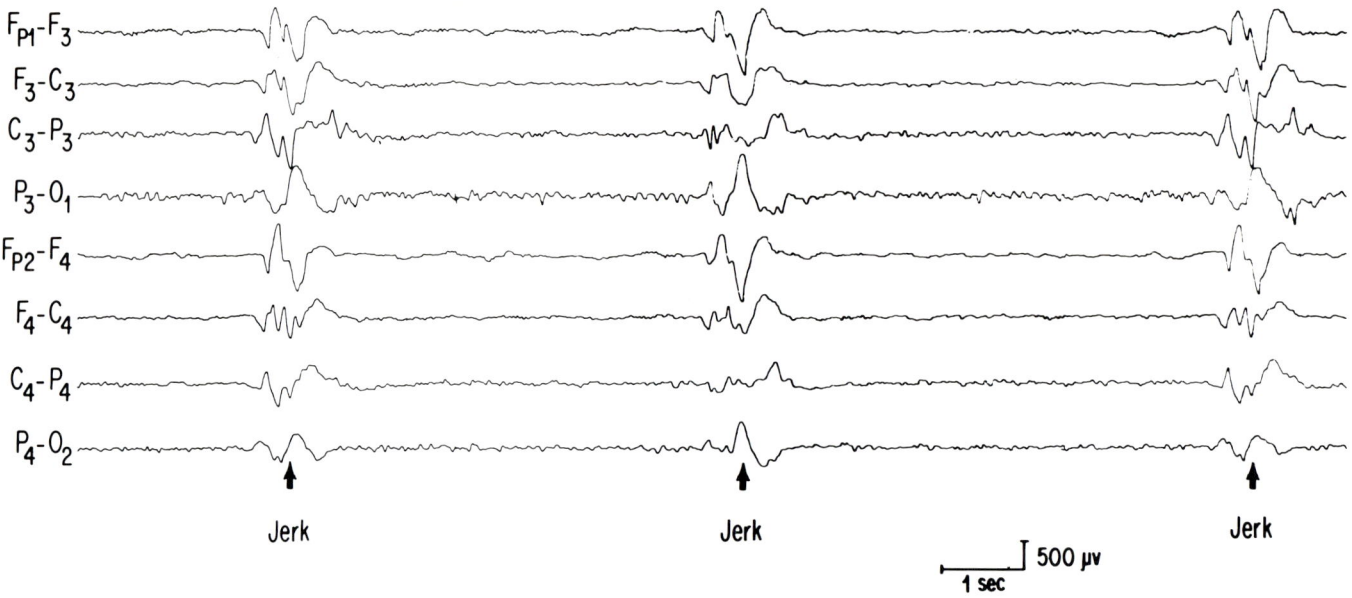

FIG. 21. Sharp and slow wave complexes recurring every 5 seconds and associated with generalized jerks of the body in a 12-year-old boy with SSPE.

pattern. In Tay-Sachs disease, the EEG shows diffuse high amplitude slow waves with multifocal spikes and sharp waves, and a prominent startle response. A distinctive EEG finding in late infantile lipoidosis (Bielschowsky-Jansky type) is the presence of high amplitude polyphasic spikes over the posterior head regions in response to low rates of flash stimuli (25) (Fig. 22).

Another distinctive EEG pattern that occurs in young children is that of hypsarrhythmia, which consists of an admixture of continuous generalized, high amplitude, irregular slow waves and multifocal spike discharges (26,27) (Fig. 23). This EEG pattern often occurs in association with infantile spasms and mental retardation and usually indicates a severe disturbance of cerebral function. The symptom complex is not a specific disease entity but reflects a severe cerebral insult or dysfunction, occurring at an early age, usually before 1 year of age (27). In about half of the patients, the cause is unknown; in other patients this symptom complex may occur as a result of perinatal or postnatal trauma or hypoxia, encephalitis, congenital defects, tuberous sclerosis, or various biochemical or metabolic de-

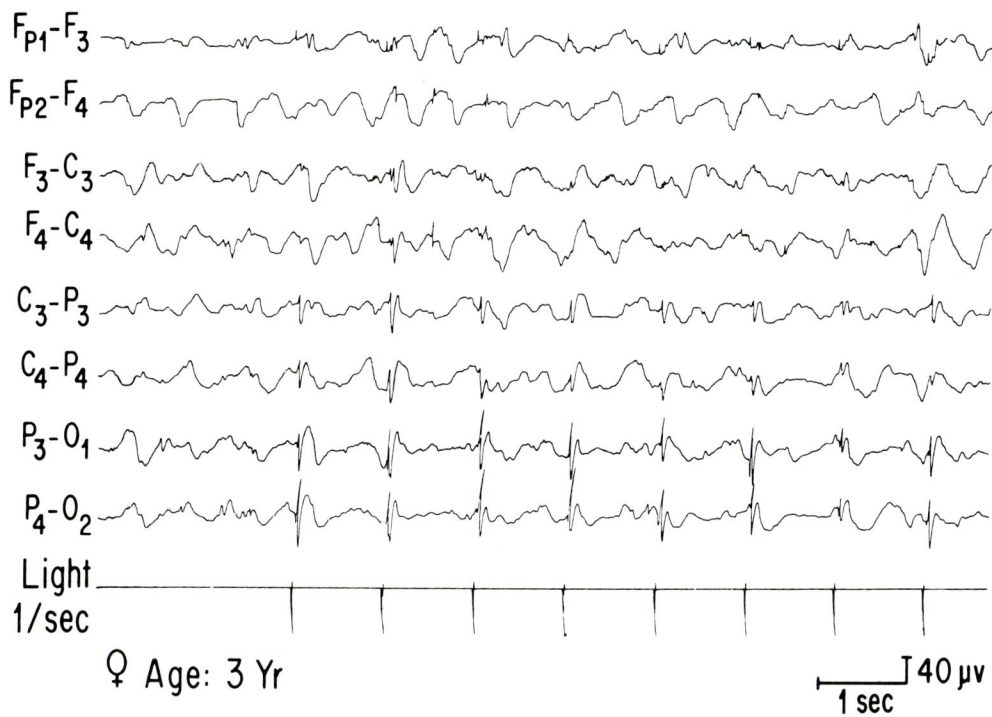

FIG. 22. Spike discharges occurring over posterior regions of head in response to each flash stimulus in a 3-year-old patient with late infantile lipoidosis.

rangements that occur in the young child, such as phenylketonuria or pyridoxine deficiency (27). In the latter condition, an intravenous injection of pyridoxine may cause dramatic improvement in the EEG pattern.

Patients with hypsarrhythmia often have myoclonic jerks or infantile spasms. The myoclonic jerks are very brief, lasting less than a second and they consist of a sudden flexion of the head, body, and extremities. The myoclonic jerks are often associated with generalized and bilaterally synchronous high amplitude spike- or multiple-spike-and-slow-wave discharges in the EEG (28). True infantile spasms, on the other hand, are of longer duration and may last from 3 to 10 sec. These often consist of a tonic flexion of the neck, body, and legs with the arms flung forward and outward (27). The EEG accompaniment usually consists of an initial, high amplitude spike and/or slow wave followed by an abrupt decrement in amplitude of activity and low voltage fast rhythms (27,28) (Fig. 24).

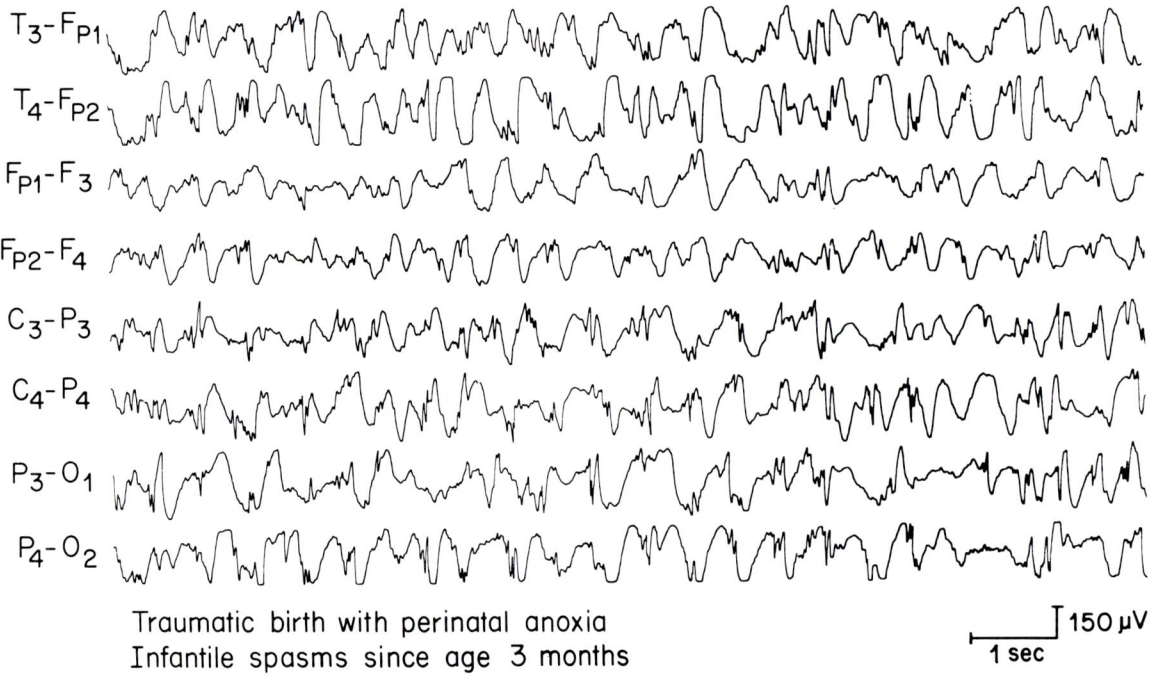

FIG. 23. Hypsarrhythmic pattern with multifocal, high-amplitude spikes and generalized slow waves occurring throughout recording in a 6-month-old girl with infantile spasms and mental and motor retardation.

INFLAMMATORY DISEASES

The EEG in acute encephalitis often shows diffuse high amplitude rhythmic and arrhythmic slow wave abnormalities (Fig. 25). The severity of the abnormalities depends on the degree of cerebral involvement, the level of consciousness, and other associated systemic or metabolic factors. Children often show more severe abnormalities than do adults. The EEG abnormalities usually diminish in association with clinical improvement but on occasion may persist for some time after apparent clinical recovery. It is generally not possible to make a prognosis of residual brain damage or to predict the possible development of postencephalitic seizures based on the acute EEG

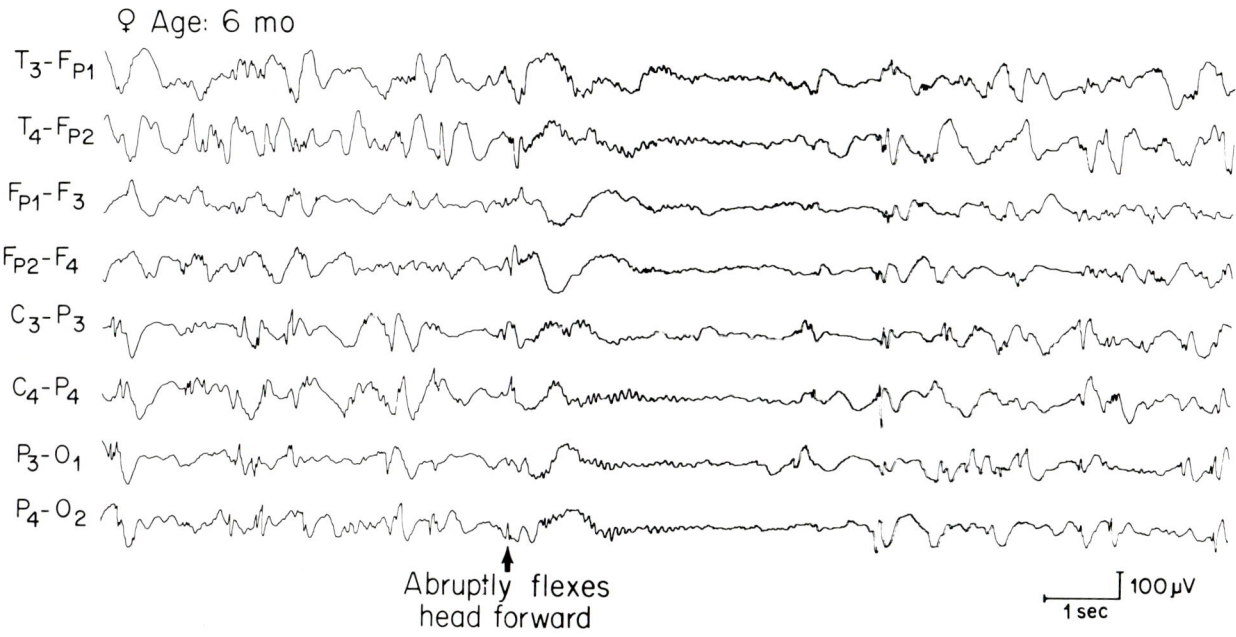

FIG. 24. Transient generalized decrement of activity in association with a flexion spasm in a 6-month-old patient with hypsarrhythmia and infantile spasms.

changes; conversely, a return to a normal EEG does not exclude the presence of residual brain damage (5).

The EEG in meningitis, particularly purulent meningitis and TB meningitis, may show diffuse slow wave abnormalities similar to those seen in encephalitis (1,5). In general, however, the changes in uncomplicated meningitis are often less severe than those seen in encephalitis, and this may be a helpful point in the differential diagnosis.

A focal slow wave abnormality should alert one to a more focal process such as an abscess, local cerebritis, or vascular occlusion. The presence of unilateral or bilateral periodic sharp waves would suggest a diagnosis of herpes simplex encephalitis (29,30) (Fig. 26).

HEAD INJURY

No specific EEG pattern is associated with head injury, and the EEG often shows a wide range of findings, depending on the degree

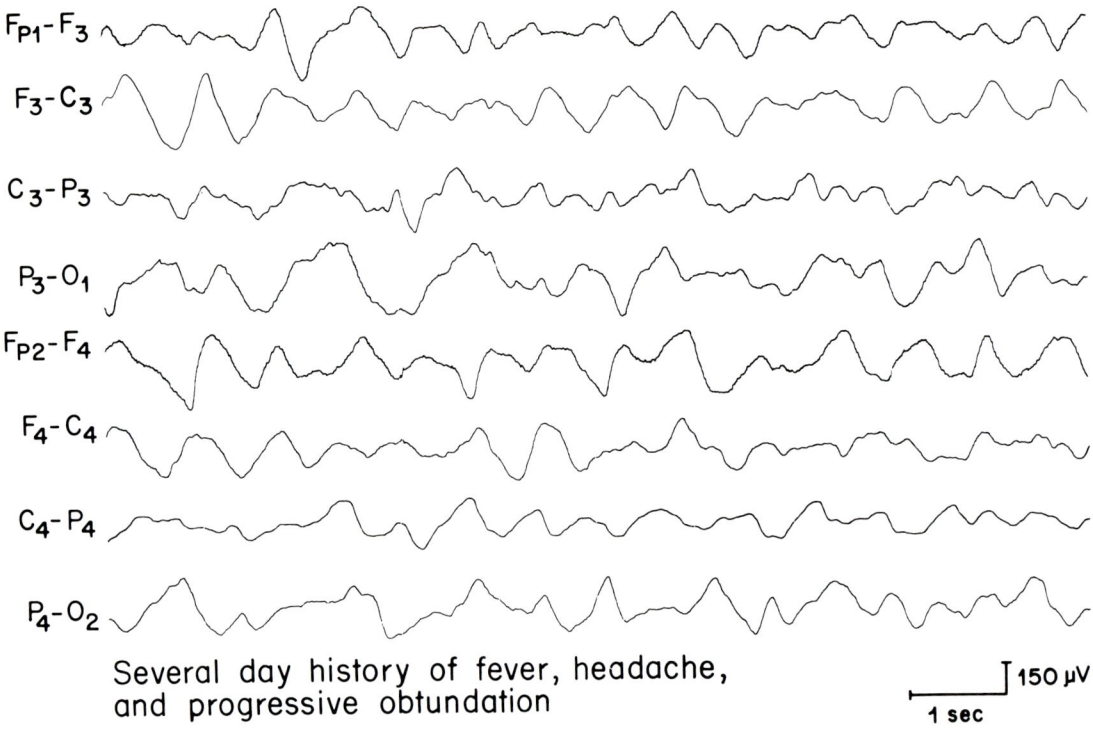

FIG. 25. Severe, generalized slow wave abnormality in a 10-year-old boy with encephalitis.

and type of injury, the age of the patient, and the individual variation of response to the injury.

Diffuse slow wave abnormalities are the most common EEG finding after a head injury. Mild slowing of the alpha rhythm or diffuse theta slowing may be present after mild or moderate head trauma; generalized arrhythmic or rhythmic delta slowing may be seen after a severe head injury. An asymmetry or suppression of activity also can be seen after a head injury. Epileptiform abnormalities, however, are uncommon shortly after a head injury, although on occasion electrographic seizure activity occurs in patients with severe head injury (31).

In children, the EEG may show more marked slow wave abnormal-

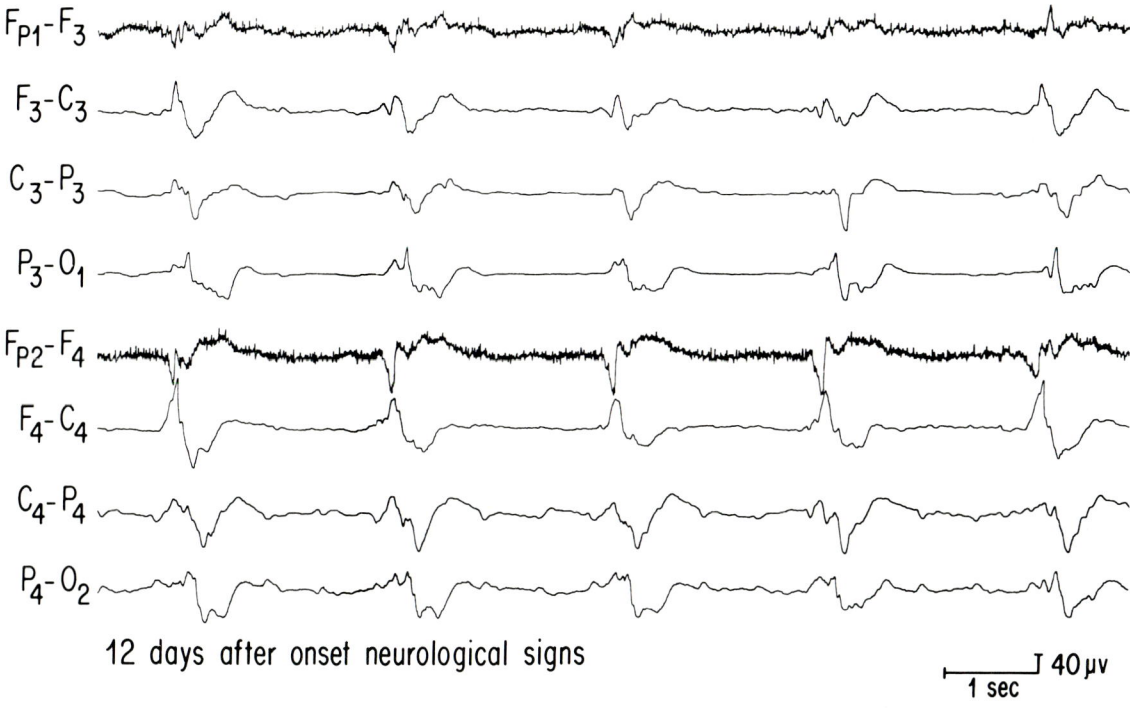

FIG. 26. Bilateral periodic sharp waves in a 64-year-old man with herpes simplex encephalitis.

ities than those seen in adults which may be out of proportion to the clinical state or the degree of head injury. The slow wave abnormalities are similar to those seen in adults but often are more severe, are of higher amplitude, are more widespread, often with maximal emphasis over the posterior regions of the head (Fig. 27), and usually take longer to resolve (32).

On occasion, less common EEG patterns may be present. One such pattern is the "spindle coma" pattern which looks like a sleep recording with spindle activity, but the patient cannot be aroused by ordinary stimuli (33). The patient, however, may show a temporary arousal response, clinically and electrographically, after an intravenous injection of methylphenidate hydrochloride (Ritalin) (Fig. 28); however, this effect is usually transient and the patient then lapses back into coma (33). The presence of this pattern or normal

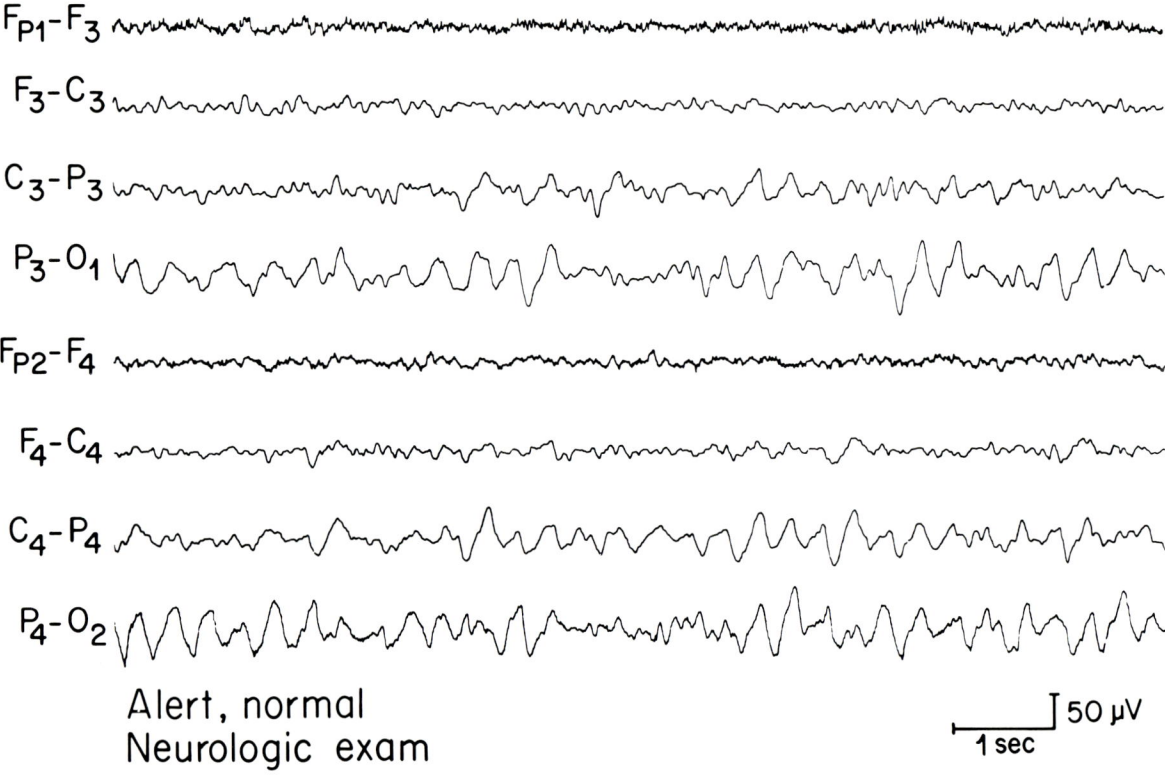

FIG. 27. EEG showing slow wave abnormalities over posterior regions of head in a 7-year-old boy one day after head trauma.

sleep cycles in a comatose patient is usually considered a favorable prognostic sign, whereas a monomorphic or unchanging sleep pattern is an unfavorable sign (34).

Another EEG pattern that often has an unfavorable prognosis is the "alpha coma" pattern described previously, in which the EEG looks like a normal awake recording with a predominance of alpha activity but is present in a comatose patient (9,35). This type of EEG pattern may be present after a severe brainstem injury, usually

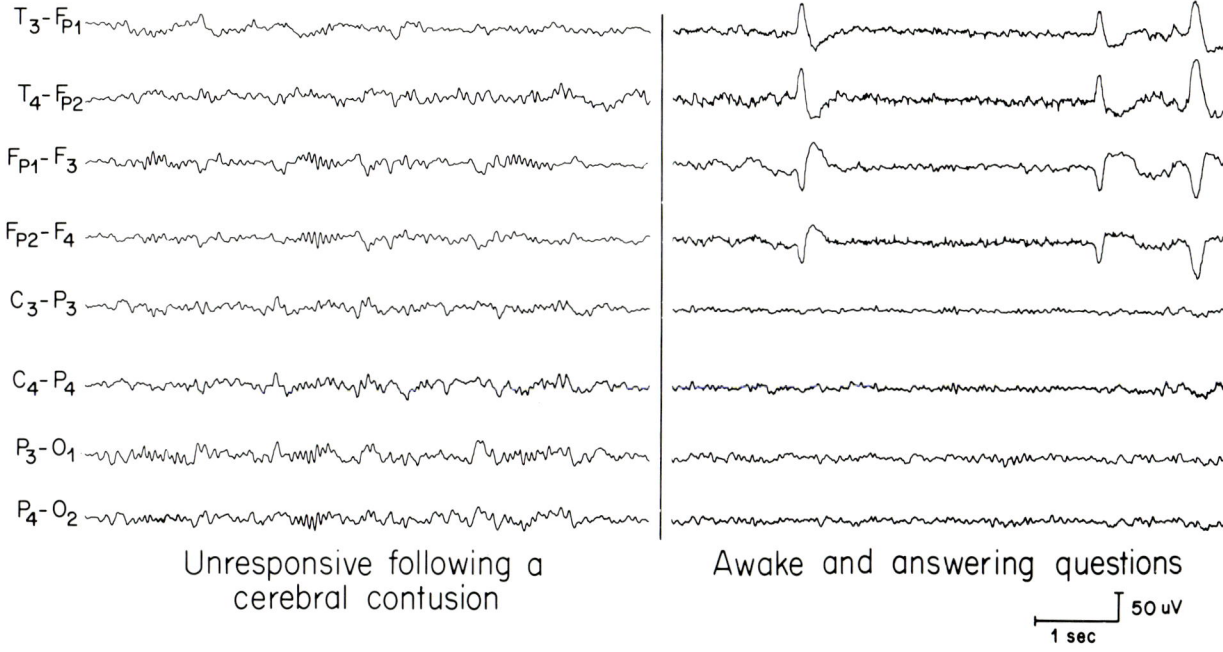

FIG. 28. Left: Before methylphenidate hydrochloride (Ritalin). Spindle coma pattern after head trauma in a 36-year-old woman. **Right:** Response to injection of methylphenidate hydrochloride. The patient aroused and was able to respond to questions, and the EEG showed an awake pattern.

at the pontomesencephalic junction (36,37), or as a result of an anoxic insult to the brain (9). Frequently the prognosis for return of useful neurologic function is poor.

One of the most common complications of head injury is a subdural hematoma. About 90% of patients with a subdural hematoma have abnormal EEGs (1,5); however, the presence of an apparently "normal" EEG should not exclude this possibility. Although correct lateralization of a unilateral subdural hematoma is possible in about three-fourths of cases, diffuse abnormalities may occur with a unilateral subdural hematoma, and especially with bilateral subdural hematomas (1,5).

During the first 2 weeks after a severe head injury, the EEG findings produced by cerebral contusion and those produced by subdural hematoma (38) are often difficult to distinguish on a single

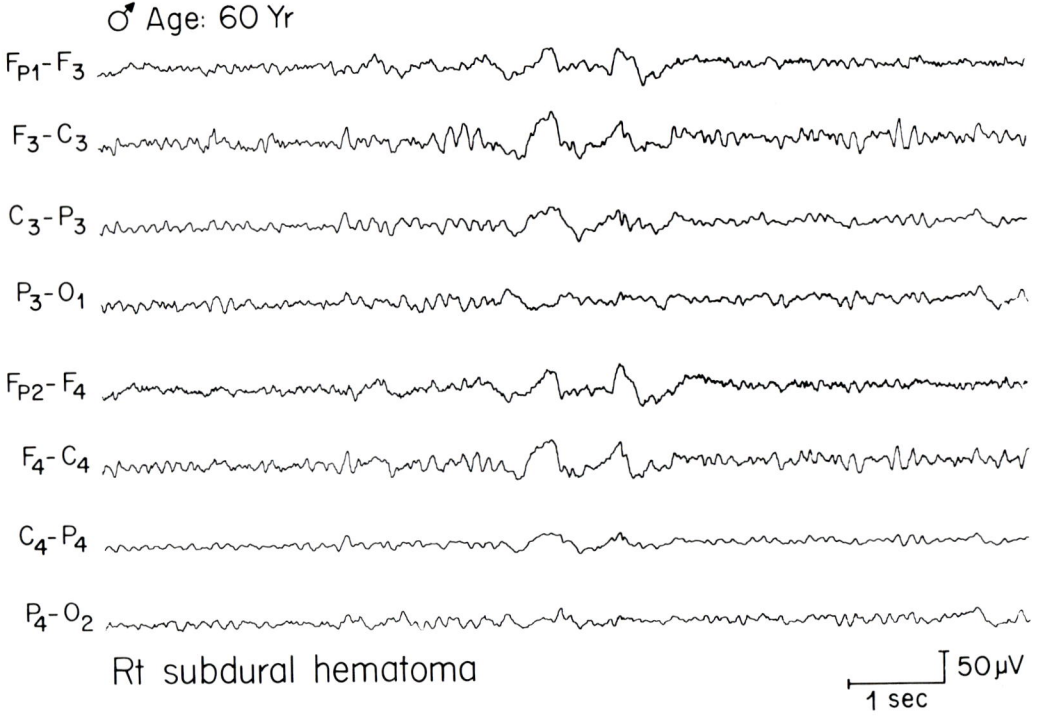

FIG. 29. EEG showing projected abnormality and asymmetry with reduction in amplitude of activity on the right in a patient with subdural hematoma on the right side.

recording. After the second week, however, a subdural hematoma should be considered if the EEG shows increased focal or generalized slowing or the combination of a focal abnormality (slowing or asymmetry) in association with a projected abnormality (38) (Fig. 29).

In uncomplicated head injuries, recovery is usually characterized by a resolution of the slow wave abnormalities, an increase in the basic frequencies, and finally, a return to more normal background activity. At times during the recovery phase, the EEG may show an enhanced reactivity as manifested by an augmented arousal response with bursts of high amplitude rhythmic and bisynchronous slow waves or generalized augmentation of the background rhythms in response to an alerting stimulus (35) (Fig. 30).

Correlation is often lacking between the type and severity of the EEG findings that are present shortly after acute trauma to the head and the subsequent course of the patient. Severe EEG abnormalities shortly after a head injury do not necessarily indicate a poor

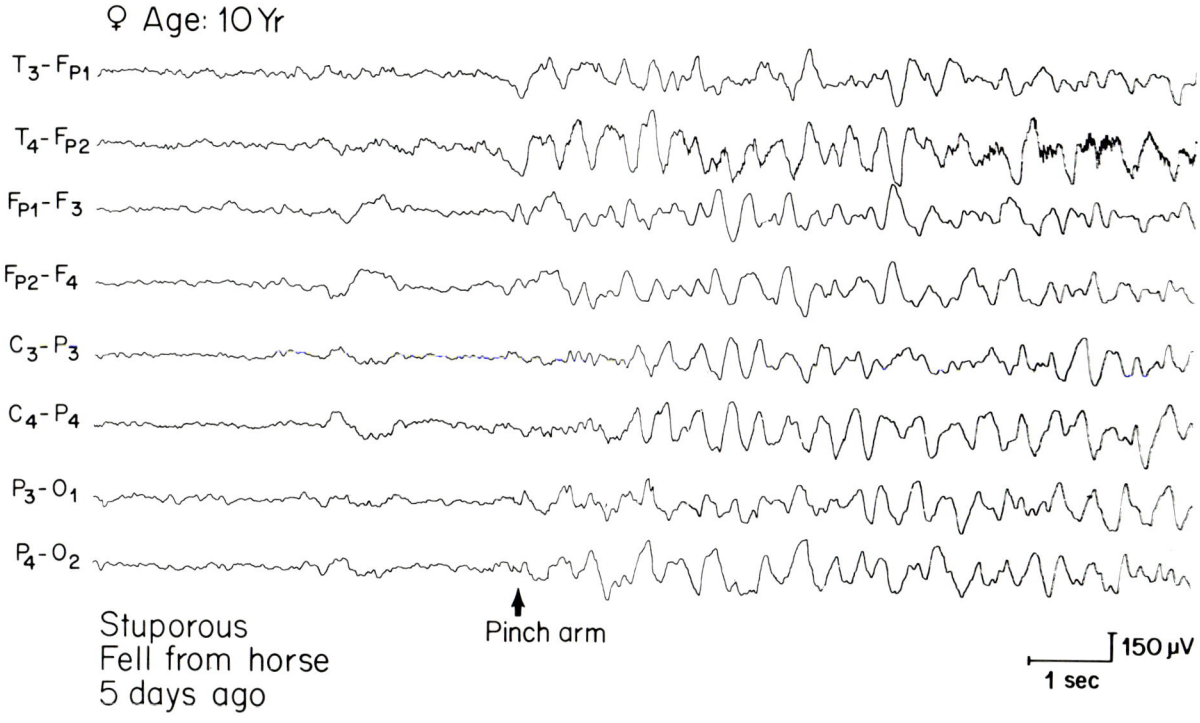

FIG. 30. Augmented arousal response in a patient recovering from head injury.

prognosis (5), and the EEG alone cannot be used for reliable prediction of the development of posttraumatic epilepsy (39). On the other hand, the return of a normal EEG pattern does not exclude a persistent neurologic deficit or the later development of posttraumatic seizures (5).

SUMMARY

With regard to the disorders that diffusely affect the brain, although the EEG often shows rather nonspecific abnormalities, the EEG can be used to:

1. document a disturbance of cerebral function,
2. determine the degree of disturbance of cerebral function,
3. monitor changes in the course of a disease process to determine whether the patient is improving or deteriorating,
4. rule out the possibility of a more focal cerebral process such as an expanding mass, and
5. establish the diagnosis in certain conditions in which a characteristic EEG pattern is present.

REFERENCES

1. Kiloh, L. G., McComas, A. J., and Osselton, J. W. (1972): *Clinical Electroencephalography,* 3rd ed. Appleton-Century-Crofts, New York.
2. Davis, P. A. (1943): Effect on the electroencephalogram of changing the blood sugar level. *Arch. Neurol. Psychiatr.,* 49:186–194.
3. Gibbs, F. A., Gibbs, E. L., and Lennox, W. G. (1939): Influence of the blood sugar level on the wave and spike formation in petit mal epilepsy. *Arch. Neurol. Psychiatr.,* 41:1111–1116.
4. Green, J. B. (1963): The activation of electroencephalographic abnormalities by tolbutamide-induced hypoglycemia. *Neurology (Minneap.),* 13:192–200.
5. Kooi, K. A. (1971): *Fundamentals of Electroencephalography.* Harper & Row, New York.
6. Singh, B. M., Gupta, D. R., and Strobos, R. J. (1973): Nonketotic hyperglycemia and epilepsia partialis continua. *Arch. Neurol.,* 29:187–190.
7. Gastaut, H., and Fischer-Williams, M. (1957): Electroencephalographic study of syncope: Its differentiation from epilepsy. *Lancet,* 2:1018–1025.
8. Saunders, M. G. (1968): EEG changes in metabolic disorders. *Am. J. EEG Technol.,* 8:41–57.
9. Westmoreland, B., Klass, D. W., Sharbrough, F. W., and Reagan, T. J. (1975): "Alpha coma": EEG, clinical, pathologic, and etiologic correlations. *Arch. Neurol.,* 32:713–718.
10. Bennett, D. R., Hughes, J. R., Korein, J. et al. (1976): *Atlas of Electroencephalography in Coma and Cerebral Death,* Raven Press, New York.
11. Reiher, J. (1970): The electroencephalogram in the investigation of metabolic comas. *Electroencephalogr. Clin. Neurophysiol.,* 28:104 (Abstr.).
12. Jacob, J. C., Gloor, P., Elwan, O. H., Dossetor, J. B., and Pateras, V. R. (1965): Electroencephalographic changes in chronic renal failure. *Neurology (Minneap.),* 15:419–429.
13. McLean, D. R., Klass, D. W., and Wakim, K. G. (1971): Factors responsible for EEG alterations in dogs undergoing hemodialysis. *Electroencephalogr. Clin. Neurophysiol.,* 31:298 (Abstr.).
14. Burks, J. S., Alfrey, A. C., Huddlestone, J. et al. (1976): A fatal encephalopathy in chronic haemodialysis patients. *Lancet,* 1:764–768.
15. Rose, A. L., and Lombroso, C. T. (1970): Neonatal seizure states: A study of clinical, pathological, and electroencephalographic features in 137 full-term babies with a long-term follow-up. *Pediatrics,* 45:404–425.
16. Allen, E. M., Singer, F. R., and Melamed, D. (1970): Electroencephalographic abnormalities in hypercalcemia. *Neurology (Minneap.),* 20:15–22.
17. Cohn, R., and Sode, J. (1971): The EEG in hypercalcemia. *Neurology (Minneap.),* 21:154–161.
18. Roseman, E. (1961): Dilantin toxicity: A clinical and electroencephalographic study. *Neurology (Minneap.),* 11:912–921.
19. Chatrian, G. E., Bergamini, L., Dondey, M., Klass, D. W., Lennox-Buchthal, M., and Petersen, I. (1974): A glossary of terms most commonly used by clinical electroencephalographers. *Electroencephalogr. Clin. Neurophysiol.,* 37:538–548.
20. Wikler, A., and Essig, C. F. (1970): Withdrawal seizures following chronic intoxication with barbiturates and other sedative drugs. In: *Modern Problems of Pharmacopsychiatry, Vol. 4: Epilepsy: Recent Views on Theory, Diagnosis, and Therapy of Epilepsy,* edited by E. Niedermeyer. pp. 170–184. S. Karger, Basel.
21. Victor, M. (1970): The role of alcohol in the production of seizures. In: *Modern Problems of Pharmacopsychiatry, Vol. 4: Epilepsy: Recent Views on Theory, Diagnosis, and Therapy of Epilepsy,* edited by E. Niedermeyer. pp. 185–199. S. Karger, Basel.
22. Gordon, E. B., and Sim, M. (1967): The EEG in presenile dementia. *J. Neurol. Neurosurg. Psychiatry,* 30:285–291.
23. Scott, D. F., Heathfield, K. W. G., Toone, B., and Margerison, J. H. (1972): The EEG in Huntington's chorea: A clinical and neuropathological study. *J. Neurol. Neurosurg. Psychiatry,* 35:97–102.
24. Cobb, W. (1966): The periodic events of subacute sclerosing leucoencephalitis. *Electroencephalogr. Clin. Neurophysiol.,* 21:278–294.
25. Harden, A., Pampiglione, G., and Picton-Robinson, N. (1973): Electroretinogram and visual evoked response in a form of "neuronal lipidosis" with diagnostic EEG features. *J. Neurol. Neurosurg. Psychiatry,* 36:61–67.
26. Gibbs, F. A., and Gibbs, E. L. (1952): *Atlas of Electroencephalography, Vol. 2: Epilepsy.* 2nd ed. Addison-Wesley, Cambridge.
27. Jeavons, P. M., and Bower, B. D. (1974): Infantile spasms. In: *Handbook of Clinical Neurology, Vol. 15: The Epilepsies,* edited by O. Magnus and A. M. Lorentz de Haas, pp. 219–234. North-Holland, Amsterdam.

28. Gomez, M. R., and Klass, D. W. (1972): Seizures and other paroxysmal disorders in infants and children. Part I. *Curr. Probl. Pediatr.,* 2:3–37.
29. Upton, A., and Gumpert, J. (1970): Electroencephalography in diagnosis of herpes-simplex encephalitis. *Lancet,* 1:650–652.
30. Smith, J. B., Westmoreland, B. F., Reagan, T. J., and Sandok, B. A. (1975): A distinctive clinical EEG profile in herpes simplex encephalitis. *Mayo Clin. Proc.,* 50:469–474.
31. Courjon, J. (1972): Traumatic disorders. In: *Handbook of Electroencephalography and Clinical Neurophysiology, Vol. 14: Clinical EEG. Part B,* edited by O. Magnus. Elsevier, Amsterdam.
32. Silverman, D. (1962): Electroencephalographic study of acute head injury in children. *Neurology (Minneap.),* 12:273–281.
33. Chatrian, G. E., White, L. E., Jr., and Daly, D. (1963): Electroencephalographic patterns resembling those of sleep in certain comatose states after injuries to the head. *Electroencephalogr. Clin. Neurophysiol.,* 15:272–280.
34. Bergamasco, B., Bergamini, L., Doriguzzi, T., and Fabiani, D. (1968): EEG sleep patterns as a prognostic criterion in posttraumatic coma. *Electroencephalogr. Clin. Neurophysiol.,* 24:374–377.
35. Bickford, R. G., and Klass, D. W. (1966): Acute and chronic EEG findings after head injury. In: *Head Injury,* edited by W. F. Caveness and A. E. Walker, pp. 63–88. Lippincott, Philadelphia.
36. Loeb, C., and Poggio, G. (1953): Electroencephalograms in a case with ponto-mesencephalic haemorrhage. *Electroencephalogr. Clin. Neurophysiol.,* 5:295–296.
37. Chatrian, G. E., White, L. E., Jr., and Shaw, C.-M. (1964): EEG pattern resembling wakefulness in unresponsive decerebrate state following traumatic brain-stem infarct. *Electroencephalogr. Clin. Neurophysiol.,* 16:285–289.
38. Gutierrez-Luque, A. G., MacCarty, C. S., and Klass, D. W. (1966): Head injury with suspected subdural hematoma: Effect on EEG. *Arch. Neurol.,* 15:437–443.
39. Jennett, B., and van de Sande, J. (1975): EEG prediction of post-traumatic epilepsy. *Epilepsia,* 16:251–256.

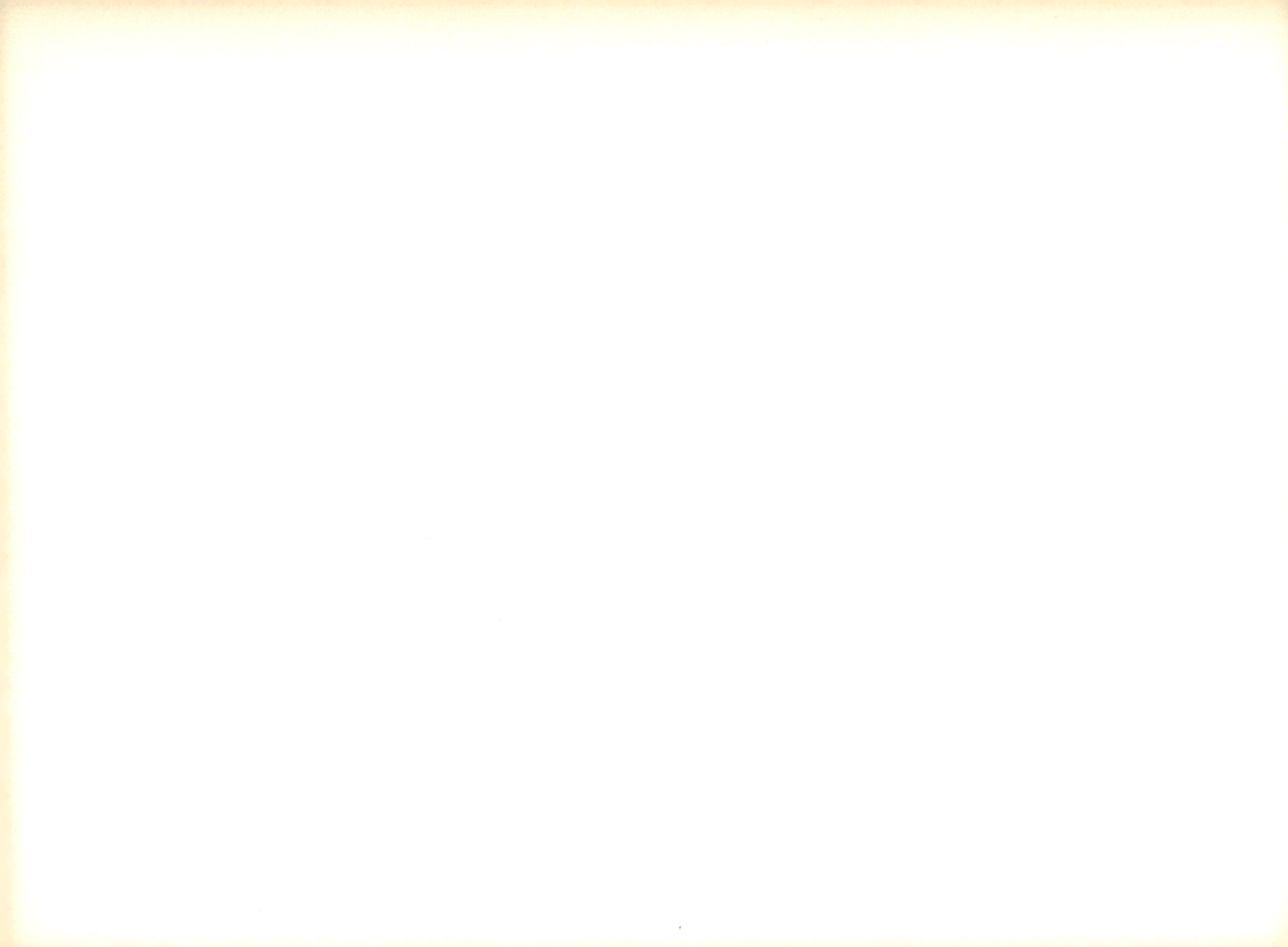

Chapter 12

EEG in the Evaluation of Headaches

Barbara F. Westmoreland

Department of Neurology, Mayo Clinic and Mayo Foundation, Rochester, Minnesota 55901

Nonorganic Tension Headache.. 383
Waveforms of Doubtful Clinical Significance 384
Migraine and Vascular Headaches.. 387
Posttraumatic Headaches... 393
References.. 393

One of the most frequent referrals to the electroencephalography laboratory is that for "headaches," and the electroencephalogram (EEG) is often used as a screening test for patients with a chief complaint of headaches.

Headaches can occur with many different conditions, and the EEG is useful in confirming the diagnosis of a suspected organic process such as that resulting from an expanding mass lesion, vascular disease, infectious process, trauma, or a metabolic, toxic, or degenerative disturbance. The EEG also may indicate the presence of a pathologic lesion when this has not been previously suspected. This situation can occur with deep-seated lesions or lesions affecting the frontal and temporal lobes of the brain in which the patient's only presenting symptom may be headaches and in which there are little or no abnormal findings on the neurologic examination (1) (Fig. 1). A persistent

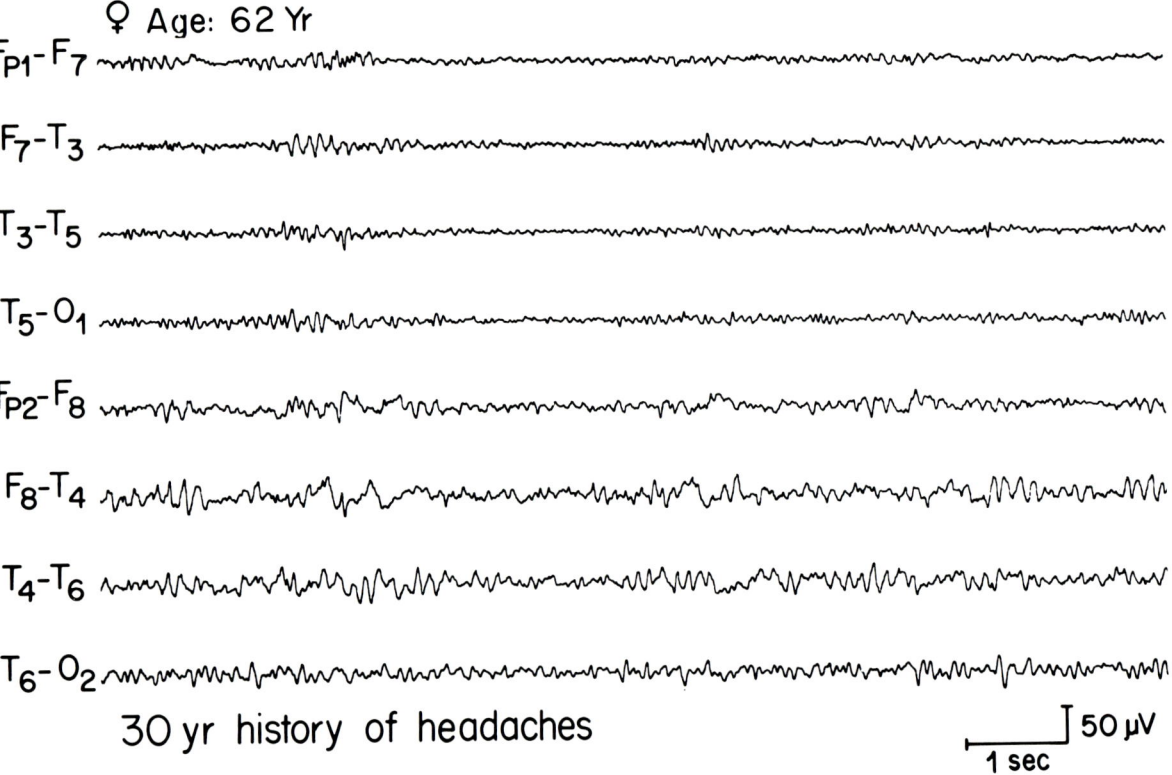

FIG. 1. EEG of 62-year-old woman who had a 30-year history of headaches and a negative neurologic examination. EEG shows focal slowing and an asymmetry of activity over right temporal lobe. Right temporal astrocytoma was found at surgery.

focal abnormality on the EEG, therefore, should be regarded as significant unless proved otherwise.

NONORGANIC TENSION HEADACHE

The EEGs in patients with tension headaches or headaches unassociated with organic disease are usually normal or contain only mild, nonspecific, and nonlocalizing abnormalities. The incidence of abnormal findings in patients complaining of headaches has been reported as 15% (2,3), and this is similar to the rate reported for the general population (3,4). Primarily, the abnormalities consist of a mild slowing of the background or an excess of theta activity occurring diffusely or maximally over the temporal regions.

At times, some of the irregularities may reflect the effect of medication, and most often, the irregularities consist of an excessive amount of beta activity (Fig. 2). In addition, medications also can produce diffuse slowing of the background, an accentuation of theta rhythms, or changes reflecting drowsiness.

Occasionally, with sudden withdrawal of medications, the EEG

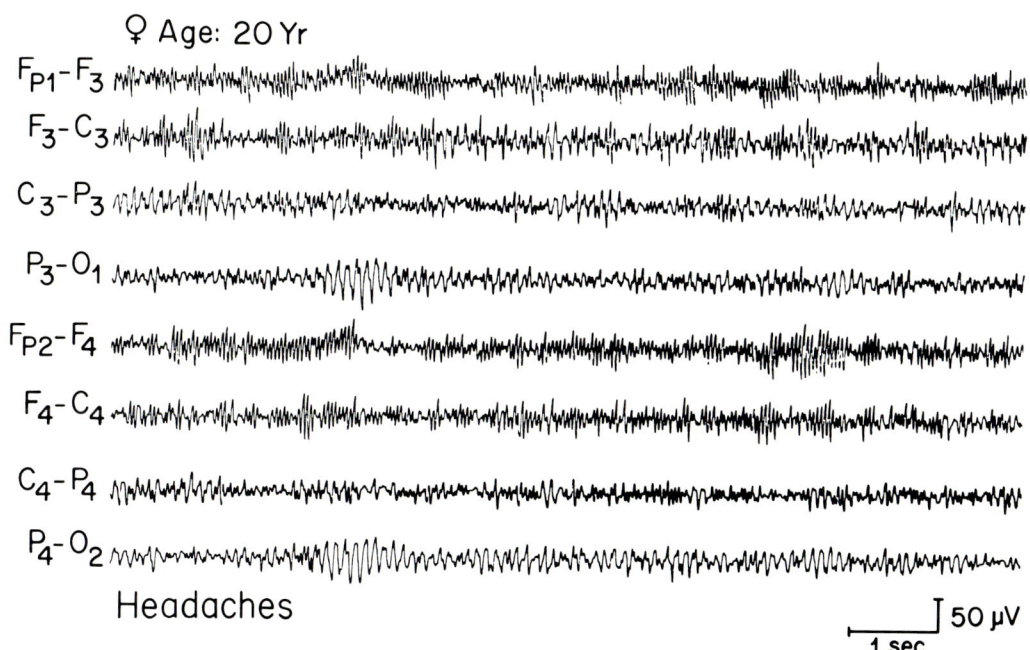

FIG. 2. EEG of 20-year-old woman with tension headaches showing an excessive amount of beta activity due to diazepam.

may show paroxysmal abnormalities or a photoparoxysmal or photomyogenic response (5). These findings do not necessarily indicate an inherent convulsive disorder and may reflect a hyperexcitable response associated with the withdrawal state. Usually, the paroxysmal abnormalities disappear after the use of the medications has been discontinued for 2 to 3 weeks. A repeat recording after this elapse of time helps assess the role of drugs in producing these changes.

WAVEFORMS OF DOUBTFUL CLINICAL SIGNIFICANCE

At times, the EEG may show incidental findings such as 14- and 6-Hz positive bursts, small sharp spikes, 6-Hz spike and wave, rhythmic temporal theta bursts of drowsiness, or the alpha-variant pattern (see also Chapter 14).

The 14- and 6-Hz positive bursts consist of rhythmic trains of arch-shaped waveforms with alternating "positive" spiky components and "negative," smooth, rounded waveforms occurring at a rate of 14 Hz or 6 to 7 Hz and usually ranging from 0.5 to 1 sec in duration (Fig. 3). Usually, these are present during drowsiness and light sleep, occurring maximally over the posterior temporal, occipital, and parietal regions and often shifting from side to side in predominance. The 14- and 6-Hz positive bursts occur mainly between 5 and 40 years of age and are most common in adolescents. The 6-Hz bursts are seen more frequently in the young child and older adult, and the 14-Hz bursts are more common in the adolescent and young adult, although both types can be seen in the same patient (6,7). In the past, this pattern has been associated with various clinical concomitants (7), including headaches, dizziness, vertigo, abdominal complaints, emotional instability, rage, violence, and "thalamic" or "hypothalamic" epilepsy. However, it has been shown that 14- and 6-Hz positive bursts can occur in asymptomatic subjects (8,9), and most electroencephalographers now regard this as a benign variant.

Small sharp spikes are usually low voltage (less than 50 μV), short duration (less than 50 msec), diphasic spikes that often have an abrupt ascending and descending limb (6,7) (Fig. 4a and b). Small sharp spikes are seen primarily in the temporal and ear leads, and provided enough recording is attained, they almost always have a bilateral representation, occurring either independently or synchronously over the two hemispheres (6). The small sharp spikes occur predominantly during drowsiness and light sleep, and most frequently occur in the adult age group (6,7).

The 6-Hz spike-and-wave (phantom spike-and-wave) pattern consists of brief bursts (usually 1 to 2 sec) of serial trains of spike-and-wave discharges that have a repetition rate of 5 to 7 Hz and occur in a bilaterally synchronous and diffuse (although at times asymmetric) fashion over both hemispheres (10) (Fig. 5). This pattern occurs during wakefulness and drowsiness and is most commonly seen in young adults (10,11).

Rhythmic temporal theta bursts of drowsiness (12)—the psychomotor variant pattern—consist of serial trains of theta waves, ranging from 4 to 7 Hz which often have a notched appearance due to superimposed faster frequencies and which occur predominantly over the temporal regions (Fig. 6). The theta bursts may occur either bilaterally or independently over the two hemispheres and, at times, may have a unilateral predominance. This pattern is seen mainly in adults and usually is present during drowsiness (7).

The alpha-variant pattern consists of activity over the posterior head regions, which has a harmonic relationship to the alpha rhythm, and shows a similar reactivity and distribution as the alpha activity. The slow alpha-variant pattern is a subharmonic of the alpha rhythm consisting of dicrotic or notched waveforms over the posterior head regions; the waveforms usually have a frequency that is one-half of

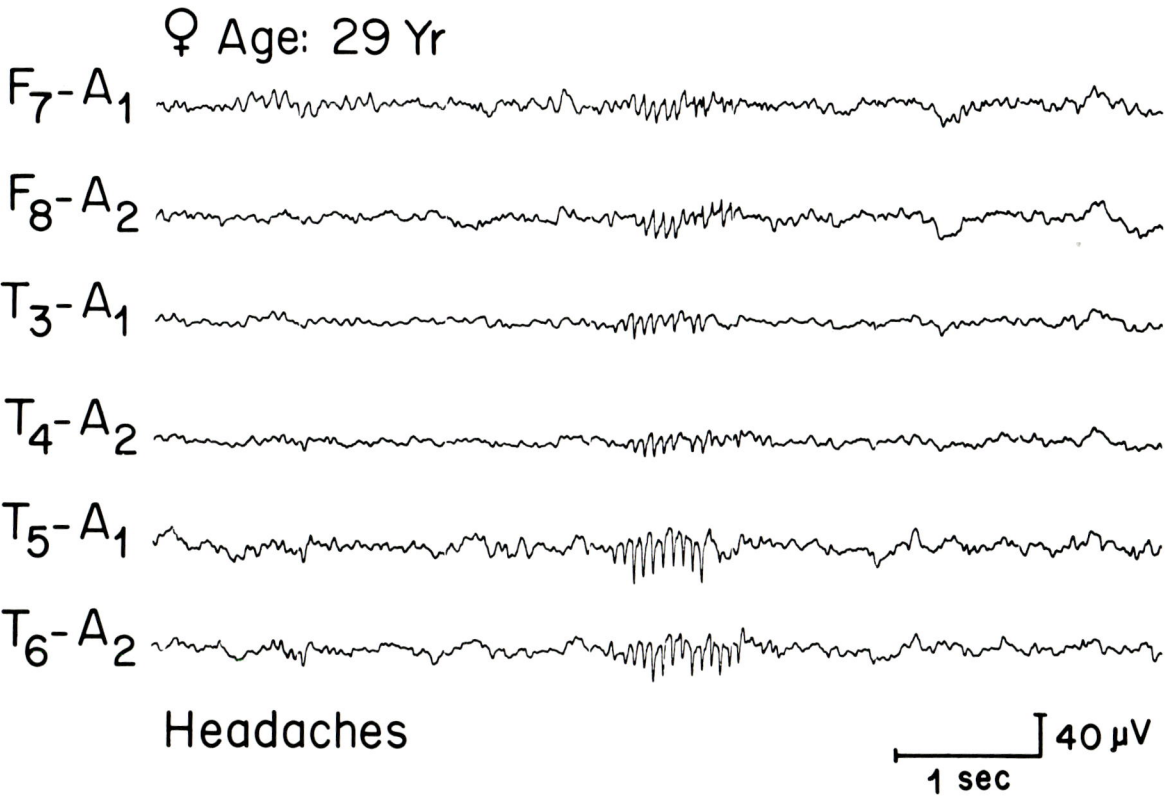

FIG. 3. Example of a 14-Hz positive burst in a 29-year-old woman with tension headaches.

the alpha rhythm, usually in the range of 4 or 5 Hz, and which may alternate or occur in association with the regular alpha activity (12) (Fig. 7). The fast alpha-variant pattern has a faster frequency, usually ranging from 14 to 20 Hz (12). These patterns are seen mainly in adults during relaxed states of wakefulness and are considered to represent a physiologic variant of the alpha rhythm.

Opinions differ regarding the significance of the above waveforms; however, these can occur in asymptomatic subjects, as well as in

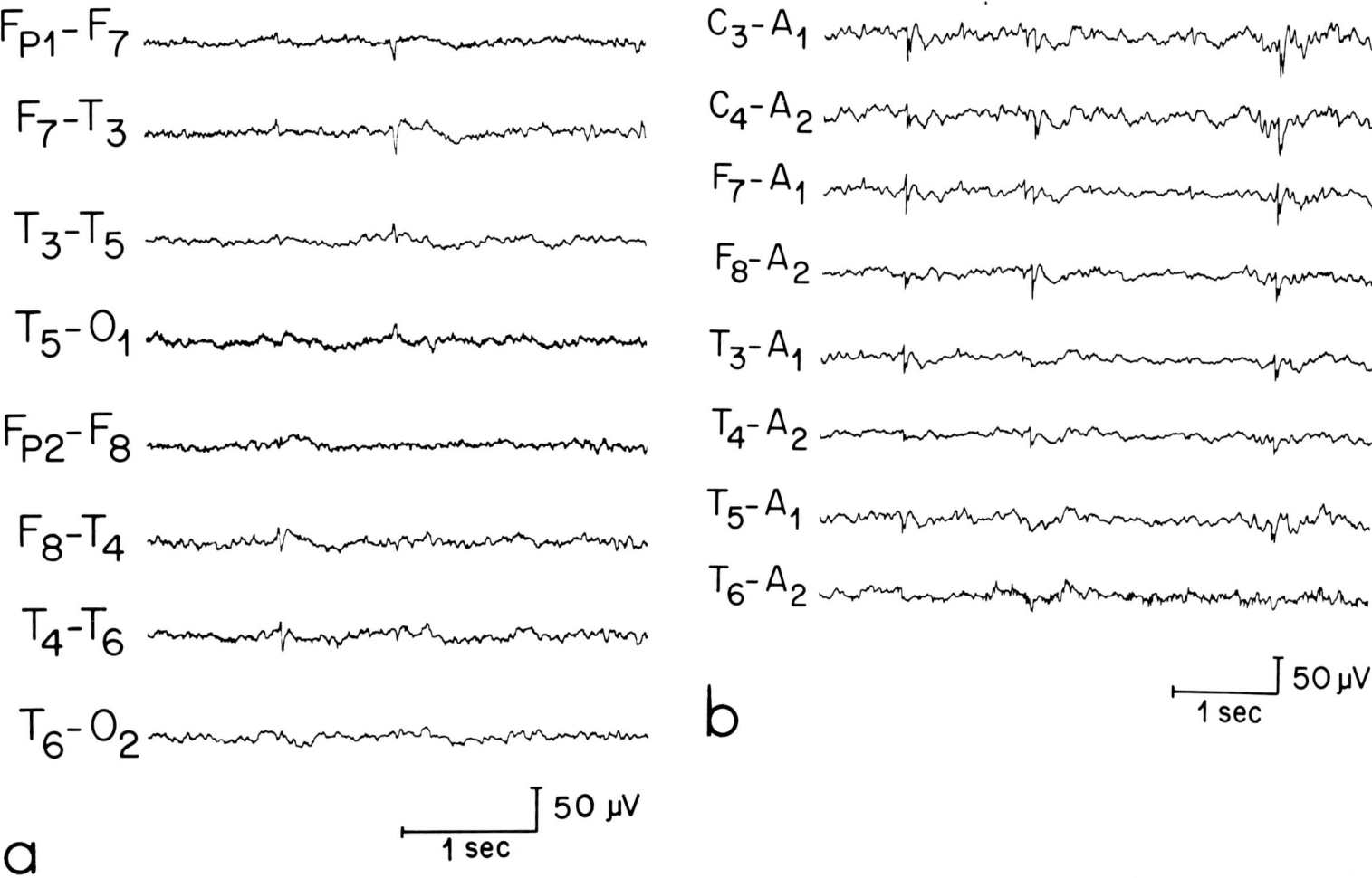

FIG. 4. Example of small sharp spikes occurring bilaterally over the temporal regions as seen on a bipolar montage (a) and on an ear referential montage (b).

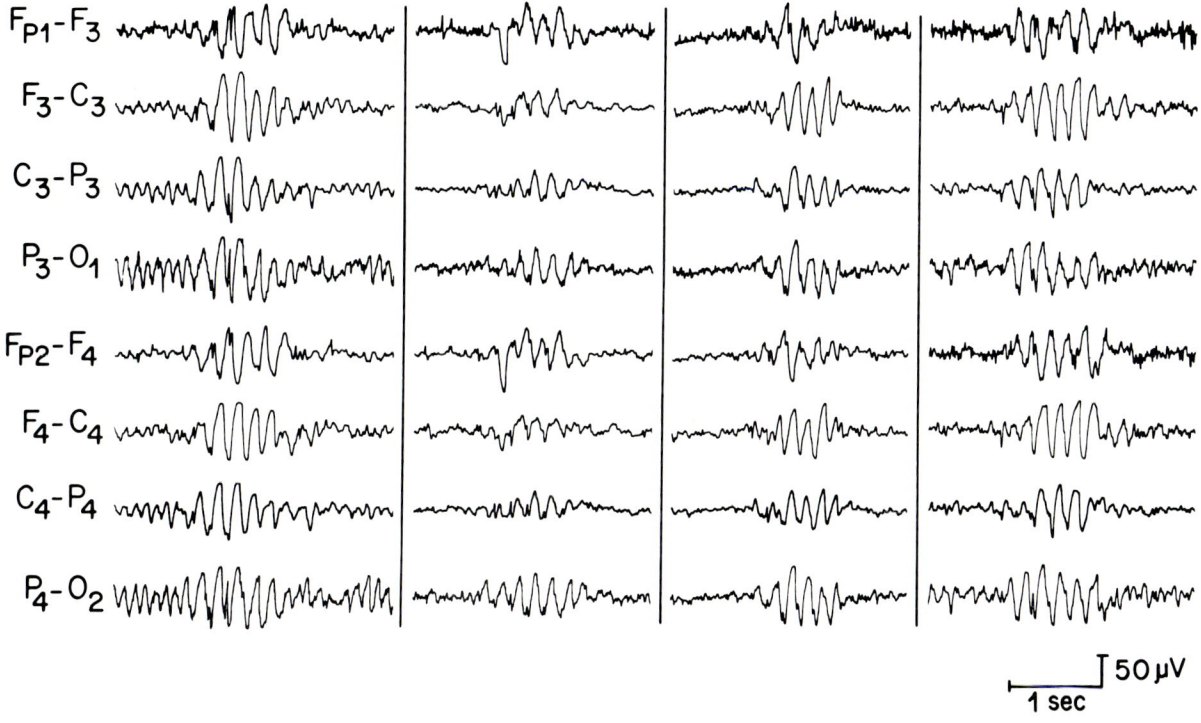

FIG. 5. Examples of 6-Hz spike and wave in a 39-year-old woman with headaches.

persons with various complaints, including headaches (6,7,10,11, 13,14). These waveforms do not correlate specifically with any one particular entity, and although they may have an epileptiform appearance, they do not have a high correlation with the presence of a convulsive disorder; and their occurrence alone is not sufficient to constitute a diagnosis of epilepsy (6,10). For the present, they probably should be regarded as waveforms of uncertain or doubtful clinical significance. A more complete discussion of these waveforms is given in Chapter 14.

MIGRAINE AND VASCULAR HEADACHES

Patients with migraine or vascular headaches have a significantly higher incidence of abnormal recordings than does the general popu-

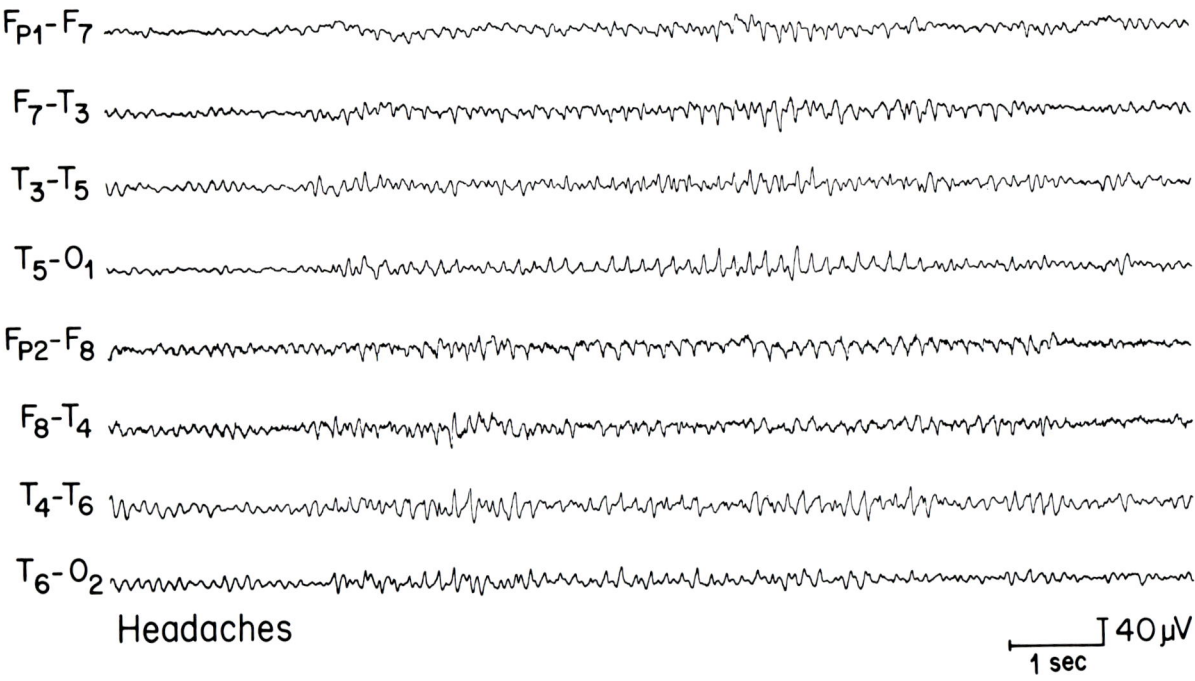

FIG. 6. Example of rhythmic midtemporal theta bursts of drowsiness (psychomotor variant) in an adult with headaches.

lation, and this incidence has been reported to range from 30 to 60% (15–19). Usually, the EEG abnormalities are nonspecific and consist of diffuse or focal slowing or an asymmetry of the background activity or a combination of slowing and asymmetry.

In the headache-free interval, the EEG may be normal or may show variable nonspecific irregularities. The most frequent finding is an excess of theta activity (15–17) occurring diffusely or having a maximal emphasis over the temporal, posterior, or anterior head regions. Diffuse bursts of theta and delta waves also may be present intermittently throughout the recording. There also may be a mild slowing of the alpha rhythms or an asymmetry of the background activity. Epileptogenic abnormalities, however, are an uncommon finding in patients with migraine headaches, and although patients with migraine may have a slightly higher incidence of epilepsy than

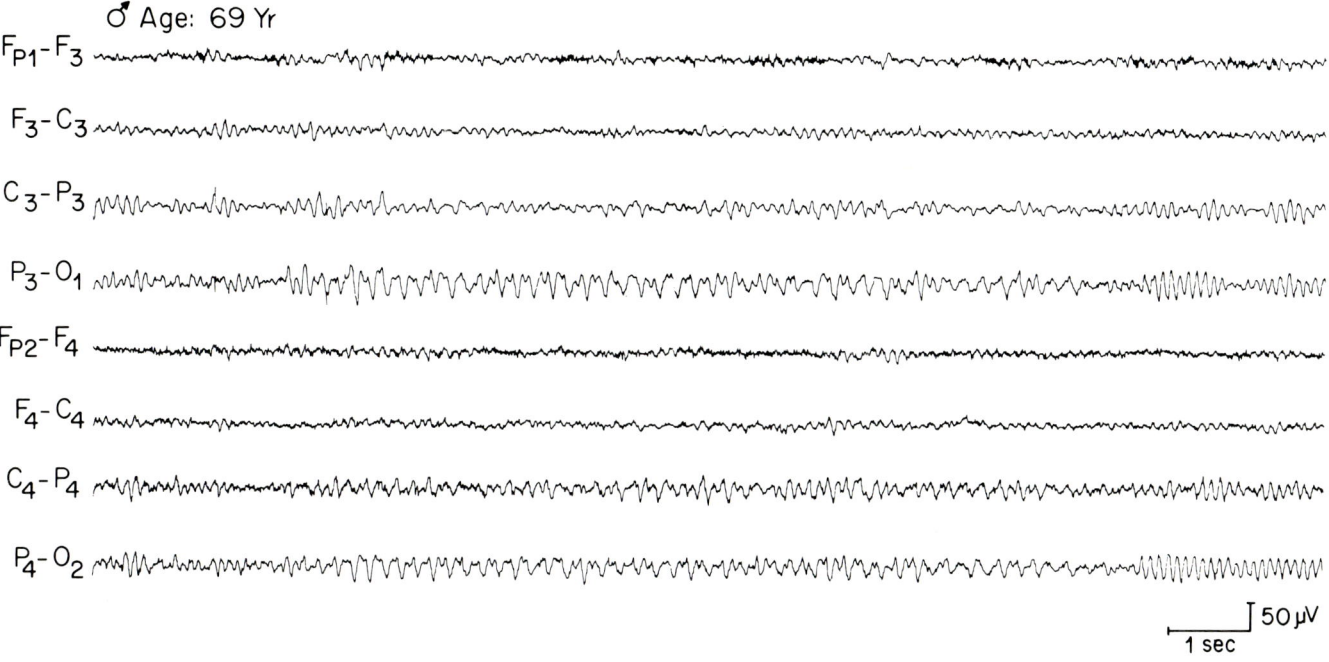

FIG. 7. Example of slow alpha-variant pattern in 69-year-old man with headaches.

patients without migraine, the association between the two disorders is debatable (15,18–23).

Other findings that have been noted in patients with migraine headaches include: A prominent driving response to photic stimulation over a wide range of flash frequencies (17,18,24), including frequencies greater than 20 Hz (the "H response") (24); an excessive response to hyperventilation (18,25); and the presence of prominent lambda waves (18) and positive occipital sharp transients of sleep ("lambdoid" waveforms) (23). These findings, however, are relatively nonspecific, as they can be seen in a normal control population and in patients with other types of dysfunction.

An EEG performed during or shortly after a migrainous episode may show focal, unilateral, or diffuse abnormalities, or it may remain unchanged.

An EEG performed during a simple migraine headache, unassoci-

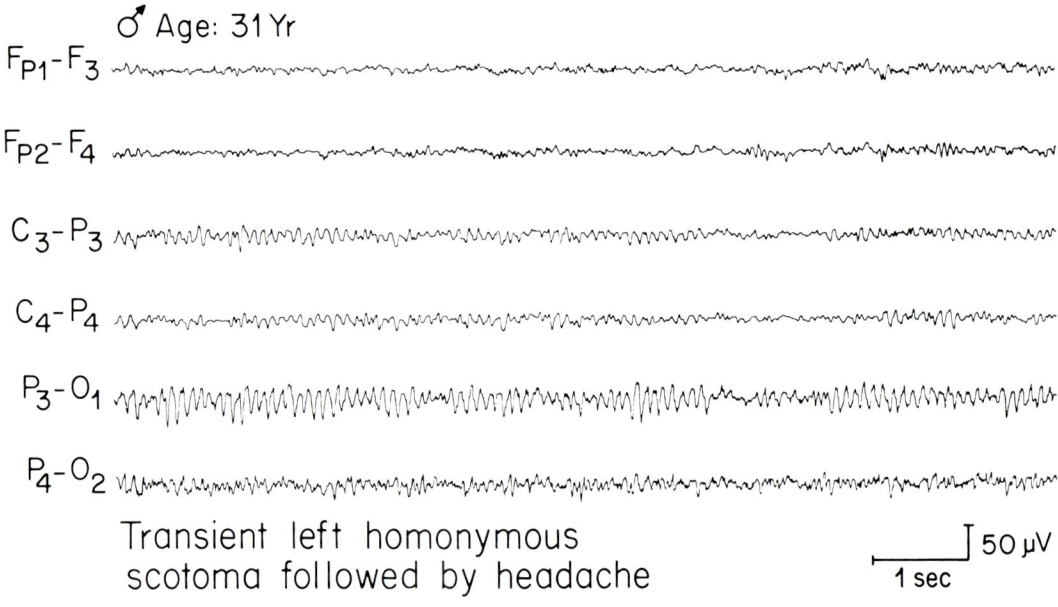

FIG. 8. EEG showing decreased amplitude of alpha activity over right posterior head region of 31-year-old man with a migraine headache preceded by a transient left homonymous scintillating scotoma and hemianopia.

ated with any aura or premonitory neurologic symptoms, may show no change, or it may show an asymmetry or slowing of the background activity. If a recording obtained during or shortly after a migraine headache shows an abnormality, a repeat recording after a headache-free interval is helpful in determining whether the abnormality is transient or persistent.

An EEG obtained during a migraine attack with a visual aura may show an asymmetry of the alpha activity (Fig. 8), a decreased reactivity of the alpha activity on the involved side, or focal slowing over the involved occipital lobe (26). At times, there may be a reflection of the slowing to the adjacent temporal regions or contralateral occipital lobe, but usually the slowing is maximal over the involved occipital lobe.

Patients with hemiplegic migraine have the highest incidence of EEG abnormalities (16,19), and the EEG often shows moderately severe slow wave abnormalities during and after a migrainous episode. Usually, the slowing corresponds to the appropriate area that gives rise to the neurologic signs (Fig. 9) (16,19); however, at times, the

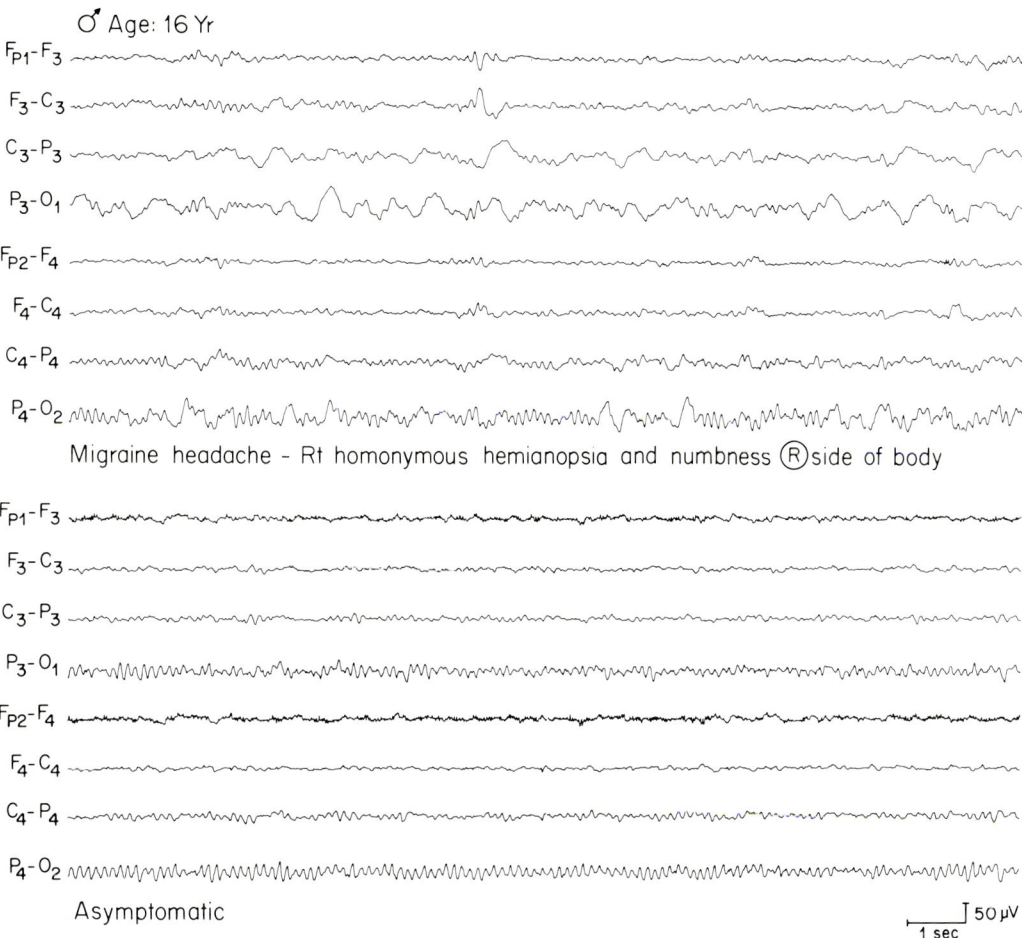

FIG. 9. EEGs from 16-year-old patient with complex migraine. Upper tracing shows delta activity maximal over left parietal and occipital regions, recorded 1 day after a transient episode of right-sided numbness and right homonymous hemianopia associated with severe headache. Bottom tracing recorded during headache-free interval shows only minimal asymmetry of activity over posterior head regions.

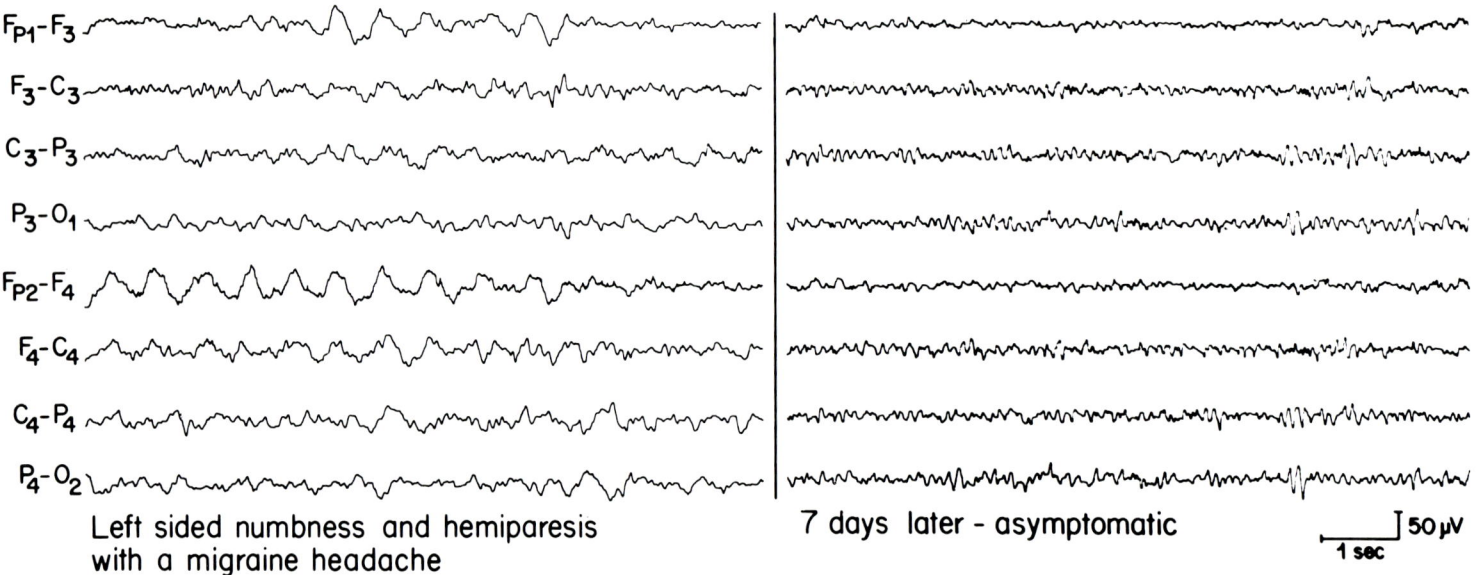

FIG. 10. EEGs from patient with hemiplegic migraine. The tracing on the left shows diffuse slow wave abnormalities, maximal over right hemisphere in 33-year-old woman who had a transient episode of left-sided numbness and weakness, followed by headache 1 day prior to recording. The tracing on the right was recorded 7 days later and shows resolution of slow wave abnormalities.

maximal emphasis of the slow wave abnormality may be over more posterior or anterior head regions, or the slowing may occur in a more widespread distribution over the involved hemisphere. On occasion, the slowing may occur in a more diffuse distribution over both hemispheres (Fig. 10). In addition, there also may be an associated asymmetry or attenuation of the background activity over the involved hemisphere.

There are only a few reports of an EEG being recorded during a basilar migraine attack. Two children who had EEGs recorded during or shortly following a basilar migraine attack showed posterior dominant, rhythmic, delta activity which resolved 1 to 2 weeks later (27). Another patient who had an EEG recorded shortly after a basilar migraine episode showed generalized delta slowing with superimposed, intermittent, high-amplitude slow waves. A repeat recording obtained 1 month later showed only some mild slowing over the posterior head region (18).

Abdominal migraine occurs most commonly during the first decade of life, and generalized slowing or paroxysmal slow wave abnormalities may be seen in the EEG of patients with abdominal migraine (28).

The EEG changes occurring with a migraine attack are usually transient. The EEG abnormalities may disappear as the neurologic deficit resolves, or the EEG abnormalities may persist for hours or days (16). This is particularly true with regard to hemiplegic migraine, and this persistence may be related to local brain edema occurring in response to vasomotor changes associated with the migraine attack (16). Usually, the more severe and prolonged the attack and the more severe the neurologic deficit, the more severe and prolonged are the EEG changes (29). Although the neurologic deficit usually improves within a period of a few hours to a day, the EEG abnormalities may persist for a longer time (23). In children who have had a severe migraine attack, the EEG slowing may last for 1 to 2 weeks before subsiding (29).

If a persistent focal EEG abnormality is present between attacks, the possibility of an underlying pathologic lesion such as a tumor, vascular malformation, or aneurysm should be considered; however, focal EEG abnormalities can be present in patients with migraine headaches in the absence of a structural lesion (19). Also occasionally, a persistent EEG abnormality and neurologic deficit may be present after a migraine attack, suggesting that permanent tissue damage such as an infarct has occurred secondary to the migrainous episode (16).

Sequential EEG recordings are useful in patients with migraine attacks because the EEG can document a transient disturbance or can help distinguish between a resolving, static, or progressive process. The EEG also can be helpful, particularly if a recording is obtained during an attack, in differentiating the transient symptoms of a migrainous episode from that of a seizure, a syncopal episode, or hysteria.

POSTTRAUMATIC HEADACHES

In general, no definite conclusion can be made concerning the relationship of posttraumatic headaches and the EEG findings on the basis of a single recording (30,31); an abnormality in the EEG does not definitely indicate an organic basis for the patient's complaint; on the other hand, a normal recording does not preclude a persistent neurologic deficit (30). The difficulty of assessing the significance of the EEG findings is further compounded by the lack of a pretraumatic recording for comparison. Sequential tracings are more helpful than a single recording in documenting a resolving disturbance, particularly if the initial recording was performed shortly after the head injury (31). Diffuse abnormalities are less significant than focal findings, and temporal abnormalities are less significant than other focal abnormalities (31). One should be aware that drugs and medications also can contribute to some of the irregularities seen in an EEG (31). In children, one should consider the role of maturational effects on the EEG (31). If there is doubt about the clinical significance of an EEG pattern, particularly with regard to epileptiform abnormalities, additional family studies may be of benefit in determining whether this may be a genetic or acquired disturbance (31).

Finally, the EEG may be helpful in detecting the presence of a subdural hematoma (see also Chapter 11). A combination of a bisynchronous and intermittent slow wave abnormality (projected rhythm) and focal delta slowing or an asymmetry (or both), if present more than 2 weeks after a head injury, should alert one to the possibility of an underlying subdural hematoma (32).

REFERENCES

1. Klass, D. W. (1970): Value of the EEG to the clinician. *Neurol. Neurocir. Psiquiatr.*, 11:197–201.

2. Ulett, G. A., Evans, D., and O'Leary, J. L. (1952): Survey of EEG findings in 1000 patients with chief complaint of headache. *Electroencephalogr. Clin. Neurophysiol.,* 4:463–470.
3. Kiloh, L. G., McComas, A. J., and Osselton, J. W. (1972): *Clinical Electroencephalography,* 3rd ed. Appleton-Century-Crofts, New York.
4. Sections of Neurology and Section of Physiology, Mayo Clinic and Mayo Foundation (1963): *Clinical Examinations in Neurology,* 2nd ed. pp. 297–310. W. B. Saunders Company, Philadelphia.
5. Wikler, A., and Essig, C. F. (1970): Withdrawal seizures following chronic intoxication with barbiturates and other sedative drugs. In: *Modern Problems of Pharmacopsychiatry, Vol. 4: Epilepsy,* edited by E. Niedermeyer, pp. 170–184. S. Karger, Basel.
6. Reiher, J., and Klass, D. W. (1968): Two common EEG patterns of doubtful clinical significance. *Med. Clin. North Am.,* 52:933–940.
7. Gibbs, F. A., and Gibbs, E. L. (1964): *Atlas of Electroencephalography, Vol. 3: Neurological and Psychiatric Disorders.* Addison-Wesley Publishing Company, Reading, Mass.
8. Lombroso, C. T., Schwartz, I. H., Clark, D. M., Muench, H., and Barry, J. (1966): Ctenoids in healthy youths: Controlled study of 14- and 6-per-second positive spiking. *Neurology (Minneap.),* 16:1152–1158.
9. Wiener, J. M., Delano, J. G., and Klass, D. W. (1966): An EEG study of delinquent and nondelinquent adolescents. *Arch. Gen. Psychiatry,* 15:144–150.
10. Thomas, J. E., and Klass, D. W. (1968): Six-per-second-spike-and-wave pattern in the electroencephalogram: A reappraisal of its clinical significance. *Neurology (Minneap.),* 18:587–593.
11. Olson, S. F., and Hughes, J. R. (1970): The clinical symptomatology associated with the 6 c/sec spike and wave complex. *Epilepsia,* 11:383–393.
12. Chatrian, G. E., Bergamini, L., Dondey, M., Klass, D. W., Lennox-Buchthal, M., and Petersén, I. (1974): A glossary of terms most commonly used by clinical electroencephalographers: Appendix B. *Electroencephalogr. Clin. Neurophysiol.,* 37:538–548.
13. Hughes, J. R., and Cayaffa, J. J. (1973): Is the "psychomotor variant"—"rhythmic mid-temporal discharge" an ictal pattern? *Clin. Electroencephalogr.,* 4:42–49.
14. Small, J. G., Sharpley, P., and Small, I. F. (1968): Positive spikes, spike-wave phantoms, and psychomotor variants. *Arch. Gen. Psychiatry,* 18:232–238.
15. Selby, G., and Lance, J. W. (1960): Observations on 500 cases of migraine and allied vascular headache. *J. Neurol. Neurosurg. Psychiatry,* 23:23–32.
16. Camp, W. A., and Wolff, H. G. (1961): Studies on headache. *Arch. Neurol.,* 4:475–485.
17. Smyth, V. O., and Winter, A. L. (1964): The EEG in migraine. *Electroencephalogr. Clin. Neurophysiol.,* 16:194–202.
18. Slatter, K. H. (1968): Some clinical and EEG findings in patients with migraine. *Brain,* 91 (Part 1): 85–98.
19. Hockaday, J. M., and Whitty, C. W. M. (1969): Factors determining the electroencephalogram in migraine: A study of 560 patients, according to clinical type of migraine. *Brain,* 92:769–788.
20. Lees, F., and Watkins, S. M. (1963): Loss of consciousness in migraine. *Lancet,* 2:647–649.
21. Lance, J. W., and Anthony, M. (1966): Some clinical aspects of migraine. *Arch. Neurol.,* 15:356–361.
22. Barolin, G. S. (1966): Migraines and epilepsies: A relationship? *Epilepsia,* 7:53–66.
23. Niedermeyer, E. (1972): Cardiac and vascular disorders. In: *Handbook of Electroencephalography and Clinical Neurophysiology,* Vol. 14, Part A, edited by A. Rémond, pp. 73–76. Elsevier, Amsterdam.
24. Golla, F. L., and Winter, A. L. (1959): Analysis of cerebral responses to flicker in patients complaining of episodic headaches. *Electroencephalogr. Clin. Neurophysiol.,* 11:539–549.
25. Towle, P. A. (1965): The electroencephalographic hyperventilation response in migraine. *Electroencephalogr. Clin. Neurophysiol.,* 19:390–393.
26. Engel, G. L., Ferris, E. B., Jr., and Romano, J. (1945): Focal electroencephalographic changes during the scotomas of migraine. *Am. J. Med. Sci.,* 209:650–657.
27. Lapkin, M. L., French, J. H., Golden, G. S., and Rowan, A. J. (1977): The electroencephalogram in childhood basilar artery migraine. *Neurology,* 27:580–583.
28. Lerique-Koechlin, A., and Mises, J. (1964): L'EEG dans une manifestation paroxystique non-épileptique de l'enfant: La migraine. *Electroencephalogr. Clin. Neurophysiol.,* 16:203–204.
29. Gomez, M. R., and Klass, D. W. (1972): Seizures and other paroxysmal disorders in infants and children. Part 1. *Curr. Probl. Pediatr.,* 2 No., 6:1–37.
30. Courjon, J. (1972): Traumatic disorders. In: *Handbook of Electroencephalography and Clinical Neurophysiology,* Vol. 14, Part B, edited by A. Rémond. Elsevier, Amsterdam.
31. Rodin, E. A. (1967): The EEG: A tool of limited courtroom proof. *Trauma,* 9:3–45.
32. Gutierrez-Luque, A. G., MacCarty, C. S., and Klass, D. W. (1966): Head injury with suspected subdural hematoma. *Arch. Neurol.,* 15:437–443.

Chapter 13

Evaluation of Psychiatric Disorders and the Effects of Psychotherapeutic and Psychotomimetic Agents

Morton D. Low

Departments of Medicine (Neurology) and Physiology, University of British Columbia, and Department of Electroencephalography, Vancouver General Hospital, Vancouver, B.C., Canada

EEG in Psychiatry	396
Organic Brain Disease	397
Seizure Disorders	398
Perceptual, Behavioral, and Learning Problems in Children	399
Drug Intoxication States	401
Pyschotropic Agents	402
Phenothiazines	402
Barbiturates	402
Benzodiazepines	402
Amphetamines	404
Monoamine Oxidase Inhibitors	404
Central Anticholinergic Agents	405
Tricyclic Antidepressants	405

Other Psychotherapeutic Agents	405
Psychotomimetic Agents	405
Serotonin Analogs	405
Cannabis Derivatives	405
Analgesics	405
Narcotics	405
Propoxyphenes	405
Anticonvulsants	406
Hydantoins	406
Primidone	406
Oxazoladinediones	406
Succinimides	406
Sulfonamides and Derivatives	406
Antihistamine Derivatives	406
Effects of Physical Treatments on the EEG	406
ECT	406
EEG Patterns Associated with Classical Psychiatric Diagnoses	406
Psychoneurotic States	406
Affective Disorders	409
The EEG in Schizophrenias	409
So-called Specific Electrographic Abnormalities in Psychiatric and Behavior Disorders	409
Acknowledgments	410
References	410
General References	410

EEG IN PSYCHIATRY

It must be stated at the outset as a major point of this chapter that, with reference to the specific classification of primarily or strictly psychiatric disorders, the routine electroencephalogram as it is now employed has no diagnostic value. One cannot distinguish, on the basis of routine EEG findings, a patient with disorder of behavior or personality, a neurosis, an affective disorder, or schizophrenia from a normal individual. Although it is true that psychiatric patients as a group do have more EEG abnormalities than the general population, none of these abnormalities is sufficiently correlated with psychiatric disorder *per se* to be useful in evaluating any given individual case.

In spite of this fundamental difficulty, the EEG can be shown to have significant practical use in the evaluation of patients whose clinical symptoms are primarily mental ones. I have (obviously, arbitrarily) divided the field into four main areas in which EEG studies have proven useful in providing some diagnostic information. These four areas are:

1. Mental and behavioral disturbances due primarily to organic/structural brain disease;
2. Behavioral and mental symptoms due primarily to seizure disorder;
3. Perceptual, behavioral, and learning problems in children; and
4. Mental symptoms due primarily to drug intoxication.

Deferred for later consideration in this chapter are descriptions of the EEG patterns reportedly associated with particular, strictly psychiatric disorders. Because there is no general agreement in the literature regarding the significance of these reported findings, their discussion is left until after a consideration of the four areas listed above in which EEG studies can provide useful differential diagnostic information.

ORGANIC BRAIN DISEASE

It is important to qualify the use of the phrase "organic brain disease." I believe that the mind does not exist apart from the brain, and yet traditionally in our clinical work we categorize diseases either as neurological or psychiatric, suggesting perhaps that so-called functional disturbances dealt with by psychiatrists are really reversible behavior and thought disorders with no correlation to biological or structural alteration. This traditional division of diseases into neurological or psychiatric groups obscures the fact that thoughts, feelings, and memories are much the result of brain activity as are sensation, speech, and movement. Furthermore, it is true that a great many "functional" disturbances of behavior and mentation resulting from or apparently markedly influenced by environmental factors can be quite permanent and irreversible (1).

In my view, traditional medicine has done itself a disservice in too strictly conceptualizing patients and their diseases as either psychiatric or neurological, with either functional or organic disorder. All behavior is organic in origin, and there is reason for continuing hope that as the techniques of electrophysiology become more refined, we will be able to demonstrate more specific correlations between electrographic patterns and behavior as such, both normal and abnormal.

With this reservation about the use of the term organic brain disease, the second major point to be made in this chapter is that a great many disease states are associated with disturbances of mentation and behavior, and may produce more or less definite EEG abnormalities. Vascular disease, space-occupying lesions, central nervous system infections, metabolic and electrolyte disturbances, and exogenous toxins all can produce personality changes and thought disorders, and to some degree all of these may mimic the picture of a primary psychosis (1). It is in the role of assessing the true or nonpsychiatric origin of such symptomatology that clinical EEG still makes its most useful contribution in this field. Along with a careful clinical evaluation of the patient's neurological and mental status, the EEG can assist in obtaining the earliest, safest, and least expensive indications of the true origin of the patient's clinical symptoms.

SEIZURE DISORDERS

Ictal or epileptic–psychic, perceptual, and experiential symptoms may be mistaken for purely psychiatric or functional disorders (2). There are two main points to be emphasized in this regard. The first is that it is sometimes difficult to distinguish the behavior of a patient having a seizure (or immediately before or after) from episodic disturbances of behavior that are hysterical or truly psychotic in origin.

The bizarre behaviors sometimes associated with seizures are sometimes difficult to recognize as ictal events. Certainly they are less obvious and less dramatic than the tonic–clonic stages of a grand mal attack. In seizures of temporal lobe origin for example the patient may exhibit automatisms which are repetitive, often consisting of oral activity such as lip smacking, chewing, gagging, retching, or swallowing. To an experienced neurologist these may be adequate clues, but some patients during the seizure may perform a variety of complicated acts that seem to blend with normal behavior to produce inappropriate actions. The verbal repetition of a phrase over and over again or stereotyped buttoning and unbuttoning of clothing are common manifestations. Some patients with psychomotor seizures may have bizarre postures resembling those of catatonic schizophrenia, and these positions may be held for variable periods of time.

Although outbursts of directed, aggressive behavior are extremely rare in psychomotor epilepsy, when such outbursts do lead to violence they often present difficult and serious medicolegal questions concerning the responsibility of that individual for his actions. It is important to remember that although the behavior of patients during psychomotor seizures tends to be automatic, it is often influenced by environmental situations.

In distinguishing between ictally determined and primarily psychotically determined behavior, the EEG in the context of the patient's medical history can be very useful. In establishing a diagnosis of seizure disorder as the origin of the patient's symptoms, the following six questions should be asked concerning the patient's history. Some or all of them are very commonly manifestations of epilepsy and are much less common in true psychosis (1):

1. Has the patient had other episodes in which he engaged in nearly identical behavior? In psychomotor epilepsy, during an attack, motor activity tends to be quite stereotyped.
2. Does the patient report changes in feeling or moods that are typical in seizures of temporal lobe origin?
3. During the episode does the patient's behavior include characteristic automatisms?
4. During the episode was the patient obviously confused?
5. Was the patient's memory impaired for events occurring during the episode?
6. Is there any evidence of postictal depression or fatigue?

It is important to remember that in both temporal lobe epilepsy and petit mal epilepsy, a patient may experience very prolonged episodes of abnormal behavior lasting for hours or days (fugue state or ictal stupor), and the EEG can be the surest possible means of making the proper diagnosis in such cases.

In the context of a discussion of seizure disorder and psychosis, it is important to emphasize the second main point here that there is apparently a relationship between seizure disorder *per se* and the development of psychosis in some patients (2). The etiology of these schizophrenia-like psychoses of epilepsy is not known, but from available studies there are two outstanding factors that are very common in reported cases. These factors are: (a) the use of anticonvulsive medication over long periods of time; and (b) poorly controlled seizures. A history of either or both of these factors precedes the development of the psychosis in virtually every case. It must be emphasized, however, that the specific role of these factors is as yet unclear. It is possible that chronic anticonvulsive therapy may have a toxic effect on mental functioning, which is either direct or indirect, mediated by some mechanism such as depression of vitamins or enzymes. Drug toxicity seems unlikely as a major factor in most cases of epileptic psychosis since the amount of medication taken by the patient rarely has any relationship either to the incidence or severity of the psychosis. In addition, it has been established that such psychoses can develop even in untreated epileptics.

Another possibility is that the psychosis in such patients is a psychological reaction to years of seizure episodes in which clouded consciousness and periodic disturbances of sensation and perception have finally led to a confusion of reality with internal or purely subjective experience. It has been hypothesized that the schizophrenia-like psychosis of epilepsy may result from abnormal electrical activity in limbic structures presenting at times as either psychomotor seizures or psychotic behavior or both.

In any given patient's case, it may be very difficult to differentiate ordinary schizophrenia from the schizophrenia-like psychosis of epilepsy. A family history and a positive medical history of epilepsy do provide important distinguishing clues. In ordinary schizophrenia there is a very high incidence of serious psychopathology in the immediate family. On the other hand, the incidence of schizophrenia in the family of patients with epileptic psychosis is no greater than in the general population. The major distinguishing feature is a history of epilepsy; such a history is present in epileptic psychosis and absent in ordinary schizophrenia. The EEG may be of some help in the differential diagnosis since EEG abnormalities, particularly involving temporal or frontotemporal regions are very common in epileptic psychosis. One should be aware, however, that abnormal EEGs are seen in schizophrenics more commonly than in normal individuals so that EEG by itself is of relatively limited value.

PERCEPTUAL, BEHAVIORAL, AND LEARNING PROBLEMS IN CHILDREN

As with most other psychiatric disorders, the exact nature of the minimal cerebral dysfunction syndrome (MCD) in children is unclear. In fact, some clinicians question the existence of such a diagnostic entity.

However unclear the etiology may be, and in spite of the confusion resulting from studies using poorly defined criteria, differences in patient population, and poor controls, it has been well established that if one starts with a group of children meeting a carefully defined descriptive profile including hyperkinetic impulsive and compulsive behavior, distractibility, short attention span, possibly outbursts of sudden unprovoked and destructive acts, learning difficulty, neurological soft signs, etc., this group of children will show a very high incidence of EEG abnormality as compared to normal controls (on the order of 40 or 50% abnormal records in the MCD children) (3). The EEGs taken from these children most commonly show an excess of slow activity, which is usually posterior dominant (Fig. 1). They may however have other EEG abnormalities such as generalized spike-and-wave bursts, asymmetries, or spike foci.

It is as yet unclear what these EEG abnormalities mean with regard to the pathophysiology of the clinical disorder. The poor performance of the children may be the result of several possible conditions, one of which is central nervous system immaturity or delayed maturation. This is the view favored by the French school led by Gabrielle Lairy. Support for this concept exists in the nature of the primary EEG abnormality, i.e., the records often look just

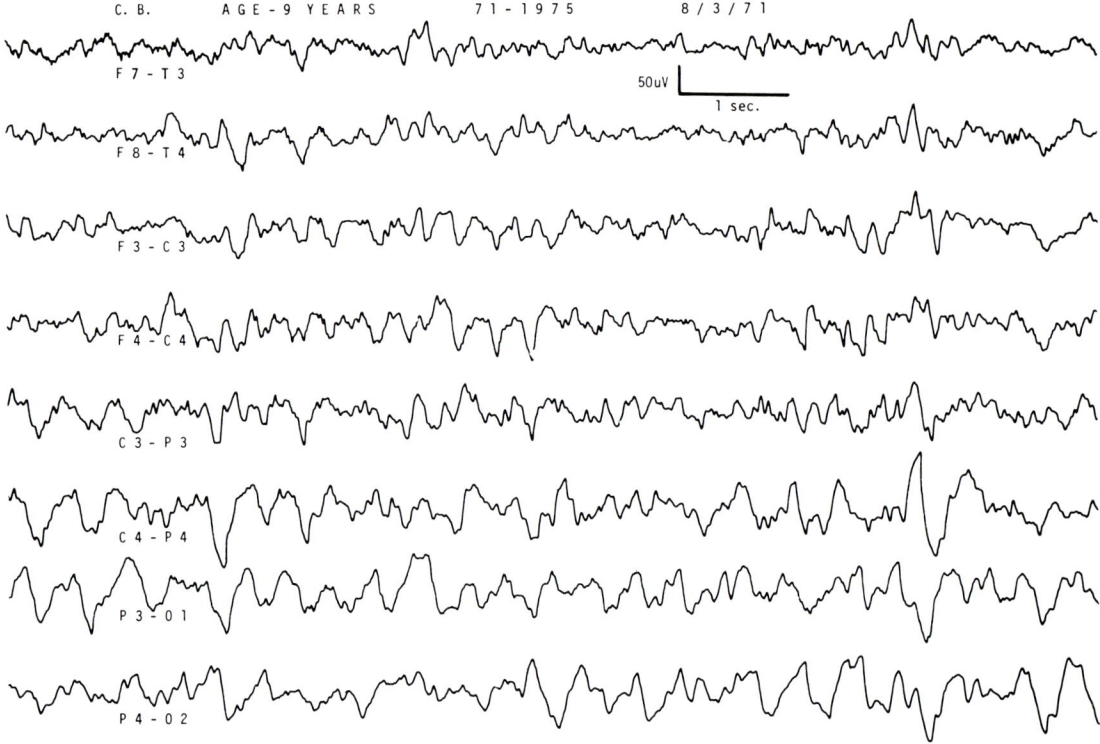

FIG. 1. Diffusely slow record. Child with MCD.

too slow for the patient's age. Some workers have demonstrated that sensory evoked potential parameters may parallel the EEG findings in such children; that is, auditory evoked potential latencies and amplitudes are longer and lower respectively than would be expected for the age of the child (4). The common observation that such children often outgrow the behavior and performance problems whether or not they are specifically treated lends some support to this view (3).

On the other hand, the poor performance of the children may result from the presence of a brain lesion with destruction of neural tissue and resultant functional disturbance in that system (which may ordinarily be involved in the normal integration of learning, communication, etc.). There may be an irritative functional disturbance which co-opts these neural systems into abnormal discharging patterns, with the result that such brain regions are prevented from normal participation in integrated motor or sensory function.

It may be that in a given population of children with the so-called MCD syndrome there is a mixture of etiologies, and this nonhomogeneity of cause may be a factor in the diagnostic and therapeutic confusion in this area.

The importance of EEG abnormalities in understanding a complex problem such as the MCD syndrome lies in their ability to provide a guide in the diagnostic and prognostic consideration of such patients. The presence of an EEG abnormality of any type in such a child should provoke a reconsideration of the possible primary role of emotional disturbance, lack of motivation, or poor inherited intellectual capacity in the child's problems. Recognition of subtle disturbances of cerebral function revealed by the EEG is important because the attitudes of the physician, parent, and teacher can be changed through realization that the child has an organic cerebral disorder.

In such children, usually the standard techniques of punishment and reward for performance are ineffective, and pressure exerted by parents and teachers may further compound the problem by producing tensions and emotional upset both in the child and other members of the family. This is likely to result in still worse school performance and behavior because these children often react to such pressures by exaggerated behavioral responses. Then the initial organically determined behavior problem may be complicated by behavior disorder of true psychogenic type.

DRUG INTOXICATION STATES

A large number of drugs now are used in the treatment of a wide variety of symptoms. It is at times difficult to determine whether new symptoms that a patient develops while on medication are due to a psychological disturbance, to an organic brain disease, or to an idiosyncratic response to or overdose of the drug being used in therapy. Often, drugs are prescribed indiscriminantly. The dose the patient is given or decides to take himself may be excessive, at least for that particular patient. The pharmacology and mode of action of many of the ataractic or psychotropic agents are poorly understood, and toxic symptoms are quite variable and often bizarre. The recognition of drug intoxication as the cause of a patient's bizarre or unusual mental status can be greatly facilitated by the use of the EEG (see also Chapter 11). In an extreme case of toxic reaction to such drugs (i.e., attempted suicide by ingestion), a prompt diagnosis may determine the difference between recovery and permanent injury or death, and it is well to keep in mind the potential value of EEG recording in such cases.

Because of the importance of recognizing drug effects when drugs are given in therapeutic, toxic, and potentially fatal doses, and because drug therapy is by now the mainstay of most psychiatric treatment programs, it is important to review some of the known effects on the EEG of commonly used drugs including psychotherapeutic and psychotomimetic agents.

Table 1 lists some drugs in common use with their principal EEG effects. It should be emphasized that these electrographic changes may occur singly or in any combination. The patterns seen depend on the electrode placement, characteristics of the subject population (patient versus nonpatient, etc.), dosage and route of drug administration, and the baseline or initial electrographic patterns prior to drug

TABLE 1. *The principal EEG effects of some drugs in common use*

Drug	Principal EEG effects
Psychotherapeutic agents	
Phenothiazines	Increase slow activity
	May induce paroxysmal slow bursts
	Diminish % time beta and sigma
Barbiturates	Increase % time beta activity
	Induce beta and sigma activity
Benzodiazepines	Induce persistent beta activity
Amphetamines	May increase % time beta activity
	May decrease postictal slowing
MAO inhibitors	May increase slow activity
Central anticholinergic agents	May diminish alpha abundance
	May decrease postictal slowing
Tricyclic antidepressants	Induce diffuse slow activity
	May induce paroxysmal slow bursts
Lithium	May induce marked and complex episodic activity
Psychotomimetic agents	
Serotonin analogs	May reduce % time alpha
LSD-25	May markedly diminish postictal slowing
Mescaline	
Psylocybin	May diminish EEG "synchrony"
Cannabis-containing drugs	May induce very slight slowing
Analgesics	
Narcotics (opiates)	Increase slow activity
Propoxyphenes	Induce beta activity
Anticonvulsants	
Hydantoins	May decrease alpha frequency
	May decrease % time alpha
	May induce diffuse slowing
Primidone	May induce beta activity
Oxazoladinediones	Usually no effect
Succinimides	Usually no effect
Sulfonamides and derivatives	Usually no effect
Antihistamine derivatives	May induce diffuse slowing

ingestion or injection. What follows here is only a brief and general discussion of the effects of various classes of drugs on the EEG.

Psychotropic Agents

Phenothiazines

All of the phenothiazines may alter the dominant frequencies of the EEG. The alpha rhythm may slow by 1 Hz or more, and there may be appearance of or an increase in slow wave activity. In fact, some of these drugs, particularly chlorpromazine, may induce high voltage paroxysmal slow activity and even seizures in some susceptible individuals. In patients with postconvulsive slowing, phenothiazines actually increase the amount of slow activity already present. The phenothiazines also diminish the percent time of beta activity present, including diminution in amplitude and persistence of sleep spindles.

Barbiturates

Barbiturates produce an increase in percent time beta activity in the EEG, and beta rhythms and spindling may appear as new wave forms in the record (Fig. 2), particularly marked during sleep induced by barbiturate administration.

Benzodiazepines

The benzodiazepine derivatives appear to be particularly potent in provoking the appearance of beta activity (Fig. 3). Such beta activity may persist in the EEG for as long as 2 weeks following the last oral dose of one of these agents.

Anticonvulsants

Hydantoins

All of the hydantoins decrease the frequency of the alpha rhythm if given in sufficient quantity. The percent time alpha is reduced, and at toxic levels the EEG shows diffuse slowing.

Primidone

Primidone (Mysoline) very commonly induces generalized but frontal dominant beta activity.

Oxazoladinediones

The diones usually have no effect on the resting EEG in therapeutic doses.

Succinimides

The succinimides usually have no effect on the EEG in therapeutic doses.

Sulfonamides and Derivatives

Acetazolamide (Diamox) produces no consistent EEG changes.

Antihistamine Derivatives

Carbamazepine (Tegretol) in therapeutic doses usually produces no EEG changes, but in doses approaching toxic levels it induces diffuse slowing.

EFFECTS OF PHYSICAL TREATMENTS ON THE EEG

ECT

ECT induces generalized slowing in the record. After a single treatment, the EEG usually resumes its pretreatment appearance in a relatively short time. As successive treatments are given, however, the generalized delta and theta activity (usually frontal dominant) may become persistent (Fig. 4).

There is a marked individual variation in the sensitivity of the EEG to ECT. In some patients, the record may show very little change after 10 to 12 convulsions, whereas in others a marked degree of persistent abnormality may be obvious after only two or three seizures. The spacing of treatments influences the severity of the EEG abnormalities produced. There may be some persistence of generalized frontal dominant theta activity for several months following the last treatment in the series of 10 to 12 convulsions, or the EEG may return to its pretreatment state within 2 to 4 months.

EEG PATTERNS ASSOCIATED WITH CLASSICAL PSYCHIATRIC DIAGNOSES

Psychoneurotic States

The EEG has been studied in psychoneurotic states including anxiety, hysterical disorders, and obsessive compulsive disturbances. During anxiety and tension, there is reportedly a relatively high incidence of low voltage fast or beta activity and a lesser incidence of well-organized alpha (Fig. 5). Photic stimulation reportedly shows less posterior recruiting than would be expected within the range of eight to ten flashes per sec but more recruiting than normally would be

Central Anticholinergic Agents

The central anticholinergic compounds may result in a decrease in abundance of activity in the EEGs of patients with a high percent time alpha, and the drugs may also diminish postconvulsive slowing.

Tricyclic Antidepressants

All of the tricyclic antidepressants can induce an increase in slow activity in the EEG and may produce paroxysmal slowing. Such episodic slowing is very commonly seen after 7 to 10 days of drug therapy.

Other Psychotherapeutic Agents

Lithium is now being used commonly in the treatment of depression. Lithium can induce EEG changes that are similar to those produced by any other metal, i.e., diffuse continuous slowing, paroxysmal generalized (usually frontal dominant) slowing, and even focal slow EEG abnormalities. These drug-induced EEG changes may be very pronounced, and may be mistaken for abnormalities due to organic brain disorder.

Psychotomimetic Agents

Serotonin Analogs

Drugs such as LSD, mescaline, and psylocybin may produce a decrease in EEG synchrony or a decrease in abundance of dominant activity (diminution in percent time alpha). These drugs may also markedly decrease the amount of slow activity present following electroconvulsive treatment (ECT) or due to organic disturbance.

Cannabis Derivatives

Marijuana, hashish, etc., contain Δ^9-THC as the main active ingredient. In carefully controlled studies, the acute administration of Δ^9-THC by smoking produces no visible effect on the EEG. Frequency analysis may show some slight changes in dominant frequency range, particularly a very slight slowing of the alpha rhythm and a slight increase in theta activity.

Analgesics

Narcotics

All opium derivatives can induce slowing in the EEG, usually first indicated by a decrease in alpha frequency and an increase in alpha amplitude. Large doses can produce diffuse moderate slowing in the EEG. Morphine and meperidine hydrochloride (Demerol) given over long periods of time have somewhat different effects. Chronic meperidine hydrochloride administration induces slowing of the alpha rhythm, and this slowing persists for as long as the meperidine hydrochloride remains in the patient's system. With chronic morphine administration, however, the alpha rhythm first slows, then returns to normal frequency; and with long term administration, the alpha rhythm may even increase in frequency.

Propoxyphenes

Compounds containing propoxyphene hydrochloride (Darvon®) can induce beta activity, most prominent in anterior head regions. If the dosage approaches toxic levels there is a mixed slow and fast pattern in the EEG.

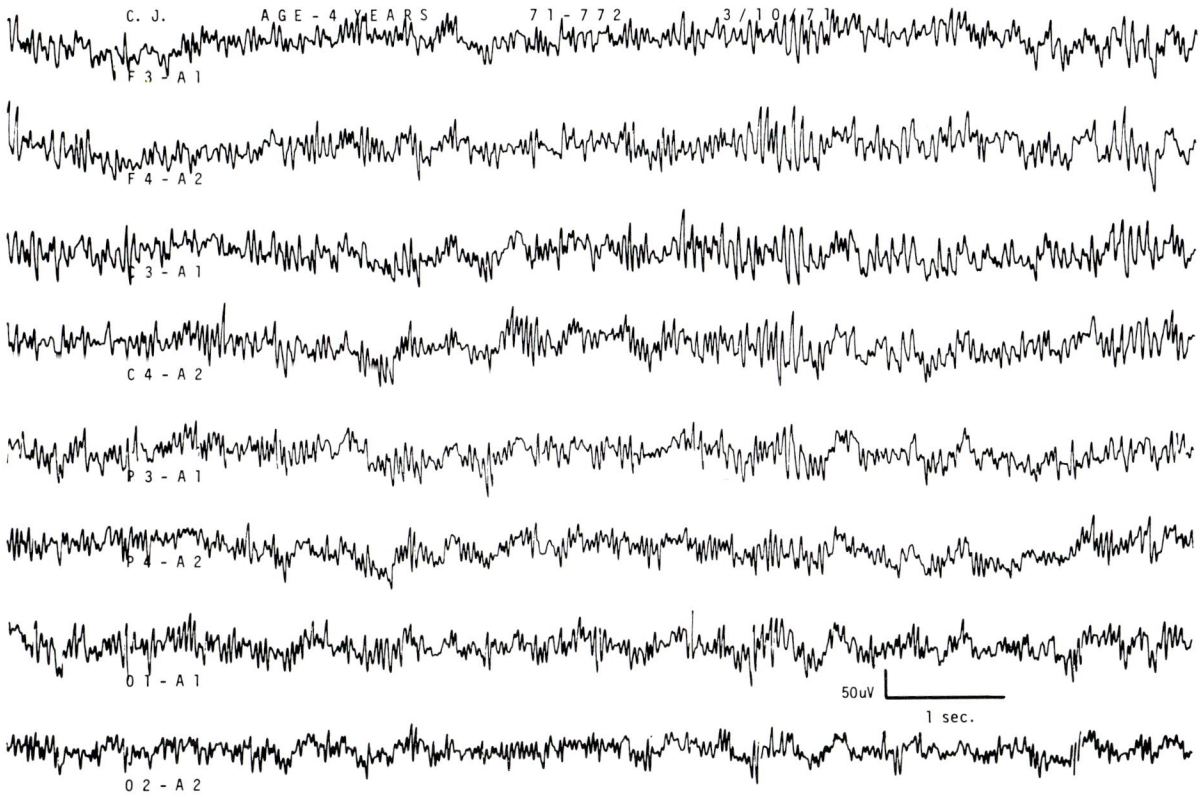

FIG. 3. Diffuse fast activity commonly associated with diazepam medication.

Amphetamines

These drugs may produce an increase in percent time beta activity. They may also decrease the amount of pathological slow activity present in the ongoing EEG.

Monoamine Oxidase (MAO) Inhibitors

These drugs have varying effects on the EEG, but agents such as iproniazid (Marsilid®) may induce some increase in abundance of slower frequencies.

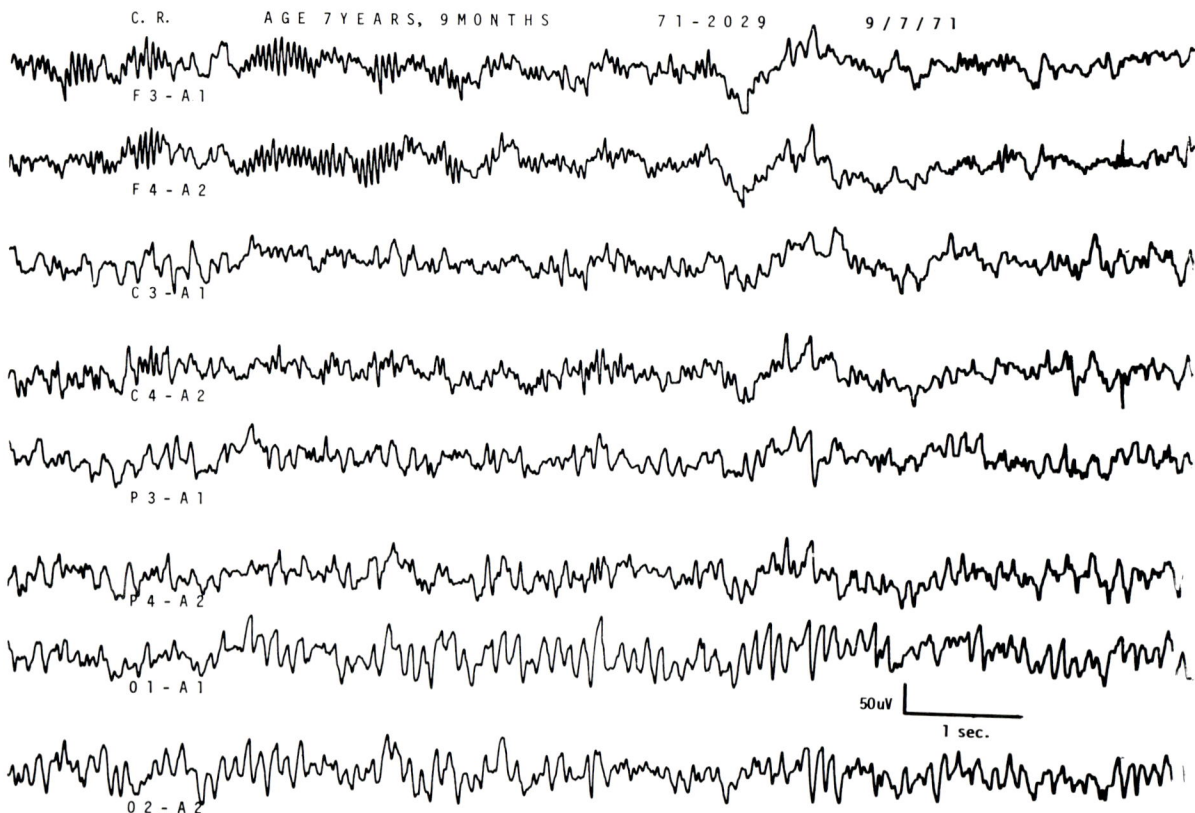

FIG. 2. Mild frontal fast activity induced by barbiturate in therapeutic dosage.

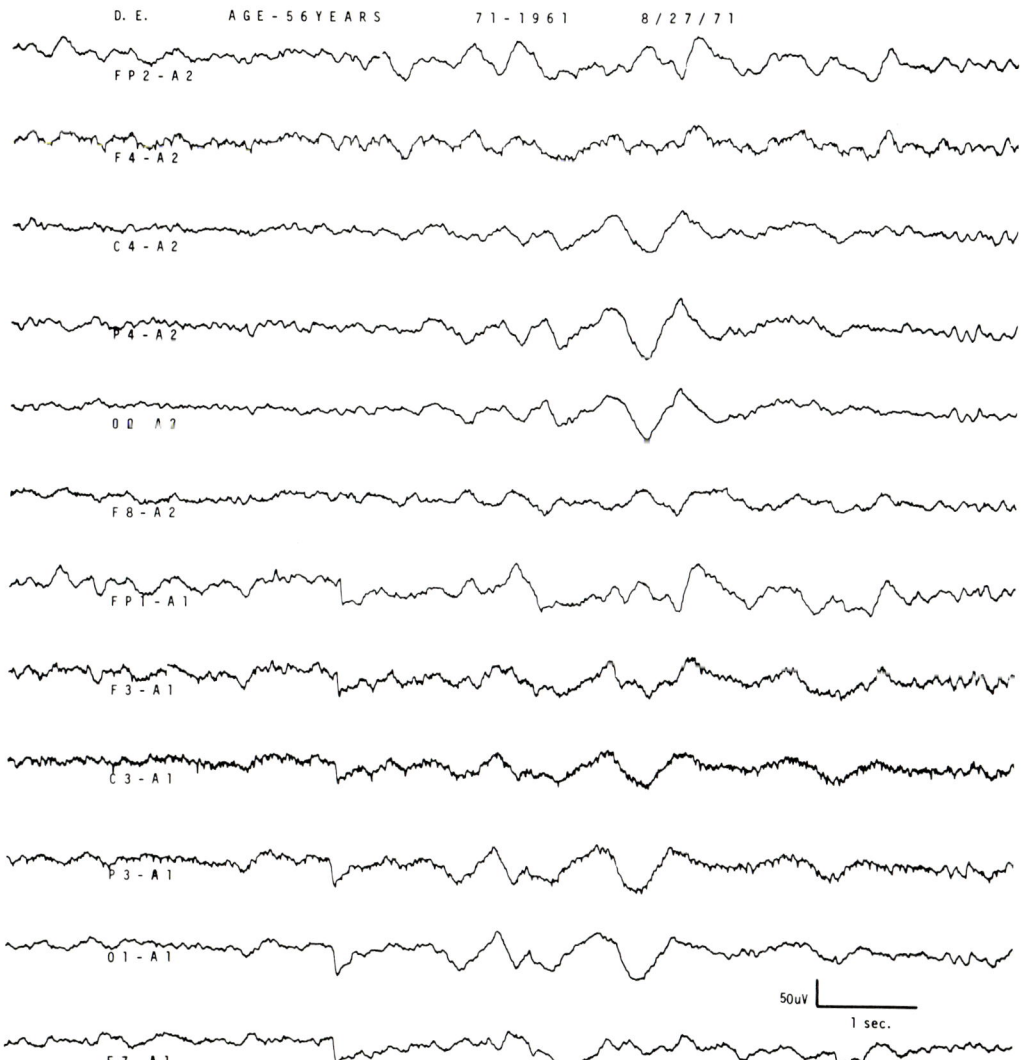

FIG. 4. Episodic, frontal dominant delta and theta activity, 3 weeks after last ECT (series of eight).

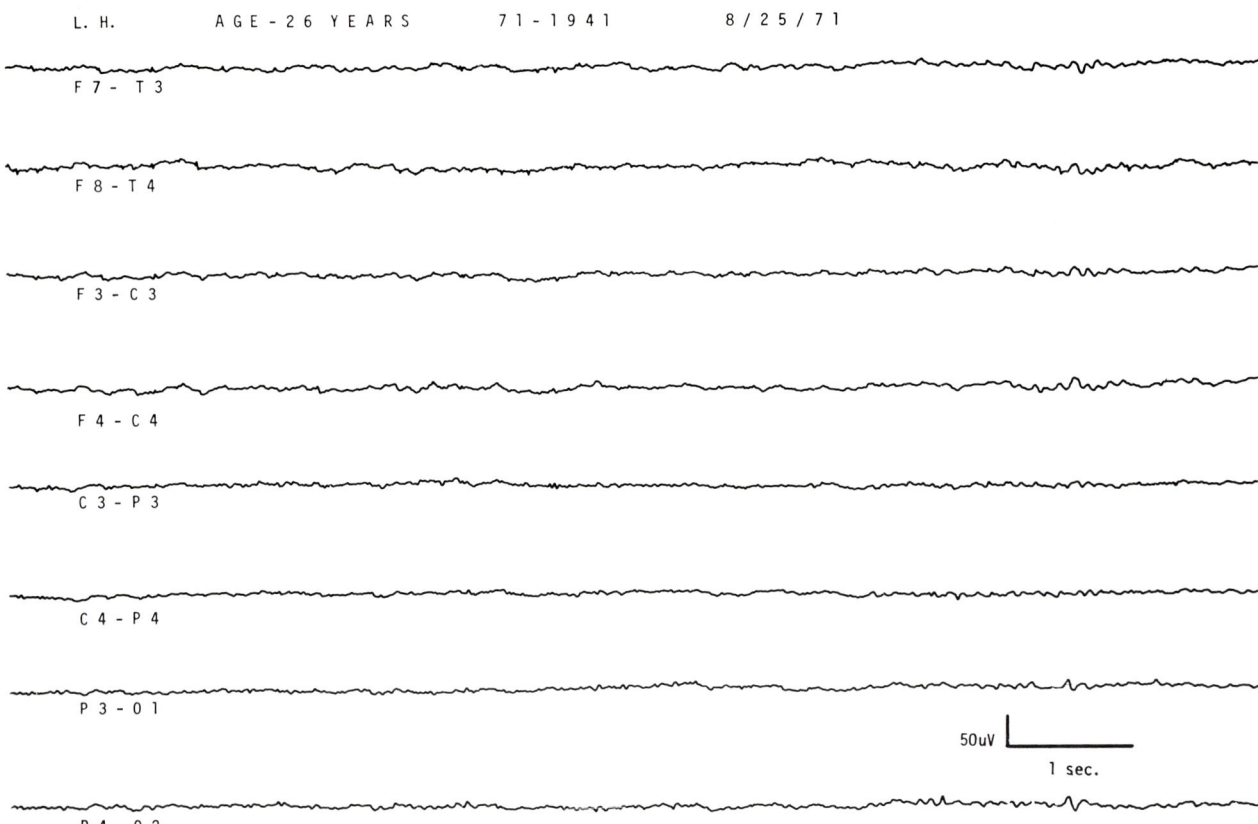

FIG. 5. Low voltage EEG, common in anxious patients.

expected with slower and higher flash frequencies. In addition, an increase in anxiety and other symptoms may be experienced by the patient during photic stimulation.

Affective Disorders

In the affective disorders (such as manic depressive psychosis), there are no significant alterations reported in EEG patterns except for a somewhat wider range of alpha frequencies than normally encountered. Shagass (5) has described a technique of determining the sedation threshold, which is a method of producing anterior dominant fast activity in the EEG by intravenous injection of amobarbital. He describes a low threshold for production of fast activity in organic psychotic states and high thresholds in schizophrenia. Similarly, he describes a high threshold in neurotic depression with a low threshold in endogenous depressive states. These results have not been generally accepted because of difficulty in replicating the findings.

The EEG in Schizophrenias

The EEGs of truly schizophrenic individuals do not show any specific abnormality and may be within the normal range. However, various reports in the literature have indicated that schizophrenic patients have a higher incidence of EEG abnormality (20 to 60%) as compared to nonpsychiatric patients of similar age (6). These abnormalities consist chiefly of excessive amounts of theta activity, and the incidence of such abnormalities is highest in patients with catatonic schizophrenia.

The relatively high incidence of occurrence of EEG abnormality in patients with schizophrenia as compared to those with affective psychoses, for example, has been cited by some investigators as further evidence that, like so-called idiopathic petit mal epilepsy, schizophrenia may occur as a result of an interaction of genetic factors (with definite age penetrance) and acquired brain damage. There are other possibilities, of course, but in considering the most obvious alternative, i.e., that the behavior disorder itself somehow changes neural activity so that EEG abnormalities develop, one is confronted with the classic dilemma of which comes first, the neuronal abnormality or the behavioral one.

Hill (7) has reported epileptiform abnormalities in 20 to 25% of his schizophrenic subjects. These abnormalities chiefly consist of fast spike-and-wave complexes in the 4 to 5 Hz range and bilaterally synchronous episodic slow wave discharges. As discussed above, it is necessary to evaluate such patients in great detail clinically because of the possibility that in some of them, the schizophrenic state might be a reflection of an underlying seizure disorder that actually has produced the EEG abnormality.

SO-CALLED SPECIFIC ELECTROGRAPHIC ABNORMALITIES IN PSYCHIATRIC AND BEHAVIOR DISORDERS

Lastly, I would like to mention four electrographic patterns that have at various times been reported to indicate more or less specifically the presence of some psychiatric or behavioral disturbance. These are the Mitten pattern of Gibbs, the exceedingly or rare fast pattern of Gibbs, the "choppy" EEG pattern, and the 14 and 6 Hz positive spikes. It is beyond the scope of my undertaking here to discuss these patterns and their significance in detail (see Chapter 14). It should be sufficient to warn the reader that none of these patterns has been proved to have any specific association whatever with any particular clinical entity, psychiatric or otherwise.

ACKNOWLEDGMENTS

The author is indebted to Frances Burton and Pat Dakin for their assistance in manuscript preparation.

REFERENCES

1. Pincus, J. H., and Tucker, G. J. (1974): *Behavioral Neurology,* p. 205. Oxford, New York.
2. Flor-Henry, P. (1972): Ictal and interictal psychiatric manifestations in epilepsy. *Epilepsia,* 13:773–783.
3. Klonoff, H., and Low, M. D. (1974): Disordered brain function in young children and early adolescents: Neuropsychological and electroencepahlographic correlates. In: *Clinical Neuropsychology: Current Status and Applications,* edited by R. M. Reitan and L. A. Davison, pp. 121–165. V. H. Winston, Washington, D.C.
4. Satterfield, J. H., Lesser, L. I., Saul, R. E., and Cantwell, D. P. (1973): EEG aspects in the diagnosis and treatment of minimal brain dysfunction. *Ann. NY Acad. Sci.,* 205:274–282.
5. Shagass, C. (1954): The sedation threshold, a method for estimating tension in psychiatric patients. *Electroencephalogr. Clin. Neurophysiol.,* 6:221–233.
6. Struve, F. A., and Honigfeld, A. (1971): Routine electroencephalograms of psychiatric patients awake and asleep. *Clinical EEG,* 1:3.
7. Hill, D. (1963): Psychiatry. In: *Electroencephalography,* 2nd ed. edited by D. Hill and G. Parr. Macmillan, New York.

GENERAL REFERENCES

Glaser, G. H. (editor) (1963): *EEG and Behavior.* Basic Books, New York.
Wilson, W. P. (editor) (1965): *Applications of Electroencephalography in Psychiatry.* Duke University Press, Durham.

Chapter 14

EEG Patterns of Uncertain Diagnostic Significance

Robert L. Maulsby

Department of Neurology, Wayne State University School of Medicine, Detroit, Michigan 48201

Historical Perspective	411
Fourteen-and-Six per Second Positive Spikes	412
The Six per Second Spike and Wave Pattern	414
The Psychomotor Variant Discharge	414
Small Sharp Spikes	417
Summary	418
References	418

This chapter comments on 14 and 6/sec positive spikes, 6/sec spike-and-wave, psychomotor variants and small sharp spikes specifically. In general, these comments pertain to any uncommon pattern which is not an expected finding in the "ideal" normal record, yet not definitely abnormal or, at least, poorly correlated with pathophysiology. The purpose of this chapter is mainly to suggest possible ways of dealing with these patterns in EEG reports and practice.

HISTORICAL PERSPECTIVE

One wonders why, after all of these years, we still have EEG patterns of uncertain diagnostic significance. Perhaps it has to do with the fact that some patterns occur infrequently, but I think the main answer lies in the quality of what is called clinical EEG research.

Much of it has been poorly done in the past and continues to inspire uncertainty.

Here is an example for perspective: A certain pattern was first distinguished and popularized in the 1950s. It was said to correlate with seizures, headaches, emotional instability, hyperactivity, autonomic lability, aggressivity, peptic ulcers, tinnitus, asthma, premenstrual tension, hypertension, hyperthyroidism, urticaria, psychiatric problems of all types, discrete involvement of structures at the base of the brain, tuberculous meningitis, obesity, narcolepsy, enuresis, "chiasmatic syndrome," "posterior fossa syndrome," parasagittal tumors, irritative lesions in the Rolandic cortex, Little's disease, etc., etc. Presumably, judging from reports, many diagnoses were strengthened by this finding over a period of about 10 years until normative studies and better controls finally revealed it to be just as common in healthy people as in the ill. Interest in the pattern lagged, publication about it practically stopped, and finally textbooks began to refer to it as a normal pattern. What was this pattern? The mu rhythm (1). Now most EEGers agree that it is a normal pattern found in about 20% of the population, sometimes enhanced or rendered nonreactive by local disturbances, but, by itself, not diagnostically significant.

FOURTEEN-AND-SIX PER SECOND POSITIVE SPIKES

Another pattern with about the same incidence as mu rhythm has an even more notorious history in this country and seems to be running a similar course—the pattern of 14- and 6/sec positive spikes (Fig. 1). The reader need not be reminded about all the clinical conditions with which this pattern has been "correlated"—a totally heterogeneous collection of complaints commonly found in teenagers and children. These usually reduce to a $1/3$–$1/3$–$1/3$ mixture of symptoms: questionable seizures, headaches-abdominal pain, and behavioral disturbances. Unfortunately, a great many patients who exhibit this pattern have been told they have thalamic or hypothalamic epilepsy or "convulsive equivalent disorder." Publications on this pattern had been appearing at a fantastic rate in the 1950s and 1960s but have now dropped to a mere trickle following the normative studies of Lombroso (11) and Eeg-Olofsson (3).

The controversy over positive spikes has not yet died completely; however, I predict that within the next five years, this pattern will also be moved to the textbook chapter dealing with normal patterns. It is probably a sleep pattern which occurs normally in 20% to 50% of teenagers. But this is not to deny that, like any other normal rhythm, it may be abnormally enhanced by certain organic cerebral disorders.

Looking backward, I think the mistakes made or the over-enthusiasm exhibited can be attributed to poorly controlled EEG research. The typical EEG research strategy of the past has been as follows:

1. Search for sharp pointed waves. From experience with epilepsy, many researchers automatically equate any unusual finding in the EEG with abnormality, particularly if the discharge is sharp or spikey.

2. Distinguish this pattern from all others and collect a group of patients with it.

3. Ask the patients, "What's wrong with you?" i.e., develop a "symptom profile."

4. Equate the EEG finding with the most common symptoms or clinical diagnoses in the group.

5. Publish.

A diagnostic relationship thus established tends to build upon itself, particularly if the symptoms are common. For example, a child is referred for head injury or syncope and his EEG shows

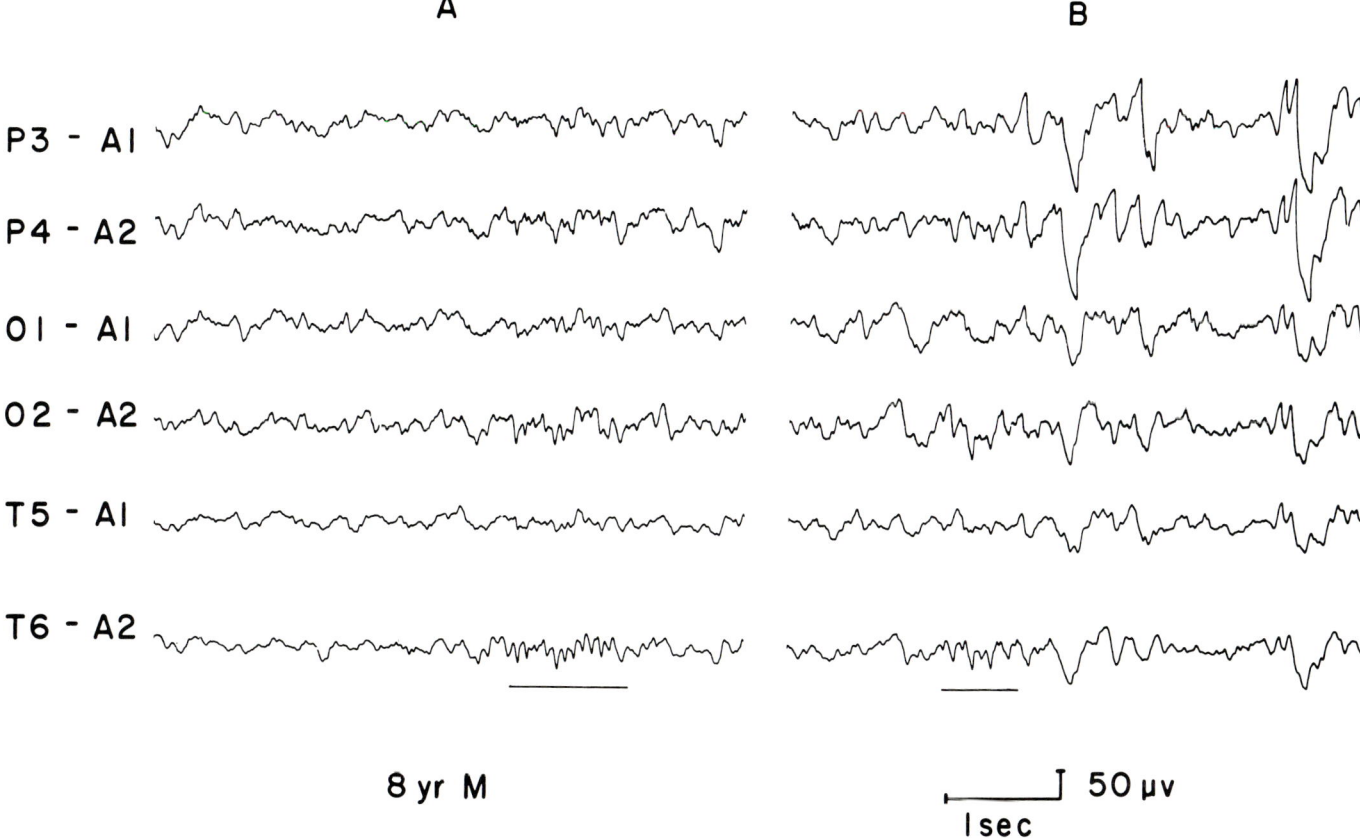

FIG. 1. Bursts of 14 and 6 Hz positive spikes in a 8-year-old boy being evaluated for poor school work. Neurological examination and neurological history were unremarkable. **A:** Illustrates the 14 Hz-positive spike burst *(underlined)* in the right posterior temporal region during stage 1 sleep. **B:** Shows 6 Hz positive spikes in the same area during stage 2 sleep.

14- and 6/sec positive spikes. The mother is then carefully questioned about headaches, abdominal pain, school difficulties, behavioral disturbance, etc. One of these will likely be found and correlations strengthened. Or, a patient may be referred primarily for headache and abdominal pain. In this case, the technicians, to please their chief, take extra care to record during drowsiness with the proper montage and then labor to elicit a few positive spikes by auditory stimulation at the right stage of sleep. Or, it is possible for the interpreter to overreact to any questionable sharp waves recorded over the back of the head, being biased by the clinical complaint.

The result of this type of research has been that nonuniversal EEG patterns, when first recognized, were often assumed to be abnormal. Papers were published and diagnoses were based on them until some skeptical EEGers finally made normative studies.

THE SIX PER SECOND SPIKE AND WAVE PATTERN

The 6/sec spike and wave pattern (Fig. 2) is much less common than 14- and 6/sec positive spikes. The incidence is usually cited in most clinical populations as less than 1% (13,14,17). However, Milstein and Small (12) found a 3.2% incidence in psychiatric hospital admissions. Gibbs and Gibbs (6) reported a 2.8% incidence in normal persons between the ages of 15 and 19, and Tharp (16) was able to induce the pattern in 30% of normal young volunteers given diphenhydramine.

The symptom profile for the 6/sec spike and wave pattern is the familiar $1/3$–$1/3$–$1/3$ mixture of headaches plus autonomic symptoms, questionable seizures, and psychiatric problems. As Thomas and Klass (17) astutely pointed out, this is the typical symptom profile for any group of patients in this age group referred for EEG. These authors conclude that "in terms of its clinical significance, the 6/sec spike-and-wave pattern in the EEG provides no proof for the presence of epilepsy, either on the basis of statistical probability or in direct relationship with the symptoms of an individual patient." In his comprehensive review of the literature on this subject, Chatrian (2) has reached a similar conclusion.

THE PSYCHOMOTOR VARIANT DISCHARGE

The psychomotor variant pattern is another rare finding (Fig. 3). Some regard it not only as an interictal sign of seizure disorder but as an ictal discharge (8). It remains dubious because a) the correlates of this pattern have a familiar ring—the same old $1/3$–$1/3$–$1/3$ mixture of symptoms, and b) normative studies have shown it to be as common in normal persons as in the sick. Gibbs et al. (7) report a 0.5% incidence of the pattern in symptomatic patients sent for EEGs; Garvin's (5) incidence was 0.28%; Lipman and Hughes' (10) was 0.33%. Normative studies are hard to find: Gibbs (7) admits only 2 out of 1,700 in his normal series; the Swedish group (17), however, found this pattern in 1.1% of their 6 to 14 year old age group, and in my own study of normal adults for NASA, there was a 2% incidence (Maulsby, *unpublished data*).[1] If these scanty figures mean anything, we can conclude that the psychomotor variant pattern is two to four times more common in normal than in patient populations. This discrepancy by itself leads me to doubt the diagnostic significance of this pattern in a patient, no matter what his complaint.

The claim that the psychomotor variant pattern is an ictal dis-

---

[1] The normative electroencephalographic data reference library: Final report.

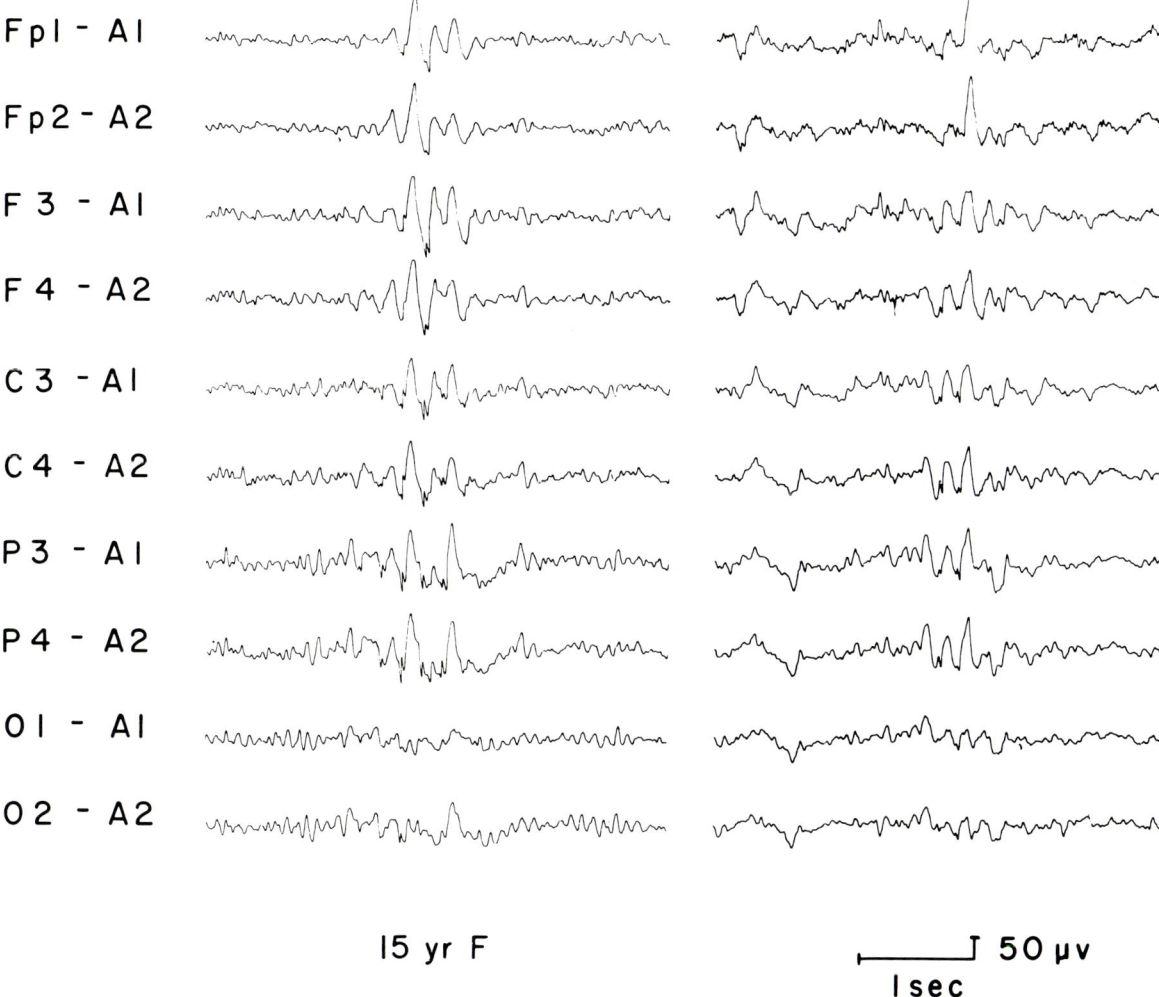

FIG. 2. Bursts of 6 Hz spike-and-wave activity in a 15-year-old girl referred for headaches. Neurological examination was within normal limits and there was no history of seizures or losses of consciousness. Spike components of the discharges are usually maximum in parietal and central leads, and are relatively low in voltage with variable polarity. The bursts are more prominent in the relaxed or drowsy state. In older patients, these discharges are often of very low voltage and are difficult to distinguish from background activity, hence, the name "phantom" spike-and-slow-wave sometimes given to this phenomenon.

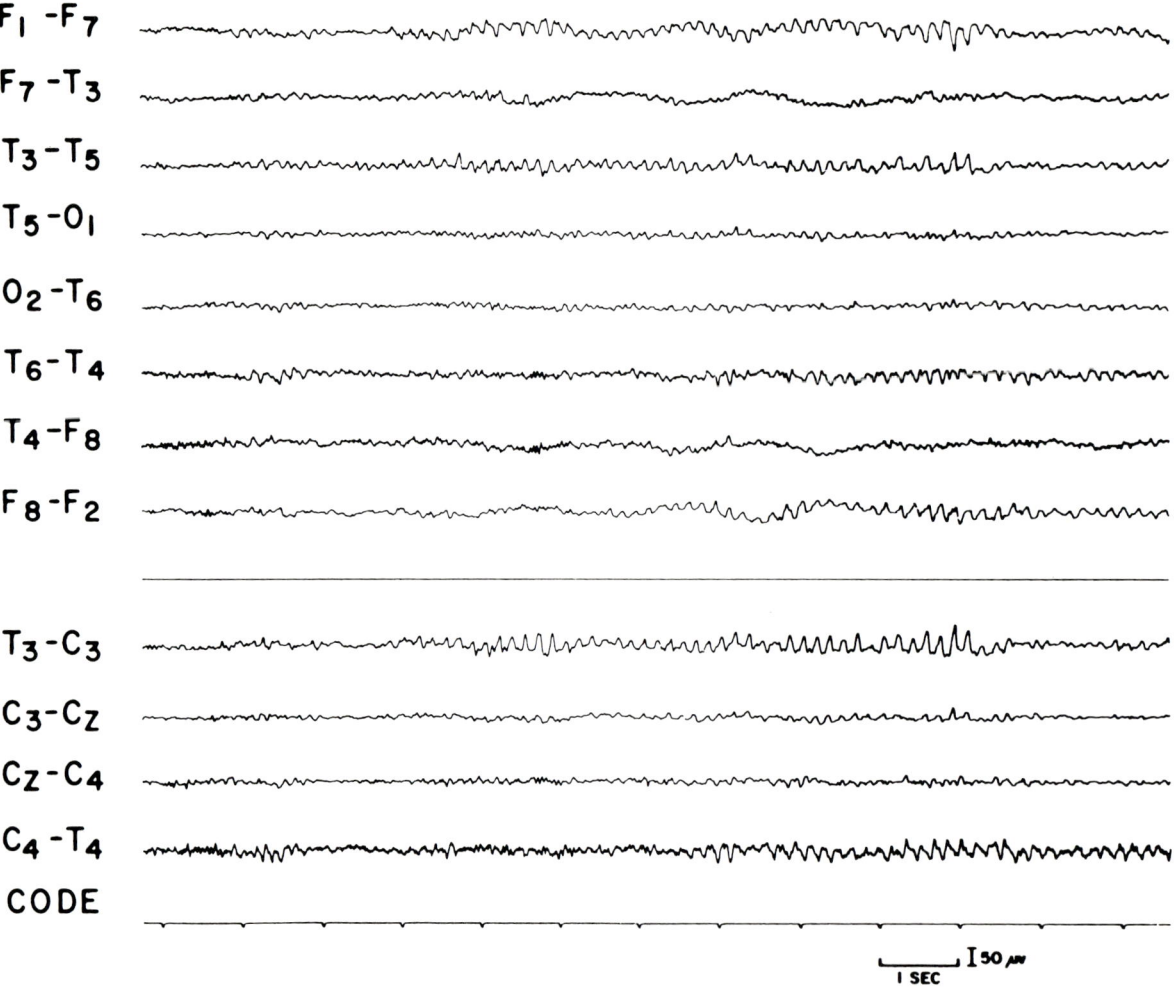

FIG. 3. The so-called psychomotor variant discharge in a neurologically normal, asymptomatic 26-year-old male (from the Baylor Normative EEG Data Reference Library). Sharp, notched theta rhythms appear in temporal leads bilaterally during drowsiness. These are approximately equipotential and maximum at electrodes F7-T3 and F8-T4. The slow potentials in this sample are artifacts caused by slow, rolling, left-to-right eye movements associated with the drowsy state.

charge rests on studies of 11 patients who showed this pattern (8). Reaction time determinations were made during the discharge and compared to reaction times of the same patients when the EEG showed no discharges; 6 of the 11 patients showed a longer reaction time during the discharge. However, this does not establish the ictal nature of the discharge because it most often occurs during drowsiness. Drowsiness is known to lengthen reaction time and control reaction times were usually taken just before the discharge appeared, i.e. probably at a higher level of vigilance.

SMALL SHARP SPIKES

For discussion of small sharp spikes (SSS) (see Fig. 4), the paper by Reiher and Klass (17) is essential. Compare this to what the Gibbses (6) say: "This pattern again is said to correlate with seizures and headaches or dizziness but not so often with psychiatric difficulty as the patterns above." Again, evidence shows that this pattern is just as common in normals as in the ill. Gibbs (6) quotes an 8% incidence in his 40 to 49-year-old normal controls.

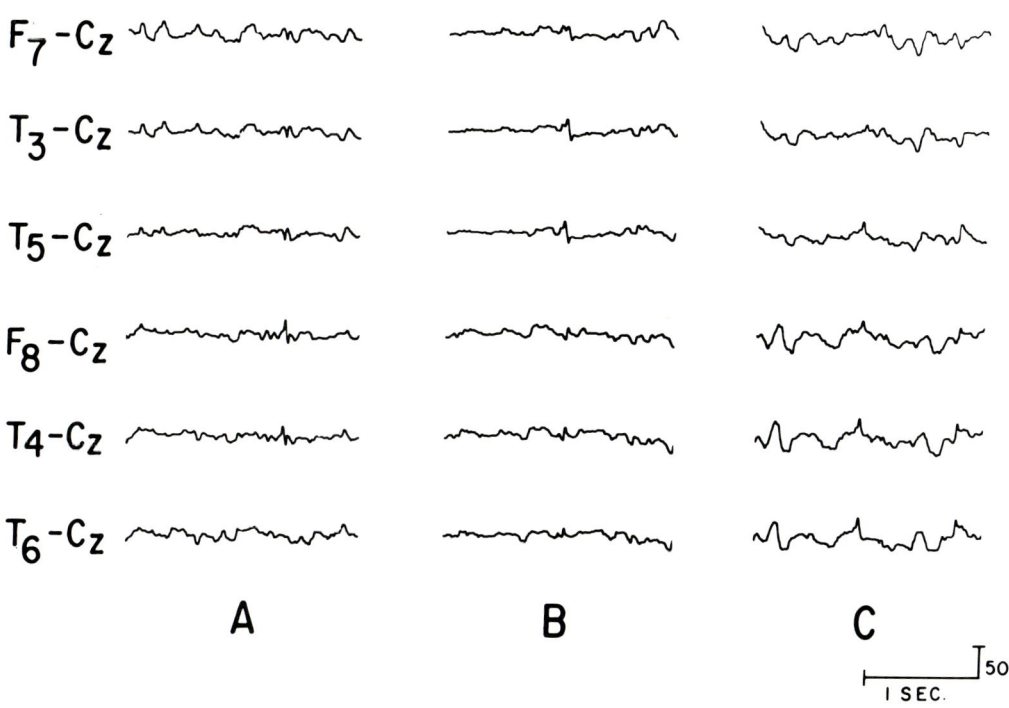

FIG. 4. Examples of small, sharp spikes in a 55-year-old man who had sensory and motor deficits of the extremities associated with cervical spondylosis. These small, sharp spikes are recorded from lateral electrodes over both hemispheres during stage 1 sleep. The waking record was normal. The patient had no signs or symptoms of cerebral disturbance. **A, B,** and **C** are sections from the record separated by several sec.

Two recent studies (9,18) are even more convincing. Lebel et al. found that there is no significant difference in the incidence of SSS between groups of patients matched for age with and without epileptic seizures (26% and 25% respectively). Furthermore, White et al. (18), in a large well controlled study, found a *higher* incidence of small sharp spikes in their group of normal volunteers (24%) as compared to their patient population (20%).

SUMMARY

What can be said the next time you encounter one of these controversial patterns? Here are the alternatives:

1. You can read all of the literature, pro and con, and then decide on the basis of the scientific merit displayed in the articles; apply statistics.
2. You can ignore the pattern and wait until all researchers agree.
3. You can call it abnormal just in case because you do not want to miss anything.
4. You can launch your own research program.
5. Toss a coin.
6. Decide on personal grounds or on the past reliability of the researcher.
7. You can equivocate, i.e., let the referring physician decide.

Obviously, all of these approaches have limitations: scientific merit is often difficult to judge; one should not ignore EEG findings; recognition of a pattern does not automatically make it abnormal; launching your own research program can be expensive, and so forth. Leaving the judgment to the referring physician through equivocation is a frequent practice, but one must realize that he is even less well-versed in these matters than the EEGer who has interest and experience. Also, consider this question: What are you going to say on the witness stand if you are called to testify in a court trial?

I think the most practical and ethical approach, realizing that you may be wrong, is to take a firm stand on the conservative side. In other words, do not call it abnormal. Records should be viewed as defendants in a trial—normal unless proved abnormal. These patterns are not proof of abnormality.

An adequate statement in the impression might be, "No definite evidence of cerebral abnormality." Then, an optional note could be added to the effect that this record shows a pattern which some authorities have considered abnormal. This view has been disputed and insufficient evidence exists to attribute any diagnostic significance to this finding. Or, more simply, "The record shows such-and-such a pattern; this is considered to be of doubtful diagnostic significance."

REFERENCES

1. Chatrian, G. E. (1976): The mu rhythm. In: *Handbook of EEG and Clinical Neurophysiology,* Vol. 6A, edited by A. Rémond and G. C. Chatrian, pp. 46–68. Elsevier, Amsterdam.
2. Chatrian, G. E. (1976): Paraoxysmal patterns in "normal" subjects. In: *Handbook of EEG and Clinical Neurophysiology,* Vol. 6A, edited by A. Rémond and G. C. Lairy, pp. 114–122. Elsevier, Amsterdam.
3. Eeg-Olofsson, O. (1971): The development of the electroencephalogram in normal children from the age of 1 through 15 years: 14 and 6 Hz positive spike phenomenon. *Neuropadiatrie,* 2:405–427.
4. Eeg-Olofsson, O., Petersen, I. and Sellden, U. (1971): The development of the electroencephalogram in normal children from the age of 1 through 15 years: Paroxysmal activity. *Neuropädiatrie,* 2:375–404.
5. Garvin, J. S. (1968): Psychomotor variant pattern. *Dis. Nerv. Syst.,* 29:307–309.
6. Gibbs, F. A., and Gibbs, E. L. (1964): *Atlas of Electroencephalography, Vol. 3.* Addison-Wesley Pub. Co., Reading, Massachusetts.
7. Gibbs, F. A., Rich, C. L., and Gibbs, E. L. (1963): Psychomotor variant type of seizure discharge. *Neurology,* 13:991–998.

8. Hughes, J. R., and Cayaffa, J. J. (1973): Is the "psychomotor variant"- "rhythmic mid-temporal discharge" an ictal pattern? *Clin. Electroencephalogr.,* 4:42–52.
9. Lebel, M., Reiher, J. and Klass, D. W. (1977): Small sharp spikes (SSS): Reassessment of electroencephalographic characteristics and clinical significance. Central Association of Electroencephalographers. St. Louis, Missouri.
10. Lipman, I. J., and Hughes, J. R. (1969): Rhythmic mid-temporal discharges. An electroclinical study. *Electroencephalogr. Clin. Neurophysiol.,* 27:43–47.
11. Lombroso, C. T., Schwartz, I. H., Clark, D. M., Muench, H., and Barry J. (1966): Ctenoids in healthy youths: Controlled study of 14-and-6-per second spiking. *Neurology,* 16:1152–1158.
12. Milstein, V., and Small, J. G. (1971): Psychological correlates of 14 and 6 positive spikes, 6/sec spike-wave, and small sharp spike transients. *Clin. Electroencephalogr.,* 2:206–212.
13. Olson, S. F., Arbit, J., and Hughes, J. R. (1971): Psychological testing in patients with the 6 c/sec spike-and-wave complex: a controlled study. *Clin. Electroencephalogr.,* 2:202–205.
14. Olson, S. F. and Hughes, J. R. (1970): The clinical symptomatology associated with the 6 c/sec spike-and-wave complex. *Epilepsia,* 11:383–393.
15. Reiher, J. and Klass, D. W. (1968): Two common EEG patterns of doubtful clinical significance. *Med. Clin. N. Amer.,* 52:933–940.
16. Tharp, B. R. (1966): The 6-per-second spike and wave complex. *Arch. Neurol.,* 15:533–537.
17. Thomas, J. E., and Klass, D. W. (1968): Six-per-second spike-and-wave pattern in the electroencephalogram. *Neurology,* 18:587–593.
18. White, J. C., Langston, J. W. and Pedley, T. (1977): Benign epileptiform transients of sleep: clarification of the "small sharp spike" controversy. *Neurology,* 27:1061–1068.

Chapter 15

Neurophysiologic Substrates of EEG Activity

Eli S. Goldensohn

Department of Neurology, College of Physicians and Surgeons of Columbia University, New York, New York 10032

The Structure of the Generators in the Cortex	422
Cortical Potentials that Generate EEG Waves	424
Cortical Potentials that Generate Epileptiform EEG Activity	425
Role of the Thalamus in Normal and Abnormal EEG Activity	428
Electrical Activity at the Cortical Surface in Experimental Epileptogenic Foci	432
Human Epileptogenic Foci	432
How the Human EEG Differs Between the Cortex and the Scalp	434
References	438

Clinical interpretation of the EEG is almost entirely empirical—we say that the waves indicate that the patient is awake or has a destructive lesion or a tendency toward epilepsy because of known correlations between clinical states and EEG patterns. The EEG record, however, contains much more information. It reflects normal organized cellular activity within the brain and indicates how it is modified by disease. This chapter discusses some of the mechanisms involved in the generation of normal and abnormal EEG activity and indicates ways in which understanding this information can be of value in clinical EEG interpretation.

It was natural that following the discovery of brain waves in man by Hans Berger (10), attempts to explain the waves were made in terms of action potentials, as investigators had already begun intensive studies on the properties of axons (21). The idea that summation of the action potentials of neurons caused EEG waves, however, was soon found to be inadequate to account for the relatively slower waves of the EEG. Two important ideas concerning the generation of EEG waves developed simultaneously in the 1940s and 1950s; one, which was rapidly accepted, was that the thalamus was capable of exerting widespread control over cortical EEG activity (8), and the other was that EEG waves are summations of graded synaptic potentials (28). The latter concept has been further strengthened by the use of intracellularly placed electrodes in living cortex (12, 19,23,27). Much is now known about the elements that generate normal and abnormal EEG waves and how they relate to each other. The EEG as seen at the scalp is generated by a complex organization of neural elements that reside solely in the cerebral cortex, although it is modified by incoming activity from other areas.

THE STRUCTURE OF THE GENERATORS IN THE CORTEX

The human cerebral cortex is a 3-mm deep covering of gray matter with six layers numbered from the subpial surface toward the depth. The lamination is best seen using stains that show cell bodies but do not stain the dendrites and axons that ramify throughout the layers. The two main types of neurons are the pyramidal cells in layers 3, 4, and 5 and the stellate cells mainly in layer 4. Intermediate types include star pyramids in the second layer and fusiform cells in the fifth and sixth layers. The star pyramids can be classified anatomically with the pyramidal cells and the fusiform with the stellate cells. Figure 1A (35) shows the cell types and their processes in the neocortex, including the vertically oriented pyramidal cells with long apical dendrites. Figure 1B (33) pictures the cortical structure in terms of operational circuits. Although oversimplified, it takes into consideration the major principles. There is no direct proof that the basket cells are responsible for the collateral inhibition indicated in the diagram, but there is much supporting indirect evidence. Cortical interneurons of the basket type contact pyramidal cell bodies with presumed inhibitory synapses (Gray type 1). In contrast, endings found on apical dendrites are presumed excitatory ones (Gray type 2) (5). Although the functional correlations of Gray type 1 and Gray type 2 synapses are not fully established, further morphologic differences between these two types have been described (2). It has been shown that the processes of the basket-type stellate cells have a wider tangential spread in the deeper cortical layers (30), suggesting greater inhibition in the deeper layers. Our intracellular electrode depth records described below also support the idea of a functional laminar distribution with excitation being greater in the more superficial layers of the cortex.

Spines on the superficially located dendrites of pyramidal cells receive what appear to be excitatory type contacts that number up to a few thousand per dendritic tree. Pyramidal cell bodies receive what seem to be inhibitory-type endings numbering only 50 to 100 contacts per cell body. Thus, excitatory impulses appear to arrive by the thousands mainly on the dendritic spines near the cortical surface, and inhibitory synapses—which are much fewer—are strategically placed more deeply on the cell body where they can prevent the generation of action potentials. Most action potentials generated in one part of the cerebral cortex go to other regions of the cortex;

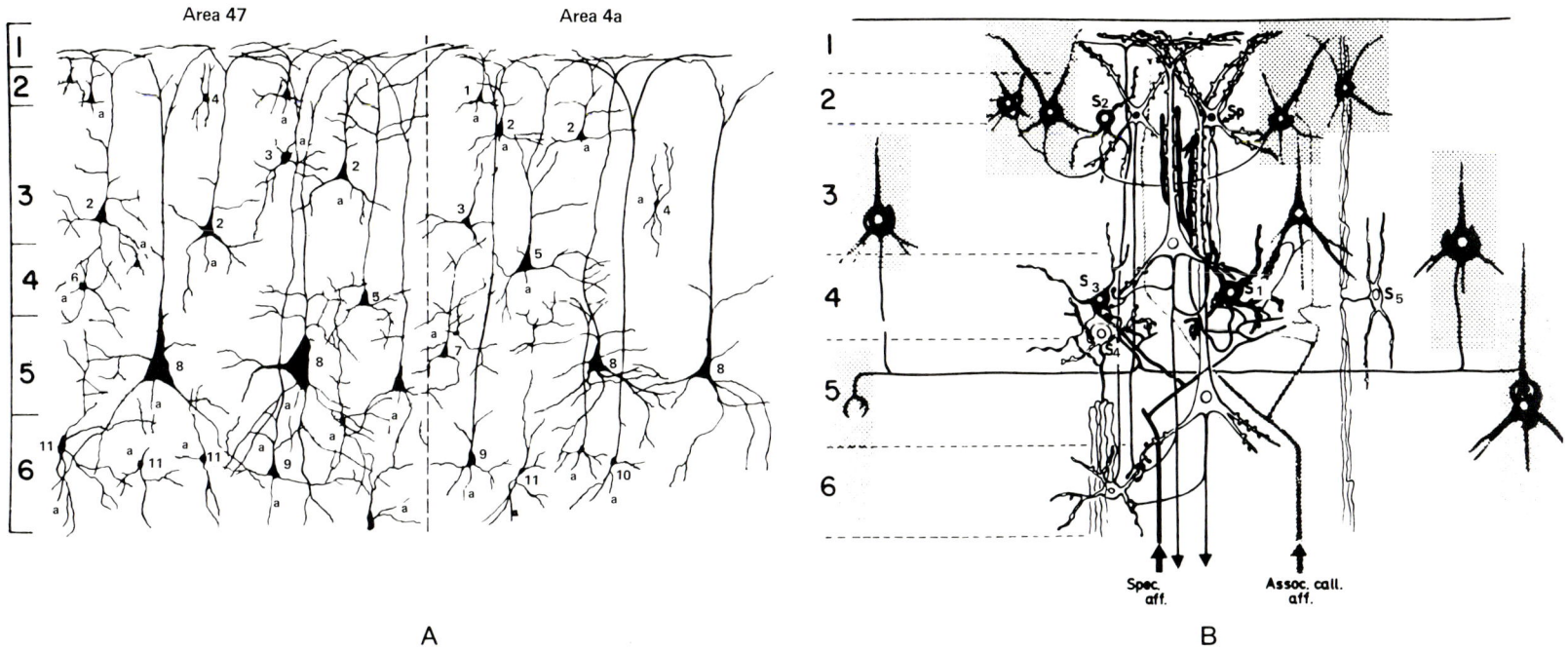

FIG. 1. A: Stratification of cells and their processes in the cerebral cortex of man. Note deeply located pyramidal cell bodies in layer 5 with their superficially located apical dendrites in layers 1 and 2. Drawn after Golgi preparations. (From Von Bonin, 1949.) **B:** Cell types in neocortex and their interconnections. Basket-type stellate interneurons (S2) have short-range pericellular connections in the second layer. Basket cells in layers 3 and 4 distribute their processes in larger areas of 500μ radius or more; in layers 5 and 6, their distribution may be still larger. If basket cells are inhibitory, this distribution would indicate greater inhibition in the deeper layers. Excitation is greatest in the superficial neuropil of layers 1 and 2 (5) (from ref. 33).

only a fraction go to subcortical areas, and many of those go to nuclei whose major output is, in turn, back to the cortex. It has been suggested that information processing occurs stepwise in successively arranged echelons of the cortex, each of which is constructed to extract some meaningful element of information (33). This concept is in keeping with the idea that the structural design of the cortex rests on complex interconnections among a tremendous number of mosaic-like units arranged in vertical columns. In Fig. 2, the presence

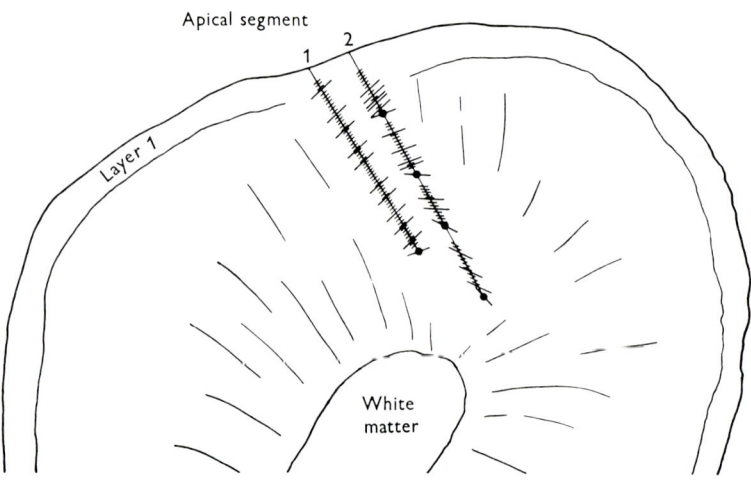

FIG. 2. Discrete, narrow columns of cortical cells which respond to restricted retinal stimuli. Reconstruction of two parallel microelectrode penetrations in the visual cortex of the cat. A given cell responds when an appropriate stimulus of specific orientation is shone on the retina. The longer lines intersecting the electrode tracks represent responsive cortical cells. The directions of the lines indicate the axes of the effective stimuli with lines perpendicular to the tracks representing horizontal orientation. Scale: 1 mm. (From ref. 15.)

of such columns in the cortex of the occipital lobe is shown (15). The hippocampus is also a layered structure with vertical orientation of its major cell processes (Fig. 3). As in the neocortex, strongly inhibitory synapses are located on the cell body (4). Thus, both the neocortex and the hippocampus seem to be organized in vertically oriented columns in which excitation occurs at dendrites predominantly near the surface and inhibition occurs predominantly near the cell body.

CORTICAL POTENTIALS THAT GENERATE EEG WAVES

The electroencephalogram and electrocorticogram measure external currents generated by differences in potential between one part of a neuron and another. The EEG waves in experimental animals and undoubtedly also in man are the result of the summation of excitatory postsynaptic potentials (EPSPs) and inhibitory postsynaptic potentials (IPSPs) that are depolarizations and hyperpolarizations, respectively, across the membranes of neurons (Figs. 4 and 5) (7,12). Currents generated by synchronous postsynaptic potentials near one or the other pole of the vertically oriented columns of neurons have relatively strong fields that are ample to generate the EEG activity. It has been estimated that a 100-μm cube in the pyramidal layer contains five to eight pyramidal cells (31). That number in columnar organization (Figs. 1 and 3) can easily generate currents of sufficient amplitude for the surface EEG activity (24).

There is little or no contribution to the EEG from the action potentials of cells and axons. It has been shown that the action potentials of large pyramidal cells have very localized electrical fields that are not evident at the cortical surface (16). An action potential does not set up a significant external potential field in spite of a large change of transmembrane potential between the inside and the outside of the cell. This is because the current flow is through all parts of the cell membrane at once. Large external electric fields are set up only when potential differences occur between two or more regions on the surface of the cell, such as occurs with postsynaptic potentials.

The role of the glial cells is not yet clarified, but as yet no strong evidence exists that they participate directly in the generation of EEG potentials.

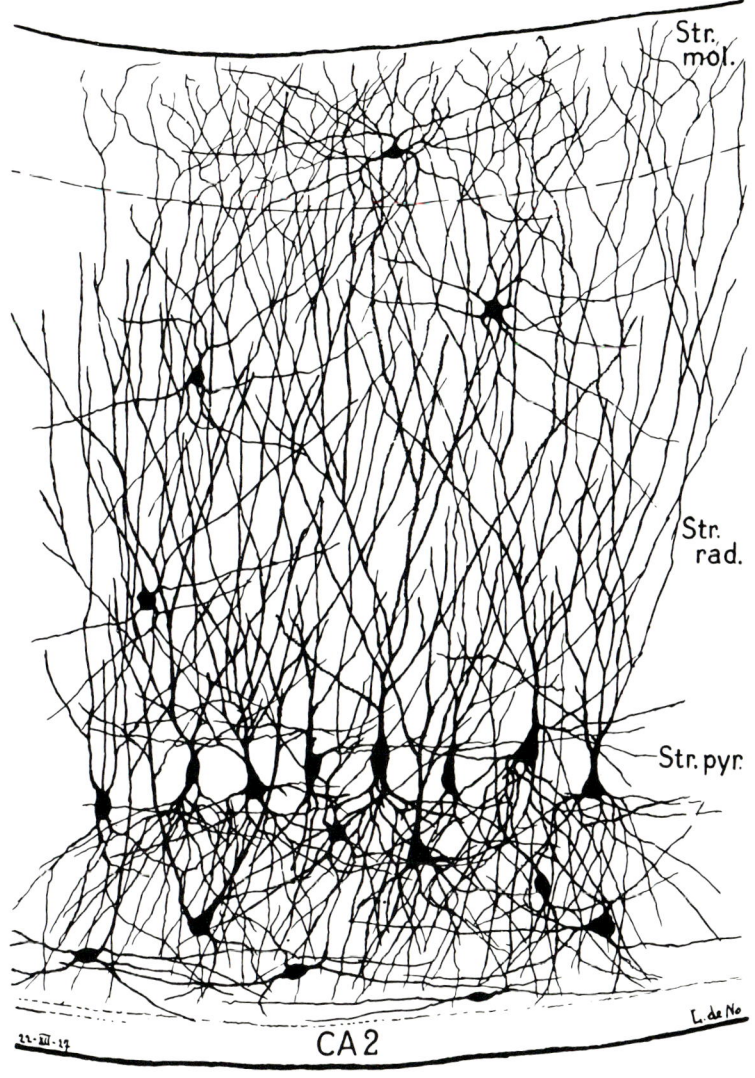

FIG. 3. Laminar arrangement of pyramidal cells and apical dendrites in field CA2 in the hippocampus of monkey (from ref. 20).

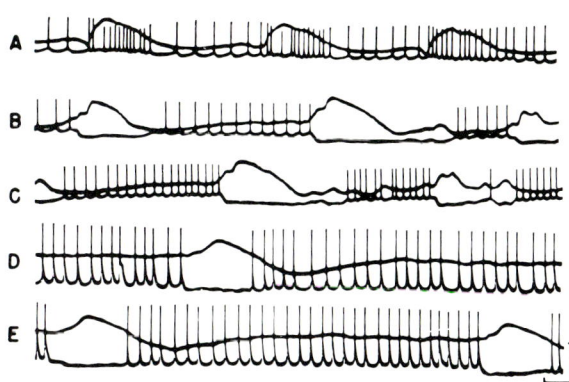

FIG. 4. Postsynaptic potentials generating paroxysmal EEG waves. *Upper trace:* recording of focal surface EEG discharge following a small focal cortical freezing lesion (negativity upward). *Lower trace:* intracellular recordings from three neurons impaled during a single penetration near the lesion (negativity downward). **A:** neuron in cortex exhibiting minimal depolarization and acceleration of firing during surface negativity. **B** and **C:** continuous recording from another cell approximately 50 μm away. Membrane hyperpolarization with inhibition of cell discharge is evident during all phases of EEG paroxysmal waves. **D** and **E:** continuous recording from cell superficial to that shown in **B** and **C**. Inhibition of cell discharge occurs only during surface negativity of diphasic low-frequency EEG paroxysmal activity. Calibrations, horizontal bar, 0/1 sec, vertical bar, 50 μV for surface EEG trace and 50 mV for intracellular records (from ref. 12).

CORTICAL POTENTIALS THAT GENERATE EPILEPTIFORM EEG ACTIVITY

During each interictal epileptiform EEG spike, neurons undergo depolarizations that are of much greater amplitude than the EPSPs of normally functioning cells. These intense depolarizations are called paroxysmal depolarization shifts (PDSs) (Fig. 6). During the PDS, the cells lose their ability to fire action potentials. As can be seen in Fig. 6A, as each PDS begins, spikes occur at increasing frequency

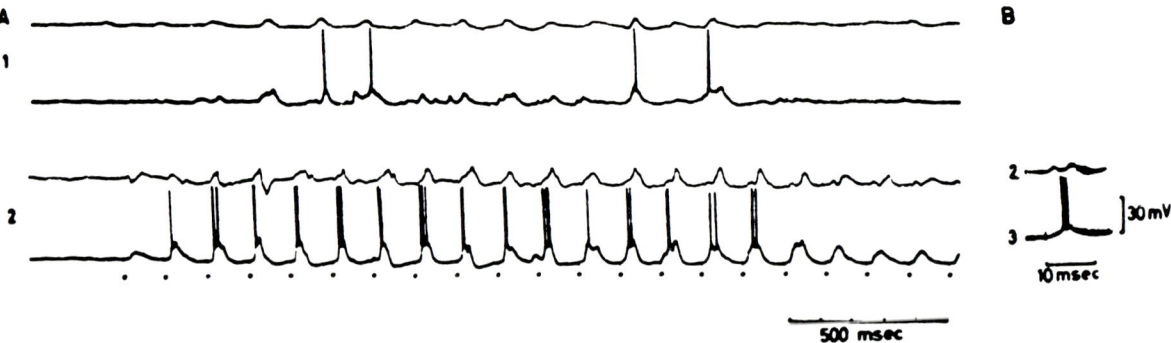

FIG. 5. **A1:** Spontaneous spindle waves *(upper trace)* during deep anesthesia. Grouped intracellularly measured EPSPs *(lower trace)* usually coincide with surface negative spindle waves. **A2:** Recruiting response during 8.5/sec stimulation in VA-nucleus of thalamus. Stimuli marked by dots. The "waxing and waning" amplitude of the EEG waves *(upper trace)* is similar to that of the amplitude changes of the intracellularly recorded EPSPs. **B:** Superimposed recruiting waves with small positive dips simultaneous with the action potentials. Cat sensorimotor cortex, nembutal anesthesia. Monopolor EEG recording, negative in top traces in **A** and middle trace in **B** (from ref. 7).

proportionate to the level of depolarization until depolarization exceeds the critical firing level and spike generation no longer occurs. Prolonged absence of action potentials is a characteristic feature. PDSs are the principal generators of negative EEG spike discharges at the center of an epileptogenic focus. Figure 6B shows the distribution of PDSs at a discrete focus (32).

PDSs, although initiated by EPSPs, may reflect intrinsic changes in the neural membrane itself or possibly an alteration of synaptic mechanisms. However, studies of cells showing PDSs have as yet failed to demonstrate changes in the fundamental physical properties of their resting membranes. In intervals between PDSs and EPSPs, action potentials appear normal and firing thresholds do not seem to be significantly altered. The fact that injection of depolarizing current cannot induce a PDS suggests that the PDS is related to alterations in synaptic mechanisms (36). The generation of PDSs is a consistent event in the epileptogenic focus. However, the molecular and structural changes that precede their occurrence are as yet unknown.

In experimental foci, the negativity of the EEG spike is greatest at a depth of about 1 mm, indicating that the spike is generated mainly in the more superficial layers. The negative spike portion of the EEG spike-and-wave complex that results from stimulation of the thalamus (see below) is also generated in the superficial layers of the cortex (25). The slow-wave portion of the thalamically induced EEG spike-and-wave complex is also surface negative but is generated differently. The intracellular correlates of the slow-wave portion appear to be IPSPs generated deep in the cortex. Thus, a negative wave is recorded at the surface of the neocortex and in the EEG

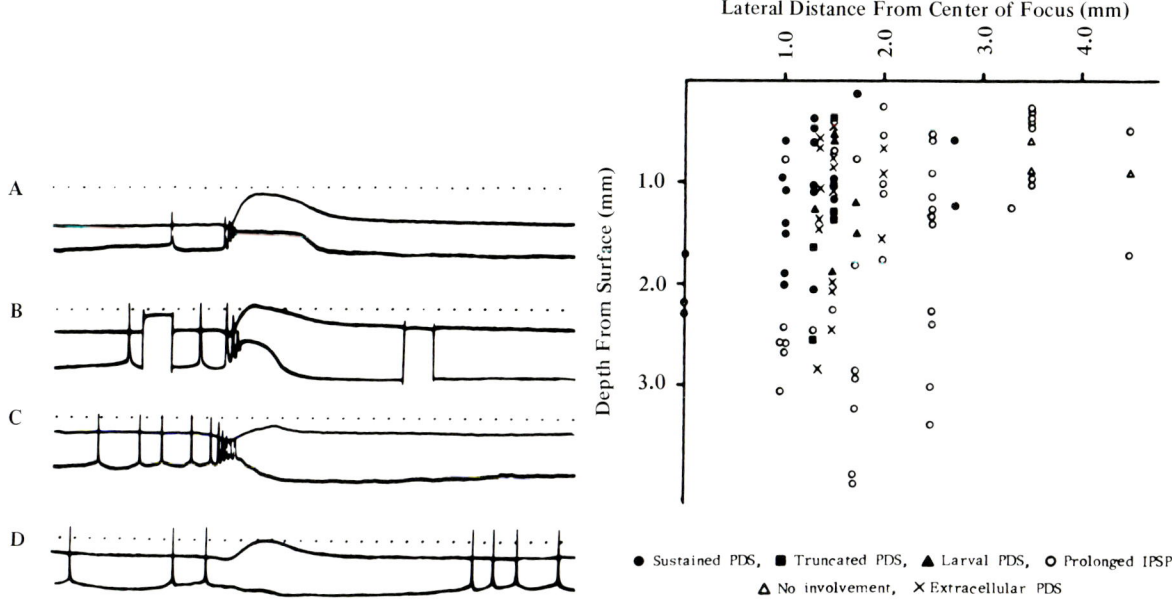

FIG. 6. *Left:* Types of intracellular activity seen during interictal EEG spiking at a penicillin-induced focus. *Upper traces:* corticogram. *Lower traces:* intracellular recordings showing **A:** sustained paroxysmal depolarization shift (PDS); **B:** truncated PDS; **C:** larval PDS; **D:** prolonged inhibitory postsynaptic potential (IPSP). Corticogram at penicillin capillary. Time marker 10 msec at DIC baseline. DC voltage calibration is shown in **B** 50 mV. *Right:* Distribution of PDSs and IPSPs during EEG spiking. Nearly all sustained PDSs are located within 1.5 mm lateral to center of focus. At 2 mm and beyond, IPSPs are preponderant.

when either the superficial apical dendrites depolarize or the cell bodies and basilar dendrites hyperpolarize (Fig. 7). Although in clinical EEG experience the preponderance of epileptogenic spikes are negative and may mainly reflect PDSs, attempts to relate the polarity and size of EEG waves seen clinically to what is occurring in different layers of the cortex have not yet been very successful. This is because each wave is the product of summation of EPSPs, IPSPs, and PDSs of many cells and their dendrites at different depths in the cortex.

Analogous electrical generation is found in the hippocampus where the principal site of IPSP generation is at the somatic portion of the neuron (4). Epileptic activity is precipitated more easily in the hippocampus than in the neocortex, which may relate to its simpler

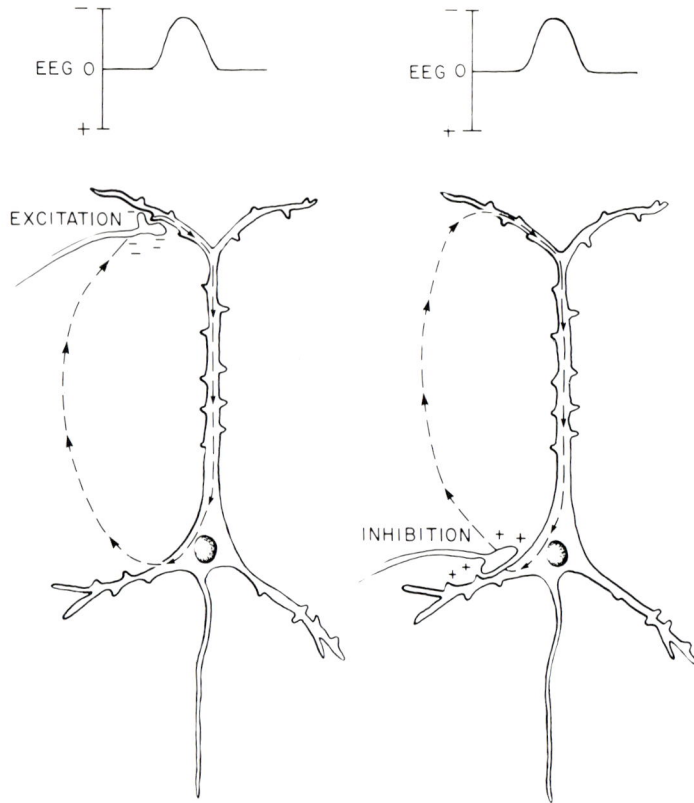

FIG. 7. Diagram shows how both excitation (EPSPs) at apical dendrites near the cortical surface and inhibition (IPSPs) at cell body deeper in the cortex can cause extracellular current flow in the same direction *(arrows)*. In either case, surface negative waves will be recorded in the EEG.

laminar structure with closely packed superficial pyramidal cell bodies and deep layer of apical dendrites (Fig. 8).

ROLE OF THE THALAMUS IN NORMAL AND ABNORMAL EEG ACTIVITY

After the thalamus is removed, the cortex does not show normal continuous or nearly continuous rhythmical activity, but rhythmical activity can still occur. Therefore, the thalamus, although not essential for the production of rhythmical activity, plays a large role in maintaining the normal rhythms seen in the EEG (3). The thalamus also appears to be involved in the maintenance and propagation of seizure discharges, but a primary role in the initiation of either focal or primary generalized seizure discharges is unproved. Bilaterally synchronous cortical spike-and-wave discharges can result from stimulation of the intralaminar nuclei of the thalamus and the midbrain reticular formation, and cortical epileptiform discharges project to the thalamus (17,18). Nevertheless, in extensive studies in the monkey, Udvarhelyi and Walker (34) experienced considerable difficulty in eliciting sustained afterdischarges with local thalamic stimulation and found that cells of the thalamus did not readily exhibit spontaneous repetitive afterdischarges. They concluded that the thalamus acts mainly as an inhibitor. The inhibitory role of the thalamus in seizures was also emphasized by Eccles (9) in his theoretical formulation on the mechanisms of rhythmicity in the EEG. Low-frequency stimulation of nonspecific thalamic nuclei that gives rise to typical long-latency recruiting responses generally does not affect cortical epileptogenic discharges, but discharging lesions of the cortex produce dramatic changes in the waxing and waning cycles of recruiting responses (11).

Present evidence appears to support the idea that the thalamic

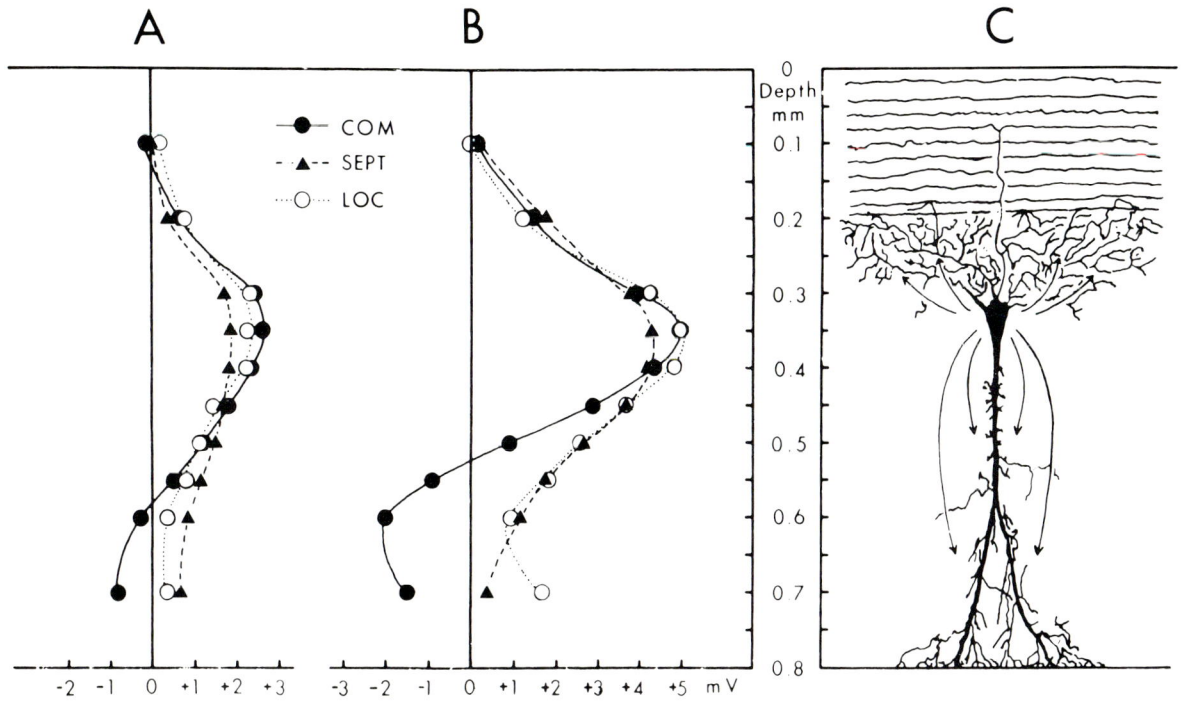

FIG. 8. Hippocampal field potentials measured at various depths. **A** and **B** are plots of the potential fields of IPSPs during two microelectrode plunges through hippocampal region CA3. Maximum positivity occurs at a depth corresponding to cell bodies of the pyramidal cells shown in **C**. Current flow direction is indicated by arrows (from ref. 4).

and midbrain structures are intimately involved in the processes concerned with maintaining, spreading, and inhibiting seizure discharges. It has been observed that complete elimination of secondary bilateral synchrony from a penicillin focus could be accomplished only after all midline structures, including the midbrain, were split. It appears that the thalamus becomes engaged early in the development of sustained cortical seizure discharges and that both inhibitory and facilitory functions come into play from both the specific and nonspecific thalamic nuclei. Both cortical and subcortical structures are clearly operating in nearly all sustained epileptic processes. Evidence suggest-

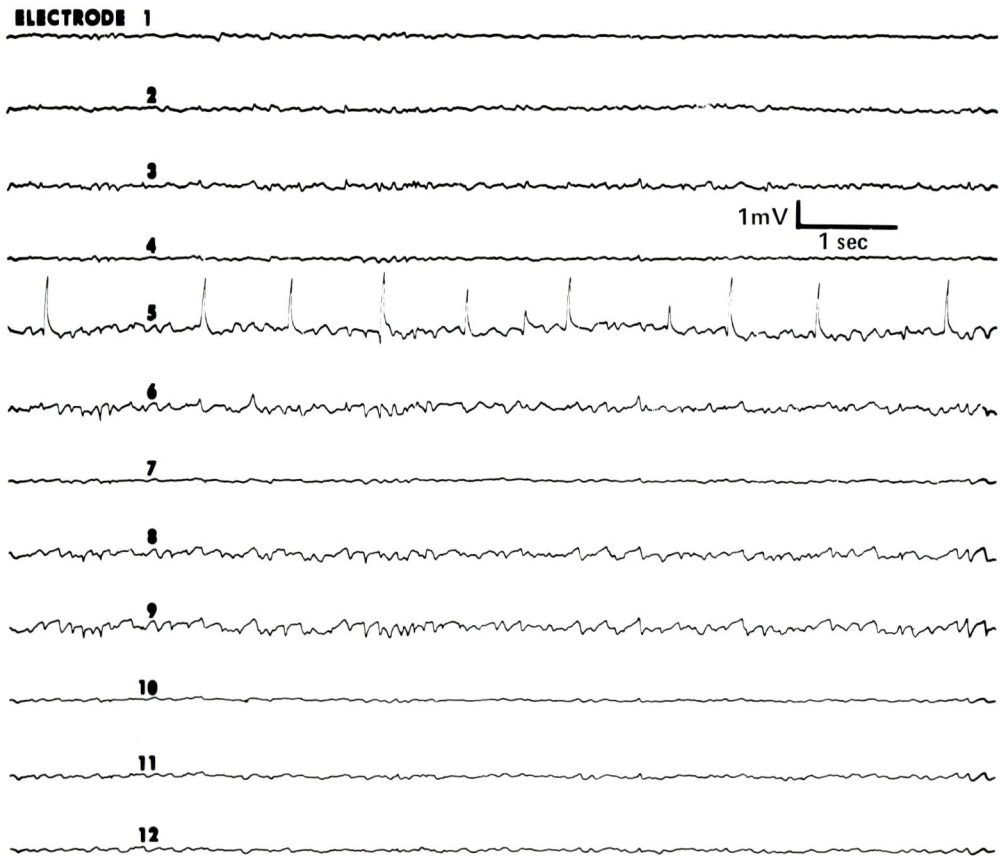

FIG. 9A: Onset of negative spiking solely at the penicillin-containing capillary (channel 5) 6 min after it was placed on the cortex. **B:** Spread of focal activity to other electrodes in the 4 × 6 mm area as recorded 43 min later. Gain in channel 5 reduced to 0.1. Electrode distribution as shown in Fig. 3. Interelectrode distances are 2 mm. Reference electrode is on neck muscle. Calibration, 1 mV, 1 sec. Negative up.

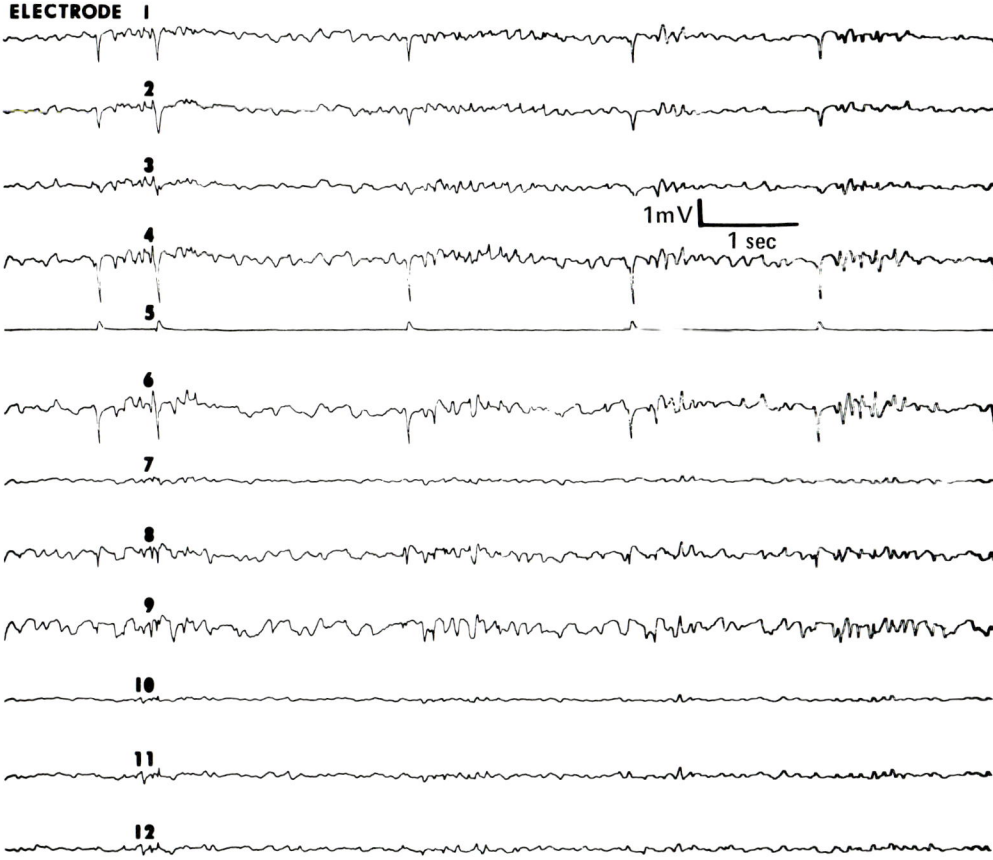

FIG. 9B. (See legend for 9A.)

ing that the thalamus initiates either focal or primary generalized seizure activity, however, is not convincing.

ELECTRICAL ACTIVITY AT THE CORTICAL SURFACE IN EXPERIMENTAL EPILEPTOGENIC FOCI

Epileptogenic foci produced by different technics vary in the rate of development and in intensity but otherwise have similar electrical characteristics (26). The earliest phenomena in a penicillin-induced epileptogenic focus in the cat are sporadic slow waves followed within a few minutes by high-voltage monophasic negative spikes limited to the area of contact with the epileptogenic agent (Fig. 9A). The negative spikes at the penicillin electrode attain amplitudes as high as 3,000 μV without any evidence of synchronous activity at nearby electrodes. As the negative spike continues to increase in voltage in a strong focus, it soon becomes surrounded by a large area of spikes whose principal polarity is positive (Fig. 9B). In weaker foci, the surrounded spikes may be essentially negative (22). The focus at this stage appears to be mainly produced by the cortex alone as similar spike foci can be produced in cortex isolated from the rest of the brain (29). The peaks of the positive spikes in the surrounding area usually appear earlier than the peaks of the negative spikes at the center of the focus. Within 30 min the activity at all electrodes becomes quite stable in wave form, and the spikes recur regularly at intervals of between 2 and 10 sec. By this time the amplitude of the negative spike at the center of the focus can become as great as 7,000 μV. The spike lasts about 100 msec, has a shorter rise time than fall time, and is usually immediately preceded by a smaller positive spike of about 30-msec duration that varies in amplitude (13) (Fig. 10).

Studies of electrical fields in the cortex in three dimension show that at the center of a spike focus a monophasic negative spike is recorded at the surface and at all depths. However, at as little as 1 mm away from the center of a strong focus, the spikes are positive at the surface and reverse their polarity between 0.2 and 0.4 mm below the surface (Fig. 11). Thus, the strong epileptogenic focus consists of a small area of repetitive negative spikes, each of which activates a larger surrounding area of independently generated mainly positive discharges. The independence of the activity at the center of the focus and at the surrounding electrodes indicates that multiple generating areas rather symmetrically located with respect to the center of the penicillin focus, contribute to the observed potential field.

HUMAN EPILEPTOGENIC FOCI

Results in man resemble those in experimental animals and also demonstrate multiple small generators in an epileptogenic area. In the humans, a single epileptogenic focus seen at the scalp overlies multiple areas of spiking at the cortical surface. Observations described here were made on human cortex prior to surgical removal for the treatment of intractable focal seizures (Fig. 12). First, widely spaced electrodes were placed on the cortex, and the most active area of spiking was located. That location was then bracketed by a linear array of six silver-chlorided ball electrodes spaced 2 to 3 mm apart. These multiple closely spaced areas often generated independent nonsynchronous high-amplitude spikes. Active spiking in the corticogram was only rarely seen in the scalp EEG, although synchronous slow waves, generated over wide cortical areas, were apparent

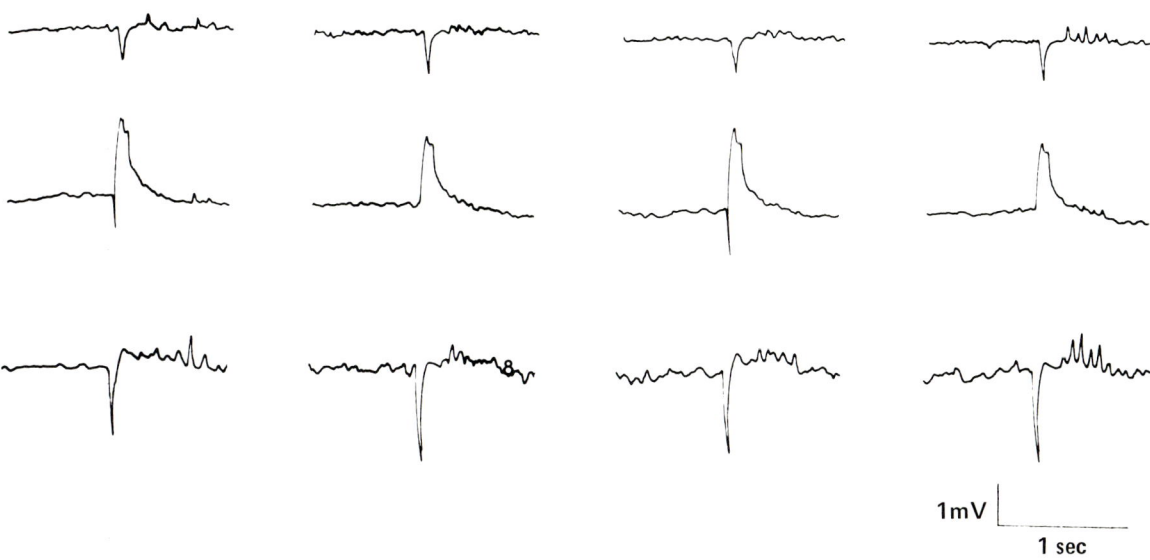

FIG. 10. Instability of the early positivity at the penicillin electrode alone *(middle row)*. Upper and lower rows, 2 mm from penicillin electrode, laterally and medially respectively. Negativity up. Note the prominent positivity prior to the negative spike in columns 1 and 3, which is absent in 2 and 4. All spikes within a 30 sec period. Calibration 1 mV, 1 sec.

in the scalp record (Fig. 12). These studies show that areas of the cortex generating focal epileptiform activity in man as well as animals are often less than 2 mm in diameter and that such spikes, in spite of great amplitude, are usually not visible in scalp recordings.

The above findings suggest that underlying a clinically evident epileptogenic EEG focus are small single or multiple spike generators usually unseen at the scalp until from time to time they provoke synaptically synchronized activity involving several square centimeters of cortex. Physical calculations (14) confirm that the smallness of the surface area occupied by a spike at the cortex is the major factor in its failure to be evident at the scalp. Observations in favor of this conclusion are seen at scalp electrodes overlying a skull defect. In Fig. 13A, a local spike from an epileptogenic lesion is seen limited to only one scalp electrode. It is located over the skull defect shown in the X-ray (Fig. 13B). Spikes with a distribution limited to one scalp electrode are only rarely found through an intact skull.

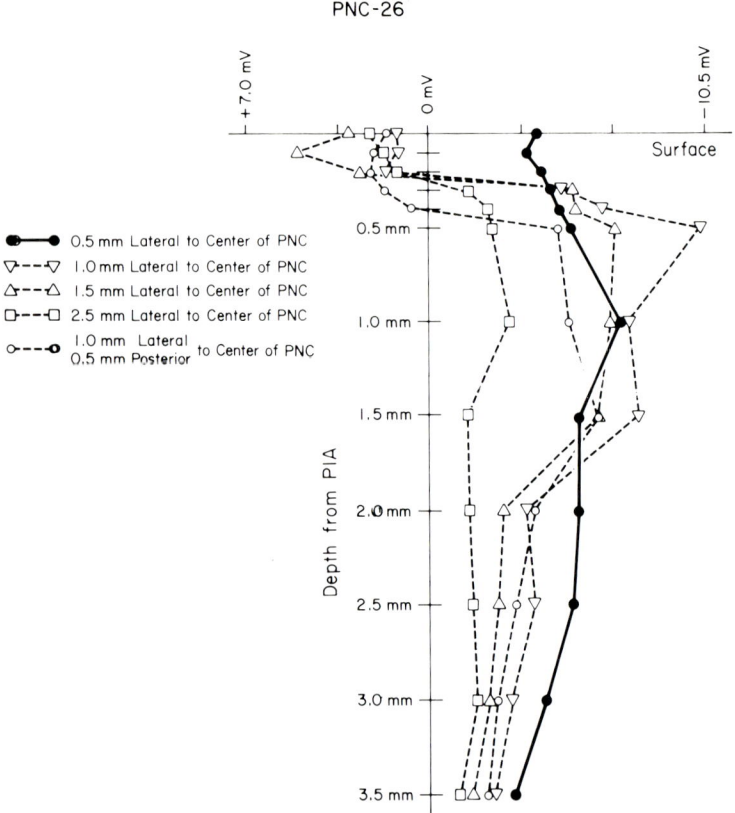

FIG. 11. Potential peak voltage distribution in three dimensions at a single penicillin spike focus. Maximal negativities and positivities are found within 1 mm of the surface, indicating superficial cortical generators.

HOW THE HUMAN EEG DIFFERS BETWEEN THE CORTEX AND THE SCALP

Experimental and human observations explain some of the previously perplexing problems in the interpretation of the EEG in epilepsy when difficulties exist in correlating what is seen at the scalp with what is actually happening in the brain. Although some authors subscribed to a general rule that the amplitude of brain waves at the scalp was attenuated from seven to 10 times compared to the cortical surface, it was always apparent that there was much more variability. Many examples of this discrepancy are seen in surgically treated patients whose preoperative EEGs from the scalp show no spikes, but whose corticograms show frequent high-voltage and often multifocal spiking. Between the cortex and the scalp some 20 to 70% of cortical spikes disappear, and the voltage attenuation of those spikes that can be seen at the scalp ranges from 2 to 1 to as high as 58 to 1 (1). Figure 12 demonstrates small spike generators at the cortex that fail to appear at the scalp.

Applying experimental data to man, it is calculated that there are attenuation factors of 600 for a highly localized spike and 60 for a generator of uniform strength over 4×6 mm area but an attenuation factor of only 1.8 for an area of 4×6 cm. Synchronous generation of spindles in the human cortex was found to extend over a distance of at least 1.2 cm (14) (Fig. 14). Cooper et al. (6) found synchronous alpha at two cortical locations 3.6 cm apart. Sources of the size indicated in these two reports can be expected to attenuate by factors of the order of 10 or less (13). It is thus evident that many cortical phenomena that do not simultaneously activate relatively large areas of cortex fail to become evident at the scalp.

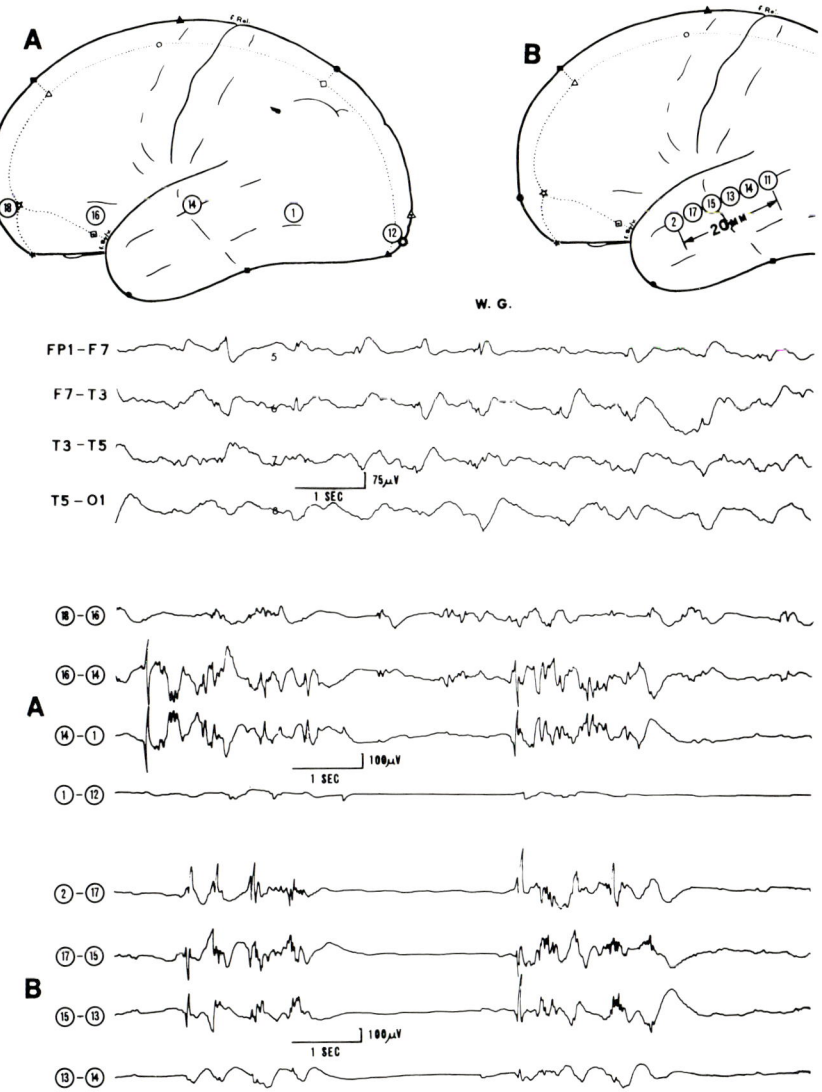

FIG. 12. Comparison of the scalp EEG with the electrocorticogram in the same patient. Uppermost four channels are EEG. Note infrequent low voltage spikes. **A:** cortical recording with widely spaced electrodes show high voltage spikes at electrode 14. **B:** cortical recording with closely spaced electrodes around area of spiking seen at electrode 14 in **A**. Note independent spikes at electrodes 2 and 15 demonstrating generation of high voltage spikes in small areas that are not apparent in scalp recording.

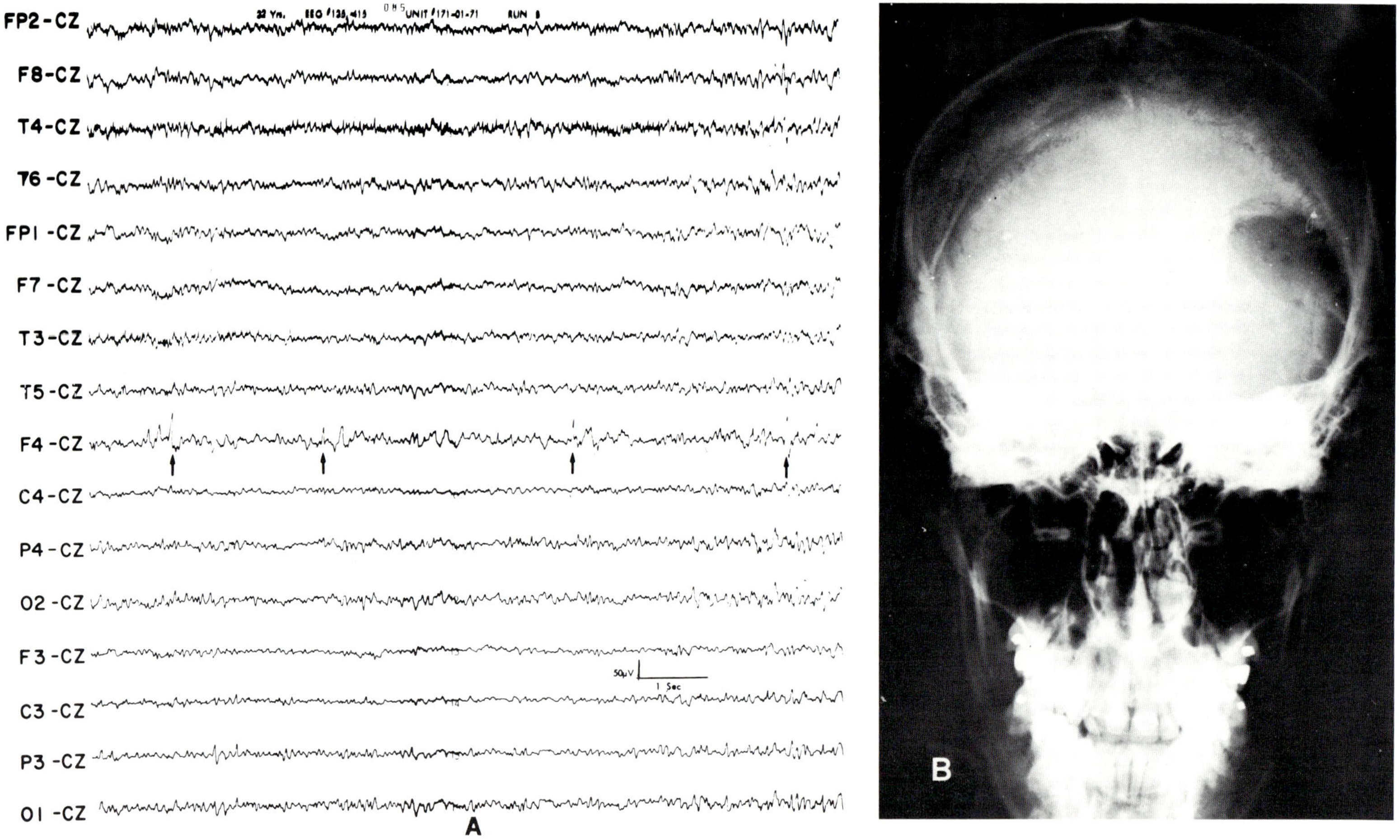

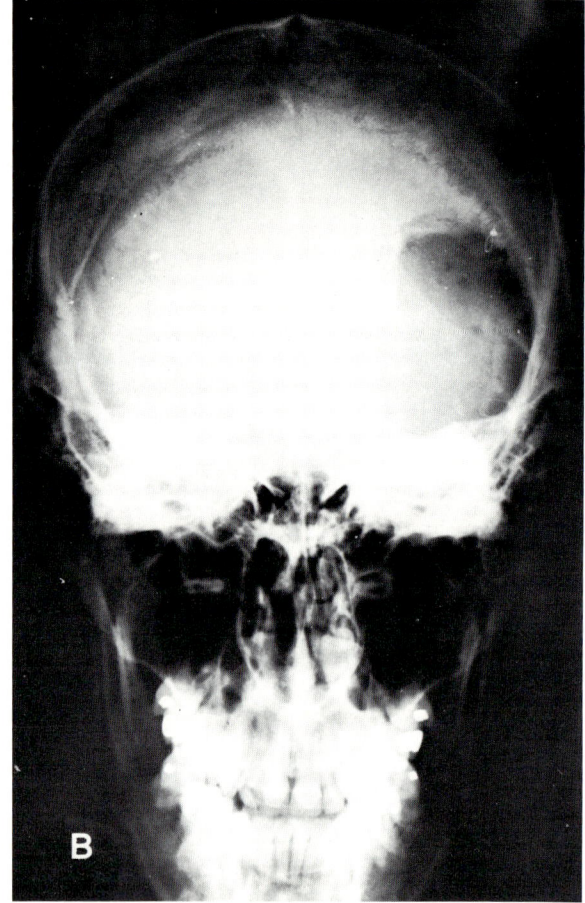

FIG. 13. **A:** EEG spike focus in man with skull defect. Spike focus limited to one scap electrode (F4) from a small cortical epileptogenic focus in **B**. **B:** X-ray of skull defect underlying electrode F4. Same patient as in 13A.

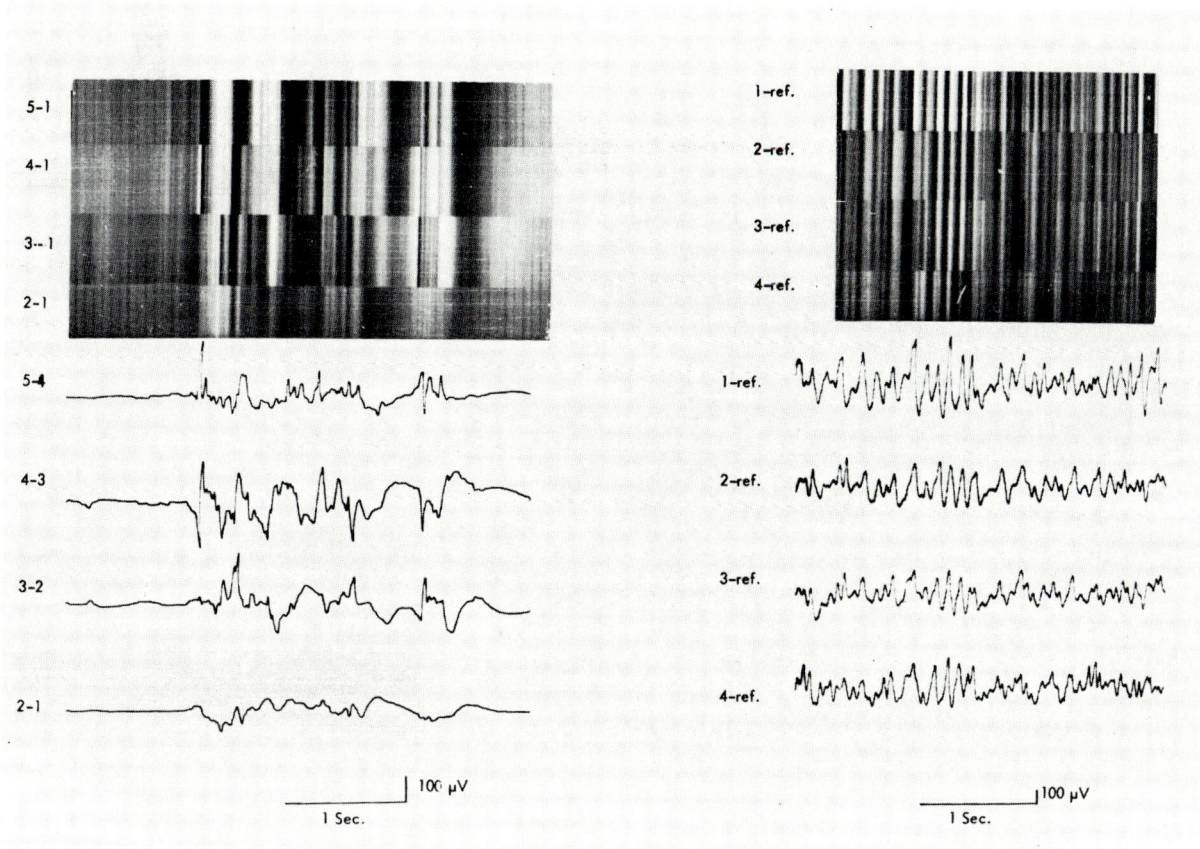

FIG. 14. *Left:* Corticogram and display of spike-and-slow-wave burst recorded from closely spaced electrodes on left medial temporal lobe of patient with left cerebral atrophy. In display, brightening corresponds to positivity. Note independent involvement at different sites 3 mm apart. *Right:* Corticogram and display of spindle activity recorded from linear electrode array with 3 mm spacing on cortex showing no lesion upon exposure. In display, brightening corresponds to positivity. Note extended region of synchrony for sleep spindles of more than 12 mm.

REFERENCES

1. Abraham, K., and Ajmone-Marsan, C. (1958): Patterns of cortical discharges and their relation to routine scalp electroencephalography. *Electroencephalogr. Clin. Neurophysiol.,* 10:447–461.
2. Akert, K., Pfenninger, K., Sandri, C., and Moor, H. (1972): Freeze etching and cytochemistry of vesicles and membrane complexes in synapses of the central nervous system. In: *Structure and Function of Synapses,* edited by G. D. Pappas and D. P. Purpura, pp. 67–86. Raven Press, New York.
3. Andersen, P., and Andersson, S. A. (1968): *Physiological Basis of the Alpha Rhythm.* Appleton, N.Y.
4. Andersen, P., Eccles, J. C., and Loyning, Y. (1964): Location of postsynaptic inhibitory endings on hippocampal pyramids. *J. Neurophysiol.,* 27:592.
5. Colonnier, M. L. (1968): Synaptic patterns on different cell types in the different laminae of the cat visual cortex. *Brain Res.,* 9:268.
6. Cooper, R., Winter, A. L., Crow, H. J., and Walter, W. G. (1965): Comparison of subcortical, cortical and scalp activity using chronically indwelling electrodes in man. *Electroencephalogr. Clin. Neurophysiol.,* 18:217–228.
7. Creutzfeldt, O., Watanabe, S., and Lux, H. D. (1966): Relations between EEG phenomena and potentials of single cortical cells. I. Evoked responses after thalamic and epicortical stimulation. *Electroencephalogr. Clin. Neurophysiol.,* 20:1–18.
8. Dempsey, E. W., and Morison, R. S. (1942): The production of rhythmically recurrent cortical potential after localized thalamic stimulation. *Am. J. Physiol.,* 135:293.
9. Eccles, J. C. (1969): *The Inhibitory Pathway of the Central Nervous System.* Charles C Thomas, Springfield, Illinois.
10. Gloor, P. (editor) (1969): *Hans Berger on the Electroencephalogram of Man.* Elsevier, Amsterdam.
11. Goldensohn, E. S. (1969): Discussion: Experimental seizure mechanisms. In: *Basic Mechanisms of the Epilepsies,* edited by H. H. Jasper, A. A. Ward, Jr., and A. Pope, pp. 289–298. Little, Brown, Boston.
12. Goldensohn, E. S., and Purpura, D. P. (1963): Intracellular potentials of cortical neurons during focal epileptogenic discharges. *Science,* 193:840–842.
13. Goldensohn, E. S., Zablow, L., and Salazar, A. M., Jr. (1977): The penicillin focus. I: Distribution of potential at the cortical surface. *Electroencephalogr. Clin. Neurophysiol.,* 42:480–492.
14. Goldensohn, E. S., Zablow, L., and Stein, B. (1970): Interrelationships of form and latency of spike discharges from small areas of human cortex. *Electroencephalogr. Clin. Neurophysiol.,* 29:32.
15. Hubel, D. H., and Wiesel, T. N. (1963): Shape and arrangement of columns in cat's striate cortex. *J. Physiol., (Lond.),* 165:554–568.
16. Humphrey, D. R. (1968): Re-analysis of the antidromic cortical response. II. On the contribution of cell discharge and PSP's to the evoked potentials. *Electroencephalogr. Clin. Neurophysiol.,* 25:421–422.
17. Hunter, J., and Jasper, H. H. (1949): Effects of thalamic stimulation in unanesthetised animals. The arrest reaction and petit mal-like seizures, activation patterns and generalized convulsions. *Electroencephalogr. Clin. Neurophysiol.,* 1:305–324.
18. Ingvar, D. H. (1955): Reproduction of the 3 per second spike and wave EEG patterns by sub-cortical electrical stimulation in cats. *Acta Physiol. Scand.,* 33:137–150.
19. Li, C., McLennan, H., and Jasper H. (1952): Brain waves and unit discharge in cerebral cortex. *Science,* 116:656–657.
20. Lorente De No, R. (1934): Studies on the structure of the cerebral cortex. II. Continuation of the study of the ammonic system. *J. Psychol. Neurol.,* 46:113–177.
21. Lorente De No, R. (1947): A study of nerve physiology (parts I and II), In: *Studies from the Rockefeller Institute for Medical Research, Vols 131–132,* Rockefeller Inst. Med. Res., New York.
22. Lueders, H., Bustamante, L., Pippenger, C., and Goldensohn, E. S. (1977): The effects of phenytoin, phenobarbital and carbamazepine on the experimental spike focus. *Neurology (Minneap.),* No. 4. 27:375.
23. Matsumoto, H., and Ajmone-Marsan, C. (1964): Cortical cellular phenomena in experimental epilepsy. Interictal manifestations. *Exp. Neurol.,* 9:286–304.
24. Pollen, D. A. (1969): Discussion: On the generation of neocortical potentials. In: *Basic Mechanisms of the Epilepsies,* edited by H. H. Jasper, A. A. Ward, Jr., and A. Pope, pp. 411–420. Little, Brown, Boston.
25. Pollen, D. A., Reid, K. H., and Perot, P. (1964): Microelectrode studies of experimental 3/sec. wave and spike in the cat. *Electroencephalogr. Clin. Neurophysiol.,* 17:57–67.
26. Prince, D. A., and Futamachi, K. J. (1968): Intracellular recordings in chronic focal epilepsy. *Brain Res.,* 11:681.
27. Purpura, D. P. (1959): Nature of electrocortical potentials and synaptic organizations in cerebral and cerebellar cortex. *Int. Rev. Neurobiol.,* 1:47.
28. Purpura, D. P. (1958): Organization of excitatory and inhibitory synaptic electrogenesis in the cerebral cortex. In: *Symposium on Reticular Formation of Brain,* edited by L. C. Proctor, R. S. Knighton, H. H. Jasper, W. C. Noshay, and R. T. Costello, p. 435. Little, Brown, Boston.
29. Purpura, D. P. (1963): Critique and review. Cortical excitability and steady potentials. In: *Brain Function.* edited by M. A. B. Brazier, pp. 281–320. Univ. of California Press, Berkeley.

30. Ramon y Cajal, S. (1911): *Histologie du Système Nerveux de l'Homme et des Vertébrés,* Vol. 2. Maloine, Paris.
31. Ramon-Moliner, E. (1961): The histology of the post-cruciate gyrus in the cat. *J. Comp. Neurol.,* 117:43.
32. Salazar, A. M., Jr., Goldensohn, E. S., and Zablow, L. (1978): Paroxysmal depolarization shifts in penicillin-induced epileptogenic foci, varieties and distribution. *(In press.)*
33. Szentagothai, J. (1969): Architecture of the cerebral cortex. In: *Basic Mechanisms of the Epilepsies,* edited by H. H. Jasper, A. A. Ward, Jr., and A. Pope, pp. 13–28. Little, Brown, Boston.
34. Udvarhelyi, G. B., and Walker, A. E. (1965): Dissemination of acute focal seizures in the monkey. II. From subcortical foci. *Arch. Neurol.,* 12:357–380.
35. Von Bonin, G. (1949): Architecture of the precentral motor cortex and some adjacent areas. In: *The Precentral Motor Cortex,* edited by P. Bucy. Univ. of Illinois Press, Urbana.
36: Walsh, G. O. (1971): Penicillin iontophoresis in neocortex of cat: Effects on the spontaneous and induced activity of single neurons. *Epilepsia,* 12:1–11.

Chapter 16

Event-Related Potentials and Their Clinical Applications

Morton D. Low

*Departments of Medicine (Neurology) and Physiology, University of British Columbia, and Department of Diagnostic Neurophysiology, Vancouver General Hospital, Vancouver, British Columbia, Canada**

Evoked Potentials	442
SEPs	442
Recording Techniques	443
Origin of Evoked Potentials	444
Applications in Assessment of Function	444
Peripheral Nerve	444
Spinal Cord	445
Cerebral Function	445
Space-Occupying and Destructive Lesions	446
Diffuse Cerebral Disease	446
Coma and Cerebral Death	447
Demyelinating Disease	447

* With the assistance of Sherrill J. Purves, Departments of Medicine and Physiology, University of British Columbia and G. Barrie Purves, Lion's Gate Hospital, North Vancouver, British Columbia, Canada.

Evoked Potential Methods in Assessment of Vision and Hearing.......................... 447
    Hearing 447
    Vision... 448
Summary and Conclusion 448
Acknowledgments... 449
References.. 449

EVOKED POTENTIALS

The relatively recent development of signal averaging techniques has made possible the precise measurement of electrical responses evoked in the nervous system by specific external stimuli. This valuable experimental neurophysiological method is currently being adapted for use in diagnostic problems by clinical investigators, and its application clinically is based on two fundamental assumptions.

1. The sensory-evoked potential (SEP) allows an objective, quantifiable assessment of the processing of sensory information by the nervous system.
2. This assessment can be at least comparable in accuracy to the reflection of structural integrity provided by contrast studies.

The pursuit of the proof of these assumptions has been extensive and complex, but it must regrettably be concluded that in spite of truly enormous deployment of talent, time, and money (a recently published review of the field of evoked potential research listed over 900 references in a selected bibliography) (1), the validity of these two assumptions remains largely unproven. Some of the reasons for this will be apparent as this chapter develops.

SEPs

The SEP is an obligatory electrical response of the brain, spinal cord, or nerve to a specific stimulus. The characteristics of this response depend upon the parameters of the stimulus itself and the state of the nervous system at the time of stimulation. Evoked responses have been elicited in man by auditory, somatosensory, visual, and olfactory stimuli as well as by electrical stimulation of afferent pathways.

Even a brief exposure to the available evoked potential literature is sufficient to illustrate one of the major inherent difficulties. Although there is some information available regarding the morphology and distribution of these responses, there are as yet no definitive studies available specifying absolute shape or distribution of any of the SEPs. The literature includes a large volume of data which are difficult to interpret and unfortunately, few comprehensive critical studies (1,2). Different investigators have found and labeled different numbers of components of evoked responses, with different latencies and sometimes a different appearance for supposedly the same component depending upon many factors, including the recording convention of whether negative or positive is up. Variations in stimulus parameters (intensity, duration, frequency, pattern) (1,2), the sub-

1 shows typical wave forms elicited by auditory, somatic, and visual stimulation. These wave forms are referential recordings (active electrode on the scalp, reference electrode on one ear) of SEPs obtained from alert adults. The levels of stimulus intensity were moderate, and the wave forms are composites of those obtained from eight different subjects using several thousand stimuli.

When stimulus and state variables are carefully controlled and the number of samples taken is sufficient to reduce the level of background EEG adequately, wave form stability within subjects can be quite high (3). By contrast, individual differences in the absolute and relative amplitudes of the various components are very marked. The latencies of the various component peaks tend to be considerably more consistent, between subjects, so that for specified stimulus conditions a "standard" evoked response wave form can be defined.

There is no universally accepted nomenclature or labeling convention for evoked potentials, and to this date generally speaking individual laboratories employ their own labeling methods.

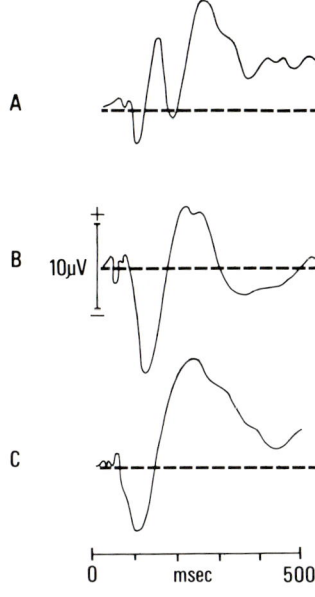

FIG. 1 Averaged evoked responses obtained from eight adult subjects to **A:** visual, **B:** auditory, and **C:** somatosensory stimulation. (From Vaughan, ref. 3.)

RECORDING TECHNIQUES

For reasons already mentioned it has been nearly impossible to compare specific details of components of event-related potentials obtained in one laboratory with those obtained in another. Generally speaking any individual investigator who wishes to use averaged evoked potentials as an aid in clinical diagnosis must either select one technique from the literature and rely on data reported using that technique as a source of normal values, or he must establish his own normative data with his own recording technique. This has been a very real and serious limitation to the application of evoked potential studies to neurological diagnosis.

ject's level of alertness, and recording electrode location all affect the configuration of the evoked response. Consequently, studies in which all of these variables are not carefully controlled are difficult to compare.

Using careful and consistent recording and stimulating techniques one can define the usual morphology of an averaged SEP. Figure

Essential components in any system for obtaining evoked potentials include differential amplifiers with sufficient gain and band-width characteristics to resolve the very low amplitude and high frequency components of evoked responses (an effective band-width of 0.5 to 3,000 Hz is required for somatosensory work although an upper-frequency response of 100 Hz is adequate for visual evoked potential recording), a signal averager with at least two channels (preferably four or more) (2,4) for processing the signals and for separating the very small evoked responses from the much larger amplitude ongoing EEG activity, stimulators appropriate for the sensory modality to be assessed, timing and switching devices for appropriate sequencing of stimuli and coordination of these with averager function, and some sort of display system for permanent recording and measurement of the obtained evoked responses. There are at this time very few commercially available packaged evoked potential systems that include all of these elements and heretofore, a clinician who wished to do evoked potential studies had to build his own system.

ORIGIN OF EVOKED POTENTIALS

The exact neuronal origin of scalp-recorded evoked potentials has not yet been established (5). The technical problems involved in obtaining such information are truly enormous. Current hypotheses suggest that for both auditory and somatosensory evoked responses one can identify specific components generated by all parts of the sensory system (including the brainstem and thalamus) from receptor to cortex (6,7).

Although some investigators have recorded and identified evoked potentials from spinal cord and brainstem (8,9,28), without the use of depth electrodes, this poses formidable technical problems that are currently beyond the capacity of most workers.

For the visual system, one can identify components generated by the retina and by the cortex using only surface electrodes, but to date no one has been able to record optic nerve, geniculate, or tract activity in intact man.

Acknowledging differences in the claims of various authors, it appears that the early components of all evoked responses (up to approximately 100 msec latency) reflect activity in specific sensory afferent pathways and primary sensory cortex, whereas later components (longer than 100 msec latency) reflect activity of both diffuse thalamocortical nonspecific sensory systems and long latency specific sensory pathways (7).

APPLICATIONS IN ASSESSMENT OF FUNCTION

Peripheral Nerve

Nerve conduction velocities can be determined quite accurately by recording the scalp response to stimuli at various positions over a peripheral nerve trunk (10,11). This technique requires more time and more complicated equipment than standard nerve conduction velocity measurements, but it has the possible advantage of being very sensitive so that estimates of conduction velocity can be made even in the presence of severe neuropathy or massive injury.

In some fortunate cases, information can be obtained regarding spinal root function (as in suspected disc protrusion) using peripheral electrical stimulation and scalp-recorded somatosensory evoked responses. Several authors have demonstrated that although peripheral nerve lesions increase the latency and duration (width) of individual SEP components, the overall form of the SEP is usually unaffected (12). In root lesions, however, in addition to latency and duration changes, the form of the SEP is distorted (this appears to be true for spinal lesions as well). Such assessments are not possible in all patients, however, for several reasons. One cannot always isolate the appropriate root by skin stimulation because of the sensory overlap of dermatomes, and it may be impossible in a given patient to identify an SEP in response to lower limb stimulation, either because of very high stimulating electrode resistance at the skin of the foot or because the cortical generators activated by such stimulation are oriented parallel to the plane of the scalp and buried on the medial surface of the hemisphere.

Spinal Cord

Some information about cord function may be obtained in a manner analogous to the assessment of peripheral nerve or root integrity using scalp recorded SEPs. Lesions of the spinal cord may cause changes in amplitude, latency, and form of the SEP. However, in cord disease resulting in disturbance of pain and/or temperature sensation only (anterior or lateral cord involvement), the SEP is quite normal (13–16). On the other hand, very abnormal SEPs can be recorded from patients with quite normal subjective sensation.

Another application of evoked potential techniques in assessing cord function is the intraoperative recording of cord potentials (16). This has a variety of potential uses (some already shown experimentally), particularly the demonstration of location and vertical extent of cord damage due to trauma (8). However, even this technique of direct recording has its limitations. In measuring latencies one must rely on the earliest negative peak since it is the least affected by anesthesia. It is also the most difficult component to resolve in averages because of its small amplitude and it may be absent from the SEP complex in 10 to 20% of all normals. Perhaps a more important limitation is imposed by the functional anatomy of the system. The posterior columns conduct virtually all of the shock-induced SEP (13,15). In other words, most of the anterior and lateral portions of the cord could be nonfunctioning, and the cord potential would appear to be normal. Some investigators are attempting to establish the reliability of recording cord responses to tactile stimuli (13), thus shifting the conducting pathway more anteriorly in the cord, but at this time the techniques are even more difficult and the results considerably less reliable than for simple electric shock stimulation.

Some progress has been made toward the recording of spinal cord evoked responses through the intact skin and spine (8). The potential value of such recording is obvious, however, the technical difficulties are enormous, consequently the procedure must still be regarded as experimental at best.

SEP recording may have possible prognostic value in cord trauma (16). D'Angelo et al. (17), and others have demonstrated a close correlation between the ultimate histological severity of experimental cord lesions in cats and the recovery of the SEP following injury. However, some clinicians feel that in human cases where SEPs can be recorded following cord trauma, there is usually some sensory sparing which can be detected on neurological examination which has the same significance. The evoked potential method would appear to be most useful in situations when the patient cannot cooperate in the usual sensory testing routines.

Finally, the recording of normal SEPs and the demonstration of normal conduction velocities in certain compensation cases or cases of suspected malingering or hysterical anesthesia can provide very useful objective data in supporting a clinical impression that may otherwise find reluctant acceptance (11).

CEREBRAL FUNCTION

As a general rule, evoked potentials do not provide useful information about the presence of disease unless the disease process directly alters the function of a specific sensory system—visual, auditory, or somatosensory (18), and of course the test method chosen must be appropriate to the sensory modality affected.

Space-Occupying and Destructive Lesions

Lesions that destroy or significantly disturb the function of primary sensory cortex, cortical afferent pathways, or thalamic sensory relay nuclei may also abolish the SEP on the side of the lesion (18). Such total abolition is uncommon, however, and it is more likely that the evoked potentials will appear to be normal or perhaps slightly asymmetrical in amplitude. Asymmetric evoked potentials are very difficult to interpret since some degree of left-right hemisphere asymmetry is encountered even in normal subjects, and in our experience, the pathology can be on the side of either the higher or lower amplitude evoked response.

Vaughan and Katzman (19) have provided a summary of the possibilities of localizing a lesion in the visual system to the retina, the optic nerve, the chiasm, the postchiasmatic pregeniculate tract, or the geniculocalcarine segment using combined visual evoked potential (VEP) and electroretinogram (ERG) recording. In our experience these tests can only very rarely contribute information of diagnostic value that cannot be found with a clinical examination in a cooperative subject, and hence are really only justified in patients in whom the latter is impossible.

These same authors used the criterion of 50% asymmetry of amplitude of the VEP as indicative of functionally significant field loss. Jonkman (20) and others have reported cases with significant field defect who have showed less than 50% amplitude difference between the left and right hemisphere VEPs, and more importantly in some patients markedly asymmetrical VEPs could be recorded in the absence of any demonstrable field defect.

In children and adults, it appears to be true that vision may return even after a period of cortical blindness during which the flash VEPs were totally absent or severely attenuated.

Diffuse Cerebral Disease

Some of the most striking changes in evoked potential configurations are caused by diffuse or multifocal disease.

Pampiglione (21) and his associates in London, have used combinations of VEP, ERG, and EEG recordings to demonstrate a reasonable degree of differentiation among the so-called neurometabolic storage disorders of childhood. In such cases, however, what one does after having made the distinction is unfortunately still an open question.

Jakob–Creutzfeldt disease may be associated with very large scalp-recorded evoked potentials to all sensory modalities. These potentials are not only much larger than usual, but they tend to show significantly shorter latency (of the peaks in 80 to 100 msec range) and greater synchronization across the scalp than responses from normals. This phenomenon is seen relatively early in the disease *(unpublished personal observations)*, while in later stages, the evoked potentials may become smaller, longer in latency, and simpler in configuration (22).

Halliday (23) has claimed that the SEP is useful in the differential diagnosis of myoclonus. He and others have demonstrated that a significant number of patients with familial, progressive myoclonus epilepsy have grossly enlarged SEPs as compared to individuals with essential or benign myoclonus. The value of this finding is tempered somewhat by the fact that the incidence of large SEPs in myoclonic epileptics appears to be correlated highly with the presence of myoclonic jerks and with the EEG abnormalities including polyspike-and-slow-wave complexes, focal spiking, etc.

Coma and Cerebral Death

Although the use of SEP recording in the differential diagnosis of coma has been attempted, in our opinion its value has not yet been demonstrated. There are theoretical reasons why newer methods of recording very short latency potentials, presumably originating in brainstem nuclei, might be more productive than the traditional techniques, but these have hardly been tried as yet.

The issue of cerebral death seems to become more complicated with time. Several investigators (24) have now reported persistence of some SEP even after cessation of all spontaneous cerebral electrical activity. Whether these sensory responses have true prognostic value or are only indicative of the already accepted phenomenon of differential rate of expiration of various components of the central nervous system remains to be proven.

Demyelinating Disease

One of the most widely celebrated and potentially useful applications of evoked response studies in neurological diagnosis was recently described by Halliday (25) at Queen's Square, and has been confirmed by others. Using a patterned stimulus (a reversing checkerboard), Halliday showed that the major positive component of the VEP (latency approximately 110 msec) is delayed by a demyelinating lesion in an optic nerve. This delay can be demonstrated in a large percentage of patients with multiple sclerosis (MS) even without clinical symptoms of visual disturbances and without visible changes in the optic disk. The assumption is that there is a relatively high incidence of plaques in the optic nerve in MS, many of which may be clinically silent, but which do cause some conduction delay detectable in the VEP. Hence, such recording may be particularly useful in differentiating between spinal cord compression and MS in a patient with progressive paraparesis but with no evidence of a separate intracranial lesion. It should be understood that the pattern VEP may be abnormal in the presence of optic neuritis from any cause, whether it be demyelination, inflammation, ischemia, or compression. Papilledema does not affect the latency of VEP components, but may cause diminished amplitude.

EVOKED POTENTIAL METHODS IN ASSESSMENT OF VISION AND HEARING

Hearing

The principle behind evoked response audiometry is based upon the assumption that if a subject "hears" a sound an evoked response will be recorded at the vertex and if the sound is not heard no response will occur. Obtaining a reasonable assessment of hearing threshold from both ears using this method is very tedious and time consuming, because hundreds of stimuli must be given at precisely specific intensities and frequencies. There is a marked moment-to-moment variability in evoked response amplitudes, and this occurs both without obvious cause in human subjects and in relation to factors such as changing levels of arousal and sleep (26).

In spite of these difficulties, the test can provide valuable information about hearing function in infants, young children, and other patients, who for one reason or another, cannot or will not cooperate in the subjective routines involved in conventional audiometry (32).

Quite recently, some investigators (9,28) have reported that recording of very early brainstem components as the indicators of hearing may significantly improve the reliability of the procedure. Another advantage of this kind of recording is that the brainstem EP components may reflect the functional integrity of individual segments of the auditory pathway in the brainstem.

Vision

Evoked potential techniques in assessing normal and disturbed function in the visual system have developed prolifically over the past 2 or 3 years. The state of the art now includes many highly refined stimulation and analysis procedures, including the use of complex patterned stimuli, phase modulated light, and Fourier analysis (1), in order to sort out electrical activity generated by the various specialized neuronal components subserving vision. There is a fast growing body of literature describing the changes in the VEP configuration to such stimulus parameters as check size (29), colors (30), intensity, and orientation of vertical lines (31). As exciting as these data have been in broadening our understanding of visual physiology, they have provided little in the way of clinically useful diagnostic information that cannot be obtained by conventional methods.

SUMMARY AND CONCLUSION

Recognizing the valuable and provocative contributions that evoked potential recordings have made to our understanding of the way in which the human nervous system processes incoming information, we believe it is worth emphasizing that at this point in time, and in all but the most experienced hands, averaged evoked potential recording is not an established diagnostic routine but is an experimental technique which is being developed for clinical application.

Anyone attempting to evaluate the literature in this field or contemplating the application of evoked potential studies to clinical diagnosis should be aware of several serious practical problems and limitations of the technique as it currently exists.

1. We do not as yet know with certainty where evoked potentials come from.

2. Such normative data as do exist tend to be useable only in the laboratory in which they are acquired because of the very marked variations from place to place in recording technique.

3. Even with the best of care and technique, not all recorded evoked responses contain all of the components expected. This is particularly true of the components in the early latency range up to 80 to 90 msec. This can be true both when recording from patients with pathology and from perfectly normal subjects.

4. Recording from patients who are ill and particularly from those who are uncooperative is always much more difficult than recording from cooperative volunteer subjects. Techniques learned with happy and comfortable volunteers are rarely directly applicable to the study of unwilling or uncomfortable patients.

5. Results of evoked potential recording are influenced by such diverse factors as age, sex, time of day, diet, state of awareness, expectancy, intelligence, and socioeconomic status (2). There is no evoked potential procedure for which such information is completely available at this time.

All of these factors limit the expectations one should have of the technique of evoked response recording. In addition, and most importantly, if such methods are to be adopted as diagnostic procedures they must be relevant to a clinical problem and must provide information that cannot be obtained more easily and more economically in other ways.

ACKNOWLEDGMENTS

The authors are indebted to Frances Burton for assistance in manuscript preparation. Some of the work reported was supported in part by Grant MT-3313 from the Medical Research Council of Canada.

REFERENCES

1. Regan, D. (1972): *Evoked Potentials in Psychology, Sensory Physiology and Clinical Medicine,* p. 328. Wiley, New York.
2. Shagass, C. (1972): *Evoked Brain Potentials in Psychiatry,* p. 274. Plenum Press, New York.
3. Vaughan, H. G., Jr. (1969): The relationship of brain activity to scalp recordings of event-related potentials. In: *Average Evoked Potentials: Methods, Results and Evaluations,* edited by E. Donchin and D. B. Lindsley, pp. 45–75. NASA Special Publication 191.
4. Desmedt, J. E., Brunko, E., Debecker, J., and Carmeliet, J. (1974): The system bandpass required to avoid distortion of early components when averaging somatosensory evoked potentials. *Electroencephalogr. Clin. Neurophysiol.,* 37:407–410.
5. Lindsley, D. B. (1969): Average evoked potentials: Achievements, failures and prospects. In: *Average Evoked Potentials: Methods, Results and Evaluations,* edited by E. Donchin and D. B. Lindsley, pp. 1–44. NASA Special Publication 191.
6. Picton, T. W., Hillyard, S. A., Krausz, H. I., and Galambos, R. (1974): Human auditory-evoked potentials. I. Evaluation of components. *Electroencephalogr. Clin. Neurophysiol.,* 36:179–190.
7. Goff, W. R., Rosner, B. S., and Allison, T. (1962): Distribution of cerebral somatosensory evoked responses in normal man. *Electroencephalogr. Clin. Neurophysiol.,* 14:697–713.
8. Cracco, R. (1973): Spinal evoked responses in man. *Electroencephalogr. Clin. Neurophysiol.,* 35:379–386.
9. Jewett, D. L., and Willeston, J. S. (1971): Auditory-evoked far fields averaged from the scalp of humans. *Brain,* 94:681–696.
10. Ball, G. J., Saunders, M. G., and Schnabl, J. (1971): Determination of peripheral sensory nerve conduction velocities in man from stimulus response delays of the cortical evoked potentials. *Electroencephalogr. Clin. Neurophysiol.,* 30:409–414.
11. Desmedt, J. E. (1971): Somatosensory cerebral evoked potentials in man. In: *Handbook of Electroencephalography and Clinical Neurophysiology,* Vol. 8, edited by W. A. Cobb. Elsevier, Amsterdam.
12. Bergamini, L., and Bergamasco, B. (1967): *Cortical Evoked Potentials in Man,* p. 116. Charles C Thomas, Springfield.
13. Nakanishu, T., Shimada, Y., and Toyokura, Y. (1974): Somatosensory evoked responses to mechanical stimulus in normal subjects and patients with neurological disorders. *J. Neurol. Sci.,* 21:289–294.
14. Perot, P. L., Jr. (1972): The clinical use of somatosensory evoked potentials in spinal cord injury. *Clin. Neurosurg.,* 20:367–381.
15. Giblin, D. R. (1964): Somatosensory evoked potentials in healthy subjects and in patients with lesions of the nervous system. *Ann. NY Acad. Sci.,* 112:93.
16. Croft, T. J., Brodkey, J. S., and Nulsen, F. E. (1972): Reversible spinal cord trauma: A model for electrical monitoring of spinal cord function. *J. Neurosurg.,* 36:402–406.
17. D'Angelo, C. M., Vangilder, J. C., and Taub, A. (1973): Evoked cortical potentials in experimental spinal cord trauma. *J. Neurosurg.,* 38:332–336.
18. Low, M. D., and Purves, S. J. (1976): Sensory evoked potentials, CNV and the EEG in patients with proven brain lesions. *Electroencephalogr. Clin. Neurophysiol. (In press).*
19. Vaughan, H. G., Jr., and Katzman, R. (1964): Evoked responses in visual disorders. *Ann. NY Acad. Sci.,* 112:305–319.
20. Jonkman, E. J. (1967): The Average Cortical Response to Photic Stimulation. Thesis. University of Amsterdam.
21. Pampiglione, G., and Harden, A. (1973): Neurophysiological identification of late infantile form of "neuronal lipidosis." *J. Neurol. Neurosurg. Psychiatry,* 36:68–74.
22. Lee, R. G., and Blair, R. D. G. (1973): Evolution of EEG and visual evoked response changes in Jakob-Creutzfeldt disease. *Electroencephalogr. Clin. Neurophysiol.,* 35:133–142.
23. Halliday, A. M. (1967): The electrophysiological study of myoclonus in man. *Brain,* 90:241–284.
24. Trojaborg, W., and Jorgenson, E. O. (1973): Evoked cortical potentials in patients with "isoelectric" EEG's. *Electroencephalogr. Clin. Neurophysiol.,* 35:301–309.
25. Halliday, A. M., Donald, W. I., and Muchin, J. (1973): Visual evoked responses in diagnosis of multiple sclerosis. *Br. Med. J.,* 661–664.

26. Low, M. D. (1973): Clinical applications of auditory evoked potentials. *Am. J. EEG Technol.,* 13:148–155.
27. Rapin, I., and Graziani, L. J. (1967): Auditory evoked response in normal, brain damaged and deaf infants. *Neurology (Minneap.),* 17:881–894.
28. Hecox, K., and Galambos, R. (1974): Brain stem auditory evoked response in human infants and adults. *Arch. Otolaryngol.,* 99:30–33.
29. Harter, M. R., and White, C. T. (1972): Evoked cortical responses to checkerboard patterns: Effects of check-size as a function of visual acuity. *Electroencephalogr. Clin. Neurophysiol.,* 33:517–519.
30. Clynes, M., and Kohn, M. (1967): Spatial VERP's as physiologic language elements for colour and field structure. *EEG Journal, (Suppl.),* 26:82–96.
31. Campbell, F. W., and Maffei, L. (1970): Electrophysiological evidence for the existence of orientation and size detectors in human visual system. *J. Physiol. (Lond.),* 207:635–652.
32. Cody, D. T. R., Klass, D. W., and Bickford, R. G. (1967): Cortical audiometry: An objective method of evaluating auditory activity in awake and sleeping man. *Trans. Am. Acad. Ophthalmol. Otolaryngol.,* 71:81–91.

Current Practice of Clinical Electroencephalography,
edited by D. W. Klass and D. D. Daly.
Raven Press, New York © 1979.

Chapter 17

Newer Methods of Recording and Analyzing EEGs

Reginald G. Bickford

University of California, San Diego, La Jolla, California 92037

Analog Methods.	452
Response Averaging.	456
Averaging Artifacts.	457
Spectral Methods.	460
The Comagram.	465
Area Display of Spectral Information.	467
Area Display of Voltage Contours.	469
Telephone Transmission Techniques.	473
Summary.	479
Acknowledgments.	479
References.	479

Although this account presents the computer techniques developed at the University of California, San Diego (UCSD), it should be noted that similar attempts at computerizing the electroencephalogram (EEG) are proceeding in many laboratories in this country as well as in Europe and Asia. Fortunately, the general topic of computer development related to clinical EEG was recently reviewed in several publications, and the reader who requires a more balanced view of computer progress in the EEG field should consult these sources (9,10).

This account emphasizes the following points.

1. Simple analog computer approaches (such as filtering, integration, subtraction, etc.) can be very successfully applied in clinical work. They have the conspicuous advantage of being quite modest in cost and adaptable for easy application to the average clinical EEG instrument.

2. In the digital computer development involving more costly instruments, our laboratory has emphasized graphic techniques because they have the dual effect of compressing EEG data and of making it more easily comprehensible.

3. Whereas graphic methods [e.g., the compressed spectral array (CSA)] transmit data between EEGer and clinician succinctly, they are less satisfactory when, for instance, fine comparisons between the spectra (e.g., those produced by a drug) are being made. Under these conditions and when decisions have to be made (as in, for instance, the administration of anesthetic in servoanesthesia), the addition of numerical data to the graphic display becomes necessary.

The questions of "Why automation?" and "What are the advantages of computer versus visual estimates?" are outlined in Fig. 1. Thus, tests in our laboratory have shown that the average EEGer's estimation of amplitude is poorly quantitated even when the descriptor is limited to "low, medium, or high." As we shall see, simple integrator systems can overcome this defect. The masking of one rhythm by another is a problem that occurs frequently in clinical practice and leads to practical difficulties (as in brain death). It is often a simple matter for the computer to solve this problem.

Referring to A3, there is certainly need for a more quantitative approach to spike classification as laboratory tests have shown a wide degree of variability among experienced electroencephalographers in their recognition of these discharges. Computer processing can at least classify them on the basis of amplitude, slope, and com-

A. DEFECTS OF PRESENT SYSTEM
  1. POOR AMPLITUDE ESTIMATES } "EYE" LIMITATIONS
  2. MASKING PROBLEMS (E.K.G.)
  3. SPIKE CLASSIFICATION } CRITERIA UNDERDEVELOPED

B. ADVANTAGES
  1. INCREASED DIAGNOSTIC ACCURACY
  2. SPEED OF READING, INTERPRETATION AND DISSEMINATION
  3. EASY COMPREHENSIBILITY
  4. DECREASED COST

FIG. 1. Automation.

plexity of components. The computer approach to this difficult problem (7) shows some promise of improving visual estimates as well as of providing a means of automatic recognition.

Figure 2 attempts to classify some of the main categories of methods that have been used for quantitating the EEG. The classification has limitations and overlaps, but gives an overall view of different kinds of approaches in use at present.

ANALOG METHODS

Let us now turn to the simplest form of EEG processing—that of channel integration seen in Fig. 3. This implies a summation of the voltages contained in all components of the trace. Expressed otherwise, it can be looked upon as a summation of the area under the curve. It is a very useful but relatively underused method of quantitating the EEG. In the example shown, all frequency compo-

1. PROCESSING METHODS — integration, subtraction, averaging, spectral analysis, spike recognition

2. DISPLAY METHODS — toposcope, compressed spectral arrays, event contouring

3. REPORTING METHODS — computer compiled report, Mayo system

4. DISSEMINATION METHODS
   - IN — telephone (data)
   - OUT — telephone (voice)
     teletype (data)
     xerox (data)

FIG. 2. Automation in EEG.

nents of the record are given equal weight or emphasis, and we see how the periodicity of sleep can be followed quite well by the recurring peaks (largely due to slow waves of stages II, III, and IV). The case of hepatic coma also shows a periodicity with about ½- to 1-hr cycle—a fact not usually apparent in the clinical EEG recording. In cerebral trauma, it has been shown that this kind of cycling indicates a favorable prognosis. It is often desirable to quantitate the number of seizures in status epilepticus and thereby detect the beneficial effects of anticonvulsant treatment. This may prove costly and difficult with a standard EEG, but it is well shown in this illustration for a patient who had a recurrent focal seizure every 15 min to ½ hr. The integrator is also useful in quantitating the course of a patient approaching brain death, and at the bottom of the figure is shown an example of a case of coma that eventually reached the state of electrocerebral silence. In the graph above, electrocerebral silence is monitored for a period of about 6 hr. Note that on integration, a common integrated microvoltage activity in electrocerebral silence is about 3 to 4 μV, which is above the International criteria for electrocerebral silence. This integrated activity results from: (a) some addition (about 1 μV) from the presence of electrocardiogram (EKG), and (b) the fact that the international criteria (2 μV) do not adequately reflect the noise level present in recording systems as they are used in the intensive care unit. Thus, a similar (2 to 3 μV) integration level is often obtained from the arm leads used as a control. The use of band-limited integration in Fig. 4 shows a series of alpha rhythms from normal subjects integrated within a bandpass of 8 to 13 Hz. The values of the alpha integration are shown with each curve.

Notice that the eye would have difficulty in recognizing any difference between the lower two curves that come from the left and right occipital regions. Thus, band integration provides not only a simple quantitation of the EEG, but also a widely applicable measure that could be used as a record descriptor when communicating information from one EEG laboratory to another. Thus, it would be quite practical to say that patient X when recorded in Y EEG lab had integrated delta values of 30 and 18 μV in tests made at 3-week intervals and that on this basis his right hemiplegia was suspected of being vascular in origin. When he comes to new lab Z, they can again perform an integration, and they may find that the value of delta activity has now fallen to six (confirming the original progressive improvement) or perhaps has increased to 30 indicating some kind of relapse. This kind of lab interchange would be very useful in the clinical field. Simple integrators that do these kinds of calculations are available or can be easily built (5,6).

Finally, another analog method, that of subtraction, can be very usefully employed in the manner illustrated in Fig. 5. Here we are attempting to remove the EKG artifact from trace #2 (FP1–A1)

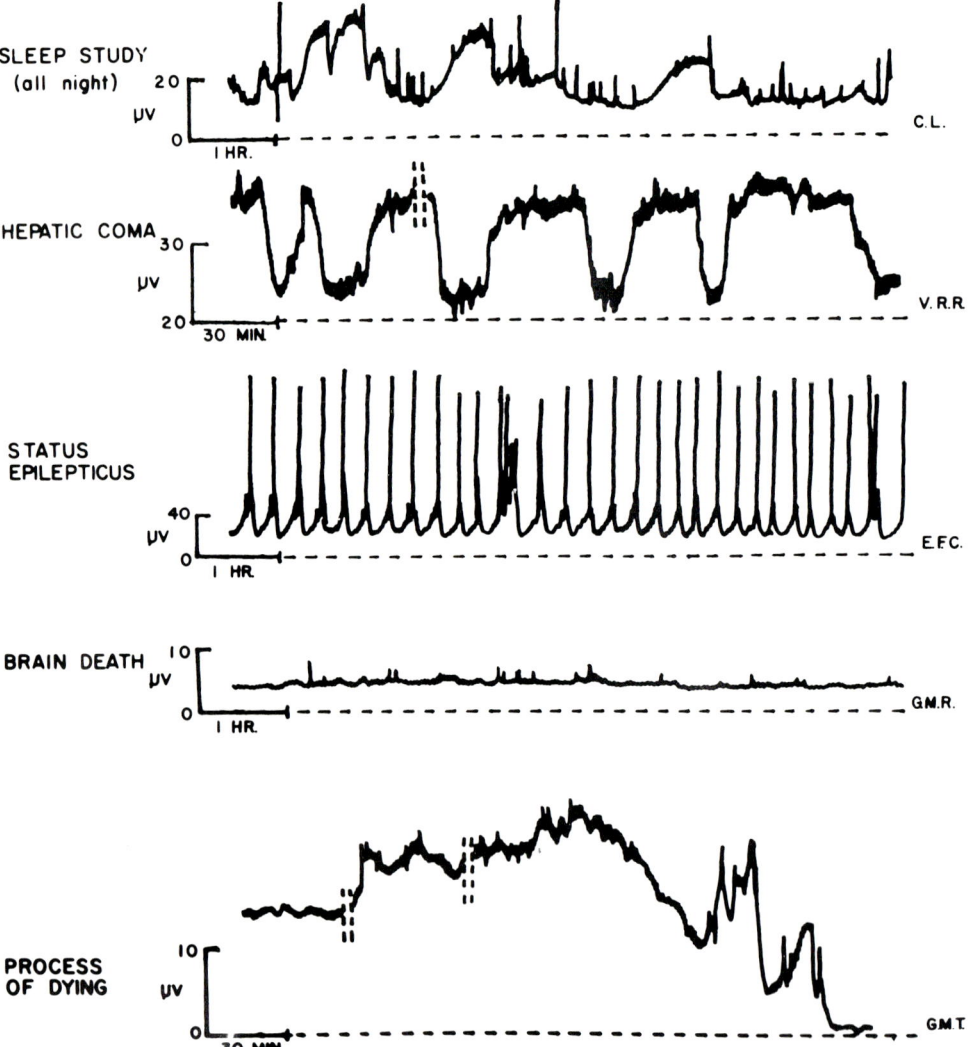

FIG. 3. Use of simple wide band integrator in clinical monitoring (see text).

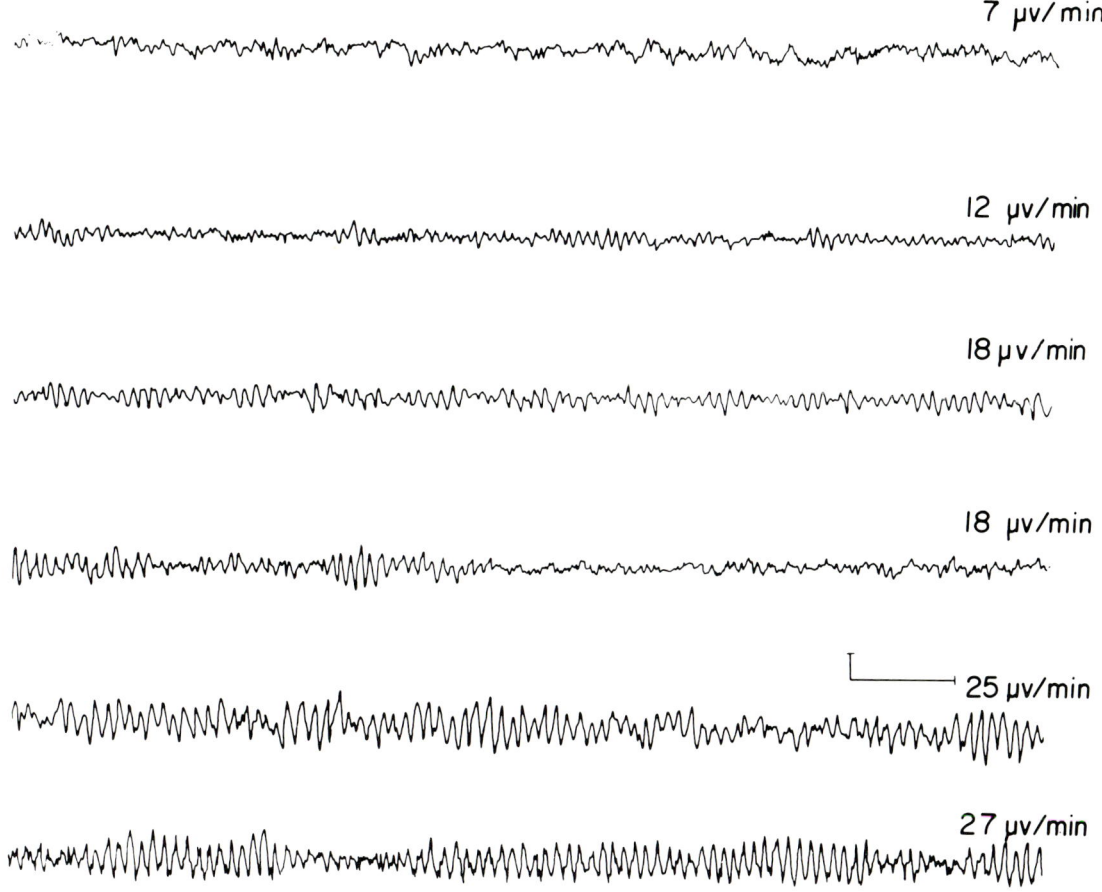

FIG. 4. Use of restrictive frequency band integration (8- to 13-Hz alpha band) using band integration computer (BIC) integrator system (5, 6). Numbers on the right indicate alpha band integration microvolts (when compared to a sine wave calibration).

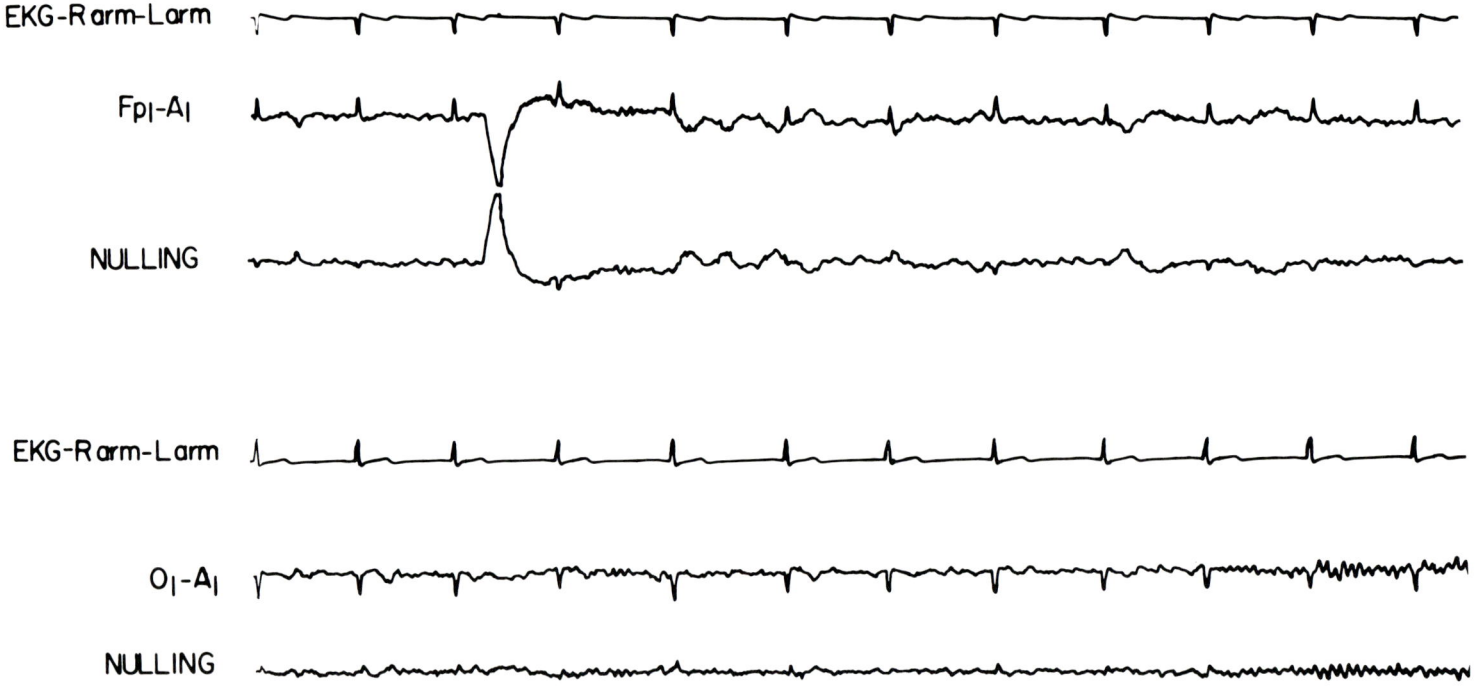

FIG. 5. Example of analog subtraction of EKG to eliminate this artifact from the EEG tracing shown for FP1–A1 above and O1–A1 below. The right arm–left arm EKG is recorded. The base of the neck is used for subtraction since this is essentially free from EEG activity. The resulting subtracted wave form is demonstrated under "nulling." It is almost free of EKG artifact in contrast to the unsubtracted EEG data. The nulled wave form can be subject to integration to produce a valid measure of brain activity in brain death monitoring.

by using a matched EKG pattern recorded from the chest. A nearly perfect removal of the EKG results as seen under "nulling." If the EEG is now submitted to voltage integration, a valuable indicator of brain viability is then available (free from the errors that would be present if the unsubtracted record were used) (4).

RESPONSE AVERAGING

We now come to consider an area of computer technique, namely averaging, some aspects of which have been discussed in Chapter 16. Response averaging is a computer method of enhancing a brain response (evoked response) to some external stimulus by the addition of a large number of responses as shown in Fig. 6. Because the signal contained in each response adds linearly (owing to its constant delay in relation to the input stimulus) and random noise such as

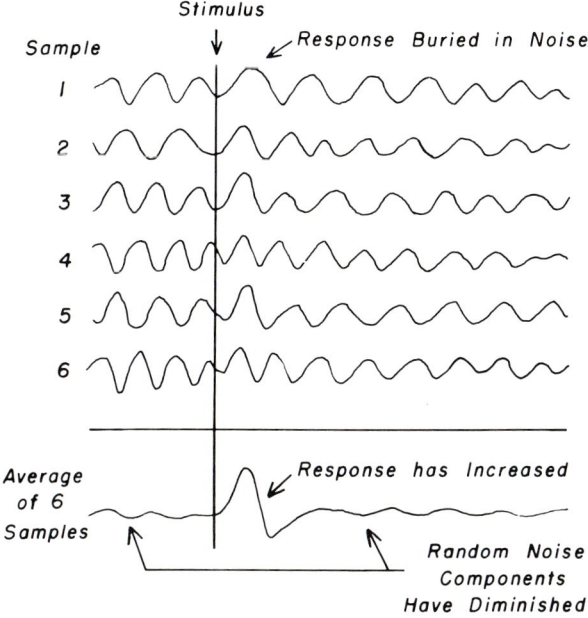

FIG. 6. A diagram of the mechanism of response averaging. It depends on the fact that in each sample the stimulus (flash, click, or shock) is followed by a response that is always at the same latency and therefore is aligned when a series of traces (samples containing the response) are added. Noise (unwanted EEG rhythms, including alpha, theta, delta, biologic, and amplifier components) tend to cancel under these conditions since they are not systematically related to the stimulus. The result of additions of six responses in the bottom trace has delineated the evoked response which is not clearly visible in any one of the single responses.

alpha rhythm, muscle, etc., is as likely to be positive as negative at any point in the summation, it trends to zero. Using this technique, very small responses, such as those from brainstem auditory evoked responses (BAERs), of 0.25-μV amplitude can still be defined so long as large numbers of responses are summated. From a clinical standpoint, evoked responses are now divided into "near field" and the recently discovered "far field" (3). The near field responses are those of the classic evoked response such as that recorded in the occipital cortex, an example of which is shown in Fig. 7. Here we see the exquisite sensitivity manifest in the evoked response pattern of an epileptic patient who was sensitive to vertical stripes (but not to horizontal). The far field responses can be recorded from the scalp surface by conventional EEG electrodes and yet represent activity originating from sequential activation of a group of nuclei and tracks in the auditory pathway. An example from a normal subject is shown in Fig. 8 in which the wave components are indicated. Note the accuracy with which the waves can be delineated. These responses provide a very important new indicator of conduction-interrupting pathology within the brainstem.

AVERAGING ARTIFACTS

Computer experts have a saying "garbage in, garbage out" indicating that the computer has very little to say about whether the data which it is fed is genuine or artifactual. This is the responsibility of the technician or interpreter. Because of the extreme sensitivity of the averaging method (evoked potential amplitudes down to $1/10$ μV can be defined) and the tendency of many extracranial generators (eyes, muscles, tongue) to be entrained by the stimulus, great care and understanding of physiologic mechanisms are needed for proper interpretation of these records. An example of a trouble-

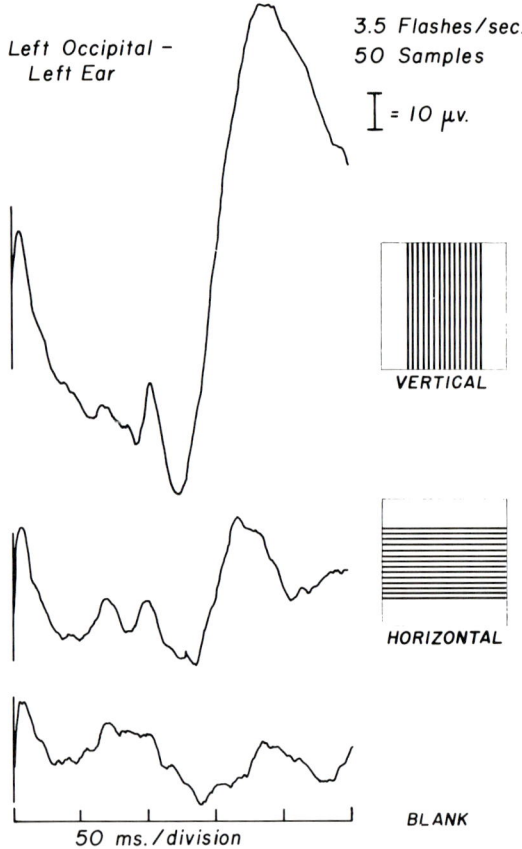

FIG. 7. An example of response averaging applied to an epileptic patient who is photosensitive and in whom spike-and-wave discharges are elicited by gazing at vertical patterns. Horizontal patterns are ineffective. Pattern was illuminated by strobe flashes (low intensity) in darkened room. In the spontaneous EEG, vertical patterns give rise to spike wave discharges. In the experiment illustrated, the patterns shown were flashed by a light placed behind the patient's head at an intensity less than that required to produce spike wave discharge. Note the large effect on the late potentials (100 to 250 msec) resulting from pattern orientation. A related pattern-shift evoked potential technique has recently been employed to detect clinically significant delays in conduction within the optic system in patients with demyelinating disease (2).

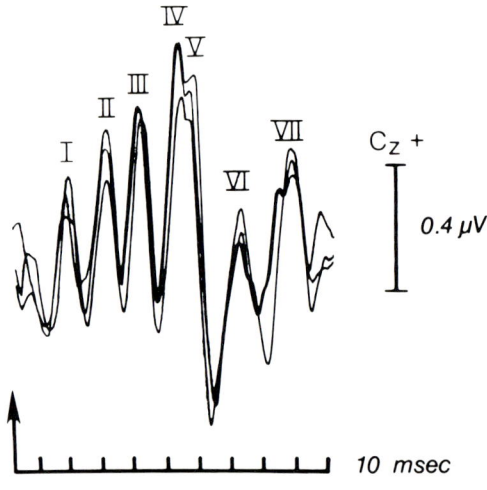

FIG. 8. Example of the far field waves (BAERs) recorded from the scalp when click stimulus is applied to the ipsilateral ear. The five waves encountered in normal subjects are thought to have the following approximate origins: wave I, eighth nerve; wave II, dorsal cochlear nucleus; wave III, superior olive; wave IV, lateral lemniscus; wave V, inferior colliculus. Note the short latency of these waves which were originally observed by Sohner and by Jewett (3). They are of considerable clinical significance in relation to neuronal maturation, detection of deafness, and in lesions of the brainstem where various waves may be prolonged in latency or eliminated. (A calibration 0.5 µV and 1.0 msec stimulus, 60 dBSL, right ear montage A_2–C_z.) (Data from Stockard and Rossiter.)

some artifact in evoked potential work is the microreflex illustrated in Fig. 9. This is a normal subject responding to strobe flashes at 2/sec. A genuine brain response is shown in the middle section from the inion electrode. On the left and the right, large potentials can be seen resembling those from the brain, but they are generated by muscle components in tension. These microreflexes (1) can be troublesome in patients who fail to relax; a knowledge of their form and

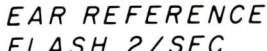

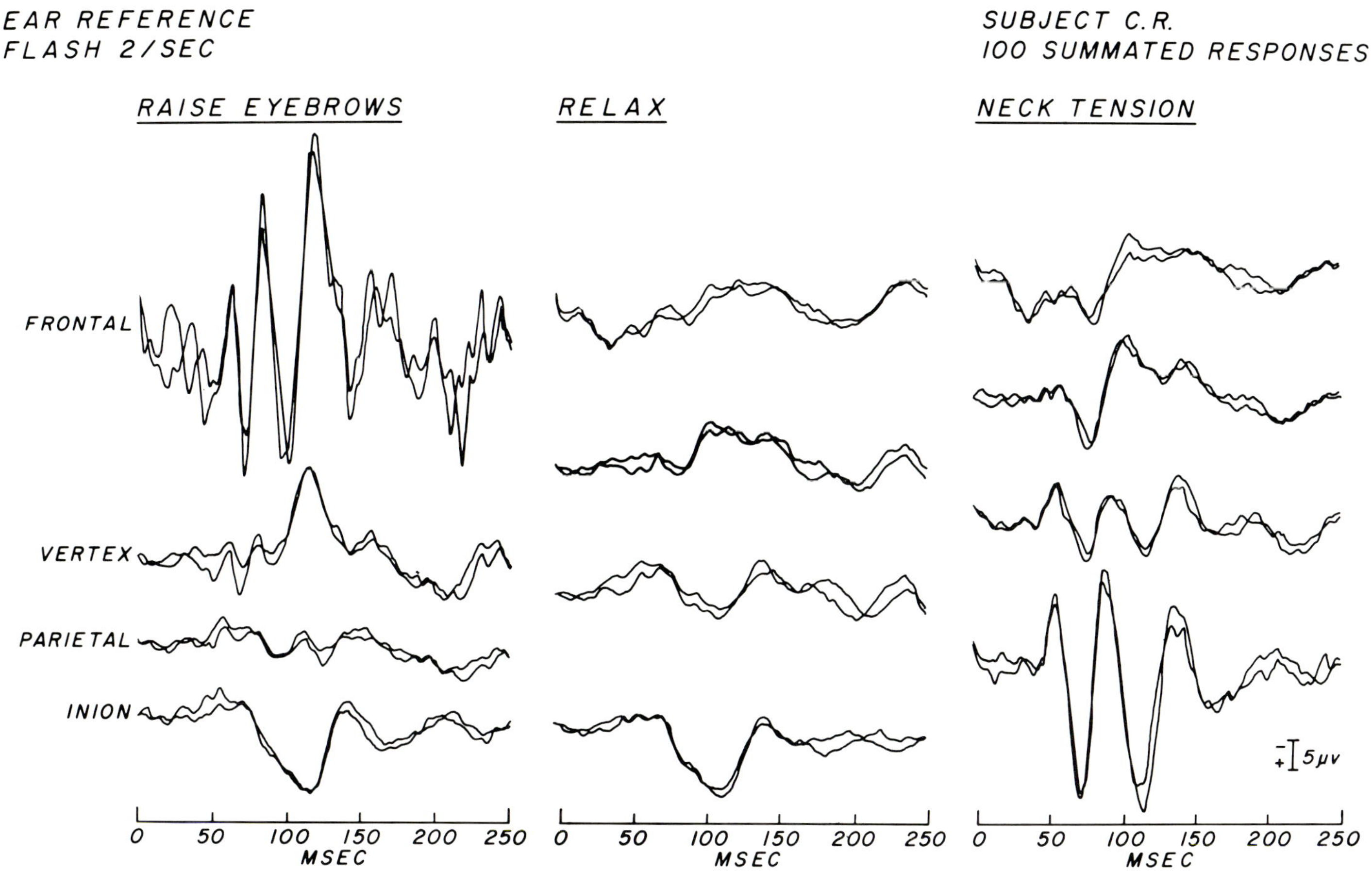

FIG. 9. Examples of contamination of an averaged evoked response in a normal subject by microreflex (myogenic) response. The genuine brain wave response is seen in the middle section when the subject is relaxed. The frontal myogenic responses are seen on the left in the frontalis muscle resulting from increasing tension and on the right in the occipitalis and neck muscles when tension is applied to the neck. Note the smoothness (unlike the muscle activity in the primary trace) of the wave form and the overall resemblance of components to those of the genuine evoked response. These myogenic artifacts appear commonly in normal subjects and can be seen in photic (as above), auditory, and somasthetic evoked potential recordings.

latency is necessary for the proper interpretation of evoked potential recordings.

SPECTRAL METHODS

Electroencephalographers have a specific interest in the frequency shifts that occur in the brain potentials in varied states of consciousness and as a result of localized or generalized pathology. Thus, it is appropriate to use computer methods that quantitate this aspect of the brain rhythms in analyzing the EEG. This is the reason for the recent popularity of spectral analysis methods in EEG. The basic theory of a spectral analysis and plotting methods is shown in Fig. 10. Note that the spectral method sorts the mixed frequencies contained in the original EEG into an orderly sequence from low to high (0.25 to 16 Hz), smooths the graph, and then packs one graph down upon another as sequential 4-sec segments of original EEG data are analyzed.

A special trick known as "hidden line suppression" is used in the compiling of more than one spectral plot. By not allowing any subsequent line to override a previous peak, a three-dimensional optical effect is produced rendering the data far more comprehensible to the eye. An example of a compressed spectral plot of this kind is shown in the bottom of Fig. 10 from the alpha rhythm of a normal subject. Note that there is some shifting of peaks in addition to the presence of subsidiary peaks at the lower end of the alpha band. Note also that in this method time rises vertically at 4 sec/spectral line, and intensity (i.e., power) is the height of peaks as they project out of the background. In Fig. 11, we see a variety of alpha spectra as they were encountered in a group of medical students. Note the great individual variability of the spectral plots and the great degree of compression of data obtained by this method.

Another example of compression of data by spectral plots is shown in Fig. 12. This is the spectra analysis of the response of the brain to a light stimulus that increases progressively in flash frequency—commencing at one flash/sec and finishing at 16. Thus, it sweeps across the frequency registers of the spectral analysis profile; and on the left the normal response to a photic sweep is seen. There are irregular series of peaks with a diagonal course, and another diagonal can be seen in the lower part of the figure representing generation of harmonics. Contrast this picture with the chaotic result of photic stimulation in a photosensitive patient. This triggers many discharges at the earlier (relatively slow flash rates), and little evidence of the basic diagonal driving response of the brain can be seen. Like response averaging, spectral analysis of the EEG also has a number of artifactual situations associated with it. Again, muscle activity often produces problems as can be seen in Fig. 13. Whereas the overall spectra of muscle are different from those of the alpha rhythm, they nevertheless contain components such as those at 10 Hz shown at the bottom of Fig. 13 which are within the alpha spectral band. Furthermore, the electromyogram (EMG) also contains a good deal of energy at the slow end of the spectrum. Therefore, it is important to monitor EEG activity entering a computing system to keep it free of this activity which may introduce many spurious peaks that are difficult to separate from the genuine components in the spectrum. Figure 14 summarizes the ways in which the graphics and numerical programs associated with spectral analysis have been developed in our laboratory. To convey general diagnostic information to the clinician, we have found the CSA, which displays individual spectra from different electrodes in their relative position on the head, to be of most significance. In contrast, EEG recording has now become important in long-term monitoring of patients during sleep, in the intensive care unit, and in coma situations. Some examples of this type of application are seen in the lower part of the

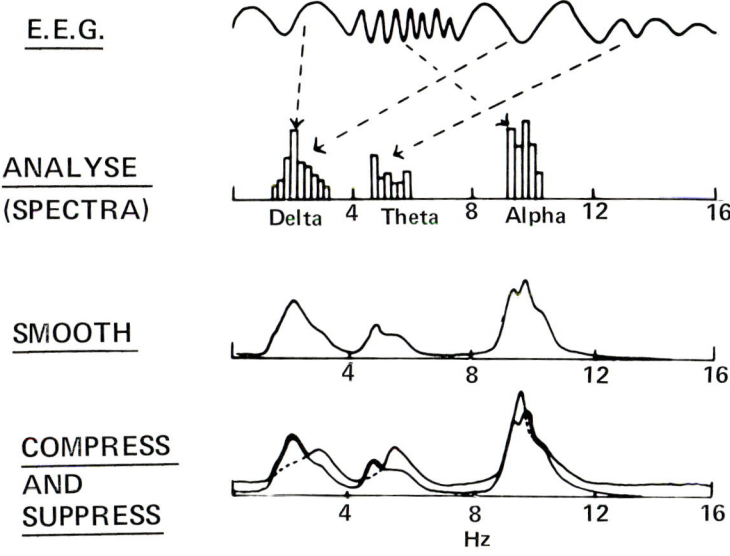

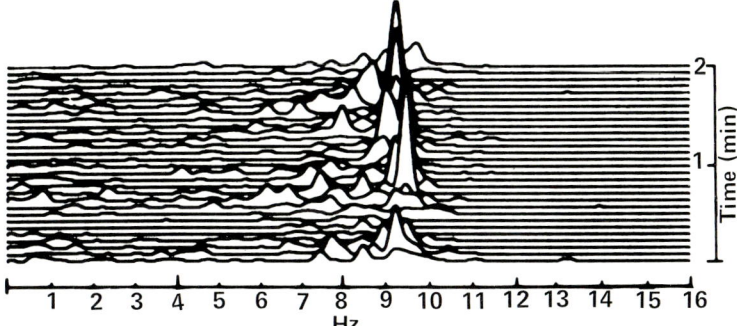

METHOD OF ANALYSIS AND DISPLAY

COMPRESSED SPECTRAL ARRAY SHOWING ALPHA RHYTHM

Fig. 10. A diagram of the mechanism of power spectral analysis used to produce the three dimensional spectral arrays. The primary EEG trace (4 sec) is shown above, and the bar spectra that results from computer Fourier Analysis is shown below. After smoothing and hidden line suppression, the final array is shown displaying a normal alpha rhythm below. In this display, time rises vertically in 4-sec line intervals, and intensity (i.e., power) is shown as the height of peaks.

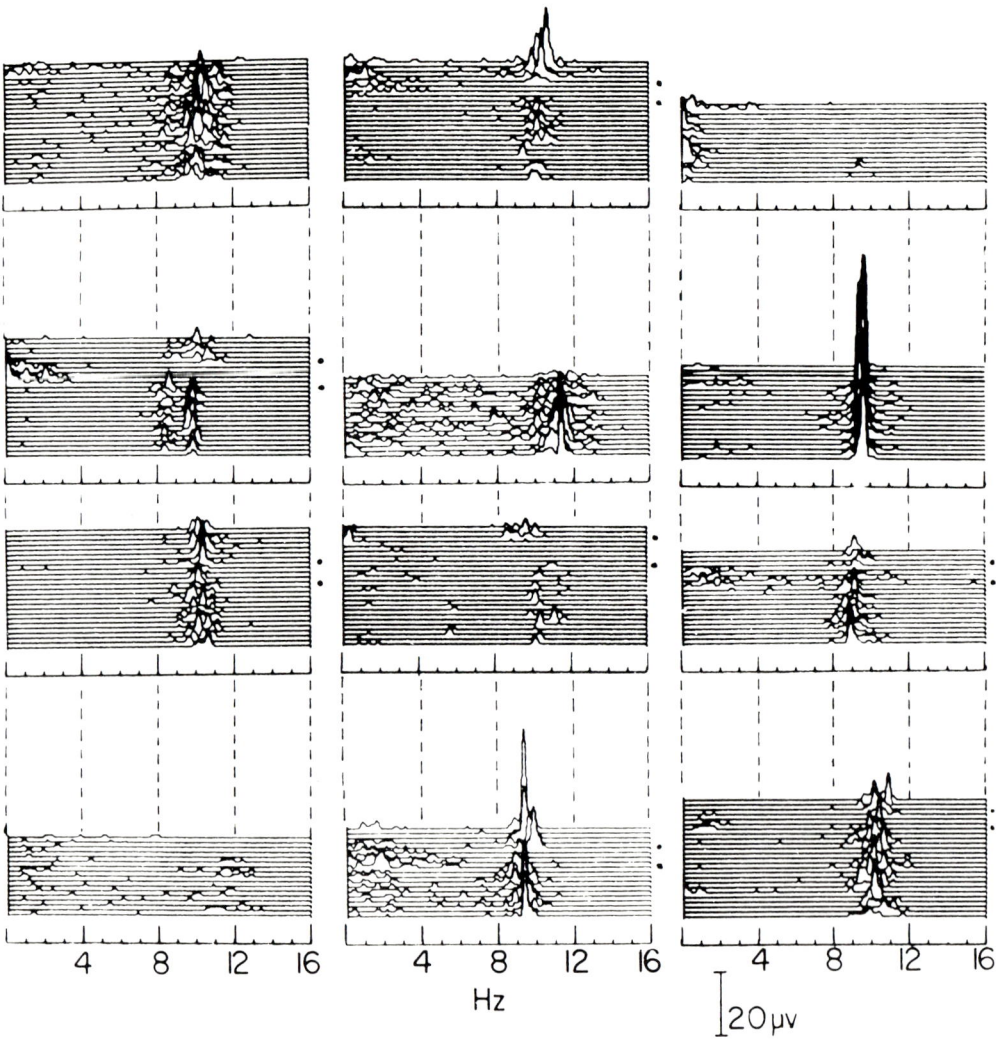

FIG. 11. Examples of the variety of alpha spectra yielded by selected examples from a class of medical students (UCSD). Note the wide variety of spectra that can be seen including some students who have little detectable alpha rhythm. One student has a high amplitude sharply tuned alpha rhythm; another shows a bimodal distribution; all recorded at standard gain.

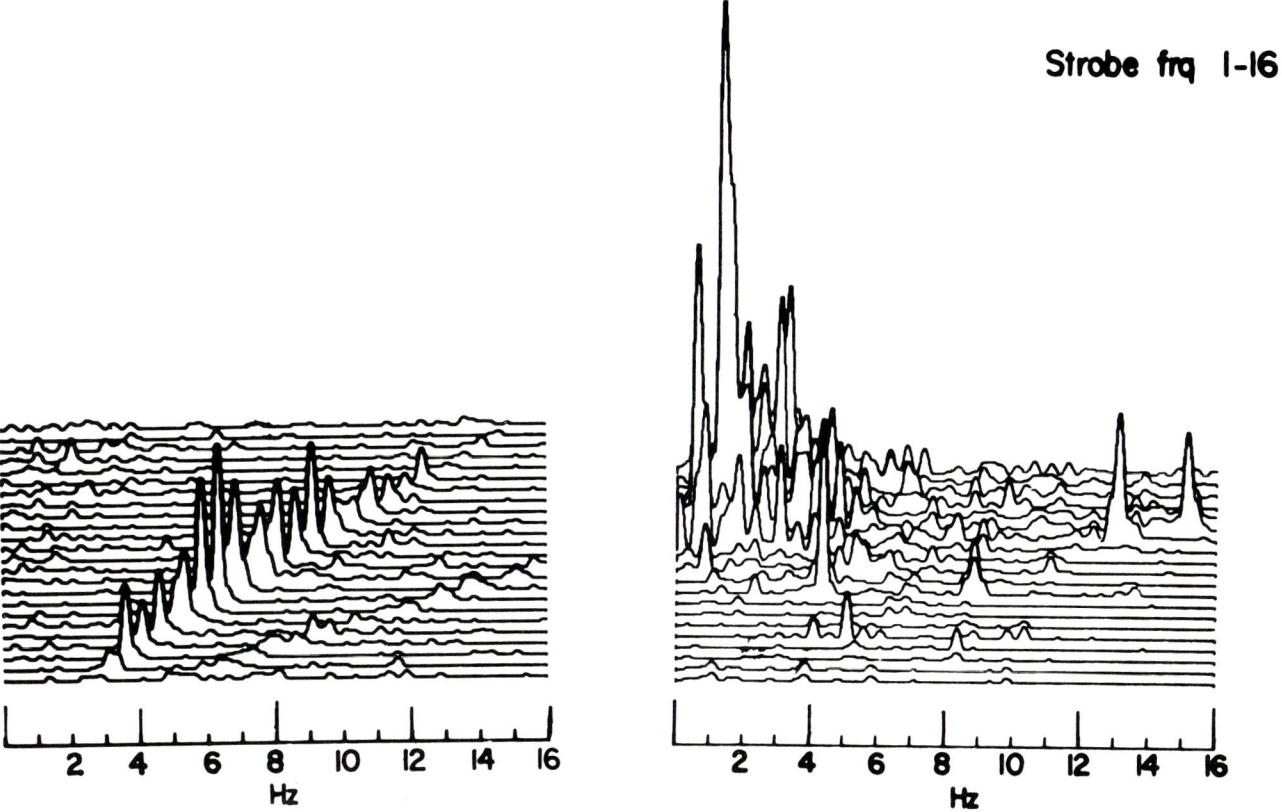

Fig. 12. On the left is shown the normal photic response when the light flash increases in rate smoothly and continuously from 1/sec on left side of display to 16/sec on the right. Note the primary driving response and below and to the right another diagonal line representing the harmonic response which is not so clearly defined. On the right is a chaotic response recorded from a photosensitive patient in whom light flash induced spike wave discharges. Identical stimulus technique is employed. Note that at lower flash rates, a relatively normal response results, but above 6 to 8/sec triggering of spike wave discharges commences giving a complex spectrum seen with maximal components in the 1- to 4-Hz band. Note that there is no exaggeration of the driving response itself; in fact, it is reduced in amplitude when compared to that seen in the normal subject on the left.

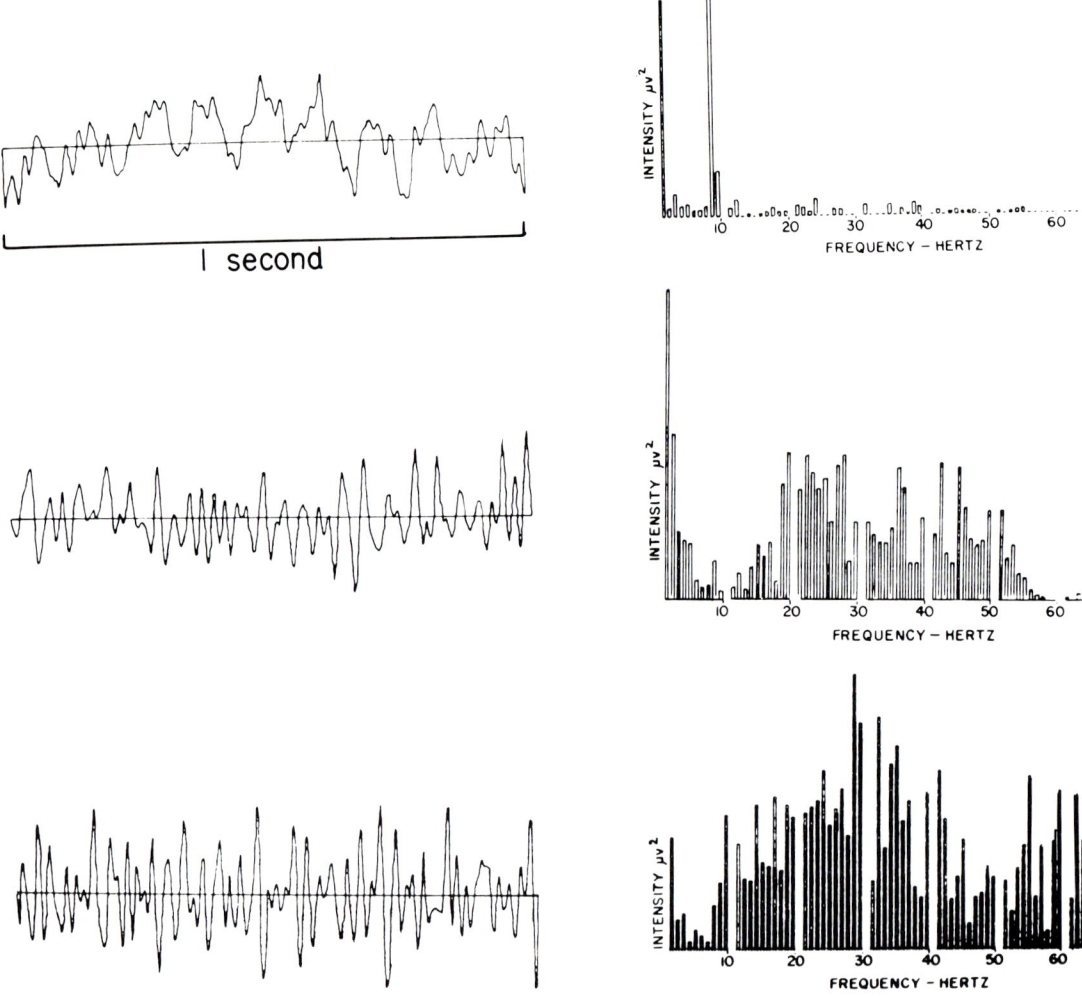

FIG. 13. The power spectra obtained from a normal subject with a clearly defined alpha peak at 9.5 Hz above. The two spectra below—forehead *(middle)* and forearm *(bottom)*—represent pure muscle spectra from EMG motor unit firing, as this is processed by a spectral analysis system. Note that in the forearm spectrum, there is a 10-Hz component that could be mistaken for alpha activity shown above. Slow waves are also present in muscle spectra, with a large component in the forehead at 1 Hz.

figure where they are represented diagrammatically. In these applications, other parameters beside the EEG are included in the display. This is well shown in the somnogram which includes EEG spectrum on the left, the integration of the EEG in the middle, the electrooculogram (EOG) on the right, and the EMG on the extreme right. The demand for quantitation of these traces and for the inclusion of evoked potentials and other parameters led to the development of what we shall call the numero somnogram. In this display, the integrated power values are plotted at intervals in the case illustrated for the delta and alpha bands. Evoked potentials are also automatically plotted as required, and the interbeat intervals that indicate heart rate are included in the display.

The somnogram, as its name implies, has been designed specifically to display the physiologic parameters (EEG, EOG, EMG) necessary for the study of sleep. Figure 15 is a diagram of the changes that take place in these parameters as a normal subject goes to sleep. Note that in the waking state an alpha peak is present, some eye movements are present, and the EMG is high. As the subject moves to stage I, there is a diminution and broadening of the alpha peak, a decrease in integrated EEG, a moderate amount of EOG due to pendular eye movement, and some decrease in EMG. Stage II is characterized by further diminution of alpha frequencies, an increase in delta activity, and the appearance of a new spectral peak due to spindles occurring at 13 to 16 Hz. Integrated EEG activity (INT) is increased by the presence of delta; EOG activity is low, and EMG has decreased. As the subject goes into stages III and IV, there is a further increase in delta activity producing an increased integration, EOG is low, and EMG is moderate. During the rapid eye movement (REM) stage, there are marked changes, including low-voltage EEG with scattered spectral activity with a low overall integration, a marked increase in EOG owing to REM, and usually a marked decrease in EMG. An example of a numera somnogram is shown on the right side of Fig. 16. This is an excerpt from a somnogram showing well-marked spindle activity interrupted on two occasions by REM. The initial burst of eye movement is caused by pendular activity characteristic of drowsiness. This was taken from a patient who claimed that she never slept more than ½ hr a night and who was suspected of having a barbiturate dependency problem. In fact, in the sleep lab she slept a full 8 hr. On the left side is a remarkable somnogram taken from a patient who suffered a severe head injury 5 years previously and who claimed not to sleep more than ½ to 1-hr per night since the accident. The correctness of this assertion is shown in the recording illustrated on the left which shows some alpha activity throughout a 6-hr period with no change in the integrated EEG, little change in eye movements, and a moderate amount of muscle. It was indeed true that the patient had become an insomniac as a result of head trauma.

THE COMAGRAM

The techniques developed for the somnogram and its extension to other parameters open up some important new fields for monitoring in which the computer output chart is used to interrelate many complex physiologic variables. This kind of recording is being employed in the newborn nursery where infants with respiratory difficulties can be studied and a decision made whether, for instance, the periods of apnea result primarily from seizure discharges, from cardiac changes, or from primary brainstem respiratory dysfunction. Likewise, in the adult coma patient, the combination of these parameters is useful in estimating the progress of patients who are unconscious from cerebral trauma. Thus, it has been shown that fluctuation and cycling of slow-wave activity, when present, improves the prognosis in comparison with those patients who show continuous, unrelent-

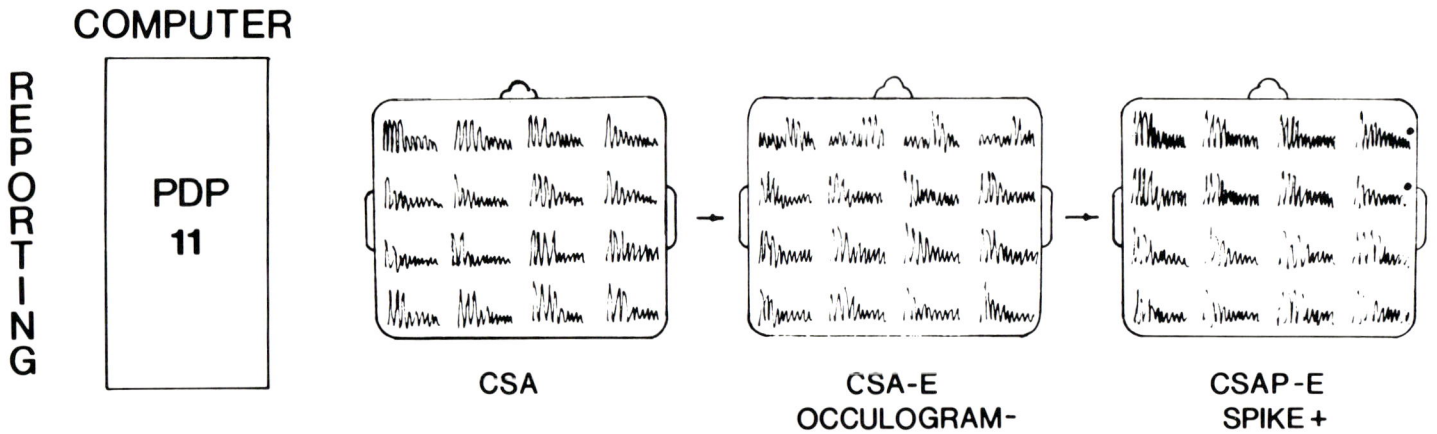
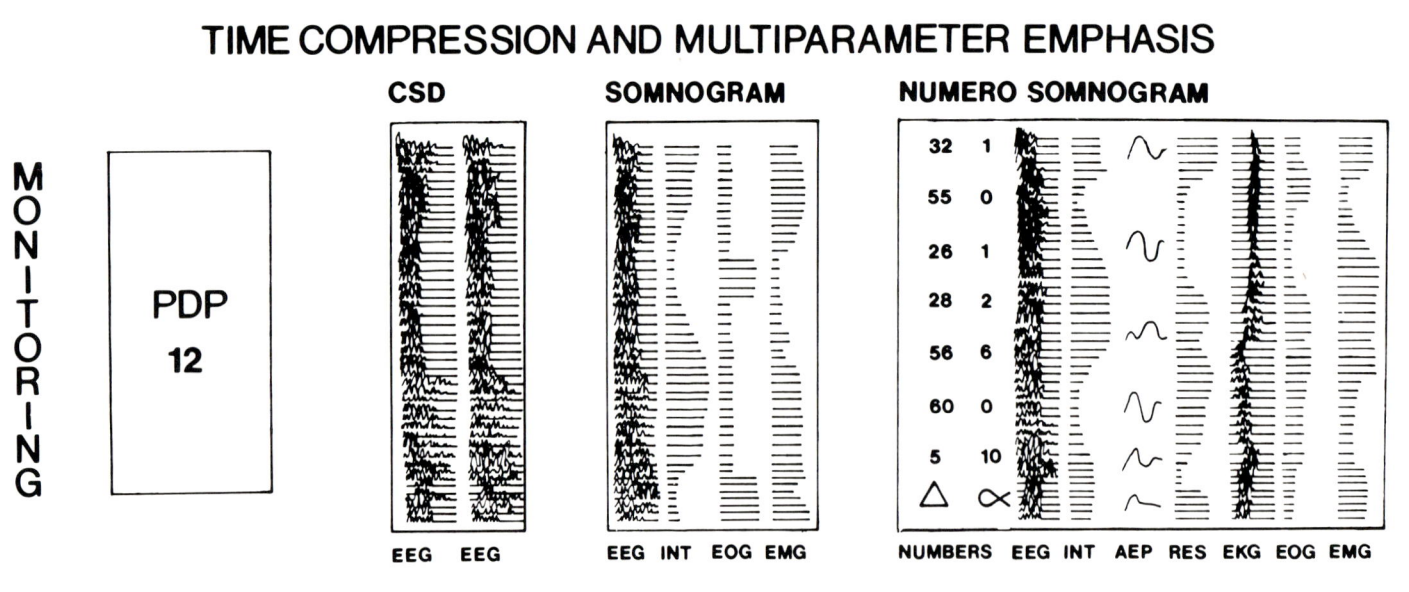

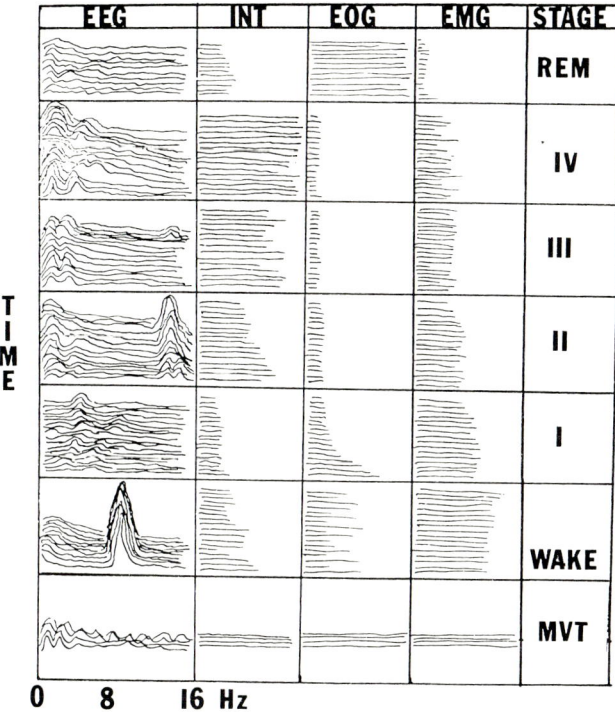

Fig. 15. Diagram of the changes seen in the CSA somnogram with the different classic stages of sleep (see text). The last trace (MVT) shows the effect of a movement artifact. INT, integrated EEG activity; REM, rapid eye movement.

ing slow-wave activity. An example of a program that depicts changes in heart rate and interbeat variability in relation to EEG changes produced by hyperventilation is shown in Fig. 17.

AREA DISPLAY OF SPECTRAL INFORMATION

We turn now from the use of spectra and integration techniques for long-term monitoring to their application to the problems of clinical EEG diagnosis. In this instance we are concerned with the multichannel displays necessary for sampling the extent of the cerebral hemispheres that are represented on the scalp surface. The technique, known as the CSA, (13) is shown in Fig. 18, which depicts a 16-channel CSA in a normal subject. Note the clarity with which the alpha mechanism can be viewed, and the absence of slow-wave activity which, if focal, could be indicative of a localized disturbance. Such an instance is indeed shown in Fig. 19 where a patient with a left temporal occipital mass lesion produced a clearly evident delta focus. This kind of display possesses such intuitive simplicity that those unfamiliar with the complexities of reading the conventional record or in fact the average clinician can see very clearly the type of abnormality manifest by his patient in a single-sheet report. For this reason, we believe that the CSA goes a long way toward bringing the EEG into the field of the general clinician so that he is as familiar with the findings as he might be with a parallel test such as the

Fig. 14. A diagrammatic representation of the computer graphics method used in the study of EEG in the UCSD laboratory. In the upper section, emphasis is on reporting methods which display topographic distribution of the spectral abnormalities. This is called a compressed spectral array (CSA). In order to reduce eye-blink artifact, occulogram subtraction programs can be employed as shown under CSA-E. In order to detect spike discharges, additional programs mark the recognition of a spike on the CSA as shown above right (CSA-E + S. See also Fig. 20). In the lower part of the illustration, methods of monitoring are illustrated. In the simplest form this consists of a compressed spectral display (CSD), and the somnogram in which components of integration of EEG, eye movement, and EMG are added. In the right diagram is an example of computer-generated spectral numbers representing activity in the delta and alpha band. Also represented is EEG integration, averaged evoked potential (AEP), respiration, EKG (heart rate), eye movement, and EMG. This numero somnogram is employed in coma monitoring.

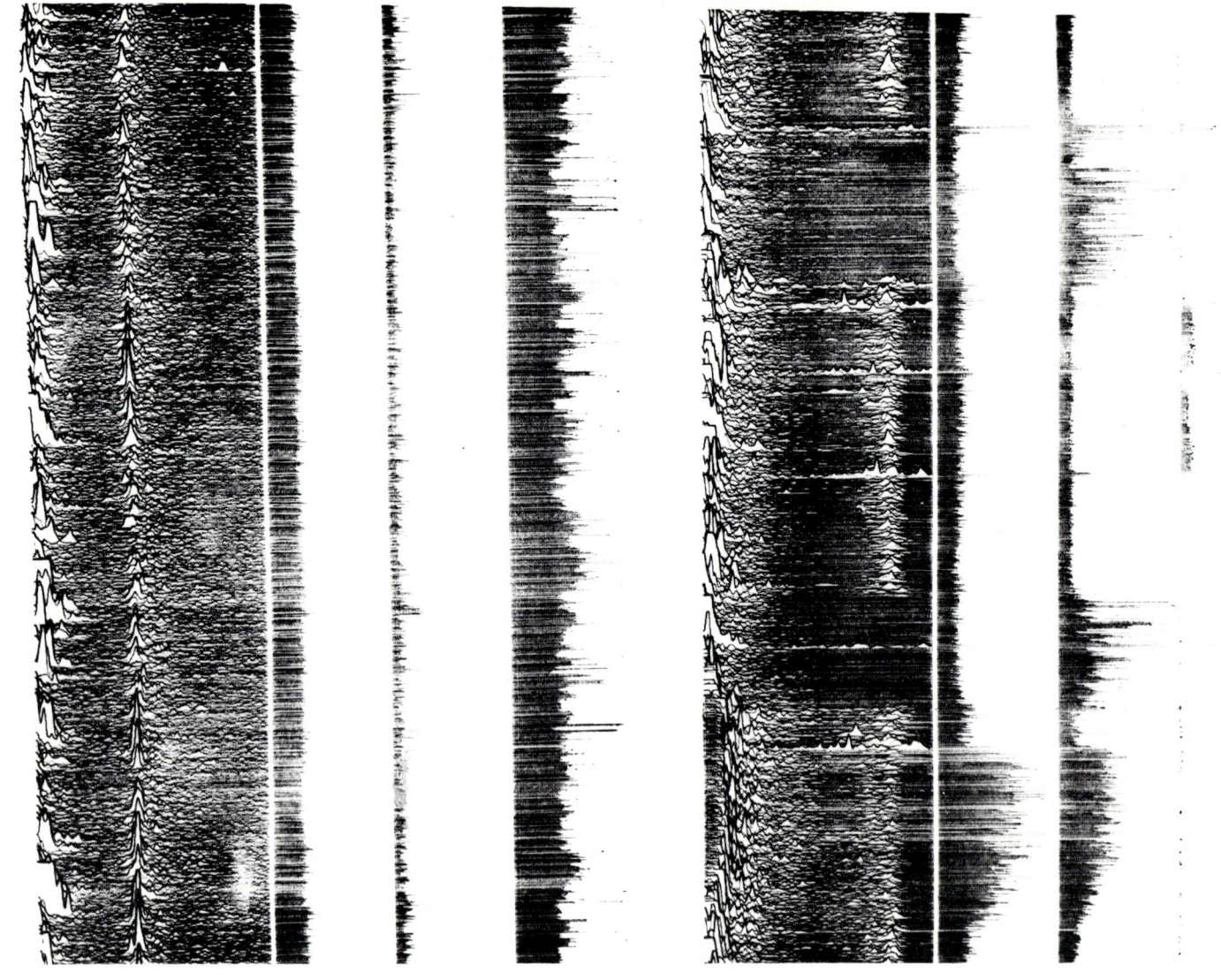

EKG. It should be noted that the CSA technique only works well for the waking record. Thus, if the patient becomes drowsy or goes to sleep, the whole display is flooded with the slow wave activity characteristic of these states and largely loses its ability to display localized slow wave abnormalities. The occurrence of artifacts can also be a problem since a single artifact, because of the nature of the memory aspects of hidden line suppression, tends to remain for a considerable period and therefore appears very conspicuous. Thus, successful application of the CSA technique requires careful control of eye movements by eye holding if necessary and elimination of other forms of artifact. Eye movements can also be removed automatically by a nulling technique which is under development.

The above discussion of the CSA has concerned its ability to display the normal EEG and localized or generalized slow wave pathology. However, a significant world of EEG is concerned with other types of pattern, such as the focal spikes and diffuse spike and wave. In techniques still under development, a spike discharge can be recognized by the computer on the basis of its amplitude and the slope of its upward and downward components (7). Figure 20 shows an example of this technique in which a focal spike in the EEG *(bottom of figure)* has been recognized by the computer and placed as a dot *(see position of arrows)* on the end of the appropriate spectral line. Spike pattern recognition becomes more difficult when carried out in the background of the sleep state in which spikes are most often encountered. This is because many of the normal sleep rhythms such as vertex waves, lambda waves, and so forth, have contours that make them difficult to distinguish from the spikes. Thus, at present the practical use of the CSA with spike recognition is confined to recordings taken in the waking state.

AREA DISPLAY OF VOLTAGE CONTOURS

A central problem for the clinical electroencephalographer is the location of events, such as spikes, that occur within the distributed sampling channels of the 16-channel recording. This difficult and sophisticated problem in the conventional recording can be greatly facilitated by the use of computer methods (8). An example of this use is shown diagrammatically in Fig. 21. Basically, the computer takes the information supplied by a square array of the primary recording electrodes, which is usually $4 \times 4 = 16$ electrodes, and by means of interpolation methods provides an equivalent of $20 \times 20 = 400$ "statistical" electrodes. When an event of interest occurs, such as a spike or an evoked potential response, a potential field map is produced of the distribution of the event across the scalp at a designated instant in time. The computer then produces a contour line plot quite equivalent to that used by the geographer to represent the irregularities of the earth's terrain. The importance of such information both in clinical EEG and in the proper understanding of evoked potential component distribution is shown in

FIG. 16. A 4-hr section of two somnograms placed side by side is shown. On the left is a patient in whom a head injury had resulted in insomnia. The EEG spectrum shows alpha rhythm present intermittently throughout the night, and the integration shows absence of the changes seen in normal sleep. The eye movement, EOG trace, and muscle are also without pattern. Contrast this with the changes shown on the right where a normal somnogram is depicted. Note the presence of spindling represented by a 13 to 14 cycle activity looking like a range of mountains which is interrupted on two occasions by REM stages indicated by bursts of high amplitude shown in the EOG channel and by inhibition of muscle activity in the EMG channel. This patient complained of extreme insomnia; yet the recording indicates that she slept normally throughout the section shown and in fact throughout an 8-hr period.

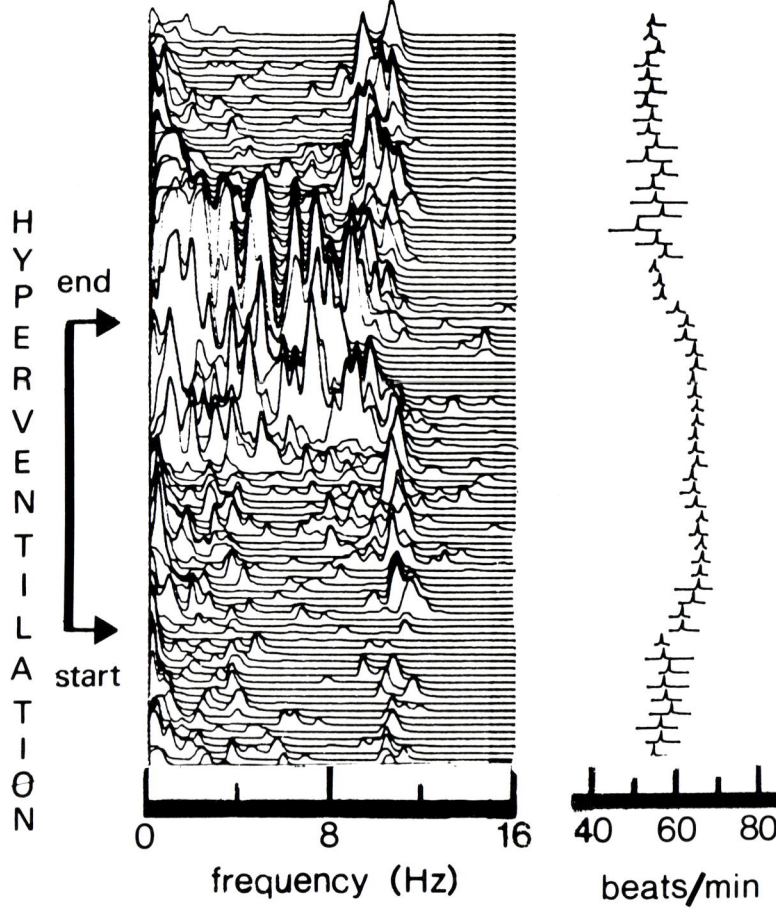

FIG. 17. The way the CSA can be combined with EKG data is shown. Normal subject (Fr1–O1) CSA shown on left, with development of slow wave activity following a period of hyperventilation. Note the intensification of alpha activity following the hyperventilation period and the shift in the major frequency component of the alpha band to a slower rate. On the right is shown the mean intervals of heart rate that occurred during a 12-sec period with the range indicated by the left- and right-hand extremes of the line. With the onset of hyperventilation there was an acceleration in heart rate and a reduction of variance of interbeat interval. At the end of hyperventilation, variance increased (vagal effect).

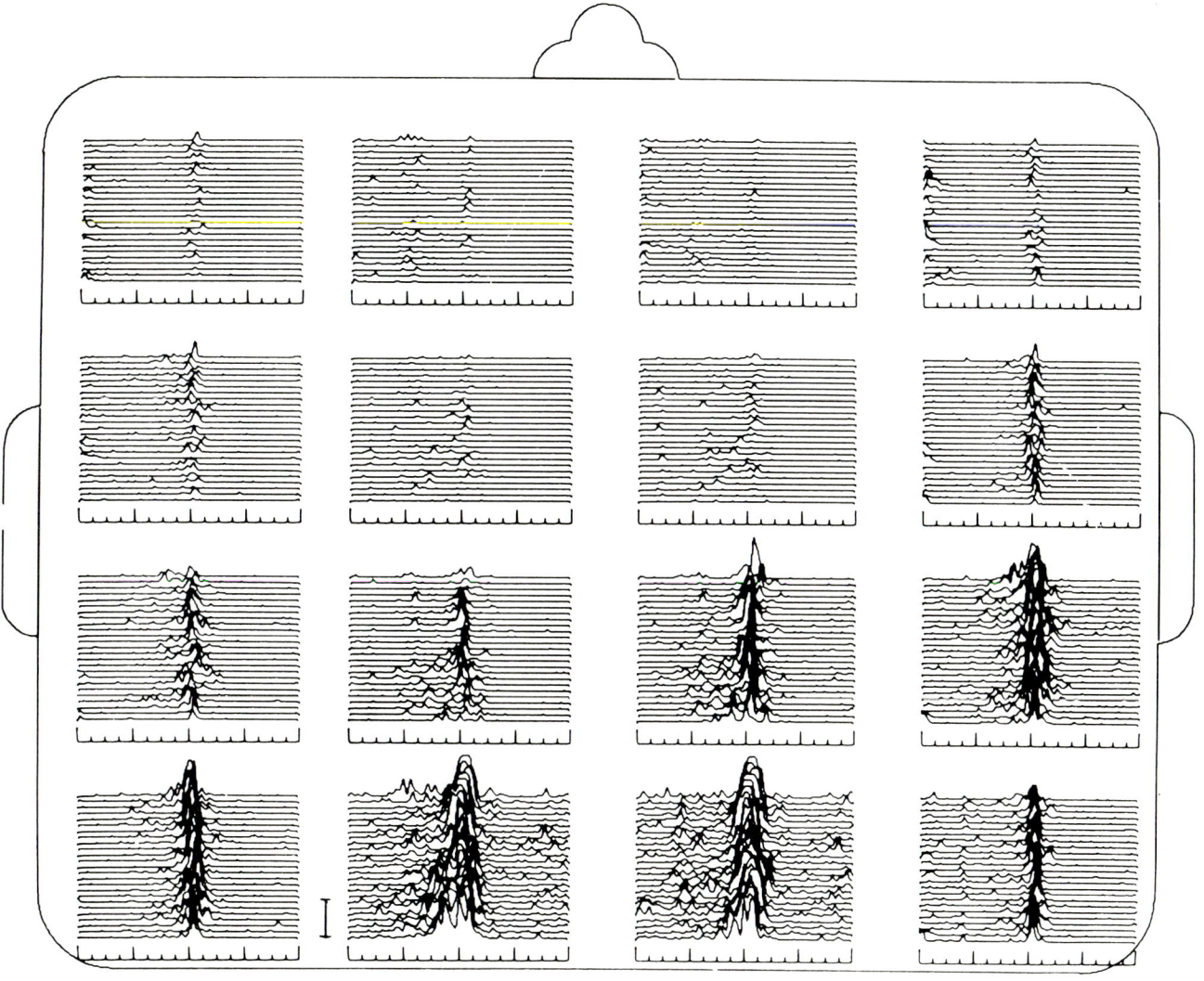

FIG. 18. The 16-channel CSA in a normal subject (bipolar recording) from parasagittal and temporal leads. Note the symmetry of the alpha rhythm and the absence of appreciable activity in the slower frequencies.

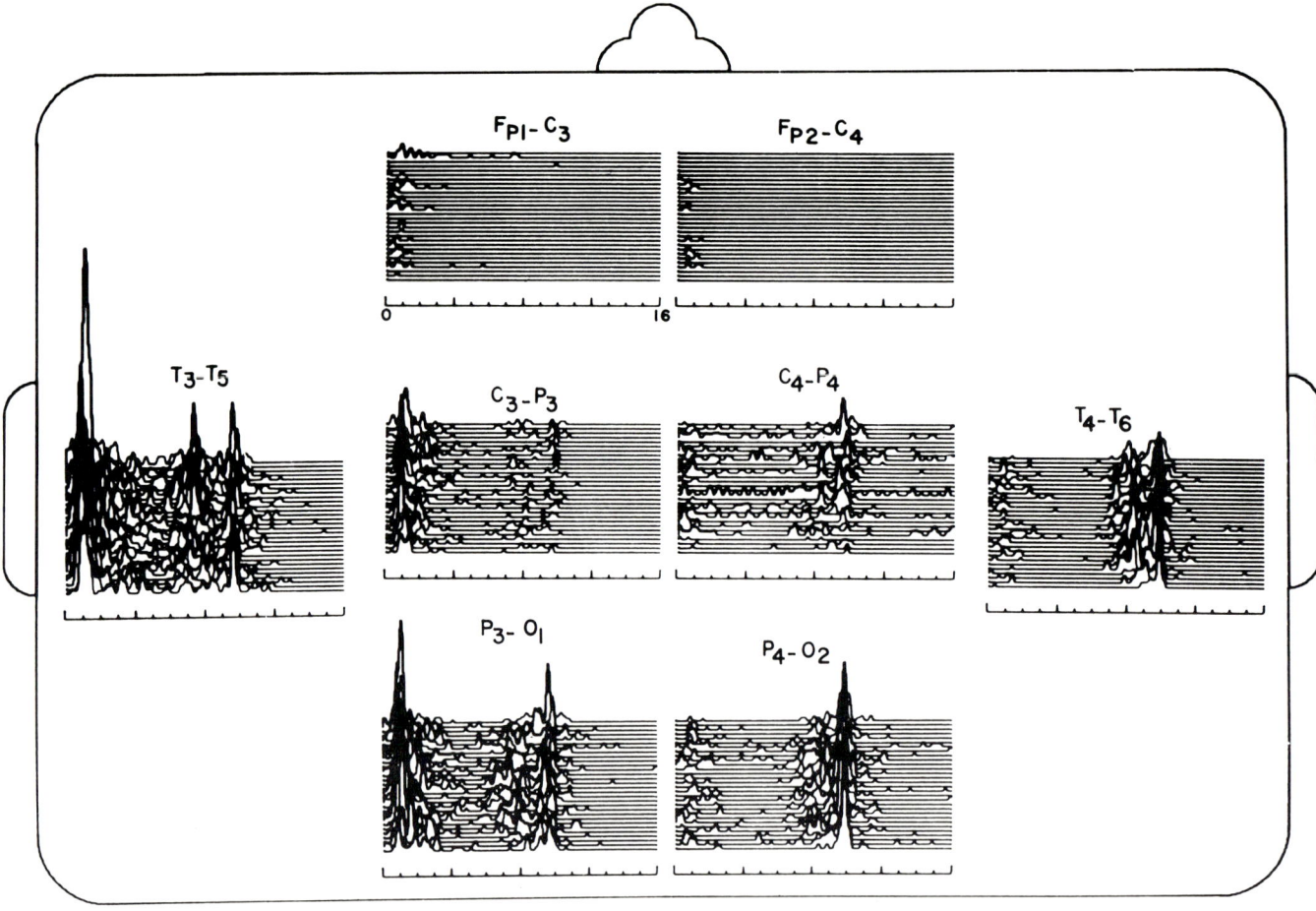

FIG. 19. Shown is an abnormal CSA (contrast with Fig. 18). Eight-channel bipolar recording shows clearly spectral changes in the left central, left parietal, and left temporal regions owing to the presence of delta activity in this area. The patient had a mass lesion in the left temporal parietal region.

Fig. 22. In this illustration from a normal subject, the 4 × 4 array in diamond shape was applied to the occipital region of the scalp where photic evoked potentials appear in maximal amplitude. In this particular subject, four peaks in the original data labeled A, B, C, and D were chosen for the display of the potential distribution across the diamond at these times. These displays are shown in the lower part of the figure. Note that the field distribution is considerably different for the different waves; this is important since it means that if only two electrodes were being used to sample each hemispheric field (as is often done in evoked potential experiments) their placement (e.g., on an isopotential line in Fig. 22A) might result in the complete disappearance of the A component from the sample. Thus, the relatively arbitrary nature of much evoked potential work appears to result from this kind of sampling difficulty. It is also evident that the field evoked by a flash does not center on the midline of the head, but in this instance is considerably displaced to the left, particularly in the later components. When an investigator uses limited electrode sampling, this normal field displacement might lead to his reporting an asymmetric evoked response and thus erroneously implying the existence of an abnormality.

TELEPHONE TRANSMISSION TECHNIQUES

The technique of transmission of EEG information across the standard telephone line has been under development for the last 10 years, and it is now possible to transmit 8-channel information with accompanying signals with good reproducibility as indicated in Fig. 23. Present transmission sysems usually have an upper limit of frequency response from 40 to 60 Hz using a standard telephone line. This results in the faster spike components being less sharp than in the original trace. Some authorities believe this reduces the electroencephalographers ability to distinguish muscle from genuine brain activity. Telephone transmission can also be the subject of intermittent noise intrusion which, although often easily recognized, at times may be troublesome and may imitate spike components, etc. Recently great interest has developed in EEG transmission networks, and there is a laboratory in San Francisco that frequently processes EEG data originating from as far away as Florida. At the present time, many electroencephalographers and some Societies have opposed the development of these techniques since it is generally believed that they are being applied in advance of proper regulation and quality control (see also Chapter 1 and Appendix). The systems to which considerable objection have been voiced have some of the following attributes.

1. They employ inexperienced technicians (often an EKG or respiratory therapy technician) to apply electrodes at the transmitting end, and it is considered that significant errors in electrode placement and consequently spurious asymmetries may result from these procedures.

2. In most instances, no recording is made at the transmitting end, which depends on monitoring carried out by a trained technician in the receiving laboratory. Some committees including that of the American EEG Society consider such a procedure unsatisfactory in the present development of technology and have called for some kind of hard copy to be provided at the transmitting end.

3. There is no regulation of the number of incoming EEGs that a single technician may monitor. It is certainly commonplace for one technician to monitor input from two labs, and it is at present unknown to what extent such activities can result in unsatisfactory recordings.

It is undoubtedly true that the centralization of facilities made possible by telephone transmission carries with it significant advan-

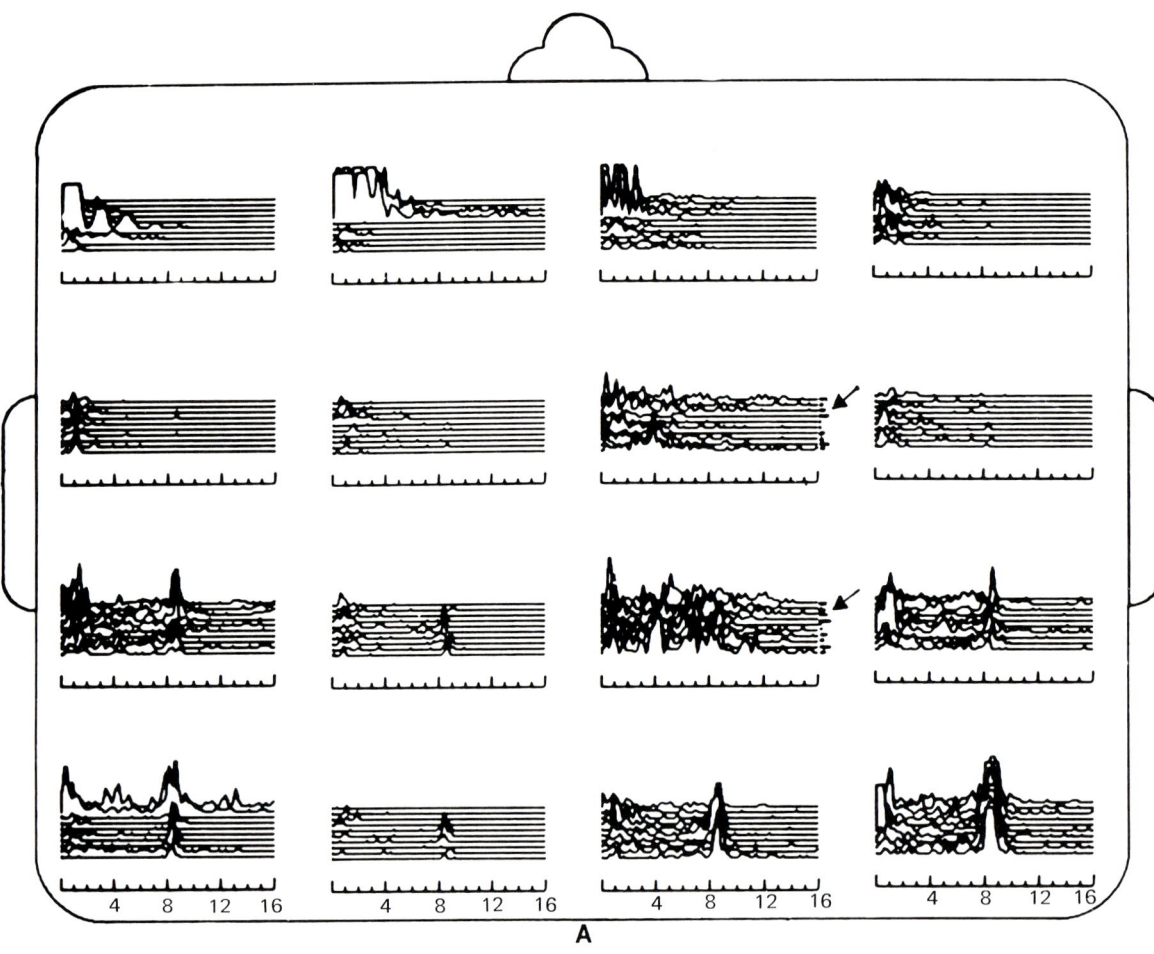

FIG. 20A. See legend Fig. 20B.

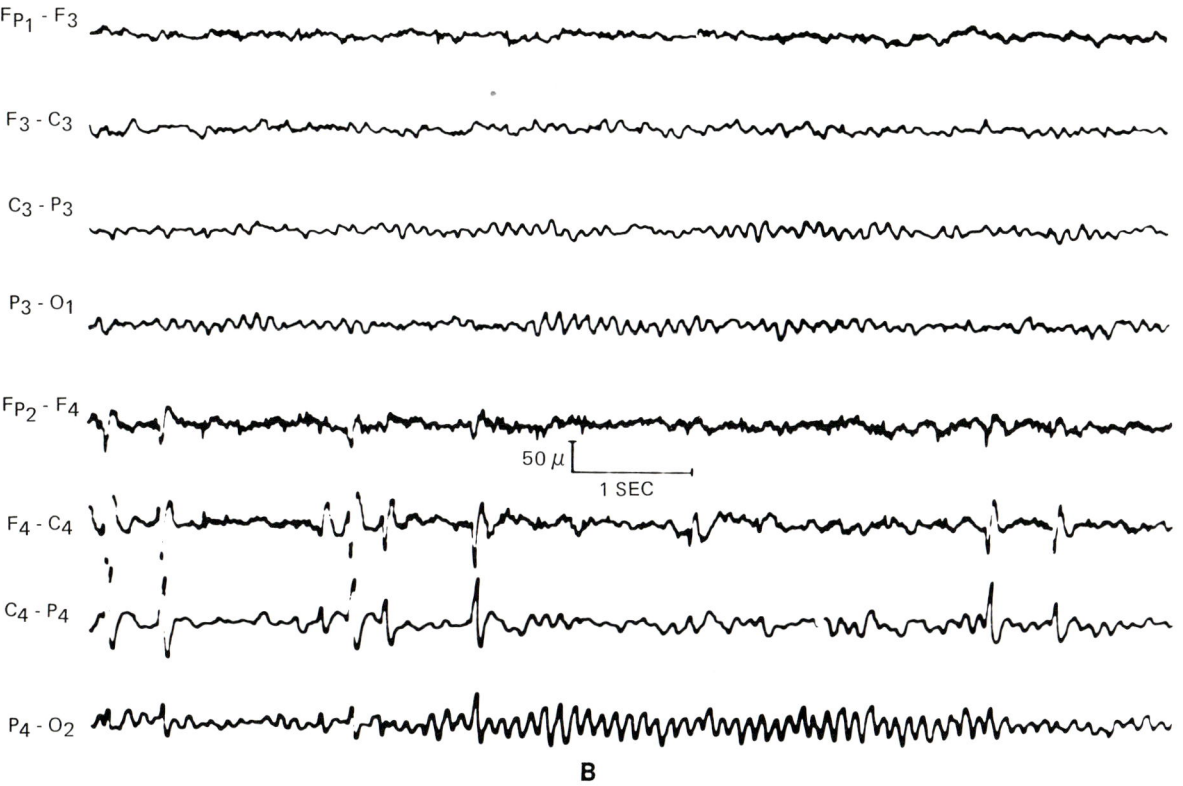

FIG. 20B. Use of combined CSA **(A)** and spike-detection **(B)** algorhythms (spike detection is dependent on amplitude slope criteria). Recognition of the spike in the primary EEG **(B)** is shown on the CSA as dots in the appropriate channel (*indicated by two arrows* in **A**).

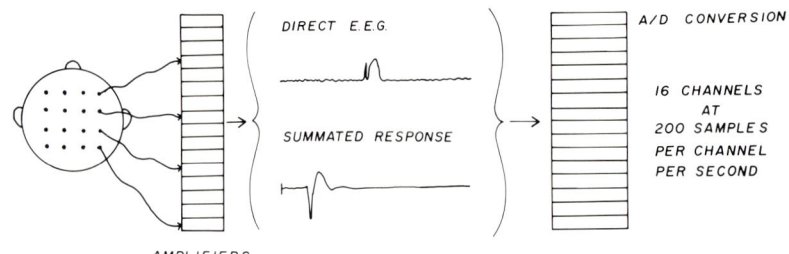
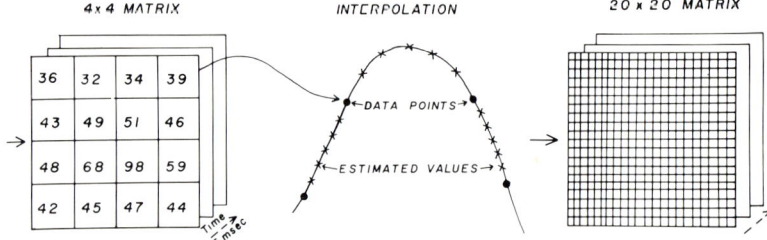
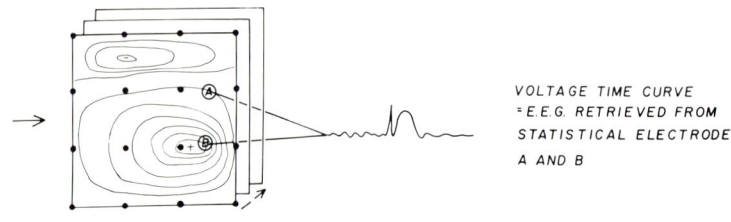

FIG. 21. Diagram of computer method employed to produce voltage contour plots of EEG events (such as spikes or evoked potential). The contour maps are made by isolating the event at an instant in time in which the voltage contours are generated by following statistical interpolation techniques necessary to produce smooth and readable contours. The method can be used to retrieve data from displays from electrode placements that may not have been employed in the original generation of the data, as shown diagrammatically *(bottom)*.

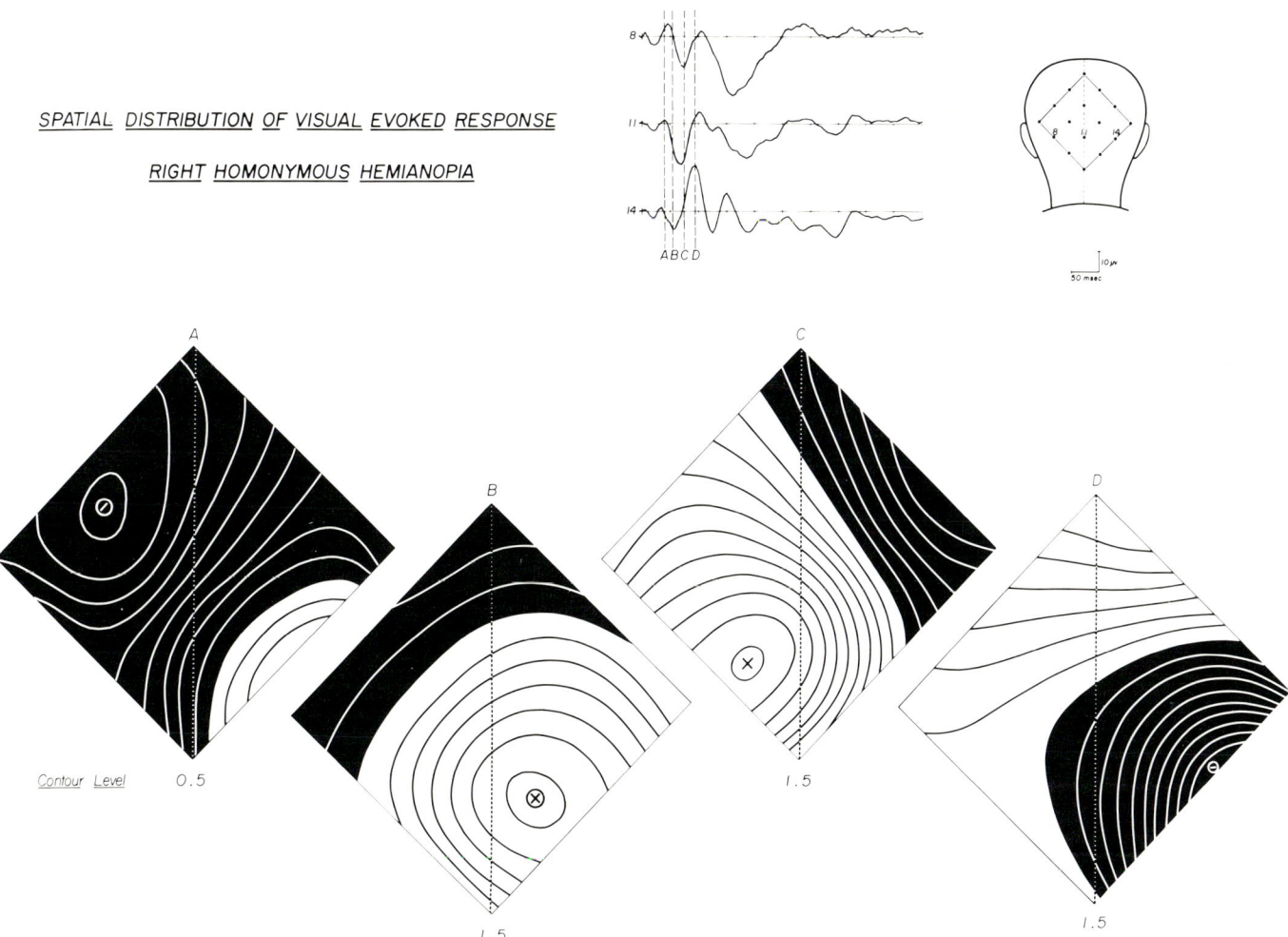

FIG. 22. Example of voltage contour distribution of evoked potentials in a normal subject recorded over a diamond *(see diagram)* arrangement of 4 × 4 electrodes in the occipital regions. Time slices of the evoked potential distribution are shown as contour maps for times A, B, C, and D when peaks occur in the primary average response (see text). In the display black is negative; white is positive.

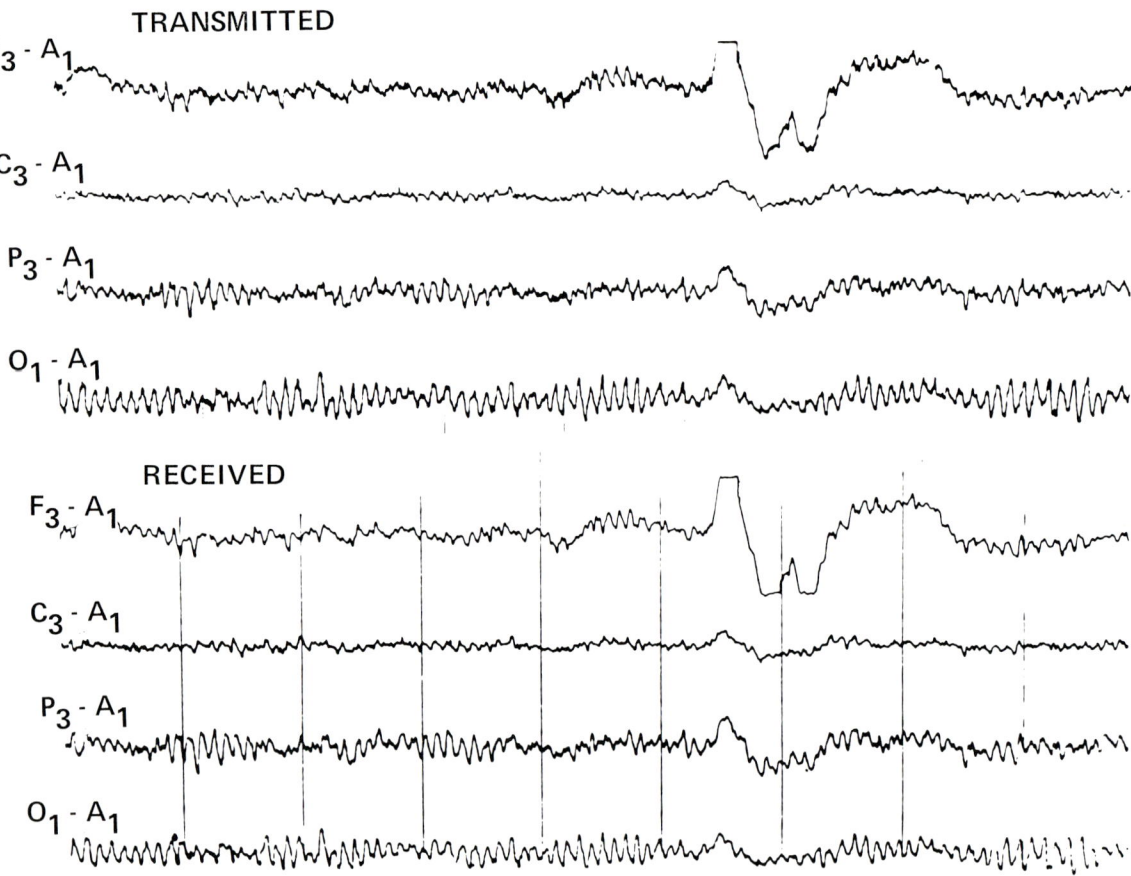

FIG. 23. The fidelity that can be obtained with commercial methods of telephone transmission of 8-channel primary EEG data is shown. Four channels of data are illustrated with a comparison of the same data before transmission *(above)* and after transmission *(below)* over a 1,000-mi telephone line. Commercial systems handling 8 channels of EEG over a standard telephone line are now available.

tages in the direction of overall economy, availability of EEG facilities over weekends, concentration of EEG interpretations, use of expertise in one area, and the ability to use additional computer techniques [e.g., averaging (16)], which might not be available in all peripheral laboratories. However, it is also true that a number of technical developments in the direction of continuous impedance monitoring and computer checking of alpha asymmetry, etc., need to be instituted in these systems before they can be regarded as satisfactory. Nevertheless, it seems likely that EEG technology will develop in the direction of centralization because of some of the advantages discussed above.

SUMMARY

The clinical electroencephalographer in office practice is unlikely in the near future to have access to the more sophisticated kinds of computer systems that can produce the CSA, the somnogram, and the area display of individual events. These techniques may become available to him via the centralization provided by telephone transmissions, but such systems have not yet been organized. However, the simpler analog systems described at the outset, such as integration, subtraction, and even response averaging, which allow simple quantitation to be applied to existing instrumentation, could with advantage be employed by the forward-looking clinical electroencephalographer (the cost of these additions amounts to less than 50% of an EEG instrument). By doing so he would add a good deal of accuracy to his record interpretation, he would prepare himself for the more sophisticated techniques that are on the way, and his technicians would benefit by exposure to techniques involving greater accuracy and the use of measurement in EEG.

ACKNOWLEDGMENTS

Work described in this review was supported by the Epilepsy Foundation of America and a U.S. Public Health Service Grant (No. NS 08962).

REFERENCES

Evoked Responses (Averaging)

1. Bickford, R. G. (1972): Physiological and clinical studies of microrcflexes. In: *Recent Contributions to Neurophysiology, EEG Supplement No. 31,* edited by J. P. Cordeau and P. Gloor, pp. 39–108. Elsevier, Amsterdam.
2. Halliday, A. M., McDonald, W. I., and Mushin, J. (1973): Visual evoked responses in diagnosis of multiple sclerosis. *Br. Med. J.,* 4:661–664.
3. Jewett, D. L., and Williston, J. S. (1971): Auditory-evoked far fields averaged from the scalp of humans. *Brain,* 94:681–696.

Brain Death Monitoring

4. Bickford, R. G., Sims, J. K., Billinger, T. W., and Aung, M. H. (1971): Problems in EEG estimation of brain death and use of computer techniques for their solution. *Trauma,* 12:6:61–95.

Analog Devices

5. Brittain, D., Allen, B. A., Berger, E. L., Nelson, B., and Bickford, R. G. (1975): Application of an EEG band integration computer (BIC) in clinical EEG. *Proc. San Diego Biomed. Symp.,* 14:31–36.
6. Emde, J. N., and Shipton, A. W. (1974): A dual purpose integrator for EEG studies. *Electroencephalogr. Clin. Neurophysiol.,* 37:185–187.

Computer Processing: General

7. Gose, E. E., Werner, S. S., and Bickford, R. G. (1974): Computerized EEG spike detection. *Proc. San Diego Biomed. Symp.,* 13:193–198.

8. Harris, J. A., Gordon, M. M., and Bickford, R. G. (1969): Computer-controlled multidimensional display device for investigation and modeling of physiologic systems. *Comput. Biomed. Res.,* 2:519–536.
9. Kellaway, P., and Petersen, I. (editors) (1973): *Automation of Clinical Electroencephalography.* Raven Press, New York.
10. Remond, A. (editor) (1972): *Handbook of Electroencephalography and Clinical Neurophysiology,* Vol. 4, Part B. Elsevier, Amsterdam.

Spectral Analysis

11. Gotman, J., Skuce, D. R., Thompson, C. J., Gloor, P., Ives, J. R., and Walter, F. R. (1973): Clinical applications of spectral analysis and extraction of features from electroencephalograms with slow waves in adult patients. *Electroencephalogr. Clin. Neurophysiol.,* 35:225–235.
12. Walter, D. O., Rhodes, J. M., Brown, D., and Adey, W. R. (1966): Comprehensive spectral analysis of human EEG generators in posterior cerebral regions. *Electroencephalogr. Clin. Neurophysiol.,* 20:224–327.

CSA

13. Bickford, R. G., Brimm, J., Berger, L., and Aung, M. (1973): Application of compressed spectral array in clinical EEG. In: *Automation of Clinical Electroencephalography,* edited by P. Kellaway and I. Petersen. Raven Press, New York.
14. Hanson, K., Stockard, J., Kalichman, M., Brimm, J., and Bickford, R. (1974): CSA somnogram—a multiparameter spectral sleep display. *Proc. San Diego Biomed. Symp.,* 13:545–548.

Telephone Transmission

15. Bennett, D. R., and Gardner, R. M. (1974): Current status of EEG telephone telemetry. *Clinical Electroencephalogr.,* 5:8–23.
16. Ray, C. D., Bickford, R. G., Walter, W. G., and Remond, A. (1965): Experiences with telemetry of biomedical data by telephone, cable and satellite: Domestic and international. *Med. Electron. Biol. Engng.,* 3:169–177.
17. Schear, H. E., Rowe, W. J., and Pori, J. R. (1974): Telephonic transmission of electroencephalograms. *Clin. Electroencephalogr.,* 5:24–33.

Appendix

American Electroencephalographic Society
GUIDELINES IN EEG—1976*

Preface 481

Standards of Practice in Clinical Electroencephalography 484

Recommended Job Descriptions for Electroencephalographic Technologists (issued jointly with the American Society of Electroencephalographic Technologists).. 486

Minimum Technical Requirements for Performing Clinical Electroencephalography 488

Minimum Technical Standards for EEG Recording in Suspected Cerebral Death 492

Provisional Recommendations for Telephone Transmission of EEGs (issued jointly with the American Society of Electroencephalographic Technologists) 496

PREFACE

In the period 1970–1975, the American Electroencephalographic Society issued a series of five Guidelines in EEG, two of which were issued jointly with the American Society of Electroencephalographic Technologists. Each of the series of Guidelines grew out of reports of the respective Ad Hoc Committees appointed to consider particular aspects of electroencephalography.

---

* Reprinted with permission of the American Electroencephalographic Society.

The membership of the original Committees with their dates follows, listed in the order in which the respective individual Guidelines of the series were issued.

Minimum Technical Standards for EEG Recording in Suspected Cerebral Death (1970):
Daniel Silverman, M.D., Chairman
Charles E. Henry, Ph.D.
Richard L. Masland, M.D.
Michael G. Saunders, M.D.
Robert S. Schwab, M.D.

Minimum Technical Requirements for Performing Clinical Electroencephalography (1970–71):
Michael G. Saunders, M.D., Chairman
John R. Hughes, M.D., Ph.D.
Donald W. Klass, M.D.
Robert L. Maulsby, M.D.
Jean Reiher, M.D.

Standards of Practice in Clinical Electroencephalography (1970):
Robert J. Ellingson, M.D., Ph.D., Chairman
Charles E. Henry, Ph.D.
Donald W. Klass, M.D.
John R. Knott, Ph.D.
Michael G. Saunders, M.D.
Richard D. Walter, M.D.

A partial revision was carried out in 1975 by a Subcommittee of the Committee on Training and Education:
Richard H. Mattson, M.D., Chairman
Donald W. Klass, M.D.
James W. Prichard, M.D.
Barry R. Tharp, M.D.

Recommended Job Descriptions for Electroencephalographic Technologists (1972) (issued jointly by the American EEG Society and the American Society of EEG Technologists):
Gian E. Chatrian, M.D., Chairman
Joanne Chastain, R.EEGT.
Charles E. Henry, Ph.D.
John R. Knott, Ph.D.
Mary Jo Martin, R.EEGT.

Provisional Recommendations for Telephone Transmission of EEGs (1974–75) (issued jointly by the American EEG Society and the American Society of EEG Technologists):

American EEG Society
B. Joseph Wilder, M.D., Chairman
John S. Barlow, M.D.
Donald R. Bennett, M.D.
Dorothea M. Brittenham, R.EEGT.
William H. Everts, M.D.
Peter J. Seaba, M.S.
Ernst A. Rodin, M.D., ex officio

American Society of EEG Technologists
Dorothea M. Brittenham, R.EEGT., Chairman
Charles E. Henry, Ph.D.
Hector Lettich, R.EEGT.
Mary Jo Martin, R.EEGT.
Thomas W. Billinger, R.EEGT., ex officio
John R. Knott, Ph.D., ex officio

The widespread and continuing demand for these Guidelines is adequate testimony that they fill a need for guidance in electroencephalography.

The decision in April of 1976 by the Council of the American EEG Society for the series of Guidelines to be issued as a single booklet offered the opportunity for all of them to be reviewed for possible updating. Accordingly, many of the members of the committees for the earlier Guidelines were asked for comments and suggestions. In addition, other members of the American EEG Society were contacted concerning areas in which they had special expertise.

A list, which can hardly be complete, of those who made suggestions for this edition of the Guidelines series includes the following:

Donald R. Bennett, M.D.
Reginald G. Bickford, M.D.
Dorothea M. Brittenham, R.EEGT.
Gian E. Chatrian, M.D.
Robert J. Ellingson, M.D., Ph.D.
C. William Erwin, M.D.
Charles E. Henry, Ph.D.
John R. Hughes, M.D., Ph.D.
Peter Kellaway, Ph.D.
Donald W. Klass, M.D.

George Klem, R.EEGT.
John R. Knott, Ph.D.
Julius Korein M.D.
Cesare T. Lombroso, M.D.
Mary Jo Martin, R.EEGT.
Richard L. Masland, M.D.
Jean Reiher, M.D.
Milton Tarlau, M.D.
Fernando Torres, M.D.
Barbara F. Westmoreland, M.D.

From the resulting generous response, a draft for a revised edition of each of the Guidelines was prepared and circulated back to those who had made suggestions, for possible further comment. At the same time, copies of the drafts of the entire series were circulated to the Council of the American EEG Society. After further changes, the new edition of the Guidelines was approved, with some modifications, by the Council at the Annual Meeting of the American EEG Society in Dearborn, Michigan in September 1976. Concurrently, those of the series that are being issued jointly with the American Society of EEG Technologists were approved by its Board.

In this edition an attempt has been made to use the terminology recommended in the Glossary of the International Federation of Societies for Electroencephalography and Clinical Neurophysiology (**Electroenceph. clin. Neurophysiol.**, 1974, 37:538–548), or, where a different terminology is used, to include also the equivalent terms from the Glossary.

Since good electroencephalography is dependent in the first instance on the competence of the electroencephalographer and of the EEG technologist, and also on the quality of the equipment in the laboratory, the first two of the Guidelines series in this booklet are devoted to these aspects: Standards of Practice in Clinical Electroencephalography, and Recommended Job Descriptions for Electroencephalographic Technologists. The technical aspects of the EEG examination then follow: Minimum Technical Requirements for Performing Clinical Electroencephalography, Minimum Technical Standards for EEG Recording in Suspected Cerebral Death, and Provisional Recommendations for Telephone Transmission of EEGs. (Committees of the American EEG Society have been appointed for 1976–77 to formulate additional Guidelines for a minimum set of montages, and for pediatric EEG, respectively.)

This edition of the series of Guidelines in EEG represents the work of a large number of people; it is hoped that it will make a commensurate contribution toward excellence in electroencephalography.

John S. Barlow, M.D., Editor
President, American EEG Society, 1975–76

GUIDELINES IN EEG — 1976

STANDARDS OF PRACTICE IN CLINICAL ELECTROENCEPHALOGRAPHY

INTRODUCTION

These Guidelines were originally prepared in response to frequent requests from all parts of the United States for information about the establishment and proper operation of clinical EEG laboratories. The Guidelines were drawn up by an ad hoc committee appointed by the President of the American EEG Society, and were subsequently approved and adopted by the Council and the Membership of the Society. They represent the accumulated experience of the Members of the Society, and derive from the work of the Training and Education Committee and the Ad hoc Committee on Techniques, as well as the American Board of Qualification in Electroencephalography (ABQEEG) and the American Board of Registration of Electroencephalographic Technologists (ABRET).

It is hoped that these Guidelines will assist in the improvement of clinical EEG practice. If the standards set forth here cannot be met, it would be well to consider **not** operating an EEG laboratory. Bad electroencephalography is worse than no electroencephalography at all.

A. QUALIFICATIONS OF CHIEFS OF EEG LABORATORIES

The minimal qualifications for chiefs of laboratories in large metropolitan hospitals and university medical centers are those set forth by the American Board of Qualification in Electroencephalography (ABQEEG) as requirements for admission to examination, and are as follows: three or more years of postdoctoral training in electroencephalography and allied fields, including one full year of formal training, or its equivalent, in a major EEG laboratory under a competent electroencephalographer. An additional year of more independent experience is also recommended. Allied fields include neurology, pediatric neurology, neurosurgery, psychiatry, and the basic neurosciences. After January 1, 1978, ABQEEG certification itself should be strongly recommended, if not required, particularly at institutions having training programs in EEG.

B. MINIMAL QUALIFICATIONS OF A CLINICAL ELECTROENCEPHALOGRAPHER*

1. The electroencephalographer should be a physician with three or more years of postdoctoral training in neurology, pediatric neurology, neurosurgery or psychiatry. The physician should preferably be board certified in his specialty.
2. Training should have included not less than a year of experience in reading and interpreting EEGs, with the initial six months assigned full time or the equivalent to a major EEG lab which performs EEGs on a wide variety of medical problems in adult, pediatric and psychiatric patients. Such a laboratory should do not less than 1500 EEGs annually.
3. Physicians beginning training after January 1, 1978 should do so in a program directed by an EEGer certified by ABQEEG.

---

* These standards are proposed for individuals entering electroencephalography after 1978. Many highly competent electroencephalographers, currently providing EEG interpretative service, do not meet the above standards. In particular, some competent electroencephalographers are not physicians, but as a result of long experience are among the leaders in the field.

C. **QUALIFICATIONS OF EEG TECHNOLOGISTS AND TECHNICIANS** (See also **Recommended Job Descriptions for EEG Technologists,** p. 486.)
   1. Minimal qualifications for senior or chief technologists in large metropolitan hospitals and university medical centers are that they be eligible for Part II of the examinations of the American Board of Registration of Electroencephalographic Technologists (ABRET). Eligibility includes one year of formal training plus one year of additional experience *or* six months of formal training plus 18 months of additional experience, including evidence of personally recording at least 1,000 EEGs after the end of training. (For further details, see **The American Journal of EEG Technology,** Training and Registration issue, Vol. 8, No. 4, Dec. 1968.) Optimally, and after Jan. 1, 1978, in any event, they should hold the ABRET registration certificate, especially if they are chief technologists in large metropolitan hospitals, university medical centers, and other teaching laboratories.
   2. Minimal qualifications for junior technicians and for technicians or technologists working independently in smaller centers are that they be eligible for Part I of the ABRET examinations. Eligibility includes one year of experience, including at least 6 months of formal training. Optimally, they should have had 2 years of experience, including one year of training.
   3. In no case should technicians with less than 6 months full-time (or equivalent) training under an ABRET-certified technologist and/or an ABQEEG-certified (at least after Jan. 1, 1978) electroencephalographer be allowed to operate independently. Such a person should preferably be designated as "EEG technician trainee."

D. **LABORATORY ORGANIZATION**
   1. The chief electroencephalographer should have primary control over the selection of other staff electroencephalographers and EEG technologists, and over the selection of equipment, and the designation of techniques and procedures.
   2. All EEGs should be analyzed by an electroencephalographer, and official reports involving clinical interpretations written (dictated) or reviewed by him. Under no circumstances should a technologist, however well qualified and experienced, have primary responsibility for clinical interpretation of EEGs. A technologist may, however, particularly if ABRET-certified, give a descriptive technical report of the record.
   3. Referring physicians should have the right, and may designate the right, to examine the EEGs of, and any records pertaining to, their own patients.

E. **EQUIPMENT**
   1. Equipment should meet the latest equipment standards of the American EEG Society or the International Federation of Societies for EEG and Clinical Neurophysiology.
      The latter standards are published following each quadrennial International EEG Congress, e.g., **Electroenceph. Clin. Neurophysiol.,** 1974, 37:549–553.

In the absence of a qualified chief electroencephalographer, advice concerning equipment purchases and equipment problems should be sought from a Board-certified electroencephalographer at another institution. The inadvisability of using locally constructed or assembled equipment is strongly emphasized.

   2. Sixteen-channel equipment is encouraged. In no event should an instrument of less than 8 channels be used.
   3. For ordinary clinical purposes, electrical shielding is unnecessary with modern equipment in the vast majority of locations, and need not automatically be installed unless local considerations warrant it.
   4. All laboratories should have a photostimulator capable of delivering brief intense light flashes at frequencies of 1 to 30 flashes per second.
   5. High quality electrodes are available from several manufacturers, and are generally to be preferred to home-made electrodes, but some technologists and electroencephalographers can make quite excellent electrodes and may prefer to do so. Silver-silver chloride or gold-plated electrodes are preferred. Needle electrodes are not recommended for general use (see also **Minimum Technical Requirements for Performing Clinical Electroencephalography,** Section 9.1).

F. **LABORATORY TECHNIQUE AND PROCEDURES, INCLUDING SPECIAL PROCEDURES** (See **Minimum Technical Requirements for Performing Clinical Electroencephalography,** p. 488.)

RECOMMENDED JOB DESCRIPTIONS FOR ELECTROENCEPHALOGRAPHIC TECHNOLOGISTS

These job descriptions are intended for directors of EEG laboratories and to provide guidelines for federal and state agencies and hospital administrations concerned with classification of personnel.

CLASS SPECIFICATION
TITLE: Electroencephalography Technologist-Trainee
SUMMARY: Receives training in Electroencephalographic Technology.
DISTINGUISHING CHARACTERISTICS:

The Electroencephalography Technologist-Trainee receives training under the direct supervision of the laboratory technical and professional staff.

Optimally, the trainee would be under an AMA-accredited educational program for EEG Technologists.

EXAMPLES OF DUTIES:

Learns functions of electroencephalography technologist by group and/or individual teaching, observation, assigned reading and practical application under the direct supervision of laboratory staff. To this effect:

1. Acquires basic knowledge of normal brain anatomy and function, disease states encountered in EEG practice, electrical patterns of the brain in normal and pathological circumstances, other diagnostic aids and operating principles of pertinent electronic instrumentation.
2. Learns to accurately record electrical impulses from the brain with increasing independence through practice. This entails the acquisition of knowledge and skills necessary to:
   a. Apply suitable electrodes on predetermined measured positions on the patient's head and check their performance.
   b. Calibrate and adjust the EEG apparatus.
   c. Select predetermined electrode combinations as well as special combinations made necessary by the case under study; take standard recordings; recognize artifacts and take appropriate steps to eliminate them; describe normal and abnormal clinical manifestations observed during the test; use activating procedures such as hyperventilation, photic stimulation and sleep; obtain the patient's cooperation for the best performance of these procedures; monitor on the same apparatus other variables such as electromyograms, electrocardiograms, electro-oculograms, respiration, etc., when indicated by the circumstances of the EEG recording.
   d. Abstract relevant information from the patient's clinical record and obtain additional information by questioning.
   e. Keep equipment in a clean operating condition, detect instrument malfunction and make minor maintenance adjustments or report need for minor repairs.
3. Files and/or microfilms recordings.
4. Performs other related duties as required.
5. Attends teaching seminars and conferences, completes formal reading assignments and demonstrates acquisition of knowledge and skills through oral, written and practical examinations by supervisory staff.

MINIMUM QUALIFICATIONS:
1. Completion of one year of college or university with emphasis on physical or biological sciences,
OR
2. High school graduation with emphasis on physical or biological sciences.

CLASS SPECIFICATION
TITLE: Electroencephalography Technologist I
SUMMARY: Under supervision of senior staff conducts electroencephalographic examinations.
DISTINGUISHING CHARACTERISTICS:

The technologist in this class is responsible for the preparation of the patient, the conduct of various electroencephalographic examinations and the collection of information pertinent to the interpretation of the tests.

EXAMPLES OF DUTIES:
1. Applies suitable electrodes on predetermined measured positions on the patient's head and checks their performance.
2. Calibrates and adjusts the EEG apparatus.
3. Selects predetermined electrode combinations as well as special combinations made necessary by the case under study. Obtains standard recordings, recognizes artifacts and takes appropriate steps to eliminate them. Describes all abnormal clinical manifestations observed during the test. Uses activating procedures such as hyperventilation,

photic stimulation, and sleep. Obtains the patient's cooperation for the best performance of these procedures. When indicated by the circumstances of the EEG recording, monitors on the same apparatus, other variables such as electromyograms, electrocardiograms, electro-oculograms, respiration, etc.

4. Abstracts relevant information from the patient's clinical record and obtains additional information by questioning.
5. May perform the above work in the laboratory or at the patient's bedside and in Intensive Care Units.
6. Keeps equipment in a clean operating condition, detects instrument malfunctions and makes minor maintenance adjustments or reports need for major repairs.
7. Files and/or microfilms recordings.
8. Fills and forwards charge slips for billing purposes as required.
9. Assists in the instruction of technologist-trainees.
10. Performs other related duties as required.
11. Continues education by participating in conferences and technical meetings.

MINIMUM TECHNICAL QUALIFICATIONS:
1. Eligibility for or successful completion of Part I (written) examination for certification by the American Board of Registration of Electroencephalographic Technologists or equivalent following:
2. Successful completion of a traineeship of the duration of one year following:
3. Completion of one year of college or university with emphasis on physical or biological sciences,
   OR
4. High school graduation with emphasis on physical or biological sciences. Experience as a research or clinical assistant in a scientific laboratory is an advantage.

OPTIMAL TECHNICAL QUALIFICATIONS:
Graduation from an AMA-accredited educational program for EEG technologists, in addition to the above minimal qualifications.

PERSONAL QUALIFICATIONS:
1. Maturity and ability to establish good rapport with patients, public and staff.
2. Capacity to deal with severely ill patients.

CLASS SPECIFICATION

TITLE: Electroencephalography Technologist II

SUMMARY: Performs standard and complex electroencephalographic recordings under minimum direction and/or serves as senior technologist with responsibilities for work assignment and in-service training instruction of junior personnel.

DISTINGUISHING CHARACTERISTICS:
The technologist in this class is responsible for obtaining standard as well as special procedure EEG recordings and for monitoring additional physiological phenomena by means of appropriate techniques. Provides training and participates in research.

EXAMPLES OF DUTIES:
1. Serves as an in-service training instructor for technologist-trainees and junior personnel.
2. Assists in supervising junior technologists in diagnostic and research procedures.
3. Prepares the patients, including those under intensive care; applies a variety of bio-potential electrodes as required.
4. Assists in obtaining recordings in the operating room, including those from the exposed brain during neurosurgical procedures.
5. Makes the appropriate calibration procedures of the EEG apparatus for standard and special recordings; inspects and assures proper maintenance of EEG and related equipment.
6. Adapts procedures to particular clinical circumstances. This implies the ability to add electrodes in non-standard locations and to devise the appropriate recording techniques with minimal assistance.
7. Recognizes and eliminates causes of electrical interference.
8. Abstracts relevant information from the patient's clinical record and obtains additional information by questioning. Observes and notes clinical phenomena occurring during the patient's test.
9. Assists medical staff during special procedures.
10. Participates in research by collecting and processing data.
11. Fills and forwards charge slips for billing purposes as required.
12. Files and/or microfilms recordings as required.
13. Performs other related duties as required.
14. Participates in conferences and technical meetings.

MINIMUM TECHNICAL QUALIFICATIONS:
1. Certification by the American Board of Registration of Electroencephalographic Technologists or equivalent.
2. Successful completion of a traineeship of the duration of one year followed by not less than one year of full-time experience in EEG laboratory following:
3. Completion of one year of college or university with emphasis on physical or biological science,
   OR
4. High school graduation with emphasis on physical or biological sciences; experience as research or clinical assistant in a scientific laboratory is an advantage.

OPTIMAL TECHNICAL QUALIFICATIONS:
Graduation from an AMA-accredited educational program for EEG technologists in addition to the above minimal qualifications.

PERSONAL QUALIFICATIONS:
1. Maturity and ability to establish good rapport with patients, public and staff.
2. Capacity to deal with severely ill patients.

CLASS SPECIFICATION
TITLE: Electroencephalography Technologist III
SUMMARY: Qualifies to serve as chief technologist and to supervise the technical operation and training activities of the laboratory.

DISTINGUISHING CHARACTERISTICS:
The person in this class is distinguished by a high degree of sophistication in the field of EEG technology; is responsible for the technical operation of laboratories performing clinical and/or research work; directs related clerical activity; supervises, plans and helps develop training activities.

EXAMPLES OF DUTIES:
1. Plans laboratory schedules; assigns priorities according to the work load and clinical urgency.
2. Supervises, plans and reviews the work of the technical staff and performs their duties when required. When necessary, takes corrective action or suggests technical innovations.
3. Supervises or performs particularly difficult and/or unusual recording procedures.
4. Keeps inventory and initiates purchasing of laboratory supplies.
5. Arranges for maintenance and repairs of equipment.
6. Takes part in the recruiting, selection and evaluation of technical staff and trainees.
7. Performs other related duties as required.
8. Organizes and participates in conferences and technical meetings.

MINIMUM TECHNICAL QUALIFICATIONS:
1. Certification by the American Board of Registration of Electroencephalographic Technologists or equivalent.
2. Bachelor's Degree or its equivalent and three years of experience in EEG technology **OR** five years of experience.

OPTIMAL TECHNICAL QUALIFICATIONS:
Graduation from an AMA-accredited educational program for EEG technologists in addition to the above minimal qualifications.

PERSONAL QUALIFICATIONS:
1. High degree of leadership, organizational and teaching talents.

MINIMUM TECHNICAL REQUIREMENTS FOR PERFORMING CLINICAL ELECTROENCEPHALOGRAPHY

INTRODUCTION

Although no single best method exists for recording EEGs under all circumstances, the attached standards are considered the **MINIMUM** for the usual clinical recording of EEGs in all age groups except the very young. (Special procedures for use in suspected electrocerebral silence are included in **Minimum Technical Standards for EEG Recording in Suspected Cerebral Death,** p. 492.)

Recording at minimum standards should give no pride to the EEG department working at this level and cannot insure a satisfactory test. Minimum standards provide barely adequate fulfillment of responsibilities to the patient and the referring physician.

To the minimum standards have been added recommendations to improve standardization of procedures and also facilitate interchange of recordings and assessment among laboratories in North America.

1.1 **Sixteen channels of simultaneous recording of the EEG are encouraged. In no event should less than 8 channels be used.**

To find the distribution of EEG activity, it is necessary to record simultaneously from as many regions of the scalp as possible. Inadequate simultaneous recording can lead to erroneous knowledge of the brain areas producing abnormality.

Minimal experience in EEG analysis demonstrates that the chances of error increase enormously with the fewer channels used simultaneously. The chances decrease with the more channels used. This is particularly true for transient activity.

Eight channels of simultaneous recording are the minimum number required to show the areas producing most normal and abnormal EEG patterns.

2.1 **The full 21 electrodes and placements recommended by the International Federation should be used (except in premature infants with small heads). These placements include: frontal polar, frontal, central, parietal, and occipital areas, the inferior frontal or anterior temporal area, the middle and posterior temporal areas, the auricular (ear) or mastoid region (all bilaterally) and mid-line regions in the frontal, central (vertex) and parietal areas. Except in Intensive Care Units (ICUs) in which other electrical equipment is attached to the patient, a grounding electrode should be added but not connected to any other electrode.**

An adequate number of electrodes is essential to insure that EEG activity having a small area of representation on the scalp is recorded, and to analyze accurately the distribution of more diffuse activity. Occasionally, additional electrodes placed between those representing the standard placements are needed in order to record very localized activity.

The 10-20 system, which is well described and well defined, is the only one officially recommended by the International Federation of Societies for EEG and Clinical Neurophysiology (IFSECN). It is the most commonly used existing system, and it should be used universally. (See Jasper, H. H. The ten-twenty electrode system of the International Federation, **Electroenceph. clin. Neurophysiol.**, 1958, 10:371–373.)

Those EEG departments not using the 10-20 system should at least define the relationships between their electrode placements and those of the 10-20 system.

The use of the term "modified 10-20 system" is undesirable when it means that head measurements have not been made and placements have been estimated. In this case the term "estimated 10-20 placement" is more appropriate.

2.2 **Inter-electrode impedances should be checked as a routine pre-recording procedure. Ordinarily, electrode impedance should not exceed 5 k ohms (for needle electrodes in suspected electrocerebral silence (ECS) recordings, higher impedances may be encountered). (See 9.1.)**

While it may not always be possible to check electrode impedances, this procedure should definitely be done when any doubtful pattern is seen in the record which might be artifactual.

3.1 **BOTH scalp-to-scalp (bipolar) and referential montages should be used.**

Two basic types of electrode connections or montages are used in the majority of EEG laboratories. The two types are frequently referred to as bipolar or scalp-to-scalp, and referential or scalp-to-reference. (The term "monopolar" as a synonym for the latter is discouraged.)

Since the EEG records voltage difference between two electrodes, all recordings are theoretically bipolar. However, in the scalp-to-scalp montages, which characteristically link scalp electrodes so that adjacent derivations or channels from the same electrode chain have an electrode in common, the EEG is a record only of the voltage differences between adjacent areas. The referential montage using one electrode common to many channels shows the voltage differences between the respective areas and the reference electrode. The patterns seen from the two types of recording may be very different since the scalp-to-scalp montage rejects or reduces activity common to many electrodes and emphasizes differences. The scalp-to-reference records better the patterns common to all or many electrodes and makes inter-areal differences less noticeable.

Use of the two types of montages becomes mandatory to extract the maximum amount of information from the EEG. The two types of montages are complementary. Use of only one can result in inadequacy of information and incorrect interpretation. Simultaneous use of bipolar and referential montages during a part of the recording is often additionally helpful.

3.2 **The electrode connections for each channel should be clearly indicated at the beginning of each montage.**

Although this may appear self-evident, it is too common practice to mark the record with some cryptic code such as "Run A" or "Run #2." The use of Master switches encourages these codes. The use of these codes, if unidentified on the record, is deplored since they can only be meaningful to a few members of the EEG department using them and to no one else.

The electrode designation, with proper input relationships, for each channel, should be accurately noted at the beginning of each different montage and whenever electrode selection is changed.

3.3 The activity from electrodes on the left and right hemispheres should be clearly specified on the tracing.

When comparison is made between EEG activity of similar areas of left and right hemispheres, it is the more common practice in North America for the left hemisphere channel or channels to precede the right. That is, for montages with block derivations, all activity from the left hemisphere is at the top of the record and from the right hemisphere at the bottom. For montages alternately comparing channels, the first channel is left; the second is right; the third is left, and so on.

This arrangement is contrary to a report of IFSECN (International Federation of Societies for EEG and Clinical Neurophysiology), which recommended right-sided precedence over left, a common practice in European laboratories. Although a number of EEG departments in North America have complied with the IFSECN recommendation, the great majority of departments still use the left-right precedence and are likely to continue to do so. Since widespread conversion is not readily feasible and not of major importance, no recommendation on change is presently offered. However, to avoid confusion, there must be clear identification of the laterality and connections of every montage employed.

3.4 The patterns of electrode connections or montages should be made as simple as possible. They should run in lines and the interelectrode distances kept equal.

At least three or four montages should be very simple in arrangement, easy to describe, and easy to interpret. Examples are frontal-central-parietal-occipital, or inferior frontal-mid-temporal, posterior temporal-occipital linkages. The recommendation in no way indicates preclusion of other montages since some activity cannot be defined by these montages alone. At least 2 minutes of a given montage should be recorded.

It is strongly suggested that the montages should be easily comprehended by any interpreter, by students and by physicians examining records of their own patients.

The use of anteriorly placed electrodes in the upper and posteriorly placed on the lower part of the record should be employed in all possible circumstances.

It is very desirable to have some of the montages comparable between all EEG Departments. A partial revision was carried out in 1975 by a Subcommittee of the Committee on Training and Education: Richard H. Mattson, M.D., Chairman.

4.1 The recordings should include periods when the eyes are open and when they are closed.

Proper EEG recording requires examination of reaction of EEG activity to stimuli. Comparison between the eyes-open (passively if necessary) and the eyes-closed condition constitutes one important means for assessing reactivity. Some rhythms can be masked by the alpha activity and visible only when the alpha rhythm has been attenuated by eye-opening. Certain forms of eye movement may appear to be frontal delta or theta activity but eye-opening and closing helps differentiation. Sometimes paroxysmal activity may appear only when the eyes are opened or only when the eyes are closed or at the time these conditions change. Failure to record with eye-opening and closing as a routine procedure can reduce chances of obtaining potentially important information. The procedure is so simple it is unjustifiable not to use it actively whenever patient cooperation permits, passively, when it does not.

5.1 Calibration should be recorded at the beginning and end of every EEG recording. At the outset, all channels should be adjusted, if necessary, to respond equally and correctly to the calibration signal.

The calibration is an integral part of every EEG recording. It gives a scaling factor for the interpreter, and tests the EEG machine for sensitivity, high and low frequency response, noise level, and pen alignment and damping. It also gives much information as to the competence and care of the technologist.

5.2 When instrument settings (sensitivities, frequency filters, paper speed) are changed during the recording, the settings should be clearly identified on the record at the time of change. The final calibration(s) should include EACH sensitivity and filter setting used in the recording, and should include calibration voltages appropriate to the sensitivities actually used.

This is also of fundamental importance. It is especially important to record calibration signals at very high sensitivities when these settings have been used.

5.3 The sensitivity of the EEG equipment for routine recording should be set in the range of 5 to 10 microvolts per mm of pen deflection (i.e., 5 to 10 μV/mm).

Sensitivity is defined as the ratio of input voltage to pen deflection. It is expressed in microvolts per mm (μV/mm). A commonly used sensitivity is 7 μV/mm, which for a calibration signal of 50 microvolts results in a deflection of 7 mm. With this sensitivity, the amplitude of most EEG activity of known significance is not too low or too high on the record.

If the sensitivity is **decreased** (for example, from 7 µV/mm to 10 µV/mm), the amplitude of the write-out of a given EEG on the paper also **decreases.** Conversely, if the sensitivity is **increased** (for example, from 7 µV/mm to 5 µV/mm), the amplitude of the write-out of a given EEG **increases.***

When the sensitivity is less than 10 µV/mm (for example, 20 µV/mm), significant low amplitude activity may become indiscernible. If the sensitivity is greater than 5 µV/mm (for example, 3 µV/mm), normal EEG activity may overload the system, causing a squaring off of the peaks of the write-out onto the paper.

During calibration for routine recordings, the recorded signals should be undistorted but large enough to permit measurement to better than ± 5% between any of the signals on the different channels.

No matter which sensitivity within the above limits is chosen prior to the recording, appropriate adjustments should be made whenever the EEG activity encountered is of too high or low amplitude to be recorded properly. These changes should be marked on the EEG record.

5.4 When doubt as to correct functioning of any amplifier exists, a calibration run should be made, followed by a recording with all channels connected to the same pair of electrodes.

Taking a record from an electrode pair common to all channels can demonstrate malfunction of the EEG equipment not necessarily noticed in the calibration. For this purpose, an antero-posterior (fronto-occipital) derivation should be used, since it can include fast and alpha range patterns as well as eye movement activity in the delta range.

5.5 Except for specific and identifiable reasons, recording of the lower frequencies should be such that 1 Hz activity is not attenuated by more than 30% of the activity in the alpha range (8–13 Hz). Recording of the higher frequencies should be such that 50 Hz activity is not attenuated by more than 30% of the activity in the alpha range.

Use of the low frequency filter (shortened time constant) routinely to "clean up" artifacts in the record is deplored, especially when slow-wave abnormalities are suspected. Vital information is lost by doing this when pathologic patterns in the delta range are present. Similarly, use of the high frequency filters to "clean up" the record can distort spike activity and other discharges into unrecognizable forms, or can render them invisible. Production of a "pretty record" which has lost important information is poor medical practice.

It must be emphasized, however, that use of the low or high frequency filters—with annotation of this on the record—can emphasize or clarify certain types of patterns in the record. These filter controls, therefore, should be used selectively and carefully.

6.1 The record should have written on it as a MINIMUM the name of the patient, the age and the date and time of recording, a list of all the medications the patient is on, the time of the last food taken. The type, quantity, and time of administration of any sleep medication or other medication should also be noted on the record.

Identification should be made at the time of recording. Failure to do so may permit mix-ups that can be catastrophic both medically and legally. Various medicines can alter the EEG, as can relative hypoglycemia. A Basic Data Sheet, permanently attached to every record, which compacts such information—together with montage data—can be very helpful.

7.1 Not less than 20 minutes of effective recording should be made for awake recordings. Longer recordings are often more informative.

The EEG is a sample in time from a patient's life—a very short sample, in fact. Within reasonable limits, the longer the recording, the better the chance of recording abnormality or demonstrating variability of abnormality. Experience in many centers shows that a very minimum of 20 minutes of artifact-free recording is necessary. It must be emphasized that with addition of photic stimulation, hyperventilation, and especially sleep—which should all be done whenever possible—the amount of recording time must be increased considerably.

7.2 Overbreathing should be used routinely unless some medical or other justifiable reasons (e.g., a recent subarachnoid hemorrhage, intracranial hem-

---

* Note that a sensitivity of 5 µV/mm means that to obtain a pen deflection of 1 mm, a 5 µV input voltage is required (and correspondingly, to obtain a 10 mm deflection, an input of 50 µV is required). If the sensitivity is **decreased** to 10 µV/mm, the same 1 mm pen deflection now requires a **larger** input, i.e., 10 µV rather than 5 µV (and correspondingly, a 10 mm pen deflection now requires an input of 100 µV rather than 50 µV). Thus as the sensitivity is **increased** its numerical value **becomes smaller.** Conversely, as the sensitivity is **decreased** its numerical value **becomes larger.** This perhaps seemingly paradoxical relationship is actually a logical consequence of the definition of sensitivity as input voltage per unit of pen deflection, i.e., input voltage required to give a particular pen deflection (e.g., 1 mm).

orrhage, or significant cardio-pulmonary disease) contraindicate it. It should be performed for a minimum of three minutes with continued recording for at least one minute after cessation of overbreathing. To evaluate the effects of this activation technique, at least one minute of recording with the same montage should be run before overbreathing begins.

Unfortunately, overbreathing is rarely performed adequately. Even without exact quantification, however, enough abnormality can be produced from time to time to make it a simple and useful additive procedure when the patient can cooperate. It is often helpful to record EKG directly on one EEG channel during this and other parts of the recording, particularly if spike or sharp activity, or pulse or EKG artifact, are in question. With an additional (e.g., 17th) channel, the EKG can be monitored continuously.

7.3 **Sleep recordings should be taken whenever possible but not to the exclusion of the waking record.**

It is increasingly evident that considerable additional information of normal or abnormal significance can be added by recording during drowsiness and sleep. Some departments use sleep recording routinely but this is not always possible in all departments. Sleep recording is usually essential for patients with suspected or known convulsive disorders.

8.1 **The state of the patient, as awake, drowsy, sleeping or comatose, and any change thereof, should be noted by the technologist on the EEG recording. Any commands or signals to the patient, and any movement or clinical seizure activity or absence thereof, should also be noted on the recording if appropriate.**

It is the responsibility of the interpreter to recognize the patterns usually associated with different states of consciousness. However, observation by the technologist about the status of the patient can be of considerable interpretative value, particularly when discrepancies or unusual correlations occur.

9.1 **Needle electrodes are not recommended for use under ordinary laboratory conditions. They should only be used when completely sterilized and when the technologist who employs them has been taught the exact techniques, as well as the disadvantages and hazards of their use. Antero-posterior alignment of the needles is important and misalignment may cause amplitude asymmetries or distortions.**

There is no perfect electrode. Experimental evidence suggests that the silver-silver chloride disc and pad held on by collodion is the best, but other electrodes using electrode pastes have been effectively used. Many other types exist but only the needle electrode is inserted into the skin and is thus a potential carrier of disease. Unless the needle electrode is properly sterilized, the user is exposing the patient to unjustifiable medical risk and himself to possible legal action.

It is rarely appreciated that the proper use of needle electrodes requires more care and expertise than for any other type of electrode.

However, needle electrodes can be effectively utilized in comatose patients, in whom pain responses are usually minimal or absent, and who are in medical settings requiring efficient recordings with a minimum of delay.

10.1 **Special procedures which are of some risk to the patient should be carried out only in the presence of a qualified physician, only in an environment with adequate resuscitating equipment, and with the informed consent of the patient or responsible relative.**

10.2 **The recording of EEGs to be used in the evaluation of cessation of cerebral function ("cerebral death") requires special procedures and extraordinary precautions.** (See Minimum Technical Standards for EEG Recording in Suspected Cerebral Death, below.)

MINIMUM TECHNICAL STANDARDS FOR EEG RECORDING IN SUSPECTED CEREBRAL DEATH

INTRODUCTION

The 1970 report of the American EEG Society's Ad Hoc Committee on EEG Criteria for the Determination of Cerebral Death filled an urgent need for guidance in EEG. Such EEG studies are no longer confined to major laboratories—some of which have now had over a decade of experience in this area. Even small hospitals may have Intensive Care Units and EEG facilities. The need for such minimal standard guidelines has thus increased.

The earlier (1970) edition of **Minimum Technical Standards for EEG Recording in Suspected Cerebral Death** reflected the state of the art and the technique of the latter 1960's. Substantially improved electroencephalographic instrumentation is now available. Equally important, there is now a much larger number of competent EEG technologists. A collaborative study of cerebral death that was being planned in 1970 has been completed and published in part (Bennett, D. R., Hughes, J. R., Korein, J., Merlis,

J. K., and Suter, S. **An Atlas of Electroencephalography in Coma and Cerebral Death.** Raven Press, 1976, 244 p.).

The present edition includes an updating of the criteria that reflects what has been learned since the first appearance of these standards.

The survey in the late 1960's by the American EEG Society's Ad Hoc Committee on EEG Criteria for the Determination of Cerebral Death revealed that out of 2,650 cases of coma with presumably "isoelectric" EEGs, only three whose records satisfied the committee's criteria showed any recovery of cerebral function. These three had suffered from massive overdoses of nervous system depressants, two from barbiturate and one from meprobamate. Many of the reported "isoelectric" records were, on review, either low voltage records or run with techniques inadequate to bring out low voltage activity—that is, inadequate technique alone gave the graphs the apearance of being "flat." Hence, the 1970 committee recommended dropping non-physiologic terms such as "isoelectric" or "linear" (the word "flat" should likewise not be used) and renaming the state "electrocerebral silence." ("Electrocerebral inactivity" is the term recommended in the Glossary of the International Federation of Societies for EEG and Clinical Neurophysiology, published in **Electroenceph. clin. Neurophysiol.,** 1974, 37:538–548.)

Electrocerebral Silence (ECS), or Electrocerebral Inactivity, is defined as no electrocerebral activity over 2 μV when recording from scalp or referential electrode pairs 10 or more cm apart with inter-electrode resistances under 10,000 ohms (or impedances under 6,000 ohms), but over 100 ohms.

Twelve recommendations for EEG recordings in cases of suspected cerebral death, with the rationale for each, are set forth and illustrated below.

Recommendation No. 1: A Minimum of Eight Scalp Electrodes and Ear Lobe Reference Electrodes

The major brain areas must be covered to be certain that absence of activity is not a focal phenomenon. The use of a single channel instrument such as is made for EEG monitoring of anesthetic levels for the purpose of determining ECS is therefore to be deplored. The frontal (frontal pole electrode), parietal (central electrode), occipital and temporal areas of both hemispheres are recommended; in terms of the International 10-20 system this would be: F_{p1-2}, C_{3-4}, O_{1-2}, and T_{3-4}. Inclusion of the frontal electrodes (F_{3-4}) is also suggested because of the frequent projection of deep potentials to this area and of the vertex electrode (C_z) as well as the ear lobe (A_{1-2}) or non-cephalic references. A grounding electrode should be added but not connected to any other electrode; however, for recordings in Intensive Care Units, a ground electrode should **NOT** be used if other electrical equipment is attached to the patient.

Since, prior to the recording, one **does not know** whether the record will be one of ECS, it is desirable to use a full set of electrodes on the initial examination, i.e., the International 10–20 system (see **Minimum Technical Requirements for Performing Clinical Electroencephalography,** 2.1). In any event, the initial study should not use less than the routine coverage standard for the particular clinical laboratory. A full set of electrodes includes midline placements (F_z, C_z, P_z), which are useful for the detection of residual low-voltage physiologic activity and are relatively free from artifact. Since the EEGs of patients with suspected ECS may actually be abnormal in a complex way, the use of more complete, rather than less complete, electrode coverage is further justified.

Recommendation No. 2: Interelectrode Impedances Under 10,000 OHMS but over 100 OHMS

Very high electrode impedances attenuate brain signals; on the other hand, very low interelectrode impedances approach the situation of a shunt or short-circuit by virtue of a salt bridge that also attenuates signals. When one electrode has a relatively high impedance compared to the second electrode of the pair, the amplifier becomes unbalanced and is prone to amplify extraneous signals unduly. This is one reason for the pick-up of 60-Hz interference or other artifact wave forms, often of high amplitude, and emphasizes the fact that situations of low cerebral input and high instrumental sensitivity demand scrupulous electrode application. There is a marked drop-off of potentials with impedances below 100 ohms and, of course, no potential at 0 ohms. This could be one possible reason for a false ECS record, which would be obviated by a simple test of interelectrode impedances to assure that they are of a proper magnitude.

Stable, low-impedance electrodes are absolutely essential for all bedside (i.e., away from the laboratory) studies.

Although not recommended for general use, needle electrodes have been effectively used in suspected ECS recordings. The greater impedances which they may have are offset by a greater probability of similar values among different electrodes, so that the likelihood of artifactual pickup is not increased. (See also **Minimum Technical Requirements for Performing Clinical Electroencephalography,** Paragraph 9.1.)

Recommendation No. 3: Test the Integrity of the Entire Recording System

Calibration tests the operation of the amplifiers and writer units, but it does not exclude the possibility of shunting or an open circuit at the electrodes, electrode board, cable or input of the machine. If, after a test run on one montage at increased amplification, an EEG suggesting electrocerebral silence is found (almost invariably, an EKG artifact will be present), the simplest test of integrity is to touch each electrode of the montage gently with a pencil point or cotton swab to create an artifact potential on the record. This test verifies that the electrode board is connected to the machine; records made with the electrode board inadvertently not connected can sometimes resemble low-amplitude EEG activity. The test further proves that the selector switch settings match the electrode placements.

Recommendation No. 4: Interelectrode Distances of at Least 10 Centimeters

In the International 10–20 system the average adult interelectrode distances are between 6 and 6.5 centimeters. Hence, with scalp montages double distances electrode linkages are recommended (e.g., F_{p1}-C_3, C_3-O_1, etc.) or referential runs; if the ears are used, crossed ear-references montages give the maximum distance. This important recommendation is often overlooked; the reason for it is that the increase in potential difference between electrodes is proportional to the square of the distance, up to roughly ten cm. An experiment with a normal subject was performed to show the effect of distance on amplitude. Electrodes were placed at the following distances anterior to the right occiput (O_2): 1 cm, 2 cm, 3 cm, 6.5 cm (P_4), 9 cm, 13 cm (C_4), 19.5 cm (F_4), and the ear reference (A_2). It was observed that opening the eyes, thereby attenuating the alpha rhythm, produces a pseudo-ECS record at the two shortest distances from the occiput. A record taken with average interelectrode distances at ordinary sensitivity may suggest electrocerebral silence; however, when recorded at long interelectrode distances, obvious potentials may be seen in the tracing. In addition to the amplitude effect, the electrical field from deep structures is more likely to be recorded from widely spaced electrode pairs than from electrodes at average distances.

The appreciable EKG contamination often encountered with the opposite ear as reference may be somewhat reduced by recording to combined ears ($A_1 + A_2$) as well as by judicious positioning of the head. A C_z reference may also be useful. The authors of the Atlas cited in the Introduction agreed that among the ones they used, the best montage was: F_{p2}-C_4; C_4-O_2; F_{p1}-C_3; C_3-O_1; T_4-C_z; C_z-T_3, with one channel EKG and one channel noncephalic (hand). (See Recommendation 7.) Occipital leads, however, are more difficult to attach in immobilized patients and are particularly susceptible to movement artifact induced by artificial respirators. The combinations of F_7-T_5, F_3-P_3, F_z-P_z, F_4-P_4 and F_8-T_6 may therefore yield a better record.

None of the foregoing should imply that the usual preselected laboratory montages may not be used.

Recommendation No. 5: Sensitivity Increased from 7 (7.5) μV/mm to 2 μV/mm During most of the Recording with Inclusion of Appropriate Calibrations

This is perhaps the most important and the most often overlooked parameter. One only has to remember that at a sensitivity of 7 μV/mm a signal of 2 μV cannot be seen because the average pen ink line is ¼ mm in width, i.e., greater than the signal one desires to see. The signal should be just visible at 3 μV/mm and certainly so at 2 μV/mm.

Modern equipment readily permits extended recording with a sensitivity of 1 μV/mm. It is recommended that a sensitivity of 2 μV/mm be the **absolute minimal standard** for evaluation of ECS. Obviously all (or virtually all) of the tracing should be run with at least this much sensitivity (see also Recommendation 9 and comment for Recommendation 7).

Adequate and appropriate **calibration** procedures are essential. Calibration with a 10, 5 or even 2 microvolt (μV) signal is required for verification of high sensitivity. (A 50 μV calibration signal at a sensitivity of 2 or 1 μV/mm is useless since the pens bloc.) A good rule of thumb is to calibrate with a signal near the size or value of the EEG signal that has been recorded; thus for electrocerebral silence, a calibration of 2 μV (preferably) is appropriate.

Recommendation No. 6: Use of Time Constants of 0.3 to 0.4 Seconds During Part of the Recording

It is well known that short time constants attenuate slow potentials. In the situation approaching electrocerebral silence, there may be potentials in the theta and delta ranges, so every effort should be made to avoid attenuation of these low frequencies. Whenever possible, high frequency filters should be set at a minimum of 30 Hz to avoid attenuation of low voltage fast activity.

Recordings with such extended time constants are usually feasible with good electrode technique, although their use is not a prerequisite for establishing ECS. There need be no hesitation in the use of the 60-Hz or notch filter, if need be.

Recommendation No. 7: Use of Monitoring Techniques

The EEG record is actually a composite of true brain waves, other physiological signals, and artifacts, either internal or external to the machine, of mechanical or of electromagnetic and/or electric field origin. When sensitivities are increased, such artifacts are also accentuated and therefore must be monitored so that they can be mentally subtracted from the tracing to give the true brain wave. Since one rarely sees a record of this type without varying amounts of EKG artifact, an EKG monitor is **essential**.

Frequently an additional monitor is needed for other artifact emanating from the patient or for artifact induced from the surroundings. The most convenient for this purpose is a pair of electrodes on the dorsum of the right hand separated by about 6 to 7 cm. Machine noise and external interference may be conveniently checked by a "dummy patient," i.e., a 10,000 ohm resistor between input terminal 1 (G_1) and input terminal 2 (G_2) of one channel. If respiration artifact cannot be eliminated, it may be monitored by a chest strain-gauge transducer, or the respirator can be stopped momentarily.

The previously cited **Atlas of Electroencephalography in Coma and Cerebral Death** should be consulted for information about a wide range of artifacts. The best insurance against these is a stable, low-impedance electrode system. It is now quite clear that some EMG contamination can persist in patients with ECS recordings. If EMG potentials are of such amplitude as to obscure the tracing, it may be necessary to reduce or eliminate them by use of a neuromuscular blocking agent such as pancuronium bromide (Pavulon) or succinyl-choline (Anectine). This procedure should be performed under the direction of an anesthesiologist or physician familiar with the use of the drug.

Even with good technique, however, recording the EEG at the increased sensitivities recommended above can at times leave the electroencephalographer who interprets the recordings with considerable difficulty. An attempt must be made to subtract from the record both the EKG artifact (which masks other rhythms) and the ongoing noise level of the complete system in the particular ICU as indicated by the recording from the hand. An estimate must then be made of whether or not the remaining activity exceeds 2 microvolts amplitude. Since this may be impossible, the electroencephalographer may be limited to making a statement such as the following: "There was a noise level in the recording system of approximately 2 to 3 microvolts as indicated in the hand monitor. Recordings from the scalp reflected a similar noise level but did not show activity in excess of this amount; therefore, it is concluded that no cerebral activity in excess of noise exists and that a state of electrocerebral silence is present." For still higher irreducible noise levels, obviously no statement can be made about ECS.

Recommendation No. 8: Tests for EEG Reactivity to Intense Stimuli Such as Pain (e.g., Pinch), Loud Sound, and (Optionally) Strong Light (Stroboscopic if Available)

There should of course be no EEG reactivity, i.e., no evidence of cortical function. Any apparent EEG activation resulting from these stimuli and any others (airway suctioning and other nursing procedures can be potent stimuli) must of course be carefully distinguished from artifacts resulting from their use. For example, an electroretinogram can still persist in response to photic stimulation when there is ECS.

Recommendation No. 9: Recording Time of at Least 30 Minutes

Periods of ECS are not uncommon in low voltage records and therefore a single recording should be long enough to be certain that short periods of low voltage activity are not missed. The necessity of running at high sensitivity (see Recommendation 5) is therefore reiterated.

To go through the necessary montages and carry out stimulation procedures is likely to require 30 minutes or more in any event.

Recommendation No. 10: Recordings to be Made Only by a Qualified Technologist

Great skill is essential in making recordings in suspected ECS, which are frequently made under difficult circumstances at best and which include many possibilities for artifact in the recording. Elimination of most artifact and identification of all others can be accomplished by a qualified technologist.

Qualifications for a competent EEG technologist for ECS recordings include the requirements of **supervised instruction and recordings in ICU settings and working under the direction of a qualified electroencephalographer.**

Recommendation No. 11: A Repeat EEG if There is Doubt About Electrocerebral Silence

In the Collaborative Study of Cerebral Death cited in the Introduction, there were no patients who survived for more than a short period after an EEG showed electrocerebral silence, provided that overdose of depressant drugs (or significant hypothermia) was excluded. This finding confirmed the results of the earlier survey which were summarized in the Introduction. It is evident therefore, that a single EEG showing electrocerebral silence is a highly reliable confirmatory procedure for the clinical impression of cerebral death. (For guidelines to assist physicians in the determination of brain death, reference is made to the most recent recommendations of the Inter-Agency Committee on Irreversible Coma and Brain Death; reports of the Committee are published in the Transactions of the American Neurological Association.)

In the event that technical or other difficulties lead to uncertainty in the evaluation of the question of ECS, the entire procedure should be repeated after an interval, for example, after 6 hours.

It should be pointed out, however, that the above-mentioned Collaborative Study of Cerebral Death did not include young children and infants and hence the comparable data on which to base recommendation for this young age group do not exist at present. There is thus clearly a need for systematic study of ECS of the age group under 3 years. In infants, apparent ECS can, for example, be associated with bilateral subdural hematoma or with serious metabolic derangements (electrolyte, blood gas alterations—hence the need for accurate determinations of the latter at the time of the tracing).

Recommendation No. 12: Telephone Transmission of EEG not to be Used for Determination of Electrocerebral Silence

At the present time, telephone transmission of EEG cannot be used for determination of electrocerebral silence in the diagnosis of brain death because of the inherent and unpredictable electrical noise present in telephone networks relative to the very low signal amplitudes in the EEG recording itself, in ECS.

Should technical advances eliminate or substantially alleviate this problem, the American EEG Society will formally review its Guidelines at that time. (See also **Provisional Recommendations for Telephone Transmission of EEGs,** below.)

PROVISIONAL RECOMMENDATIONS FOR TELEPHONE TRANSMISSION OF EEGs

1. The basic standards for clinical EEG, defined in **Minimum Technical Requirements for Performing Clinical Electroencephalography** (p. 488)

should be followed in the transmission of clinical electroencephalograms by telephone.

2. The statements set forth in **Standards of Practice in Clinical Electroencephalography** (p. 5) and in **Recommended Job Descriptions for Electroencephalographic Technologists** (p. 8) are reaffirmed for telephone transmission of EEGs. These standards define the basic level of competence of the EEG technologists at the transmitting and at the receiving sites, as well as the competence of the electroencephalographer who interprets the record. Under no circumstances should the technologist at the transmitting laboratory be less qualified than one who works independently under a laboratory director who is based outside of a hospital. Indeed, the responsibilities falling upon the EEG technologist staffing a telephone transmitting laboratory are greater than those of a technologist working under relatively direct supervision in a hospital or office laboratory.

Technologists staffing a receiving facility, who should be skilled and experienced, should be specifically trained in EEG telephone transmission, including recognition of artifacts that are peculiar thereto, familiarity with which is essential in EEG telephone transmission. The technologist at the transmitting laboratory, because of its remoteness from the receiving center, should be well trained, especially in EEG telephone transmission, irrespective of any limited utilization because of size of referral load, and should be acquainted with the receiving laboratory. In view of the isolation of the transmitting laboratory, provisions for continued education and updating of information are essential to maintaining the skill of the transmitting technologist. A program of continuing education should also be available for the technologist at the receiving laboratory.

3. There should be an original ("hard copy") EEG recorded at the transmitting end of the circuit, so that the technologist can correlate ongoing EEG events with ongoing behavior changes or activities of the patient. This recommendation necessitates that a complete electroencephalograph be employed at the transmitting site.* Voice or other signaling capabilites should be incorporated in the telephone-EEG system, from transmitting to receiving stations, to identify such correlations as they occur, with minimal interference with the EEG record. Such on-line correlation will assist in avoiding misinterpretation (e.g., muscle artifact being regarded as spikes, etc.). There should be adequate identification appearing on both the original ("hard copy") transmitted record, and the received record to identify the latter as being a copy of the former; this identification should include patient ID, all calibrations and changes in instrument controls and of montages used, and of patient behavior and activity (see paragraphs 5.1, 5.2, 6.1, 7.1, and 8.1 of **Minimum Technical Requirements for Performing Clinical Electroencephalography**). The use of a standard code for transmitting such information should be required. "Fail-safe" indication of difficulties due to line losses or other transmission or receiving problems should be included in the transmitting-receiving system itself. (Assistance from the telephone companies themselves with general information concerning identification of artifacts generated within the telephone systems could be most helpful.) Signal checks of equipment at both the transmitting and receiving laboratories should be introduced preceding and following each recording, i.e., prior to the initial calibration and subsequent to the final calibration.

4. The technical specifications for received recordings should be not less than those defined in **Minimum Technical Requirements for Performing Clinical Electroencephalography,** paragraph 5.5; within these specifications, the tracings written out at the transmitting and at the receiving sites should be essentially identical.

5. Manufacturers should provide frequency response, noise and cross-talk data operating conditions, so that consumers can make intelligent comparisons. Periodic checks of equipment at both the transmitting and the receiving laboratories should be carried out.

6. Provided that all of the above and previously approved procedures are followed, and that there is a qualified technologist both at the transmitting and receiving terminals, and that a qualified electroencephalographer interprets the received EEG, with the capability of a "hard-copy" original at the transmitting site for back-up comparison (a provisional recommendation, as noted above), no ethical problem in the use of telephone systems for expediting interpretation of EEGs should arise.

7. If the previously adopted Guidelines are not carried over to cover the telephone transmission of EEGs, and if users are not aware of the characteristics of ancillary equipment used in telephone transmission of EEGs, the installation of a telephone transmission system may well cause a degradation of the quality of practice of clinical electroencephalography.

8. At the present time, telephone transmission of EEG cannot be used for determination of electrocerebral silence in the diagnosis of brain death be-

---

* This is an interim recommendation, and may be modified if adequate data indicate that a reliable alternative to a "hard copy" will suffice.

cause of the inherent and unpredictable electrical noise present in telephone networks relative to the very low signal amplitudes in the EEG recording itself, in ECS. Should technical advances eliminate or substantially alleviate this problem, the American EEG Society will formally review its Guidelines at that time. (See Recommendation No. 12 in **Minimum Technical Standards for EEG Recording in Suspected Cerebral Death,** p. 496.)

9. Reference for further information is made to the portions of the **Handbook of Electroencephalography and Clinical Neurophysiology** concerning Telephone Transmission of EEGs (Vol. 3A, Section E, and Vol. 3B, Section IV), and to the recommendations of the Committee on EEG Instrumentation Standards of the International Federation of Societies for Electroencephalography and Clinical Neurophysiology (IFSECN), **(Electroenceph. Clin. Neurophysiol.,** 1974, 37:552).

Discussions

DISCUSSION OF CHAPTERS 1 TO 7

Daly: To begin, in the matter of electrocerebral silence, there are documented instances of survival, and all of these have been in patients who have had significant amounts of depressant drugs in the blood. So the mere demonstration of electrocerebral silence does not mean that the brain is dead.

Question: Dr. Saunders, why cannot the electrode paste alone without collodion, be used for scalp electrode placement, especially in the small premature infant who tolerates manipulation or handling very poorly?

Saunders: It can be. Bentonite paste and other pastes are often used as a mixture of the sticky substance to hold the electrode in position and also as the electrolyte. Commerical pastes are less likely to be irritating than bentonite.

Knott: Some commerical "creams" are also irritative. Calcium chloride mixed with betonite can be dangerously irritative. Read the label on the container. Do not use homemade pastes.

Question: Dr. Saunders, would you comment on the effect of different interelectrode distances on amplitude.

Saunders: The closer the electrodes are together, the lower the amplitude of the response. This is a very difficult question to answer very briefly because, in fact, you'd have to go into mathematical analyses. Generally speaking, the amplitude of activity increases with the square of the distance as you get further away from the reference electrode. If you have two electrodes a long way apart you get bigger voltages which get smaller and smaller as you bring the electrodes closer together.

Question: Dr. Henry, first, would you discuss the concept of overloading of the amplifier and how this is manifest in EEG recording? What do you mean by overloading of the amplifier?

Henry: It's not always the amplifier that is overloaded; sometimes it's the write-out system. Mostly, all you see is the pen blocking with high amplitude activity.

Question: Second, in your example of spontaneous spike-wave discharge and high-voltage hyperventilation response, why do you need hyperventilation at all?

Henry: I suppose we don't. You can justify it in other ways. If, following appropriate treatment, such a youngster had no spontaneous discharges, we would regard a follow-up tracing (he had them the first time, he did not 4 months later on anticonvulsant medication) as improved. On the other hand, the discharges might still be present if we did hyperventilation. Furthermore, you may bring out with hyperventilation a little focal emphasis that is not evident otherwise, just as you may with a sleep recording.

Question: Dr. Henry, could you comment on the removal of ECG artifact from cerebral death records?

Henry: Fortunately, we have an expert on removal of this activity. Dr. Bickford has designed a way of doing this. I should say, however, that his removal system is not without some financial cost, but it works. Dr. Knott has described a simple no-cost procedure wherein two pages of EEGs are superimposed. When transilluminated, the ECG and its related ballistocardiogram can thus be subtracted out by visual analysis.[1]

Question: Does using an ipsilateral ear lead constitute a basis of reference?

Henry: Yes, it is a reference. Any time you use a single electrode in common with several channels, it is a reference recording. We have for

---

[1] Knott, J. R. (1976): Identification of EEG-related artifacts in very low voltage EEG records. *Am. J. EEG Technol.*, 16:129–130.

the last few years been playing with something that is surprisingly useful if the record has sufficiently high voltage. This is a low cervical reference, probably on C6 or C7. It works quite well at times, and it is worth a try. Nose or chin reference may be helpful, and we have even tried an electrode tucked into saline-soaked cotton and tucked in the mouth along the jaw. Any such point can be your reference. We are still looking for a first-class, indifferent, noncontaminating reference in electroencephalography; even all channel or average reference is not without pitfalls. Can we ask those present, Who uses exclusively reference or exclusively bipolar recording and never the other?

Klass: Each of us here uses both. Dr. Daly, since you raised the point about drug intoxication producing a record of electrocerebral inactivity that is recoverable, let me direct this question to you. What is the time or for how many days would you wait until you declare cerebral death?

Daly: Some of you may be familiar with a collaborative study sponsored by NINCDS.[2] This study analyzed 503 patients over the age of 1 year admitted to study because they were comatose and apneic. If one omits patients with drug-induced coma, no patient recovered after having an EEG that showed no electrocerebral activity (electrocerebral silence) during a 30-min recording. The study concluded that the criteria for cerebral death should be: coma with cerebral unresponsivity, apnea, dilated pupils, absent cephalic reflexes, and electrocerebral silence. All these should have been present for 30 min at least 6 hours after the onset of coma and apnea. Obviously if not all of the circumstances preceding the onset of coma are known, specifically, the possibility of drug intoxication, the period of observation must be extended by an appropriate time.

Let me point out that determination of electrocerebral silence is not always easy, particularly if the electroencephalographer has not had a large experience. In the collaborative project, concurrence between the electroencephalographers and the review panel was approximately 97%. However, the electroencephalographers were highly competent, and the review committee had the opportunity to evaluate over 1,000 EEGs. My personal view is that evaluation of electrocerebral silence in smaller community hospitals can pose major problems. I believe that the EEG should be paralleled by an independent technology. At the present time the use of a radioisotope bolus to evaluate intracranial blood flow offers such a technology.[3]

Saunders: The big problem is not really a question of electrocerebral silence, but did the patient have drugs or not, and how do you find out? I have been a witness on a number of these cerebral death cases, confronted by a very clever prosecuting attorney, and these are the questions you are asked: Are you absolutely sure that this patient was not on drugs? What methods did you take to demonstrate that this person had not had drugs without your knowledge? There are all sorts of new exotic methods for drug determinations that often aren't available in the small centers. It's a very complicated problem.

Ellingson: Of course, it makes a lot of difference if a patient has been brought in and you don't know the history or if a patient has had a cardiac arrest during an operation and has been in the hospital and worked up immediately.

Kellaway: Dr. Klass, I'm concerned—if I understood Dr. Henry correctly—when he said that he wasn't called upon to do EEGs on patients with isoelectric EEGs in infants. The impression was given that a single EEG in time, say 30 min or even an hour in duration, is definite indication whether the electrical activity of the brain is gone or the recovery of cerebral function will occur. I think that a single EEG run for 30 min, even in the absence of drugs, does not tell you the whole story. This seems to be age related. Far from just one EEG to go on, you have to have at least four or more. We have had infants whose EEGs have remained flat for many hours, and they improved. So I think that in multiple recordings time is extremely important and that this is age related.

Daly: Yes. Let me reemphasize that the collaborative study did not accept any children under 1 year of age, so what I said applies only to children over 1 year.

Question: Dr. Daly, could you comment on the criteria for body temperature and electrocerebral inactivity?

---

[2] Walker, A. E. (1977): An appraisal of the criteria of cerebral death. *JAMA*, 237:982–986.

[3] Korein, J., Braunstein, P., George, A., Wichter, M., Kricheff, I., Lieberman, A., and Pearson, J. (1977): Brain death: I. Angiographic correlations with the radioisotopic bolus technique for evaluation of critical deficit of cerebral blood flow. *Ann. Neurol.*, 2:195–205.

Daly: I think that most of the time this is not a relevant factor. Many patients with severe anoxic encephalopathies begin to lose control of autonomic functions as death approaches, and their body temperature begins to fall.

Klass: It has been asked whether you or your colleagues use succinylcholine or any of the muscle-relaxant drugs in the determination of electrocerebral silence? I count nine who do of the 10 who are present.

Knott: I would like to make the comment that when you are using this, unless you use a continuous drip method as described by Suter, you may be interpreting EEGs at considerably less than half an hour in length.

Question: Dr. Ellingson, may a persistent, two-cycle activity in the first week or two be considered normal?

Ellingson: No, I would not consider that normal. I assume "persistent, two-cycle activity" means invariant monorhythmic slow activity.

Question: Dr. Ellingson, please clarify again the four characteristic patterns, exclusive of *tracé alternant,* seen in awake, drowsy, active, and quiet sleep of the newborn full-term.

Ellingson: I assume that the question refers to the low-voltage irregular, mixed, and high-voltage slow patterns and that the question is, Can any of those be seen during wakefulness and/or drowsiness and/or quiet sleep? Yes, in a given infant you may see only one of the patterns, and you may see it during all of those stages, although the low-voltage irregular pattern is unlikely during quiet sleep. Further, the *tracé alternant* pattern is not always seen during a recording. Sometimes an infant will cycle beautifully through wakefulness to quiet sleep but never show *tracé alternant* during quiet sleep in a given recording, only the high voltage-slow or the mixed pattern.

Question: Is your Class A premature pattern a suppression-burst pattern or not? I'm not clear about your position. I would conclude that the suppression-burst pattern in a 35-week-old conceptional age newborn is not abnormal per se.

Ellingson: That depends on what you mean by "suppression-burst." It also depends on what you mean by *"tracé alternant."* Literally, if you take *tracé alternant* to mean an alternating pattern, all of these patterns could be called *tracé alternant.* Likewise, if you use the term suppression-burst in a literal sense, any of them can be called a suppression-burst. I use the term suppression-burst, however, with the connotation of a pathological type of activity distributed in time as bursts with lower voltage or flat tracings in between. In this sense, the very early premature record is not a suppression-burst pattern.

Question: How long can the "suppression areas" last in a "normal" tracing of your EEG Group A?

Ellingson: In very young prematures they sometimes last for many seconds, 15, 20, 30 sec, or even longer. The younger the infant, the longer the period. There has been discussion about an upper limit for the periods of flattening beyond which they might be considered abnormal. There are still not sufficient data on which to base a conclusion.

Goldensohn: I wonder whether the definition of suppression-burst ought to be gone into a bit, in view of the question. How do you define "suppression-burst?"

Klass: The reason Dr. Goldensohn raises this question, of course, is that the term has been used in many different ways. Some would confine its use to high-amplitude activity alternating with very low-amplitude activity seen in deeper stages of anesthesia, and there have been other uses of it. There was a difference of opinion among members of the last Terminology Committee of the International Federation when drawing up its glossary.[4]

Goldensohn: It seems to me that if you want suppression-burst to have some special meaning other than the fact that there has been a paroxysm that recurs now and then, then the activity that we see between the bursts should be at a considerably lower voltage than the rest of the background.

Kellaway: I would like to comment on what I think is the fastest way of clarifying this. I know exactly what Dr. Ellingson is saying. Some of the confusion relates to the factor of what one sees with changing age. I think a good concept is to think about it in terms of the fact that in the nonviable, very immature infant, the electrical activity of the brain is discontinuous and, in fact, we might say silence is the rule. A burst of activity of polymorphic character, generally asynchronous, is the only kind of activity one sees in babies this premature. The continuity of the electrical activity of the brain begins first with increasing age in REM sleep. The continuity

---

[4] Chatrian, G. E., Bergamini, L., Dondey, M., Klass, D. W., Lennox-Buchtal, M., and Petersen, I. (1974): A glossary of terms most commonly used by clinical electroencephalographers. *Electroencephalogr. Clin. Neurophysiol.,* 37:538–548.

is next reached in the awake state, which would be about 37 weeks, and last in so-called quiet or stage 4 sleep. Therefore, in determining normality of the full-term newborn, one expects continuity of activity throughout the entire record except when the baby is in quiet sleep. I would like to differ a little bit from Dr. Ellingson in reserving the term *tracé alternant* for the episodes of slow-wave activity in quiet sleep. Now, quite different from, and generally not seen in premature babies but in term infants, is that which he is referring to as suppression-burst activity. This, in its grossest form, consists of episodes of silence lasting 5 or 6 sec followed by a generalized, more or less synchronous, polymorphic bursts that may contain sharp and slow waves and fast components that you don't normally see, alternating quiescence and burst activity. Sometimes in the relatively quiescent periods there may be some low-voltage activity present so that one might ask, Is this *tracé alternant?* But the important thing, of course, is that no baby with suppression-burst activity has any degree of consciousness. It is a sign of a comatose infant, so age and state are the important factors besides the morphology of the activity.

Klass: I think that some of this confusion relates to the fact that there needs to be some objective and quantitative descriptions of these patterns to help make the distinctions. So often they're given a descriptive term in a qualitative way, but we need more accurate specifications of the amplitude relationships between the higher amplitude phases and the lower amplitude phases, the duration of each phase, the components of morphology and synchrony—all of the things that we try to do in objectively describing other patterns.

Kellaway: One last comment concerning a locus. I really hate to see shadows cast on the walls of a cave, but the system given to us from the sleep-cycle people as a way of looking at the EEG, that is, the use of respiration, eye movements, and one EEG derivation, doesn't tell us anything about the brain. The shadows on the wall are the expressions of brain activity that we see in respiration, eye movements, and so on. One needs to look at the total electrical activity, and one doesn't need very many electrodes to do this in the newborn because the patterns do not show narrow areas of differentiation. But, for example, I think that one can clearly stage an infant's sleep and can also make decisions regarding age and so on if one has the proper electrode placements and appropriate montages. I would disagree with some of the conceptional ages that Dr. Ellingson shows, including the 32-week infant, because the EEG is not consistent with that particular age. One of the questions I would like to ask him is, How was the decision made that the baby was 32 weeks old?

Ellingson: I agree with Dr. Kellaway that the term *tracé alternant* as it is usually used, and as we should continue to use it, refers only to the alternating tracing pattern of the full-term newborn during quiet sleep. What I said earlier was that, taken literally, it could mean any alternating tracing. Dr. Kellaway's question about age ranges is cogent. Whenever one sees a pattern different than that expected for a given conceptional age, the first thing to do is question whether there is a mistake in the estimated age. The baby might be, for example, 4 weeks younger.

Question: Isn't it an oversimplified mistake that prematures beneath 33 weeks CA show no changes in the EEG pattern related to this status of waking and sleep? Haven't Parmalee and his group clearly shown interaction between the EEG patterns and states of consciousness below CA 33 weeks as well as above it? Isn't it judicious use of this interaction that enables some electroencephalographers to give gestational age of the subject accurately to within 2 weeks, i.e., to differentiate from EEG a 24-week from a 26-week gestation?

Ellingson: If one obtains extensive recordings in addition to the EEG, including polygraphic variables and a full wakefulness-sleep cycle, then one can often come within 2 weeks, plus or minus, of the conceptional age of the baby. With regard to wakefulness-sleep cycle changes in the EEG under 33 weeks CA, I pointed out that there are some correlative changes in some babies, mostly consisting of simple amplitude shifts, with higher amplitudes and slower waves occurring when the baby is quiet. This is a very controversial area, and some even maintain that there is no such thing as a wakefulness-sleep cycle analogous to that which occurs at birth and beyond.

Question: Dr. Ellingson, are there differences in the EEGs of newborns presumably at normal gestation, 40+ weeks, between those born to anesthetized mothers and those born to nonanesthetized mothers, and also what about the effects of cesarean section?

Ellingson: In recording an EEG a day or two after birth, I have not been impressed with EEG changes associated with maternal anesthesia or analgesia or with cesarean section, assuming an otherwise normal baby. Few workers have done recordings soon enough after birth to be able to examine these questions. Rosen has shown prompt EEG pattern changes in fetuses *in utero* upon administration of anesthesia to the mother, but these effects are not long lasting.

Klass: There have been reports of withdrawal seizures in infants born to mothers who were addicted to narcotics. Have you had an opportunity to record interictally or ictally from such infants?

Ellingson: One or two cases. Some such babies can be very irritable. Some show withdrawal syndromes. Other than the withdrawal convulsions themselves, and I've only seen a couple of cases, I have not seen anything very striking.

Question: How useful are visual and auditory evoked responses in the newborn?

Ellingson: At least as useful as they are in older individuals.

Question: Dr. Kellaway, how do you read the pattern of intermittent posterior runs of bilaterally symmetric monorhythmic theta in an otherwise normal record of a 35-year-old female said to have epileptic seizures, the last one 3 years ago, and now on phenytoin (Dilantin®) and phenobarbital? What can you say generally about posterior rhythmic slow activities in adults?

Kellaway: First of all, the question of posterior slow activity in adults, rhythmic in character, has been studied by several different groups, and there does not seem to be any specificity, that is; rhythmic low-voltage four to five per sec activity occurring as a subharmonic of the alpha and interrupting the alpha has been seen in patients with diverse symptoms such as peptic ulcer (in which Petersén found a higher percentage of this than anything else) and vertebral-basilar insufficiency. The presence of any kind of slow activity of a rhythmic sort in an EEG of a patient suspected of having seizures, I think, does not make any kind of a differential factor to help the diagnosis, and one would then have to seek out a means to prove the existence of epileptic activity in the EEG. If the patient was having seizures, sleep deprivation, 24-hr recording, many different ways of demonstrating, although a little bit more arduous, are certainly more reliable than trying to make any diagnostic significance out of a pattern like this in relation to epilepsy.

Klass: There are two questions that relate to some frequencies you referred to—one regarding rhythms below 8 Hz and the other one specified as 3½ Hz "alpha" waves in infants. They're wondering, since alpha is a frequency between 8 to 13 Hz, "How do you know that these are really alpha waves, other than by their sinusoidal appearance?"

Kellaway: The sinusoidal appearance doesn't help me at all. The point I was trying to make is that at the age of 3 to 4 months occipital rhythmic activity of a sustained type first appears that is reactive to eye opening or is increased by forcing the baby to keep his eyes closed. If one follows that baby consistently from month to month, as we did years ago, one sees that that same rhythm (I do not mean the same waves, I have no guarantee of this) seems to just increase in frequency and become more rhythmic, more consistently reactive to eye opening, and we say that this is the precursor of the occipital alpha rhythm.

Question: Do you consider the number of slow fused transients in children in considering whether it's normal or abnormal, i.e., the percent time and/or the number of transients in a row?

Kellaway: Well obviously, if it occupied 100% of the time, one would have to assume that it was an abnormal rhythm. I was trying to make clear the differentiation between random and rhythmic occipital slow activity, because if you have activity as slow as 0.5 cycles/sec occurring as a random occipital fused wave, it may have no significance, but put that in a rhythmic sequence and you move out of the normal range, assuming you know a lot of factors about the patient's state and so on.

Question: If a nonspecific response, that is, diffuse or symmetric bisynchronous delta and theta that you would consider normal during hyperventilation is elicited, at what point in time posthyperventilation do you consider its persistence abnormal—1,2,3 min—and is there a difference between children, adults, and adolescents?

Kellaway: I think one can say that the normal evolution is for the high-voltage rhythmic slow activity to gradually diminish with time after the first postoverventilation period of 60 sec. But persisting slow activity may go on in the record beyond this time, and we have no way, without measuring the CO_2 in the blood, of knowing whether or not one has reached an equilibrium state, so there is no way in which one can precisely use this information. However, in practice, I think a prolonged response to overventilation is often a sign of a breakdown of the autoregulatory mechanisms in the brain; we see it in postinjuries, postencephalitis, many different things, and so if I see it I'm concerned that this is a sign of abnormality. But I must say that I have rarely seen a prolonged overventilation response without the presence of something else.

Saunders: In children, the most common cause of a prolonged overbreathing response is that the child continues overbreathing. It's not always easy to stop this. In adults, this is a very different matter. I expect it to return in about 30 sec or a minute maybe. If it persists longer than that, it may reflect some vasomotor instability. You seem to see these prolonged responses more commonly in people with headaches. I don't think there is any specific neurological or neuronal fault.

Klass: Dr. Daly, do you have another comment?

Daly: I was going to say the same thing; but, while I've got the chance, I'll say something else. One must also think about whether the patient has been fasting when he hyperventilates. If the blood sugar gets down to around 60 mg/dl or lower, slowing will persist a little longer. If you then give i.v. glucose, the EEG will very quickly return to normal.[5]

Question: Dr. Maulsby, where is your work on the normative data for the NASA study published?

Maulsby: It is an unpublished report submitted to NASA entitled *The Normative Electroencephalographic Data Reference Library Final Report,* prepared under contract no. NAS9–1200 by Baylor University College of Medicine and the Methodist Hospital, Houston, Texas.

Question: Dr. Kellaway, how much does the matter of asymmetry that's persistent influence you in judging it normal or abnormal?

Kellaway: I think one has to recognize that these waves are not always bilaterally symmetrical. They often are higher in voltage and are more constant on the right side, and unless this was a gross asymmetry or only occurred on one side, we would consider them normal. One has to realize that just because one does see slow waves in normal individuals, abnormal conditions make similar diffuse waves in a patient who doesn't normally have them, and that is why we in our laboratory never use the term "normal electroencephalogram." We always say it is within the range of normal variation, because actually it may be an abnormal EEG for that particular patient.

Question: Dr. Kellaway, can you describe what the significance is of the Kellaway frontal modification of the infant electrode placement?

Kellaway: It grew out of our interest in children, particularly babies. Since 1948 we've done 1,000 normal infants using the simplest montages possible and we've stuck to this intermediate frontal placement because there was less contamination from eye movements. If I go on further, we will get into a discussion about what I believe is the minimum number of electrodes in order to characterize the EEG in all the patients, and I don't want to get to that point.

---

[5] See also Chapter 9 and discussion of Chapters 8 to 14.

Klass: Dr. Goldensohn, did you have a comment?

Goldensohn: I don't think that the relationship between distance and sets of electrodes has anything per se to do with voltage.

Klass: Perhaps you'd like to go on and explain that further.

Goldensohn: What I want to say is simply that it's hard to get a good reference, that most references do take part in the events going on beneath the stigmatic electrodes, and that the only reason that a drop in voltage occurs is because of in-phase cancellation of potentials under both electrodes that are happening with similar magnitude and phase.

Saunders: It's a very complex problem. I've simultaneously recorded from the same areas of the head and used four different montages. You can see very marked differences in the patterns coming from the same electrodes. Obviously, if you have two electrodes far apart, in effect you use one as your referential electrode and the other as the active electrode. One doesn't know which is which. Whereas, when you bring them closer and closer together, then, in effect, you may or may not have mathematical cancellation of the signal; because if it's a montage with electrodes very close together, you can pick up very localized changes which you missed, because of the size of the electrical field. If you have a discharge of 2 cm in diameter, it doesn't really matter where the other electrode is. It could be on the ear, or some other place, and it makes no difference; but if you have a big field over the head, then it does make a difference.

Daly: Let me point out that one of the bitter battles in the field of EEG was over 14 and 6/s positive transients. Some people were using closely spaced electrodes thus virtually sitting on the top of the mesa-like generator. Other people were using widely spaced electrodes, so that one of them was off the generator. If everybody had realized that, many tempers would have been spared.

Klass: There is a question about the significance of the frontal bilateral sharp synchronous activity in light sleep without concomitant central parietal vertex activity, that is, the frontal sharp transients.

Kellaway: The only pattern I know of that is like this is the so-called FST or frontal sharp wave transients seen in the newborn. Is that what the question is about? Frontal sharp wave transients are of brain origin and haven't any remote resemblance to vertex transients. The so-called FSTs, by the way, are extremely useful in determining the age of an infant, seeing as how they have a rather specific ontogenesis. They appear around the gestational age of 35 weeks, and they last until about the end of the first

4 to 6 weeks postterm. These are often mistaken for eye movements, and recently I heard somebody giving a discussion of this as a sign of rapid eye movement. They don't occur in rapid eye movement sleep; they occur in transitional sleep and are not at all associated with eye movements.

Low: I agree with that entirely. We have seen them appear very prominently in early stages of sleep in newborn infants. FSTs, we find, often are the earliest manifestations of drowsiness in infants.

One technical point is worth emphasizing. I would estimate that about 20 to 30% of EEGs we do on very young babies will show sleep activity while the baby's eyes are wide open. Rather than relying on the technician's written comments on the record, the best our technicians can do to help you decide what's going on is to put an EMG lead on the chin and EOG leads for eye movement. You will get very good clues from eye movements and EMG amplitude about whether the child has gone to sleep.

Saunders: Another thing is that children go to sleep very suddenly. I first noticed that with my own children. One actually went to sleep in the middle of a sentence. Of course, this gives a paroxysmal appearance to the tracing. In a very, very brief period of time they just drop off to sleep.

Klass: Does anyone have any other comments?

Bickford: I would like to raise a couple of points. There's one artifact that doesn't come into mention any more which I think is one of the commonest ones that occurs, and it's also not even mentioned in a recent textbook. Yet I see it all the time in my own lab. I don't make any vast apology for that; I suspect it occurs in all your labs. I think it's one of the commonest and probably one of the most important ones, as a matter of fact. It's the ground lead recording, and it's part of the problem of increased electrode resistance and can be extremely misleading to people if they don't know about it. I'm sure members of this panel know about it, but it hasn't been mentioned. Anyway, the concept perhaps is not known to the majority of people, and it's this—that amplifiers really have three inputs to them, not only two as we have been hearing about. They have a ground, and the ground you can forget most of the time, but you can't forget it if the amplifier switches over to a ground lead recording when the resistance of one of the input leads becomes high enough (in the order of 100,000 Ω on either G1 or G2). Then the amplifier starts to record between the remaining good electrode and your ground electrode if that happens to be good (otherwise you get a more complex situation). But now it's very important to know where your ground lead is located because what you get when you switch to a ground lead recording is dependent on where your ground lead is situated. Some people put it frontally near the eyes, and, therefore, when their occipital lead becomes of high resistance they will see what appears to be eye blinks coming from the occipital region. This should tell them that there's trouble with that electrode. And when you fill that O1 or O2 electrode, you'll find that the eye blink disappears because you've switched from the ground lead, which was a frontal one, to a true occipital recording. Now at my old home at the Mayo Clinic we used to put the ground lead on the mastoid, and many people probably do this, so when you get a ground lead recording under those circumstances you often see alpha rhythm appearing in unusual places like the frontal region. If the resistance of the frontal lead goes up and you switch from either G1 or G2 to ground, your alpha rhythm starts to appear and there are some other changes that can occur, such as the eye blinks themselves becoming inverted. It's a very complex story, but it surely ought to be dealt with in some detail, because if you suffer from increased resistance in your leads, as we all do, you will see ground recordings. You can't avoid them, and whether you recognize them will depend a little bit on whether you happen to have your ground lead in the frontal region or in some other region that has some particular signature, so I thought perhaps we should mention that.

Henry: It's absolutely true, and the problem is going to get worse because 20 years ago, when we had equipment which was a lot more vulnerable to bad electrodes, if one saw 60 cycle artifact, assuming you had a bad lead, then you had to do something about it. Now the lead can practically fall off the head before you get any 60 cycle, and the old tipoff is missing. The higher the amplifier impedance, and it keeps going up and up, the more permissive such equipment is, and this is probably going to be with us for some time.

Klass: Dr. Low, did you have a comment?

Low: I think Dr. Henry has covered it just about completely except that I think, as Dr. Bickford knows, this sort of problem is more obvious with some machines than others. People who have been using EEG machines with transistorized input circuits won't run into this problem and won't see a ground reference recording until the active electrode or the reference electrode resistance gets extremely high. What Dr. Henry has said works both ways. The new machines are going to make it easier for technicians to get by with a good looking recording, even though their electrode resistances are perhaps too high, but, at the same time, they're going to make it possible for us to get good EEG recordings in noisy areas even with relatively high-resistance electrodes. The cure, of course, is to know what your electrode resistances are.

Klass: There's one further extension of that, Dr. Low, in that the electrode may, in fact, be detached from the head, and, with that kind of equipment, you can get a misleading record. There are several questions directed to Dr. Henry.

Question: Why are reference runs always alternating with channels left-right, left-right?

Henry: Sheer perversity, but I prefer it that way. It does not bother me if they go the other way—right-left, right-left.

Question: Using an active reference, you noted a paradoxical disappearance of activity in some channels; if the electroencephalographer is aware of this, can't the absence of an event be a good localizing sign?

Henry: Yes, indeed it can, but you have to be a pretty fair EEGer to take advantage of the disappearance of a phenomenon to prove that the phenomenon exists. It seems just a little bit illogical. This has gone on in some laboratories for a long, long time. I submit it's an awkwardness and almost an embarrassment to have your residents come in to learn EEG and have to say to them, "Now watch, as soon as you don't see something in this part of the head, this means that it's an abnormality or it's abnormal." I'd rather take the positive approach.

Question: Under what circumstances is Cz a useful reference?

Henry: It's excellent for looking at any type of abnormality that is not too close to it. Even, believe it or not, as active as the vertex can be in sleep and loaded with spindles and other activity, it's not a bad way to look at anterior and midtemporal spike discharges because you can generally differentiate them from the ongoing vertex activity. The main thing to do is to get far enough away from the abnormality you wish to study.

Question: Why do you use a reference lead on the body?

Henry: We played around a little bit, running with what we used to call a "blue sky reference" where you dial your selector switches to a position that does *not* have an electrode on it at all, and then I suppose in some way the entire chest is part of the reference. It's a treacherous, unstable thing to work with.

Question: Why do you use a reference on the head?

Henry: All you have to do is to put a reference off the head, and you will discover you get a great big, monstrous, nasty EKG signal. People have tried to work with this in various ways. A good number of years ago, there was a system for balancing a noncephalic electrode. In fact, the old Grass Model III had a little potentiometer to balance the size of the EKG pickup from a lead on the sternum and a lead on C7, which then became your reference. It was never very popular. The critical thing is to get a reference that is not involved in what you want to look at. To look at a right frontal slow focus, very often the left occiput is useful, despite the fact that it is full of alpha activity. That doesn't bother you; you're not interested in alpha in that situation. You want to use a reference that has no slow activity in it. The ideal reference and the ideal electrode have yet to be invented.

Bickford: I was just thinking, if you disconnect the reference lead, it's an example of what I was talking about—that you're getting multiple ground lead recording, some kind of averaging, possibly, in this case, between electrodes. Since you've now provided higher resistance to all G2s, each amplifier is now switching to G1 and ground. Probably what you're getting under those circumstances is a multiple ground lead recording. When I was talking about this, I forgot to mention that if any of you are skeptical about what I'm saying about ground lead recordings, you should go home and take out electrodes, one at a time. Even when they are disconnected you will not, for most of your machines, get a lot of 60 cycle. You'll get a perfectly good looking recording from each of those channels, and it will teach you in your montage what a ground lead recording looks like, how easy it is to get it, and that this is not a fiction. It's something that is happening in your labs quite often I would guess.

Klass: Why don't you use a reference lead on the big toe?

Bickford: Of course, the idea of a reference lead's being some kind of averaging device depends on the old concept of there being some kind of averaging fluid around the brain, and this works if you could take the brain out and put it in a bath of fluid and then record some distance away. You'd get an averaging effect. In the human you don't get this by going to the big toe. You can, of course, record perfectly good alpha rhythm in a recording from the left occipital to the big toe. You'll get some EKG picked up on the way. But all you're doing, really, is just using a neck connection to the brain. You're not really averaging. The brain isn't sitting in a fluid bath. You've got multiple leads going to the brain, really from the neck. So, by getting a distance away you're not really achieving very much. In fact, you could show that you get the same recording from up above the neck as you do from the big toe, so you don't really gain much by that.

There is one other point I wanted to make. Maybe this is being a maverick, I don't know. You've been told the very best techniques to use, but there is another side to this that I don't think always get mentioned. Most of the things that we've been talking about, like extra channels, produce a more costly test. I agree that the resident would like this better because it does make EEG easier, but it makes it more costly, and I think this is a side of the question that we should bear in mind, because we're costing ourselves out of the field. The economics of medicine is extremely important, and you ought to consider how much more clinically useful information you get. We can all demonstrate cases where 16 channels did a better job than 8 channels, but the thing is, on the average, does it produce a better result in the big matrix of medical tests that we have available now? I think EEGers have got to be more cost-conscious about the advantage to be gained from some of these things now. We use 16-channel instruments, but not altogether routinely. When I have to present illustrations it will be mainly on 8-channel records, because you can see these when they're put out on slides, and 16-channel records are very difficult to see. That's another aspect.

Klass: Before we get off that, however, Dr. Saunders looks very anxious to make a comment.

Saunders: I completely agree with Dr. Henry and not with Dr. Bickford. All of my instruments, except those used for portables, are 16 channels. They aren't that much more costly. Although there is a capital outlay that's nearly twice as much and you do tend to use a little more paper, the amount of information is not just doubled, it is squared. You've already said that a physician's time is his money, and you can see things better on the 16 channel; you can pluck them out quicker than you can on an 8 channel. No way are you going to do an 8 channel if you can get a 16. No way.

Klass: There is another factor here, I think, to round out the picture. Unlike automobiles, EEG instruments are not built for obsolescence. Those made by the best manufacturers work very well for a long period of time, and if you have obtained some of these instruments, what are you going to do? Throw them in the junk pile? Not at all.

Dr. Bickford, you had another comment?

Bickford: It partially applies to Dr. Saunders. If it saves him time, I think this is a bad thing. This means, I assume, that he's sampling less timewise, and I wouldn't swap spacewise sampling for timewise sampling. If you do this you get a poor sample of the patient's EEG. We get a poor enough sample anyway because, as you well know, many paroxysmal discharges are infrequent, and if he was meaning by this that he takes a shorter record, then I would be doubly against it.

Klass: Obviously, there is some divided opinion about this topic.[6]

Kellaway: I'm in disagreement, of course, with Dr. Henry and Dr. Saunders. I am solely in favor of what Dr. Bickford has to say. I think it's very important that we realize what the job to be done is. To me 16 channels represent a kind of medical and scientific elitism that is not applicable to the problems of everyday practice where there is great need for better health care delivery. Of the vast number of patients who need EEGs, those who have discrete focal abnormalities are relatively few compared to the large number of patients who really need a kind of screening EEG. One of the big applications of electroencephalography is for the patient in the acute hospital condition, and there is really no time for this type of application in those patients. When we talk about electroencephalography, we usually talk about it from the point of view of our own country, but we are really providing the basis for the type of clinical electroencephalography to be practiced in countries like India, Russia, and China. What are those people going to try to do to deliver EEG to those huge populations? I think we've got to try to develop electroencephalography of two kinds—that which is directed toward the, you might say, overall view of what the EEG shows, and the special situation where one is required to make precise localizations and determination of foci, etc.

Maulsby: This was a comment followed by an exclamation point that reminds me I said the dipole is near the center of the lesion. I didn't really mean to say that. The dipole indicates where the electrical discharge is coming from. This may be near the center of the lesion, on the edge of it, or several centimenters away. I'm localizing electrical discharges, not lesions. The electrical phenomena often arise from the side of a lesion rather than in the center of it.

Klass: In fact, most fields that we plot on the surface are generated by many closely related dipole sources that we think of and plot as an equivalent of the total as they appear on the scalp.

---

[6] See Appendix.

DISCUSSION OF CHAPTERS 8 TO 14

Klass: One of the things that Dr. Bickford previously alluded to was the importance of giving thought to the proper use of EEG, the proper indications for doing it in the first place, with a full awareness of its consequences. I think this perhaps has not been stated explicitly in our discussions so far. It's incumbent on us, and I include all of us here, to impart our knowledge and experience to our colleagues so that they, in turn, can make an appropriate selection when they refer a patient for EEG, doing it in the best possible way, weeding out the needless indications for referral, and concentrating on areas where the EEG is most likely to be of value. I think this is a service that we can render, so that the ripples of the effects of our stone dropping in the pond here can spread more widely.

Another important aspect that Dr. Bickford touched on was the need for proper training of technicians, not only in manipulating the controls on the instrument, but also in being fully aware of the implications of the patient's behavior during the time the test is in progress and of the means for properly assessing significant clues offered by the patient's behavior in association with the EEG events. It's this conjunction with behavior that makes EEG most valuable, just as is the recording of a seizure during the time of the EEG as opposed to merely recording interictal spikes. The correlation of the clinical events during the EEG discharge is perhaps the most important evidence, in my opinion, that EEG can render in the diagnosis of epileptic seizures.

The significance of spikes has been touched on by Dr. Maulsby, and I won't dwell on that except to say that for some historical reason, it was thought originally that everything in the EEG that came to a point meant fits. Well, it just isn't so. There are differences in the implications of waveforms that can be classified as spikes and sharp waves. Perhaps there are some who would not agree with this either, and I'll have to say that this is also controversial. Until you define well enough what the phenomenon is, however, I think it's foolhardy to try to say, "Well, this is significant or this is insignificant," or, "It isn't worth localizing a spike," or "It isn't worth trying to decide whether it appears only during sleep or in wakefulness or if it's modified by attention." Only when one defines the characteristics of the activity as precisely as possible can one begin to make statements about significance. That, however, poses a problem of how far to go with the investigation, and how far to go is a difficult question certainly. There is no substitute for meticulous and careful collection of the data. I can't impress on you strongly enough that without reliable data, the whole EEG is worthless. You can't even begin to talk about interpretation until you're sure that the data have been collected accurately. Then, to interpret the findings adequately requires proper education.

Dr. Daly talked about making distinctions among attacks that may be difficult to distinguish clinically. The occasions where EEG can be most helpful are the instances where clinical diagnosis is uncertain, or where the EEG can make the distinction, or where it can turn up a previously unsuspected finding.

So then, how do you limit the referrals if you're going to include times when you don't suspect that the EEG is going to turn up something significant? This has to do with Dr. Bickford's statement about photic stimulation. However, I will use a different terminology. I prefer to use the term "photoparoxysmal" for the events that Dr. Bickford referred to as "photoconvulsive." The photoparoxysmal response is a valuable finding for several reasons, one of which is its high incidence of association with clinical seizures—in our experience approximately 86%—even if the EEG at rest and during hyperventilation is nondiagnostic. Only a small proportion of patients who exhibit the photoparoxysmal response have previously been known to have their clinical seizures precipitated by light, however. If one carries out tests of responsiveness in the ways that Dr. Bickford showed and observes the patient carefully, one can often establish significant interruptions in behavior that may be clinically important. I don't want to take up more time with this and I want to give others a chance to respond, but I felt obliged to let you know that Dr. Bickford uses provocation not only in terms of EEG activation.

Knott: I would like to point out that I think there is indeed a need to examine the cost of electroencephalography. This has concerned me for a long, long time. But I also think we must be extremely careful not to deprive the individual who really needs an extensive examination because we are merely trying to streamline the procedures. I think there are many cases where sleep is extremely important. In our practice, at least, we find many of our children who show relatively normal electrical activity in a standard electroencephalogram when awake, turning up with some very interesting focal findings in stage 1 and stage 2 sleep. There are other cases certainly where sleep becomes very confusing, and you just have to know how to handle these situations. There are many cases, especially of adults, where all your information comes out in the first minute of a 16-channel EEG. You really don't need any more. You can attenuate these records if you can provide proper patient delivery into the electroencephalographic laboratory. I think also there is a need for a very close communication between the electroencephalographers and the clinicians in the medical complex or in the medical community. In this way, you can get rid of a lot of really unneeded EEGs, and you can stir up more of those than are truly needed. I think this is essentially up to you people to maintain and to try to develop these lines of communication. There is an area here where you have to make a choice—where your EEG technologist has to make a choice—and if you're going to discourage this kind of continued excellence on the part of your EEG technologist, then you're going to get poorer EEGs all around. So I think that there has got to be a very careful weighing of all of the important problems that are presented by the particular case that is now going to be examined in the laboratory.

Low: Although I disagree with some of the emphases Dr. Bickford put on some topics, I agree completely with his point that it's important, in fact essential, at this time in history, for us to try to make EEG more relevant, more efficient, and, most importantly, more useful than it has been. I would remind you of the comments of Dr. A. B. Baker who said that as far as he could judge from his experience (and, most of you will admit, he's a man of very broad experience in the field of clinical neurology), EEG was used by neurologists primarily for two reasons: first, to corroborate the diagnosis that they already had in their minds and, second, to make money. Neither of these is a particularly good reason to use EEG. That, to me, was obviously an indictment but, on the other hand, a challenge. As EEG has been constituted in the past 40 years, it turns out not always to be terribly useful. One very important point that always comes up in what Dr. Bickford says is, "There has got to be a better way to do this," and there are better ways, clearly. He will tell you about some of them later.

But I'd like to make another comment from the perspective of someone who now lives and works professionally in a country that has what amounts to socialized medicine. Those of you who live in the United States, which does not yet have anything resembling a national-level, socialized medicine scheme, had better start thinking about the very obvious sequence of events that occur when a third party, one major monolithic third party, starts paying for services. That party will eventually and inevitably get to the point of asking what it's getting for its money. Just as an example of how this can happen and what does happen when it starts asking, there are two provinces in Canada now (British Columbia, in which I work, and Quebec) that have very specific rules about accreditation requirements for performance of electroencephalography. The accreditation requirements are spelled out in detail, not only for the professional who does the interpreting, i.e., the kind of qualifications one must have in order to receive money from the medical care schemes for doing the work, but also for the running of the laboratory. This sort of thing, I think, is inevitable, and it's best to preempt the bureaucrats if you possibly can by making EEG as good and as useful as it can be.

Question: Dr. Daly, what is the mechanism of production of, and the EEG accompaniments of, micturition syncope and cough syncope?

Daly: Tussive syncope, or syncope induced by coughing. The mechanism is analogous to the cyanotic syncope of children. In other words, repetitive coughing leads to respiratory insufficiency; the patient makes repeated Valsalva maneuvers with obstruction of venous return to the heart. Eventually syncope results from reduced cerebral blood flow. Micturition syncope results from an autonomic disturbance associated with the pressures of a full bladder and subsequent voiding. Such autonomic changes also occur in spinal man in association with bladder distension. Vagal inhibitory mechanisms lead to reduced cerebral blood flow and syncope.

There's room for improvement in ordinary laboratories by extending existing technique to yield greater understanding. For example, I don't think one should get into an "either-or" approach about waking and sleeping recordings: if you find something in a waking record, you don't learn anything by doing a sleep record. I think that's simplistic. A great deal needs to be learned about the relationship between seizures, sleep, and wakefulness. Since the day of Sir William Gowers, we have known that the time at which seizures occur in the 24-hr cycle relates to the underlying pathologic process causing the seizures. It's not a happenstance relationship. Serious gaps exist in our knowledge about the relation of circadian cycles to seizures. For example, does a basic rest-activity cycle (BRAC) operate in the wakeful state and influence seizures? The few studies that have been done on this are often inconclusive for a variety of reasons, but there could be plenty of evidence that we need to understand and know a great deal more about. We also need to know a great deal more about diurnal fluctuations in body chemistry. There is evidence[1] that indicates the biotransformation and the pharmacokinetics of drugs fluctuate markedly in a 24-hr cycle. At least some of the escapes from seizure control in some patients are related to fluctuations in blood level of the drugs. I don't think we should get too negativistic about this and feel that we only have to do the simplest and most economical thing. Technology costs more, but I don't think we should become antiintellectual about it. I think, quite to the contrary, the EEG would have a great deal of promise if we push on with the evidence we have and also if we would use much more effectively the knowledge we now have.

Question: Dr. Daly, how will you interpret several (four to five) short bursts of paroxysmal 4-, 6-Hz activity in the EEG of a 54-year-old without a history of seizures? The other parts of the record are normal.

Daly: It's a little hard to answer that because there really isn't enough information. You need to know the distribution, amplitude, and reactivity of the bursts. As you know, about 10% of normal persons have some theta activity in their record.

Question: What about the percent of abnormal EEGs in common migraine versus focal hemiplegic types?

Daly: If one sees many patients with headaches, it becomes difficult to fit all into neat diagnostic boxes. The only generalization I would make is that in patients with extracranial vascular headaches without any cerebral accompaniments—and I would mention cluster headaches specifically—the EEGs look like any other population. On the other hand, patients who have some kind of cerebral accompaniment to their headaches, that is hemisensory migraines, are more likely to have some type of abnormality in the EEG. The closer in time the recording is made to a specific headache, the more likely the EEG will show focal abnormality. I don't know that this gives us any better understanding of the genesis of such headaches.

Question: Have you or any others tried treating patients who suffer from complex migraine and who have abnormalities in the interval EEGs with anticonvulsant medications? If so, what were your results?

Daly: I know of no controlled clinical trials that can answer this. The headaches of hemisensory migraine occur infrequently. If a patient's headaches decrease from three a year to one, is this chance or a significant result? I don't know why anybody should choose to treat such migraine with anticonvulsant drugs, any more than one would treat parkinsonism with anticonvulsant drugs because some of those people have abnormal EEGs.

Question: How would you interpret an EEG of a girl with migraine that contained paroxysmal delta activity?

Daly: One can't interpret an EEG in abstract. What is the type of migraine? What is the distribution, reactivity, and state-relation of the delta? In the light of some of the clinical data, it helps if one knows about family history and the time interval between headaches and EEG. Even knowing this, I think all one can say is what I've said before: there are some changes in the interval recording of this patient who has an unusual form of migraine, and I don't know what they signify.

Question: What is the pathophysiology of absence attacks, Dr. Daly, and what is the pathophysiology of migraine?

Daly: Obviously, nobody knows what the pathophysiology of migraine is. The pathophysiology of absence is only slightly less obscure.

Question: Do you have any notions about why complex partial seizures, which are a common type of seizure, rarely result in status?

Daly: Would someone like to ask a question that I could answer?

Question: Dr. Goldensohn, can you define what is mostly responsible for the mental alteration of Dr. Daly's cases, the spike or the wave, and, if both, which is more important?

Goldensohn: There is some information on this. The information is to the extent that the wave of the spike and wave does have to do with inhibition. Many years ago, Dr. Fischgold[2] did some of the studies that Dr. Bickford was suggesting we all do for reaction times and found this to be clinically so. The second thing is that I do not fully agree with Dr. Daly. I feel that when consciousness is lost or suppressed, it is a bilateral dysfunction that involves electrically, as well as otherwise, midline structures in the diencephalon or upper midbrain. I think bilateral discharges from these structures are responsible, in part, for the suppression of awareness.

Klass: I would like to add a couple of comments. Ordinarily, would you not agree, Dr. Goldensohn, that if there are myoclonic jerks, they're usually

---

[1] Halberg, F. (1974): Timing and toxicity: The necessity for relating treatment to bodily rhythms. In: *Chronobiological Aspects of Endocrinology,* edited by J. Aschoff, F. Ceresa, and F. Halberg, pp. 1–35. F. K. Schattaver Verlag, Stuttgart.

[2] Fischgold, H. and Mathis, P. (1959): Polygraphics des modifications de la conscience. *Electroencephalogr. Clin. Neurophysiol.,* 9:177.

associated with the spike component and that this is one definite association? The spike-and-slow-wave complexes, however, also need to be viewed as a whole. In the same patient you can see a generalized burst of 3-Hz spike-wave lasting 10 sec on one occasion associated with complete interruption of responsiveness, and a few minutes later a burst of the same type and duration occurs with partial retention of responsiveness that changes during the course of the burst. So there must be something other than either the individual spike or the individual slow wave that is changing.

Goldensohn: That's absolutely so. I was attempting to indicate that although we're looking at the cortex, the spike and wave may be epiphenomena, and one should be thinking of the diencephalon and the midbrain in terms of both the myoclonic effects and consciousness.

Klass: This is the reason, of course, for careful individual testing, because you can't determine the degree of interference with consciousness from just looking at the EEG. Numerous short spike-wave bursts may be a great handicap to a young child who is having frequent interruption of responsiveness when he or she should be learning to read and write in school, whereas longer bursts occurring infrequently—if responsiveness is not interfered with—may not have such dire clinical importance.

Bickford: May I make a quick comment on the concept, which perhaps has been around for a long time, that we're trying to popularize a little—that there's a third process between the discharge itself and the seizure, a gating process if you like, and that people with matched discharges who don't manifest any behavioral changes probably have some sort of conceptual neuronal gate closed, not letting the bad electricity close up the rest of the brain. The ones who have an identical discharge and a complete petit mal or other attack have the gate open.[3]

Question: Dr. Low, would you comment on the inverse relationship between exacerbations of epilepsy and exacerbations of psychosis?

Low: I know it happens and is a reliable observation. However, why this happens is really a matter for speculation, as far as I know. Some very interesting papers have been written on this problem. One could think of it as a release phenomenon. The psychiatrists used to say that if you take a neurotic's symptom, or one manifestation of his neurosis, away from him, another one will pop up. It's like pushing down on a spring that comes up somewhere else. Perhaps an overt seizure or a psychotic or schizophrenic

---
[3] See also Chapter 9.

episode in some way serves a releasing function. One or the other symptom is going to break through periodically depending on internal and external factors. When one is breaking through the other is not manifest. This implies that they're different manifestations of disturbance in a common neural system, but as yet the nature of the relationship between seizures and psychosis is poorly understood.

Question: Dr. Saunders, could you comment on the EEG in alcoholics? Have you or has anyone else noted persistent low-voltage fast activity in the records of chronic alcoholics?

Saunders: Yes, we seem to get more and more of these people coming in now that we've got a very expensive clinical control unit, a very advanced form of motel. They get fast activity, and I don't know why. They often have a tachycardia. They're tense people and do not have very high amplitude alpha activity. Whether this is an alcohol effect or not I don't know, and I don't know if anybody else here knows either. Certainly a common finding among them is a normal EEG.

Question: Dr. Bickford, how do you phrase your informed consent for pentylenetetrazol (Metrazol®) activation studies? Have there been any fatalities from such studies?

Bickford: That's a good question, and, of course, we need these for all such procedures. I think, like all other procedures, you have to state everything you conceivably think can happen. I'm not sure at this particular moment what consent form we are using because I haven't been doing this test for the last year or so myself, and Dr. Aung isn't here at the moment. I don't think the form of consent for pentylenetetrazol would be any different from any other. You'd have to mention the possible orthopedic problems and cardiovascular problems. We have had no deaths as far as I know. And, of course, you have to include the fact that many people get tense and anxious with this test and that you'd deliberately stop the test if this were so. Some people have vomiting and a variety of unpleasant vertiginous sensations.

Question: If an awake record is desired prior to a sleep record, what is the best way to obtain a sleep record in the same recording session? What is your actual procedure?

Bickford: This is a problem, of course. If a sleep recording might be appropriate (and this is the case with epileptic patients), most of our patients are told to keep off stimulants and to get tired so that they will be likely to sleep. Then the technician has the problem of keeping the patient awake.

This isn't very easy sometimes. The technician has to try to alert them. We do a number of things that perhaps relate to this, like the 100-minus-seven test. It tends to keep the patient alert while certain observations are made. If you have a delta focus, for example, you would want to know whether it disappears with alerting. Eye opening is one approach to this. You use a common sense approach to these things. The worst problem, and one which is commonly seen these days, is that of patients who are abnormally drowsy and very difficult to keep awake because of drugs.

Question: What hypnotic medications do you use to help induce sleep?

Bickford: There's a wide variety, of course. It is better, most people agree, not to use medications at all. This, however, is not always feasible. The ones that are less favorably looked on these days are barbiturates because of their tendency to induce fast activity and to produce changes in the EEG that are spike-like, leading to practical difficulties in interpreting the record. Chloral hydrate is one that many people are using. It doesn't have marked effects on the EEG, and it's probably a better choice. There are a myriad of others. They all have some minor difficulties. Chloral hydrate is probably one of the safest and best nonaddicting drugs to use.

Klass: Dr. Kellaway was one of the first to study the effects on activation of drugs used to induce sleep. Dr. Kellaway, what do you use at present?

Kellaway: We're using less and less medication as the years go by. We train our technicians that an adequate electroencephalogram, in a child anyway, is a wake and sleep record, and we get both usually without any medication. But where we feel it's absolutely necessary while the patient is still there, we give pentobarbital (Nembutal®) or secobarbital (Seconal®) in a dose which is tailored to the patient's weight. More recently, in an adult series, we've been trying flurazepam (Dalmane®) because of our broader experience with this in computer analysis, and so far it hasn't been quite as effective as the secobarbital, but here sometimes technician bias needs to be considered.

Bickford: I'd like to add something that Dr. Maulsby whispered in my ear and I think is very important. He says he uses placebo very often.

That reminds me of a study that you and I did at the Mayo Clinic many years ago in which secobarbital, placebo, and glute thimide (Doriden®) were given to alternate patients, and we measured the time of going to sleep. I don't even think that we ever published this in detail, but the important fact, as I remember, that came out is that the effects were almost equal. I think it's very important to bear that in mind.

Klass: Are there any "favorite" medications other than those that have been mentioned?

Low: One of my most "unfavorite" medications is chlorpromazine. There was a mystique that crept into the business some time ago causing some people to think phenothiazine derivatives have a special activating effect on EEG abnormalities, and some physicians like to use them routinely. We don't like such agents primarily for two reasons. First, because of the very long latency of onset, one just gives up the waking trace. By the time you start recording from the patient whom you've presedated with chlorpromazine, the EEG is full of slow activity, and you have no idea whether this slow activity is pathological in origin or induced by the drug. Second, phenothiazines diminish fast activity normally present during sleep (spindles, for example), and they also may provoke episodic activity that can look abnormal and be misinterpreted.

Klass: Occasionally we have used hydroxyzine (Vistaril®) for the hyperactive child. Do you find that useful at all, Dr. Low? You have had more experience than I in this area.

Low: Some of our people have used that, and it does work. In such cases we do go along with the referring clinician's judgment.

Ellingson: We did a study a few years ago, never published, in children comparing hydroxyzine versus chloral hydrate versus placebo. Hydroxyzine and cloral hydrate were equally effective in inducing sleep, and both were superior to the placebo.

Goldensohn: I think one thing that hasn't been mentioned yet is that we do all our sleep studies in the afternoon.

Klass: Is that on the basis of the difference in proportion of slow wave and REM sleep that has been reported for morning and afternoon?

Goldensohn: It wasn't instituted on that basis.

Question: Can spike activity associated with sleep spindles be called an epileptiform discharge or distinguished from other normal patterns?

Bickford: I didn't mean to imply that the spike discharge associated with spindles is any different from the spike occurring at any other time or at any other place. I just was pointing out the fact that the association of the two makes visual recognition somewhat more difficult. But I don't think the spikes have any different implications.

Question: What are your criteria for differentiating the spike and sharp waves associated with or resembling high-amplitude, sharp-contoured V-waves or K-complexes?

Bickford: I can't say I can tell you any exact differentiating criteria, but we are studying the capacity of people, experts in the field, to recognize spikes. As many of you know, we have put out various questionnaires giving sample spikes and we have now a spike library. There is enormous variation in what trained electroencephalographers recognize as spikes. Also, in the same rater, reliability is not very great. My own isn't very good either, I may say. Put through the same set of spikes a second time, we make, many people do, very considerable errors. That doesn't exactly answer your question, but we are trying to develop criteria, as others are, for recognizing spikes by computer. That is a very difficult area, and I can't say we have anything at the moment that's very helpful.

Question: What do you think about methohexital (Brevital®) activation, especially in temporal lobe epilepsy?

Bickford: Brevital activation we have looked at—Dr. Aung[4] has mainly done this—also in combination with pentylenetetrazol activation. It started out with a comparison study on the same patients—activate them one day by methohexital and another day by pentylenetetrazol and compare the results. I would only quote approximately. We haven't confirmed the usefulness of methohexital activation. The problem is related to the one I've mentioned before with the barbiturates; methohexital does produce a lot of spikey activity and gets you into the problem of what spikes are. In the cases that activate, and I regret I don't know the proportion of these, it depends really upon how you choose your population. There are cases that activate with methohexital, but pentylenetetrazol is about twice as effective as an activation agent. As a result of these studies, Dr. Aung started to use the two together, giving methohexital first and following it by pentylenetetrazol and thereby has reduced some of the unpleasant vertiginous effects and panic that sometimes accompany pentylenetetrazol in adults. These are markedly reduced if you use methohexital first, and yet you do not seem to lose the EEG activating effect. I should point out however, as I've tried to, that pentylenetetrazol is really a clinical EEG test. In many of the cases you want to activate with pentylenetetrazol, you indeed want to produce the seizure you're studying, so it usually isn't good enough just to produce EEG changes. This is not the case with methohexital, so in that sense they're different.

Question: Why do you think that some patients have exclusively nocturnal epilepsy? Is there some increased predisposition to abnormal discharges during sleep in these patients, and would you put more importance on the sleep record in these patients or not?

Bickford: Yes, this has been reviewed by Dr. Daly.[5] In spite of what you'd expect, the patients who have seizures at night do not necessarily activate better than those who do not. Nevertheless, it's a reasonable thing to do, an indicated thing to do—a sleep recording on patients who are having nocturnal seizures. It seems obvious.

Kellaway: I think that the problem of recording sleep really has to do with the nature of the sleep attained. In continuous recording studies that are going on in our laboratory and elsewhere, I think the evidence is clear that abnormal discharges, both generalized and focal, go through periods of increased activity during episodes of sleep. A good example of this, of course, is a classic 3/per sec spike-and-wave activity which, as Fato et al.[6] have shown and we have shown in our laboratory, is increased in stages 2 and 3 sleep, markedly depressed during REM sleep, and most markedly depressed during the rapid eye movement periods of REM sleep. It may in some patients in a 48-hr recording appear only during sleep, whether this be a nap period or during nocturnal sleep, and the first period of stage 2 or 3 sleep of the night appears to be the most active period for this kind of activity. In other words, the density of the discharge goes up by a factor, in some patients, of as much as 30. Some patients we studied had no seizure discharges at all throughout the day; other patients waxed and waned in the amount of seizure activity they showed throughout the day and throughout the night. Another group of patients had their seizure discharges exacerbated after they first aroused in the morning. We've been doing this in relationship to continuous monitoring of drug levels, so that hasn't been a factor to suggest that if the last dose were given in the evening, then 12 or 10 hr later the patient may have more seizure activity. This is true both for focal abnormalities, whether focal central or temporal discharges, and for generalized 3/sec spike and wave.

Klass: I think that there is general agreement in the literature that the number of generalized spike-wave discharges increases with progressively

---

[4] Aung, M. H. (1974): Electroencephalographic activation with methohexital in an epileptic population. *Dis. Nerv. Syst.*, 35:246–248.

[5] See Chapter 8.

[6] Fato, S., Dreifuss, F. E., and Penry, J. K. (1973): The effect of sleep on spike-waves discharges in absence seizures. *Neurology*, 23:1335–1345.

deeper stages of NREM sleep and then decreases during REM sleep. Also, the configuration and duration of the discharges change. Compared with their appearance in wakefulness, the paroxysms become shorter and contain more multispikes. I've had the same experience with temporal lobe discharges as Dr. Kellaway has, although in the literature I think there is more variance reported with respect to an increase or decrease of focal temporal discharges during REM sleep.

Bickford: In regard to the question of temporal lobe seizures in depth electrode studies, you sometimes see the discharge remaining the same in depth but spreading out to the surface as sleep occurs and then the reverse occurring as the waking state supervenes. This is one of the reasons for saying that sleep opens up synapses. Slow-wave sleep seems to allow spread of a discharge from the depth to occur.

Klass: Would you like to comment on the findings of Dr. Brazier about coherence between areas during sleep?

Bickford: Coherence is a mathematical measure dependent on frequency. The relatedness can be expressed from 0 to 1, 1 being an absolute coherence. Brazier feels that in epilepsy you need a measure not only of which discharge occurs first, but also of the general relatedness of one area to another, and so the coherence measures seem to be appropriate. Dr. Brazier feels that she can map the spread of the discharge using these techniques. The kinds of techniques that Brazier has used add quantitation to these kinds of estimates.

Question: If 3 min of hyperventilation is effective, wouldn't 4 or 5 min be better?

Bickford: Yes, there are occasions where you want to extend the hyperventilation period. Just bear in mind that you then get into a different set of criteria. If you indeed know your criteria for 5 min of hyperventilation on the normal subjects, feel free to do this, but remember, of course, that the extent of slow-wave buildup will be greater. Also, you run into the problem we mentioned already, that patients may become confused and go on hyperventilating even longer. You might get a spike discharge or even a seizure under the conditions of going to 5 min that you might not get in 3. I think there's general agreement that 3 is a sort of best average, but it shouldn't necessarily be absolute. Does anyone else have thoughts on that?

Saunders: If you don't get anything in 2 or 3 min, in 99% of cases, you won't get anything with a longer time.

Low: I more or less agree with Dr. Saunders on that. It's usually more useful not to extend a single period of hyperventilation, but to repeat the 3-min period 5 to 20 min after the first one. If you haven't produced some abnormality in a 6-year-old child, for example, whom you suspect should have 3/sec spike-and-wave bursts during hyperventilation, you will find that often you can provoke them with a second period of hyperventilation.

Question: How important is the persistence of the photoconvulsive response after the intermittent photic stimulation has been discontinued?

Bickford: This is the most important part of the criteria that differentiates it from the photomyoclonic response. Since the photomyoclonus is essentially a reflex, it ends with the last flash, and an important differential but not an absolute one for the photoparoxysmal response is that it continues after the end of photic stimulation.

Klass: But the point I think was in the photoparoxysmal. Is there a difference in the significance of those that do self-perpetuate and those that don't?

Bickford: Yes, I think the longer they last the more significant they are. Whether they are associated with detectable signs of a clinical seizure, however, also would be important.

Klass: In 1964, I carried out a study of photoparoxysmal responses, and found that indeed there was an increased significance for diagnosis of seizures if the response showed self-perpetuation.[7,8] I think that Drs. Reilly and Peters have more recently published evidence[9] for this conclusion.

Question: Dr. Bickford, regarding stimulation, would you comment on self-stimulation in epilepsy? The second part of the question is, Why do they do it?

Bickford: There are various means of self-stimulation. Waving the hand in front of the eyes, looking at the sun, and separating the fingers to increase the frequency of stimulation is a fairly common way of doing this. Some highly intelligent patients will have this phenomenon, but it's much more common, I think, in retarded children. Some pattern-sensitive patients are able to induce attacks by staring at the pattern on their skin. Self-induction

---

[7] Klass, D. W. (1964): Age variations of syndromes associated with visually provoked discharges. *Electroencephalogr. Clin. Neurophysiol.,* 17:715.

[8] Klass, D. W., and Fischer-Williams, M. (1976): Sensory stimulation, sleep, and sleep deprivation. In: *Handbook of Electroencephalography and Clinical Neurophysiology,* Vol. 3D, Section I, edited by A. Remond, pp. 5–73. Elsevier, Amsterdam.

[9] Reilly, E. L., and Peters, J. F. (1973): Relationship of some varieties of electroencephalographic photosensitivity to clinical convulsive disorders. *Neurology,* 23:1050–1057.

to seizures is used sometimes as a manipulative weapon. The pathophysiology, of course, is not really known, but the Olds model of the self-stimulating rat is a rather interesting and relevant one. With intracerebral electrodes in certain locations, the rat will self-stimulate sometimes to death, actual death. This seems to be a limbic system kind of mechanism. It's questionable I think in what detail this can be applied to self-stimulating epileptics. They usually have spike-wave disorders and not anything specifically limbic. It's rather uncommon to find any mechanisms for self-stimulation among temporal lobe patients.

Klass: Very often the motivation is entirely unconscious.

Question: The AMA committee on medical aspects of driving recommends no night driving of autos by persons with photosensitive epilepsy. Is this logical or supported by convincing data?

Bickford: It seems very logical and sensible to me. I didn't realize this was the case, but clearly, the changes in light intensity from headlights and various other lights encountered in night driving could very well set off a photoepileptic. I think it is a hazard that's real. Probably they shouldn't be driving anyway in view of the spike-wave discharge, quite apart from the photic epilepsy, if these are expressed as seizures.

Question: Would you discuss another activation technique—alcohol activation of the EEG in patients who are reported to have an excessive, often violent response to "reasonably small" amounts of alcohol? What changes can occur, and is there any relevance to the claimed clinical manifestations?

Bickford: I think Rodin and others looked into alcohol activation. It may activate some patients. I'm not sure what the yield is. I don't think the yield is very great.

Saunders: We've been doing this for about 15 to 20 years and had one doubtful case of provoking abnormalities. Just forget about doing alcohol activation.

Bickford: It might be of some negative significance, I suppose, the absence of activation with alcohol.

Saunders: If you want an involved discussion about this, you could get in the question of whether this is an hydration effect, but I won't go into this any further.

Question: Drs. Goldensohn and Low, please comment on nasopharyngeal leads.[10] Your opinions in this matter are quite different.

Goldensohn: I once knew a senator who said, "Never accuse me of the great guilt of being consistent." On this point, I am very consistent. Regarding the possibility of faulty placement, anybody can tell whether the electrodes are sticking out of the nose unequally, if they are of the same length when you get them from the manufacturer. The same thing is true if you look at your electrodes to see if the bends are the same. The other thing is when you take the right electrode, turn it clockwise, and turn the left one counterclockwise they're not going to cross each other; it's physically impossible in back of the nasopharynx. It takes exactly 5 min to teach an intelligent resident these things so that he doesn't do it wrong and you can have confidence in your electrodes. You should have a skull in your office to be able to practice where you put them. But Dr. Low is right when he said that if you can't count on them getting in the right place, you shouldn't do it, absolutely. Now the question goes beyond that, and, What is the value? Well, we find the nasopharyngeals frequently give information from an area where the surface electrodes can't. The actual distance through the nasopharynx and the bone to the mesial temporal lobe is about 2 cm. As with additional scalp leads, you're not getting closer to the brain, but you're in a different area. Especially with sleep we find discharges limited to the nasopharyngeals. However, when you see a spike in the nasopharyngeal, watch out that it's not originating somewhere else and the nasopharyngeal is only acting as a very fine reference lead. Dr. Low and I still have this difference of opinion, but I think very highly of nasopharyngeal leads. On the other hand, I agree with Dr. Low about the value of sleep recording. I think these two things together have practically eliminated the use of sphenoidal leads in our laboratory.

Low: I think the obvious point here is that these things are useful in direct proportion to the amount of care that you're willing to put into their use, and your care will often be repaid. We don't always have as intelligent residents as they may have at Columbia Presbyterian Hospital, and we have other problems besides the resident supply. I'll only say in defense of my initial argument, which I still maintain, that I talked to a friend and confidant in Seattle[11] and said, "You know, Dr. Chatrian, Dr. Goldensohn really took me to task for saying that nasopharyngeal electrodes were easy to use but rarely useful." He replied, "Well, I would take you to task, too, for saying that." I was a little downcast because I think a

---

[10] See also Chapter 9.

[11] G. Chatrian, *personal communication,* 1972.

great deal of Dr. Chatrian's opinion, and I said, "Well, I'm sorry. Did I say the wrong thing?" He said, "Yes, you should have said that they're *very* rarely useful." They can be helpful, but they have to be used carefully, and I think that statistically the application may not be worth the amount of time that you invest.

Goldensohn: That's a very good point, because I have a great admiration for Dr. Chatrian. But the fact is that you won't find a high incidence of abnormality with nasopharyngeal electrodes when you don't have a high suspicion of seizures, and this is looked on as a last resort to find them. You're not going to find problems in people who don't have them. The selection of case material is important. If you think you're dealing with a seizure disorder of the medial temporal area, then the results are quite good.

Bickford: Can I get a word in edgewise very quickly? One of the difficulties that I have encountered with nasopharyngeal leads is the muscle twitch that occurs in the pharyngeal muscles. It looks like a spike. I think bilateral leads help you here, and sleep probably helps because the nasopharyngeal muscles are less active, but these and other artifacts are very nasty problems. They are the reasons that I sometimes dislike nasopharyngeal leads.

Goldensohn: We've found some extra diagnostic use in these things that have bothered Dr. Bickford. We have made the diagnosis of palatal myoclonus when the muscle artifact is typical. In other words, you have to know how to identify the artifacts, which are considerable.

Klass: Dr. Bickford, would you comment on a question about the requirement for bilateral depth electrode implantations and a question about whether depth leads can instigate epileptogenic spikes?

Bickford: Yes. We may want to settle the question with bilateral implantation if we don't have any definitive information about whether the seizures are arising from the left or right side. In other cases we may know already that the seizures are arising from one side only, but the precise origin is uncertain. In our experience of putting in electrodes freehand and, more recently, of putting them in stereotactically, it's better to my mind to go for a way that sows them evenly over the suspected area than to go for particular targets. There's a good research reason perhaps for concentrating on a particular target, but we think the thing to do is to sow the electrodes systematically, in 1-cm or 2-cm intervals if you can, both over the affected area and outside it because you want to know how far the epileptic process extends. That information is important to help design the limits of your excision. These are cases that are usually oriented in the direction of a cortical excision.

Klass: I think there is evidence by now that leads implanted purposely beyond the epileptogenic area don't set up new and permanent epileptogenic discharges ordinarily.

Question: Dr. Maulsby, do "small sharp spikes" occur in sleep? Are they focal by the usual criteria or bilaterally symmetrical without being focal?

Maulsby: In my experience, they occur best during drowsiness and light sleep. They occur unilaterally, and the field is usually very broad across the lateral part of the head.

Klass: Yes. They don't occur in scalp recording during wakefulness. Although each spike appears to be predominantly unilateral, most usually the spikes occur on both sides at different times in the recording of one patient.[12]

Question: Dr. Maulsby, what is the objection to calling these patterns abnormal? Abnormality per se is not, by any means, implied pathology. For example, the presence of supernumery digits, nipples, sesamoid bones, and the like, as well as many cases of dextrocardia, abberent vessels, are all anatomically abnormal but not pathological. Is it not also possible to have electrocerebral abnormalities that are nothing but coincident to a disease?

Maulsby: That's a good question. It's a matter of semantics really. A person with very high IQ is abnormal, but not necessarily pathological. I think there's a stigma attached, particularly when you're talking about the brain, to say something is abnormal about a person's brain. I think it's just best to avoid that term in any way you can because when you tell a person or a patient that his brain is abnormal, you change his whole image of himself. It's important to use the term "abnormality" conservatively in the case of EEG or anything to do with the brain.

Daly: Can I add something to that? I think that one of the problems is we have a sort of a Ford Motor Company concept of the brain; we think we're turned out on a production line and everyone ought to look like the other. Only a minority of people have the classic circle of Willis, so is it abnormal to have the normal complement of vessels? I really think that we ought to recognize there are a lot of variations in the EEG from person

---

[12] See references, Chapter 14.

to person and not demand that they all fit into some Procrustean bed of normality. I think this point hasn't been emphasized enough.

Maulsby: Maybe we should call them variants rather than abnormalities.

Question: Dr. Maulsby, you have written about the ocular compression test in children. What is your current opinion about its usefulness?

Maulsby: I don't employ it anymore because of possible complications, and I think it is not very useful diagnostically.

Question: How many of you think that 14 and 6 Hz-positive spike activity is abnormal?

Henry: Before I vote, I have to give a reason why.

Klass: Afterward. Dr. Henry is the only one of 11 who thinks they are abnormal. Now your comment, Dr. Henry.

Henry: I have been troubled by the increasing number of people we see with bad encephalopathies who have these things in their EEGs. They are occasionally seen, awake or asleep, in adults with liver disease and uremia.

Saunders: I would agree with Dr. Henry that there are such conditions when you see a 14 and 6 burst in an otherwise abnormal record.

Question: How many think that the 14 and 6 phenomenon is indicative of epilepsy?

Klass: No one here thinks so.

Question: Where can one find the International classification of seizures?

Daly: It's in *Epilepsia,* 11:102–113 and 114–119, 1970.

Question: Dr. Goldensohn, what are the implications of a normal EEG in a patient with a severe hemiplegia from a vascular accident?

Goldensohn: A very large percentage of vascular accidents cause abnormal EEGs, but there is one group that usually doesn't—lacunar lesions that occur in the depth of the brain and usually in patients with hypertension. Clinically they are usually characterized by pure motor loss.

Question: What's the current status of the kappa rhythm?

Bickford: It depends what you read. Perhaps some people here don't know about the kappa rhythm. This is an alpha-like rhythm that appears in leads near the outer canthus of the eye and is claimed by Kennedy[13] to be associated with mental calculation. In cases that we looked at, although we never said that this was always the case, oscillatory movements of the eye seemed to generate this. Such movements are common, of course, with calculations as a mannerism, and if you hold the eyelids, at least in subjects in our experience, the kappa rhythms disappear, so we regard it as an artifact caused by tremor of the eye triggered by calculations. There is some evidence in the literature which contradicts this, however, mainly from Armington.[14,15]

Question: Dr. Goldensohn, if you maintain that the delta activity from intracranial lesions emanates from the white matter, why so little change in the EEG with cerebral multiple sclerosis?

Goldensohn: I really don't know, but maybe it's not as destructive and doesn't cause as much edema. Slow-wave foci can occur with multiple sclerosis, but I really have no good explanation except for the size of the lesion and the acuteness. There is a tremendous amount of polymorphic delta activity in cases of Schilder's disease where there's considerable demyelination of the centrum ovale.

Klass: Dr. Goldensohn once asked me to lecture about the EEG and cerebral lesions at a course he organized for the American Academy of Neurology, and he has chided me ever since about a phrase that I used to incorporate all the factors that would influence the amount of EEG abnormality produced by a lesion—spatial-temporal biodynamics. The location of the lesion with respect to the external surface, the size of the lesion, the rapidity with which the lesion develops, and the time that you see the patient in the course of the development of the lesion (early or late), as well as the individual response to the lesion and its proximity to the midline ventricular axis, all are factors that need to be considered in any one case.

Daly: To get things straight now, Dr. Goldensohn, are you saying that the polymorphic delta arises in the white matter?

Goldensohn: No. I was talking about some possible mechanisms for generating this activity. One suggestion was that lesions of the white matter produce denervation of the gray matter above, and the gray matter is still functioning to create these slow synaptic potentials.

---

[13] Kennedy, J. L., Gottsdanker, R. M., Armington, J. C., and Gray, F. E. (1948): A new electroencephalogram associated with thinking. *Science,* 108:527–529.

[14] Armington, J. C., and Chapman, M. (1959): Temporal potentials and eye movements. *Electroencephalogr. Clin. Neurophysiol.,* 11:346–348.

[15] Chapman, R. M., Armington, J. C., and Bragdon, H. R. (1962): A quantitative survey of kappa and alpha EEG activity. *Electroencephalogr. Clin. Neurophysiol.,* 14:858–868.

Daly: Dr. Saunders and I just thought that some people might be confused by the way it was phrased.

Saunders: Again, in multiple sclerosis you can get slow activity in the acute phase, of course. In fact, you can get focal abnormalities.

Klass: Dr. Bickford has published on that subject.[16]

Saunders: Yes, but the point is that it's not the white matter that produces the EEG abnormality.

Klass: Here's a question for both Dr. Goldensohn and Dr. Daly. Does a slow-wave focus from a superficial tumor have a different response to sleep than the delta from a deeper lesion, and what does sleep do to polymorphic delta activity?

Goldensohn: I think that I would rather let Dr. Daly answer that.

Daly: It was originally reported that with lesions deep in the white matter, polymorphic delta activity disappeared during slow-wave (NREM) sleep. In fact, this is not a reliable differentiation. With tumors of the thalamus, polymorphic delta activity persists during slow-wave sleep. I don't know how to differentiate the superficial from the deep.

DISCUSSION OF CHAPTERS 15 TO 17

Question: Dr. Goldensohn, In your acute experiments, was the variability of the electrical responses relative to the distance from electrode 5 due only to current travel and neuronal interactions, or was it, at least in part, due to diffusion of the "spikeogenic" substance?

Goldensohn: We were very careful to observe and to make sure that there was no more diffusion than would occur for nontechnical reasons, and we are using carbon 14 in our penicillin to delineate the amount of diffusion. I think there's no question that these changes are exclusively neuronal synaptic and not electrical field effects.

Question: Does the scalp recording always reflect the *polarity* of underlying cortical surface events? There must be some kind of average, for instance in the "pussycat" cortex, with the penicillin-induced negative spike at electrode 5 with positive spikes at neighboring electrodes. What would a single scalp electrode over that area show? Which of the two polarities?

Goldensohn: That's a very good question. The discharge is seen on the scalp when all the activity that's in-phase is happening in a wide area.

Question: Could you briefly go over again what PDS is?

Goldensohn: PDS, paroxysmal depolarization shift, is observed only with intracellular electrode recording. It is a shift in the membrane potential toward depolarization in the amount of perhaps one-third or one-half of the total potential difference across the membrane, which is usually set about 60 or 70 mV outside positive so that it drops to say 30 or 40 mV outside positive. The depolarization reaching about 30% is sufficient to impair the function of the cell. So the cell is no longer able to generate action potentials, because the membrane cannot regenerate in terms of moving sodium and potassium. Therefore, a plateau of depolarization takes place until the membrane is able to start to reconstitute itself and become repolarized. This takes about 40 to 60 msec. It may be that during the time of this inactivation of the soma the axon hillock is firing rapidly using the depolarization in the cell as the source, but we don't have any data on that.

Question: What *direct* evidence is there that the surface-negative wave in the EEG is, indeed, the sum of massed PSPs rather than massed action potentials? For example, you show unidirectional surface changes whether your sample unit shows after-potentials which hyperpolarize or depolarize the membrane, and you emphasized to the group that you sampled only one unit while the surface wave is a population phenomenon.

Goldensohn: This matter was settled many years ago. Back in the late 1930s Bonnet and Bremer[1] showed that potentials from the surface of the spinal cord were postsynaptic in origin. Bremer formulated that cortical potentials were graded postsynaptic responses and not a conglomeration of action potentials.[2] One of the simplest ways of demonstrating this is simply to stretch out an EEG wave on the oscilloscope with a very fast sweep. You find that it doesn't break up into little points to indicate individual elements. The other more sophisticated reason why this is impossible is

---

[16] Jasper, H., Bickford, R. G., and Magnus, O. (1950): The EEG in multiple sclerosis. *Res. Publ. Assoc. Res. Nerv. Ment. Dis.*, 28:421–427.

[1] Bonnet, V. and Bremer, F. (1938): Relation des potentiels reactionnels spinaux avec les processus d'inhibition et de sommation centrale. *C.R. Soc. Biol.*, 127:812–817.

[2] Bremer, F. (1949): Considerations sur l'Origine et la nature des ondes cerebrales. *Electroencephalogr. Clin. Neurophysiol.*, 1:177–193.

that, when a cell body discharges completely in an action potential, the whole cell discharges all at once and the current flow is directed mainly across the cell membrane, not in the external fluid.

Question: Can you explain—and this is offering a hypothesis for your comments—surface positive spikes at a distance from the penicillin focus on the basis of the anatomy of synapses mediating IPSPs on apical dendrities, that is, are some or all inhibitory interneurons known to synapse more superficially compared to excitatory interneurons or direct axon collaterals?

Goldensohn: The evidence for the preponderance of excitatory potentials, being on the apical dendrities is very strong from electrophysiological measurements, the use of drugs, and the shape of the synaptic endings themselves. The predominant conglomeration of inhibitory synapses are deeper on the trunk and much fewer in number than the predominance of excitatory endings on the apical dendrities.

Question: You speak of the basic mechanism for the epileptic discharge as excitation, yet there are data to suggest that it is lack of inhibition that underlies the epileptic process. Will you please comment on this?

Goldensohn: I really didn't mean to differentiate between excitation and lack of inhibition. They're both going on, and I think there are some situations, as the question suggests, that lack of inhibition, especially in the chemically mediated seizure, can be the mechanism.

Question: What precisely is the role of the thalamus in the generation or perpetuation of spikes?

Goldensohn: Of course, no one knows precisely this role. In my experience seizures beginning from thalamic lesions are very uncommon. I don't think that the gray matter of the thalamus is as epileptogenic as the gray matter of the cortex. So I think the role of the thalamus is a secondary one; it's a broadcasting role rather than an initiating role.

Klass: I want to check with Dr. Bickford regarding one of his EEGs. My comment has to do with data collection and pitfalls that can creep in for the unwary. Getting back to very simple matters, regarding the receiving and transmission of four channels of the EEG with a normal record, Dr. Bickford, I would suspect that this is eye blink. Is that how you interpret it?

Bickford: Yes, I think so.

Klass: I would submit then that this must be the wrong montage, because I don't see how the amplitude of the eye blink would be less in C3 than in P3 with the ear lobe as a common reference.

Bickford: I think you're right. There's been a mistake. I hadn't noticed it. I think it should be a parasagittal bipolar.

Klass: But if someone were to take a CSA of this, for example, the results might be misleading if that person wasn't aware that the montage is incorrect.

Low: I want to bring up another matter. Since Dr. Bickford has already anticipated that what he said was going to come back to him, here it is. I would like you people to look at this. This is a telephone bill. You see the total number at the bottom is $16,186.50. This is the total bill for a telephone transmission system that we set up between Trail Regional Hospital and Vancouver General Hospital (a distance of 400 miles) in British Columbia, for approximately 6 months.

Bickford: I take it that's a digital system, isn't it? Is that using a standard telephone wire?

Low: Yes. I just want you to reflect on that number for a minute, because that represents an average of three EEGs a day for about 6 months. Divide that in your mind and decide, whether or not we're really saving money with these new techniques. That's point No. 1. The other point I'd like to make is a plug for this system that costs so much money. You'll see in some of the programs references to two commercially available analog systems. As far as I know, there are only two or three now available to purchase "off the shelf" and to use. But we have designed and built, to my knowledge, the only digital EEG transmission system that has ever been put to practical use. We've been using it virtually every working day now for something over a year. It's a 9-channel system, 8 channels of EEG plus one code channel. It has two main advantages over analog systems. First, the transmitted signal is virtually "noise" free, and, second, the signal is in an appropriate format for data processing or storage. As you have seen, digital transmission costs are very expensive at the moment, but because Canada has done extensive work in long-distance data transmission, we already have a digital "data track" network across the country and it's easy for us to access this "data track" system. We originally used the commercial data lines, but since that bill came, we switched to another system that's considerably less expensive. I think your first (United States) "data track" or dial digital network is going to go into use on the East Coast soon. So, remember, there is another system available that you don't hear about simply because we're not interested in trying to sell it yet, but it works very well.

Bickford: Could I make a quick comment? I wasn't necessarily promoting this system, mind you. I think there are economical arguments which can be made in the opposite direction, and I have not had experience with the economics of it, but the main reason I mentioned it really is to point out the very considerable difficulties it involves. Please don't think I'm promoting telephone transmission necessarily. I just want to point out that I'm glad to have these additional comments, but there are plenty of economic difficulties. Dr. Bennett has used telephone transmission in a practical way and maybe can come up with some actual figures for you.

Kellaway: Dr. Klass, could I comment? One very economical use of transmission of this type that is going to become available in the near future is the electromagnetic coupled type of transmission system that has been recently developed.[3] At the present time we're finding this tremendously useful in not having to make night calls. At the moment Dr. Frost is using it and carrying it around with a portable machine, and when technicians go to the emergency room, the ICU, or the patient's room, all they need to do is plug in the telephone and connect the telephone to the electromagnetic coupler and transmit it to me at home. I can discuss the report with the resident or whoever is doing it, and I think it's this kind of EEG that's going to be more and more important. It's relatively inexpensive and easy to use because you don't need modems at each point of transmission.

Bickford: How many channels?

Kellaway: Eight.

Question: Dr. Bickford, what do you think of the validity and use of biofeedback in the management of the severely handicapped such as quadriplegia or related disability, and maybe other aspects as well?

Bickford: I assume the question is referring to therapeutic use, probably the EMG feedback, which I think is currently of most interest in paraplegic disorders. I'm sure that this has a good effect on patients' morale. The idea, of course, is to listen to the muscles that you are trying to move, and seemingly this adds a further incentive to that of seeing some movement that you're able to make. This is used as an adjunct in the rehabilitation of patients. On the other hand, there's the technique, used by Sterman and others, of feedback of certain components of the brain rhythms, supposedly to reduce the incidence of epileptic discharges in the EEG. There are claims that this does reduce the number of paroxysmal discharges. Cruder methods, of course, with feedback of spike discharge signal have been used.

Klass: Perhaps you could tell us what you think of the results.

Bickford: I've heard Sterman[4] talk about this. I've seen graphs of seizure discharges before and after treatment, and I've seen lessening of the seizure discharges in his graphs, and that's all I can tell you. He claims that it reduces them. Of course, we all know that epileptics vary in their output of discharges over the years under constant medication. Others are more complex because the medication has been changed. I haven't been greatly impressed with the results myself, but then perhaps I'm a skeptic.

Klass: Dr. Daly?

Daly: I think somebody should challenge this because the study was ill-conceived and poorly controlled. No serum levels of antiepileptic drugs were determined on these patients; everybody knows that compliance is a major problem in patients under study. Any time you begin to study a population of epileptic patients, compliance, that is, the reliability of the patient in taking the medicine, improves and serum levels of the drug rise. So merely announcing to patients that you're going to study them is a good way to reduce their seizures. Secondly, the study did not include sham conditioning. I'm not saying that Sterman may not be correct. I'd give him the Scotch verdict of *not proved,* because of the two enormous holes in the study. Unfortunately, such reports often attract undue attention from the press. I have had a rash of phone calls from patients who want to rush out and get "hooked up and tuned up." I think this is most unfortunate.

Question: Dr. Low, Why positive up, in evoked potential studies?

Low: We don't record evoked potentials in any way that's out of the ordinary. I would turn the question around. Why negative up? Some people record with positive up; some people with negative up.

Klass: Aren't there any rational reasons for this?

Ellingson: It's a matter of history. Physiologists started using negative up many years ago. Engineers started using positive up. More recently some physiologists decided that as long as the engineers use positive up, they would too. So now some physiologists use positive up while most physiologists use negative up. It's quite arbitrary. One must examine the figure or the legend to find out which convention is being used.

Question: What is the mechanism, i.e., pathogenesis, of barbiturate-induced beta?

---

[3] NASA Contract NAS 9-12947 and NAS 9-13870.

[4] Sterman, M. B. and MacDonald, L. R. (1978): Effects of central cortical EEG feedback training on incidence of poorly controlled seizures. *Epilepsia,* 19(4):207–222.

Low: I haven't got the vaguest notion.

Question: Ceroid lipofuscinosis *is* Batten's disease or Jansky-Bielschowsky disease. I do not understand the description of how different patterns of ERG-EEG-VER differ in the same disease.

Low: I don't think I was referring to the same disease, exactly. There are two kinds of Batten's disease as I understand it. Speilmeyer-Vogt has been called juvenile Batten's, and Bielschowsky-Jansky is a late infantile form of Batten's disease. By the way, I don't think there's any terminology more complicated than that whole bag of worms in the neurometabolic storage disorders. There apparently is now recognized a 'juvenile' Batten's as opposed to a 'late infantile' form.[5]

Question: What is the usefulness of evoked potentials in the determination of cerebral death?

Low: Some people have used them, and I think that some use them more or less routinely, simply as another means of assessing residual brain function. We don't use them. We don't feel that it's necessary, but it is a matter of individual practice.

Saunders: I don't like doing them for the simple reason that you're taking a voltage generator that produces a 15,000-volt signal into an oxygen-laden atmosphere, and you haven't got certainty of the grounding techniques. You can run into trouble from the standpoint of safety, and I don't think it's worth the trouble, considering the uncertainty of significance attached to the procedure.

Bickford: There is something more important to add to this question. I agree with the answers given, but, in point of fact, both animal experiments and our own observations on the human and more recently some work from Sweden indicate that evoked potentials are more resistent to anoxia than the spontaneous potentials, thus probably raising some nasty philosophical questions. When the EEG is flat—and this has been shown quite clearly I think—evoked potentials can be obtained for a further period of time.

Question: Dr. Low, are the slow negative shifts on the left hemisphere only specific to language, that is, semantic tasks and not to phonetic or audiological tasks?

Low: As far as we know now, yes, but this has not been established with any certainty. Data have been gathered over about 2 years, and we're increasingly confident about their significance. The phenomenon, which I demonstrated in the slide, of greater negativity on the apparently language-dominant side seems to be related to the process of getting ready to speak, and although we don't know exactly what the neural basis of this negativity is, perhaps it's something that reflects the neurons preparing to do whatever they do during articulation. That's a reasonably attractive hypothesis because we know that similar shifts occur prior to movement of any sort. Just before moving your thumb, for example, you can detect a similar negative shift over the motor cortex in the appropriate place.

With regard to auditory function and hemisphere dominance, the best evidence I know of is a paper by Wood, Goff, and Day.[6] Wood and his colleagues described evoked potential configurations that were different over the two hemispheres, and the differences seemed to be related to linguistic rather than to nonlinguistic parameters of exactly the same auditory signals. There is some evidence, therefore, that one can find electrophysiological correlates of language dominance.

---

[5] The reader is advised to consult the article and reference list by G. Pampiglione (1977): In: *Current Concepts in Clinical Neurophysiology, Didactic Lectures of the Ninth International Congress of Electroencephalography and Clinical Neurophysiology, Amsterdam, The Netherlands, September 1977,* edited by H. Van Duijn, D. N. J. Donker, and A. C. Van Huffelen, pp. 23–30. N. V. Drukkerij Trio, The Hague, The Netherlands.

[6] Wood, C. C., Goff, W. R., and Day, R. S. (1971): Auditory evoked potential during speech perception. *Science,* 173:1248–1251.

Subject Index

Abscess
  cerebellar, 319,321
  cerebral, 371
Absence seizures, 244,510
  automatisms in, 241,259
  hereditary factors in, 243
  spike-and-slow-wave complex in, 241
Acetazolamide, affecting EEG, 406
Acidosis, diabetic, 349
Action potentials, of pyramidal cells, 425
Activation procedures, 269–304
  alcohol in, 515
  auditory stimulation, 284
  hyperventilation, 258–260, 272–276; see also Hyperventilation, interpretation of, 274
  and hysterical seizures, 285
  internal triggers in, 285–286,287
  method of approach in, 271–272
  methohexital in, 513
  pentylenetetrazol in, 250,291–294,295,511, 513
  photic stimulation, 260–262,277–284; see also Photic stimulation
    interpretation of, 280–284
  sensory stimulation in, 276–286
  sleep deprivation, 258,291
  sleep recording, 256–258,286–291; see also Sleep recording
    all-night monitoring in, 291
    interpretation of, 290–291
  somesthetic triggers in, 284
  startle-sensitivity triggers in, 285
Affective disorders and EEG, 142–143,409
Age factors in EEG patterns, 71,73,140–141
  and alpha frequency, 75,79–80

and arousal patterns, 119,121
and beta activity, 83
and focal spikes, 231
and hyperventilation response, 112
and ideal EEG, 102–103
and posterior slow activity, 91
and temporal slow activity, 105
and theta activity, frontal, 87
Alcohol
  and activation of EEG, 515
  withdrawal of, affecting EEG, 362
Alcoholics, EEG in, 511
Alpha rhythm, 73–82
  age factor in, 75,79–80
  and alpha coma pattern, 350–352,354,374
  asymmetry between sides, 81–82
    in mu rhythm, 83
    in temporal alpha activity, 82
  in children, 75–76,79–80
  in elderly, 76
  in eye-open periods, 18
  frontocentral, in arousal pattern, 124
  in infants, 163
  locus of, 80
  in migraine, 390
  mu rhythm, 80,81; see also Mu rhythm
  in newborn, 170
  normal parameters of, 74–75
  occipital, 80
    in drowsiness, 115
  phenothiazines affecting, 402
  in quadriplegia, 330,337
  regulation of, 77–80
  slowing of, 74–75,344
  split-alpha, 253
  temporal, 80

variant patterns in headache, 384–385,389
voltage of, 76–77
  interelectrode distance affecting, 76,77
Alzheimer's disease, 366
American Electroencephalographic Society guidelines, see Guidelines of American EEG Society
Amobarbital injections, effects of, 250
Amphetamines, affecting EEG, 402,404
Amplifier, overloading of, 499
Amplitude, affected by interelectrode distance, 499
Analgesics, affecting EEG, 402,405
Analog computer techniques, 452–456
Analysis of EEG, 27–36
  and computer use, 451–479
Anoxic periods, 349
Anticholinergic agents, affecting EEG, 402, 405
Anticonvulsants, affecting EEG, 359,363, 402,406
Antidepressants, tricyclic, affecting EEG, 402, 405
Antihistamine derivatives, affecting EEG, 402, 406
Anxiety, affecting EEG, 142–143,406,408–409
Arousal activity, 118,119–124
  in adults, 124,125,126
  age factor in, 119,121
  in children, 118,119–124
  fast component in, 120–121
  and postarousal hypersynchrony, 121
  slow component in, 120–121
Artifacts, 37–67,212
  averaging of, and computer techniques, 457–460

SUBJECT INDEX

and ballistocardiograph effect, 66
from EEG machine, 43–46
from electrocardiogram, 63,64–65,66,212 290
   analog subtraction of, 453,456
   removal from cerebral death records, 499
and electrocerebral silence, 210
in electrocorticography, 299
from electrodes, 43,44,48
external causes of, 38–39,40–42
from eye activity, 56–61
   blepharospasm, 56,57
   blinking, 56,59,505
   in CSA technique, 469,519
   nystagmus, 56
   in one-eyed persons, 56,60
   simulation in hepatic coma, 56,61
from ground lead, 505
from hyperventilation, 272–273
instrumental causes of, 39–46
from intravenous drips, 39,41
mixed causes of, 63–66
from muscle activity, 46,47,51–55,61
in neonatal EEG, 152–153
from pentylenetetrazol activation, 293
from photic stimulation, 278
physiological causes of, 46–63
from pulse, 63,65–66
from respiratory pumps, 39,66
from 60-Hz interference, 38–39,40
from skin movements, 46,47
and status of patient, 118
suppression with succinylcholine, 52,55,212
suppression-burst, 212
from sweat, 43,46,48–51
from telephone ringing, 39,42
from tics, 66
from tongue and mouth, 61,63
from tremors, 66
from vacuum tubes, 44,199
Asymmetry, 504
   in alpha rhythm, 81–82
   in beta activity, 83–84
   in fast activity during sleep, 134–135

   in lambda waves, 103
   in neonatal EEG, 166
   in positive, occipital, sharp transients of sleep, 137
   in vertex sharp-wave transients of sleep, 124
Asynchrony, interhemispheric, in newborn, 175
Audiometry, evoked response, 447–448
Auditory stimulation, and activation of EEG, 284
Automatisms, 222,223,231
   in absence seizures, 241,259

Background rhythms
   decrease in metabolic disorders, 345
   slowing in drug toxicity, 359
Ballistocardiograph, artifacts from, 66
Barbiturates
   affecting EEG, 359,360,364,402,403
   withdrawal of, affecting EEG, 361
Basket-type stellate cells, 422
Batten's disease, 520–521
Behavior disorders and EEG patterns, 141, 399–401
   correlation with spike focus, 233
   and slow waves, posterior, 90–91
   and theta activity, frontal, 87
Benzodiazepines
   affecting EEG, 359,360,402
   withdrawal of, affecting EEG, 361
Beta activity, 82–86
   age factor in, 83
   asymmetry in, 83–84
   drug ingestion affecting, 83,359,360,402
   and fast EEGs, 83,84
   frontocentral, 84
   high-voltage, 83
   locus of, 84
   in sleep, 83,84–86
Bielschowsky-Jansky lipoidosis, 368,520–521
Bilateral synchrony, secondary, 250–252
Biofeedback training, effects of, 520
Bipolar recording, 30–31
   comparison with referential montages, 9,14

simultaneous positive and negative spikes in, 33,34
Blepharospasm, artifacts from, 56,57
Blinking of eyes, artifacts from, 56,59,505
Brain death, see Electrocerebral inactivity
Brainstem auditory evoked responses, 448,457
Burst-suppression pattern
   in drug overdosage, 360
   in hypoxia, 349–350,352
   in neonatal EEG, 166,170,171
   in premature infants, 501

Calcium metabolism, disorders affecting EEG, 357–359
   hypercalcemia, 358–359
   hypocalcemia, 357,362
Calibration, 18,19,490,491
   and detection of artifacts, 46
   and sensitivity control, 199
Cannabis-containing drugs, affecting EEG, 402,405
Carbamazepine, affecting EEG, 359,406
Cardiac arrest, 350,353,354
Cataplexy, 264
Cerebellar abscesses, 319,321
Cerebral cortex
   corticograms compared to scalp EEG, 434–438
   electrodes in, 298–299
   potentials generating EEG waves, 425–426
   potentials generating epileptiform EEG activity, 426–428
   structural design of, 422–425
Cerebral death, see Electrocerebral inactivity
Cerebral functional disorders
   diffuse, see Diffuse disorders of cerebral function
   focal, see Focal intracranial lesions
Cerebral palsy, beta activity in, 85
Cerebrovascular disease, affecting EEG, 364–366, 517
   and temporal slow activity, 105–106,110
Channels for recording EEG
   adjustment to calibration signal, 18,19

for neonatal recordings, 151
number of, 7–9,10,11,488–489,507
Childhood EEG, 71,73
  alpha rhythm in, 75–76,79–80
  arousal activity in, 118,119–124
  beta activity in, 83
  drowsiness activity in, 112–119
  encephalitis affecting, 370
  focal spikes in, 231
  head injury affecting, 372–373,374
  hyperventilation response in, 109,112,142
  hypocalcemia affecting, 357
  hypoglycemia affecting, 349
  and hypsarrhythmia, 368–369
  lambda waves in, 103
  lipoidosis affecting, 367–368
  and minimal cerebral dysfunction, 399–401
  neonatal, 149–176; see also Neonatal EEG
  sleep patterns in, see Sleep recordings
  slow waves in
    anterior, 100–102
    and ideal EEG, 102–103
    posterior, 90–100
  theta activity in, frontal, 87
Chlordiazepoxide, affecting EEG, 359
Clothing, electrostatic potentials from, 39
Coma, 24, 25; see also Electrocerebral inactivity
  and alpha coma pattern, 350–352,354,374
  evoked potentials in, 447
  hepatic, 56,61,353,356
  hypoglycemic, affecting EEG, 349
  irreversible, definition of, 208–209
  spindle coma pattern, 129
  in head injury, 373,375
Comagram, 465
Computer techniques, 451–479
  analog methods in, 452–456
  and area display of voltage contours, 469–473
  averaging artifacts in, 457–460
  and comagram, 465
  and compressed spectral array (CSA), 467–469

response averaging in, 456–457
  and somnogram, 465
  and spectral analysis, 460–465
  and telephone transmission techniques, 473–479
Computerized transaxial tomograms, 316,319, 331–339
Consciousness, state of, affecting EEG, 71,73
Coronary Care Unit, and causes of EEG artifacts, 39
Cortical structure, see Cerebral cortex
Costs of electroencephalography, 507,508
  for telephone transmission, 519
Cough syncope, 509
Creutzfeldt-Jakob disease, 252,367,446

Decerebrate rigidity, artifacts in, 52
Degenerative conditions, affecting EEG, 364–370
Delta activity
  in drug toxicity, 359
  in focal intracranial lesions, 310,326,328
  in head injury, 372
  in hypoxia, 349
  in infants, 163
  low frequency filters affecting, 203,206
  in metabolic disorders, 346
  in migraine, 388,391
  monorhythmic paroxysmal, 253
  in newborn, 170
  in perinatal EEG, 159
  polymorphic, 517
    and arrhythmic slowing, 344,345
    flat, 311
    in focal intracranial lesions, 308–310
    localized, 235,238
  in renal disease, 357,358
  spindle bursts in premature infants, 157,168
  and time constant, 25
Dementia syndrome, in dialysis patients, 357, 361
Demyelinating disease
  affecting EEG, 517
  evoked potentials in, 447

Dendrites of pyramidal cells
  in hippocampus, 425
  in neocortex, 422
Depolarization shifts, paroxysmal, 426–427, 518
Depressant drugs, electrocerebral silence from, 499
Depression, affecting EEG, 409
Depth electrography, 296,300–303,516
Deviations from norm
  and patterns of uncertain significance, 384–387,409,411–418
  significance of, 139–143
Dexamethasone, affecting EEG, 316,319,322, 331
Diabetes, affecting EEG, 349
Dialysis
  affecting EEG, 357,360
  and dementia syndrome, 357,361
Diazepam, affecting EEG, 359,383,404
Differential method of recording, 30–31; see also Bipolar recording
Diffuse disorders of cerebral function, 343–378
  in degenerative conditions, 364–370
  evoked potentials in, 446–447
  in head injury, 371–377
  in inflammatory diseases, 370–371
  in metabolic conditions, 141, 345–359
  slow-wave abnormalities in, 344
  in toxic states, 359–364
Diphenylhydantoin, see Anticonvulsants
Display of EEG activity, 179–220
  instrumental controls in, 197–204
  montages in, 179–197; see also Montages
Documentation of data, 24,491
  in electrocerebral inactivity, 213,215,220
Drowsiness, 112–119,287
  monorhythmic slow activity and, 112–115,116,117
  in newborn, 159,176
  paroxysmal slow activity in, 115–119
  and patterns in headache, 384,388
Drug effects on EEG, 359,383
  and alpha rhythm, 75

and beta activity, 83,85—86
dexamethasone, 316,319,322,331
and electrocerebral silence, 499,500
in overdosage, 359—360,364
psychotropic agents, 359,402—405
and sleep, 85—86,133—134,512
spindling from, 132
Drug use with EEG
for activation, *see* Activation procedures
pancuronium for elimination of EMG artifact, 199,203
for sleep induction, 512
succinylcholine for artifact suppression, 52, 55, 212
Drug withdrawal affecting EEG, 361—362, 365,366,383—384
alcohol, 362
antiepileptic drugs, 255—256
photosensitivity in, 284
Dysmature EEG patterns, 175

Elderly persons, EEG in, 73
alpha rhythm in, 76
temporal slow activity in, 103—109,110
Electrical fields, 28—35
construction from recordings, 31—32
graphic representation of, 29
localization of, 32—35
recording methods for, 29—31
Electrocardiogram, and artifacts in EEG, 63—66,202,290
analog subtraction of, 453,456
removal from cerebral death records, 499
Electrocerebral inactivity, 204,208—220,352, 355
and artifact production, 210
criteria for cerebral death, 500—501
in newborn, 163
and definition of irreversible coma, 208—209
documentation of data in, 213,215,220
from drugs, 499,500
and evoked potentials, 447,521
number of electrodes needed for, 210
and photic stimulation, 280,281

and standards for EEG recording in suspected cerebral death, 492—496
Electroconvulsive therapy, affecting EEG, 406,407
Electrocorticography, 298—299
artifacts in, 299
compared to scalp EEG, 434—438
Electrodes
artifacts from, 43,44,48
collodion technique with, 209
cortical, 298—299
identification for each channel, 12,15,489
impedances of, checking of, 9,13
implanted, in depth electrography, 296,300—303,516
interelectrode distances, 12,16,489,504
affecting amplitude, 499
and alpha rhythm voltage, 76,77
and lambda wave voltage, 103
nasopharyngeal, 297—298,515—516
needle, use of, 25,492
number of, 180,489
for ECS studies, 210
pastes for scalp placement in infants, 499
patterns of connections, 12,16
placement positions, 9,12,489
in neonates, 150—151
special types of, 294—303
sphenoidal, 298
Electroencephalographers, qualifications of, 2, 484—488
Electrography, depth, 296,300—303,516
Electromagnetic fields, artifacts from, 39
Electromyogram, neonatal, 151,152
Electrooculogram, neonatal, 151
Electroretinogram recordings, 446
Electrostatic potentials, artifacts from, 39
Emotional state affecting EEG, 142—143
and theta activity, frontal, 87
Encephalitis
acute, affecting EEG, 370,372
herpes simplex, affecting EEG, 371,373
Encephalopathy
hepatic, affecting EEG, 352
uremic, affecting EEG, 357

Encoches frontales, in neonatal EEG, 166,172
Epilepsy, *see* Seizures
Epileptiform discharge, 224,225,227
in brain tumors, 311
cortical activity in, 432—434
generation by cortical potentials, 426—428
in hypoglycemia, 349
thalamus role in, 428—432
Equipment for EEG, guidelines for, 3,485
Ethosuximide, affecting EEG, 359
Evoked potentials, 441—449,520
auditory, 447—448
brainstem, 448,457
averaging artifacts in, 457—460
in cerebral death, 447, 521
in cerebral disease, 445—447
in coma, 447
in demyelinating disease, 447
in hearing assessment, 447—448
and hemisphere dominance, 521
in Jakob-Creutzfeldt disease, 446
in multiple sclerosis, 447
in myoclonus, 446—447
in optic neuritis, 447
origin of, 444
in peripheral nerve lesions, 444—445
recording techniques, 443—444
sensory-evoked, 442—443
in spinal cord lesions, 445
visual, 446
in visual assessment, 448
voltage contour distribution of, 469,473,477
Excitatory postsynaptic potentials, 425,519
Eye activity, artifacts from, 56—61,505
in CSA technique, 469,519
Eye-open periods, recording in, 17,18,490

Fast activity
in arousal reaction, 120—121
and beta activity, 83, 84
in sleep, 132—135
Flat tracings
and electrocerebral inactivity, 204,208—220
in newborn, 163,166,168,169
Focal intracranial lesions, 307—339,518

and characteristics of tumors, 312-331
and computerized transaxial tomography with EEG, 316,319,331-339
continuous polymorphic delta waves in, 308-310
epileptiform discharges in, 311
evoked potentials in, 446
extra-axial lesions, 330-331
infratentorial tumors, 312
intermittent rhythmic delta activity in, 310
intraventricular tumors, 312
metastatic lesions, 319
nonspecific changes in, 312
posterior fossa tumors, 314
serial EEG studies in, 331
in subcortical gray matter structures, 326-330
   extension from white matter lesions, 321-326
thalamic tumors, 312
and unilateral absence of background activity, 311
white matter lesions, 316-321
   extension into midline structures, 321-326
Four-to-six Hz activity, paroxysmal bursts of, 510
Fourteen-and-six-per-second positive spikes, 409,412-414,517
Frequencies
   low, recording of, 18,24
   ratio to voltage, and slow activity in EEG, 102
Frequency controls, 199-201,204
Frequency filters, 491
   high frequency, 201-202,205
   low frequency, 202-204,206-208
Frontal lobe tumors, 316-319
Frontal sharp transients, in neonatal EEG, 166,168,172,504-505
Frontocentral locus
   for beta activity, 84
   for theta activity, 74,87-90

Generation of EEG waves, mechanisms in, 422
Genetics
   and absence seizures, 243
   and EEG patterns, 140
Glial cells, and generation of EEG waves, 426
Glucose
   blood levels of, and response to hyperventilation, 112,273,274
   metabolism disorders affecting cerebral function, 347-349
      hyperglycemia, 349
      hypoglycemia, 347-349,350
Glutethimide, affecting EEG, 359
Goldman-Offner reference, 39
Guidelines of American EEG Society, 2,184, 481-498
   and minimum technical requirements, 7-25
   for qualifications of technologists, 2,486-488
   for recording EEG, 488-492
      in suspected cerebral death, 492-496
   for standards of practice, 484-485
   for telephone transmission of EEG, 496-498

Head injury, 371-377
   and alpha coma pattern, 374-375
   and posttraumatic headache, 393
   recovery phase in, 376,377
   and response to methylphenidate, 373,375
   and subdural hematoma, 375-376,393
Headache, 381-393,510
   alpha-variant patterns in, 384-385,389
   and fourteen-Hz bursts, 384,385
   migraine or vascular, 387-393
   posttraumatic, 393
   and rhythmic temporal theta bursts of drowsiness, 384,388
   and six-Hz bursts, 384,387
   small, sharp spikes in, 384,386
   tension, nonorganic, 383-384
   and wave forms of doubtful significance, 384-387
Hearing assessment, evoked potentials in, 447-448
Hematoma, subdural, 331,375-376,393
Hemisphere dominance, and evoked potentials, 521
Hemodialysis
   affecting EEG, 357,360
   and dementia syndrome, 357
Heredity
   and absence seizures, 243
   and EEG patterns, 140
Herpes simplex encephalitis, 371,373
High-voltage slow pattern, perinatal, 157,159
Hippocampus, 425
   generation of epileptic activity in, 428
Huntington's chorea, 366-367
Hydantoins, *see* Anticonvulsants
Hypercalcemia, 358-359
Hyperglycemia, 349
Hyperventilation response, 109-112,258-260,272-276,491-492
   in adults, 112
   age factors in, 112
   artifacts from, 272-273
   beta activity in, 84
   in children, 109,112,142
   glucose levels affecting, 112,273,274,348,504
   in migraine, 389
   prolonged response in, 503
   slow waves in, posterior, 100
   time required for, 514
Hypnagogic state, 113
Hypocalcemia, 357,362
Hypoglycemia, 347-349,350
Hyponatremia, 359
Hypoxia, 349-352
Hypsarrhythmia, 235,237-239,240,368-370
Hysterical seizures, 285

Impedances, electrode, checking of, 9,13
Implanted electrodes, 296,300-303,516

Infant EEG, 161–163
  in sleep, 162–163
Inflammatory diseases affecting EEG, 370–371
Inflection point, in bipolar recording, 31
Inhibitory postsynaptic potentials, 425
Injuries of head, affecting EEG, 371–377
  and posttraumatic headache, 393
Instrumental causes of artifacts, 39–46
Instrumental controls, 197–204,490
  and electrocerebral inactivity determination, 204,208–220
  frequency, 199–201,204
  high frequency filters in, 201–202,205
  low frequency filters in, 202–204,206–208
  sensitivity, 197–199,200
Intensive Care Unit, and causes of EEG artifacts, 39,66
Intravenous drips, artifacts from, 39,41
Iproniazid, affecting EEG, 404

Jakob-Creutzfeldt disease, 252,367,446
Jaw myoclonus, from reading, 285

Kappa rhythm, 517
Ketoacidosis, diabetic, affecting EEG, 349
Kidney disease, 357,358
  and effects of dialysis, 357,360,361

Laboratory organization, guidelines for, 485
Lambda waves, 103,106
  asymmetrical, 103
  high-voltage, 103,108
  in migraine, 389
Learning problems in children, and EEG patterns, 399–401
Lennox-Gastaut syndrome, 248
Lipoidosis, 520–521
  cerebral, 367
  late infantile, 368,369
Lithium, 402,405
Liver disease, 352–357
Localization of electrical fields, 32–35
Low-voltage pattern
  irregular, perinatal, 157,159
  in newborn, 163,166,167,168,169
LSD-25, affecting EEG, 402,405

Machine for EEG, artifacts from, 43–46
Manic depressive psychosis, 409
Marijuana, affecting EEG, 405
Memory recall, and seizure initiation, 285,286
Meningioma, 331,339
Meningitis, 371
Menstrual cycle, and alpha rhythm frequency, 78–79
Mental retardation
  beta activity in, 85
  sleep stage I in, 159,176
Meperidine hydrochloride, affecting EEG, 405
Mephenytoin, affecting EEG, 359
Meprobamate, affecting EEG, 359
Mescaline, affecting EEG, 402,405
Metabolic disorders
  affecting EEG, 141,345–359
  evoked potentials in, 446
Metastatic lesions, intracranial, 319
Methohexital, for activation of EEG, 513
Methylphenidate, response to, after head injury, 373,375
Micturition syncope, 509
Migraine, 387–393,510
  abdominal, 392–393
  basilar, 392
  hemiplegic, 390,392
Minimum technical requirements in EEG, 7–25
Mirror focus studies, in experimental epilepsy, 237
Mixed patterns, perinatal, 157,159
Monoamine oxidase inhibitors, affecting EEG, 402,404
Monopolar recording, 29–30,193; see also Referential method of recording
Montages, 9,12,14–16,179–197
  arrangement of, 490
  basic data in, 188–189,195,196–197
  bipolar, 489
    compared to referential montages, 9,14
  circular triangle display in, errors with, 192–193,194
  eight-channel, 9,180,181
  eighteen-channel, 189,191,196
    F run, 189,196
    I run, 196
    J run, 189,196
    K run, 189,196
  logical display of, 184,186,187
  in neonatal EEG, 151
  pitfalls and errors in, 180,182,183,185
  preselected, 189
  and problems of reference recording, 193–196
  referential, 193,489
    compared to bipolar montage, 9,14
  right/left or left/right display in, 185,188,506
  in seizure evaluation, 225
  sixteen-channel, 9,180
  small triangles for localization in, 190
    misinterpretation of, 190,192,193
  transverse, 188–189,225,250
Morphine, affecting EEG, 405
Mouth movements, artifacts from, 61,63
Mu rhythm, 80,81,412
  asymmetry of, 82
  sex difference in frequency of, 80,140
Multiple sclerosis, 447,517
Muscle
  artifacts from activity of, 46,47,51–55,61
  photomyoclonic response, 280,282,514
    in drug withdrawal, 361,365,384
Muscle relaxants, use of, 52,55,199,203,212
Musicogenic epilepsy, 284
Myoclonus, 245–248
  evoked potentials in, 446–447
  of jaw, from reading, 285
  photomyoclonic response, 280,282,514
    in drug withdrawal, 361,365,384

Narcolepsy, 264
Narcotics, affecting EEG, 402,405

Nasopharyngeal electrodes, 297–298,515–516
Needle electrodes, 25,492
  artifacts from, 25,43
Neonatal EEG, 149–176,501–502
  abnormalities in, 163–175
  asymmetry in, 166
  burst-suppression pattern in, 166,170,171,501
  and criteria for cerebral death, 163
  deviations of uncertain significance, 175–176
  dysmature patterns, 175
  excessive sleep stage I in, 159,176
  flat tracings in, 163,166,168,169
  frontal sharp transients in, 166,168,172,504–505
  in infants, 161–163
  low-voltage activity in, 163,166–169, 501
  perinatal patterns in, 157–161
  poor interhemispheric synchrony in, 175
  in prematures, 153–157
  recording techniques, 150–153
    artifacts in, 152–153
    electrodes in, 150–151
    instrumental control settings in, 151–152
    montages in, 151
    non-EEG variables in, 151
    procedures in, 152
  rhythmic patterns in, 168,170,173,174
  in seizure activity, 170,173–175
  spikes, sharp waves, and slow transients in, 166,168,172
Neoplasms, see Focal intracranial lesions
Neurophysiologic substrates of EEG activity, 421–438
  comparison of scalp EEG with corticograms, 434–438
  and cortical potentials generating EEG waves, 425–426
  and cortical potentials generating epileptiform EEG activity, 426–428
  and epileptogenic foci, 432–434
  and structural design of cortex, 422–425

and thalamus role in EEG activity, 422,428–432
Neuroses, affecting EEG, 406,408–409
Newborns, see Neonatal EEG
Normal EEG, 69–143
  alpha rhythm, 73–82
  in arousal, 118,119–124
  beta activity, 82–86
  in drowsiness, 112–119
  and hyperventilation response, 109–112
  and ideal EEG, 102–103
  lambda waves, 103,106
  and patterns of uncertain significance, 409,411–418
  in headache, 384–387
  and significance of deviations, 139–143
  in sleep, 124–138,141
  slow activity in
    anterior, 100–102
    posterior, 90–100
    temporal, 103–109
  theta activity in, frontal, 87–90
Nystagmus, artifacts from, 56

Occipital region
  alpha rhythm in, see Alpha rhythm
  lambda waves in, 103
  spikes in, 231
Occipital transients of sleep, 138
  positive sharp, 135–138,289
Occipitotemporal region, slow activity in, 90–100
Ocular compression test, in children, 517
Opiates, affecting EEG, 402,405
Optic neuritis, evoked potentials in, 447
Organic brain disease, 397
Overbreathing, see Hyperventilation
Overdosage of drugs, affecting EEG, 359–360,364
Overloading, of amplifier, 499
Oxazoladinediones, affecting EEG, 402,406

Pancuronium, use of, 199,203,212
Panencephalitis, subacute sclerosing, 252–253,367,368

Paper speed, variations in, 18,20
Parietooccipital region, slow activity in, 90–100
Parkinson's disease, 366
  artifacts from, 66
Paroxysmal depolarization shift (PDS), 426–427,518
Pastes, for scalp electrode placement, in infants, 499
Patterns of uncertain significance, 409,411–418
  fourteen-and-six-per-second positive spikes, 409,412–414,517
  in headache, 384–387
  psychomotor variant discharge, 414,416–417
  six-per-second spike and wave pattern, 414,415
  small sharp spikes, 417–418
Pediatric conditions, see Childhood EEGs
Penicillin-induced epileptogenic focus, 432,518
Pens, aligning of, 18,19,46
Pentylenetetrazol activation, 250,291–294,295,511,513
  artifacts from, 293
Perinatal EEG patterns, 157–161
  high-voltage slow, 157,159
  low-voltage irregular, 157,159
  mixed, 157,159
  in sleep, 159,161,164,165
  spindle-delta bursts in, 159
  tracé alternant, 159,501,502
Periodic discharges, localized, 233–235,326
Peripheral nerve function, and evoked potential recordings, 444–445
Pharmacological techniques, see Drug use with EEG
Phase reversal, in bipolar recording, 31
Phenobarbital, affecting EEG, 359
Phenothiazines, affecting EEG, 402
Phenytoin, see Anticonvulsants
Photic stimulation, and activation of EEG, 212,260–262,277–284
  artifacts from, 51,278

convulsive responses in, 281–282,508,514
   in drug withdrawal, 362,366,384
  driving response in, 278,280
   in migraine, 389
  in electrocerebral silence, 280,281
  interpretation of, 280–284
  myoclonic response in, 280,282,514
   in drug withdrawal, 361,365,384
   and sensitivity to light, 281–284
  photoconvulsive response, 281–282,508, 514
   in drug withdrawal, 362,366,384

Photomyoclonic response, 280,282,514
  in drug withdrawal, 361,365,384
Pick's disease, 366
Pinealoma, 328
Placement positions for electrodes, 9,12,489
  in neonates, 150–151
Polarity, 27–28,193,518
Polyphasic slow waves, posterior, 91,92,104, 105
Potentials
  cortical
   generating EEG waves, 425–426
   generating epileptiform EEG activity, 426–428
  evoked potential recordings, 441–449
Premature infants, EEG patterns in, 71,73,153–157
  intermittent burst pattern in, 166
  pattern A, 153–155,501
  pattern B, 155,156,158
  pattern C, 155,157,158,160
  ripples or brushes in, 157,168
  in sleep, 155,157,162
  spikes, sharp waves, and slow transients in, 166
  spindle-delta bursts in, 157,168
  tracé alternant in, 157,162
Primidone, affecting EEG, 359,402,406
Propoxyphenes, affecting EEG, 402,405
Psychiatric disorders, 395–410
  affective disorders, 142–143,409
  beta activity in psychoses, 84

drug-induced, 401–406
and electroconvulsive therapy affecting EEG, 406,407
and minimal cerebral dysfunction in children, 399–401
neurotic states, 406,408–409
organic brain disease, 397
schizophrenia, 409
in seizures, 398–399, 511
and so-called EEG abnormalities, 409–410
Psychomotor variant discharge, 414,416–417
Psychomimetic agents, affecting EEG, 402, 405
Psychotropic agents, affecting EEG, 359,402–405
Psylocybin, affecting EEG, 402,405
Pulse, artifact from, 63,65–66
Pyramidal cells
  in hippocampus, 425
  in neocortex, 422
Pyridoxine deficiency, affecting EEG, 369

Quadriplegia, alpha activity in, 330,337
Qualifications of EEG technologists, 2,484–488

Reading epilepsy, 285,287
Recording methods, 29–31
  computers in, 451–479
  differential, 30–31; see also Bipolar recording
  electrode placement positions in, 9,12,489
   in neonates, 150–151
  eye-open and eyes closed, 17,18,490
  instrumental control settings in, 18,21–23
   for neonates, 151–152
  left/right or right/left, 185,188,490,506
  referential, 29–30,193; see also Referential method
  in seizure evaluation, 225
  standards in, 488–492
   in suspected cerebral death, 492–496
  time span of, 491
  written data included with, 25,491
   in electrocerebral inactivity, 213,215,220

Referential method of recording, 29–30, 193,499–500,506
  compared to bipolar montages, 9,14
  and construction of field, 31–32
  problems of, 193–196
  simultaneous positive and negative spikes in, 33,34
Respirators, artifacts from, 39,66,212
Respirogram, neonatal, 151
Reticular formation lesions, 330
Rolandic spikes, 227,231

Schilder's disease, 517
Schizophrenia, 409
  and epilepsy, 399,511
Sedatives, affecting EEG, 359,360
  withdrawal from, 361
Seizures, 221–264
  absence, see Absence seizures
  activation procedures in, 256–262
  alpha rhythm voltage in, 76,78
  beta activity in, 83,84
  biofeedback training in, 520
  classification of, 222–224
  and effects of withdrawal from antiepileptic drugs, 255–256
  experimental epileptogenic foci, 432,518
  generalized paroxysmal abnormality in, 223,239–252
   multiple spike-and-slow-wave complex, 245–248
   periodic discharges in, 252–253
   secondary bilateral synchrony in, 250–252
   sharp-and-slow-wave complexes, 248–250
   spike-and-slow-wave discharge, 239–244
  hyperventilation response in, 258–260
  in hypocalcemia, 357
  in infants of drug-addicted mothers, 503
  interictal abnormality in, 225–262
  in newborn, 175
  localized continuous abnormality in, 235, 238

localized paroxysmal abnormality in, 225–235
    periodic discharges in, 233–235,326
    pseudoperiodic lateralized discharge, 233, 236
    spike-and-sharp-waves, 227–233
multifocal paroxysmal abnormality in, 235–239
    hypsarrhythmia, 235,237–239,240
    multifocal spikes, 235–237
myoclonic, 245–248
in newborn, 170,173–175
and interictal EEG, 175
nocturnal, 513
nonspecific paroxysmal discharges in, 253
normal interictal EEG in, 253–256
partial, 223
    complex, 223,510
    elementary, 223
photic stimulation in, 260–262
polymorphic delta activity in, 235,238
and pseudo petit mal, 115,117
and psychomotor variant discharge, 414, 416–417
and psychosis, 398–399,511
recording methodology in, 225
self-stimulation in, 514–515
and sleep recordings, 256–258,513–514
and slow waves, posterior, 97,100
unilateral, 223
Sensitivity control, 197–199,200
    and electrocerebral inactivity, 208–209
    increased in low-voltage recordings, 18,21–23
    ranges of, 490–491
    and spike-wave paroxysms, 199,200
Sensory-evoked potentials, 442–443
Sensory stimulation, and activation of EEG, 276–286
Serial EEG studies, in intracranial lesions, 331
Serotonin analogs, affecting EEG, 402,405
Sex differences in EEG patterns, 140
    in mu rhythm, 80,140
Sharp waves, *see* Spikes and sharp waves
Shivering, artifacts from, 52

Sigma activity, 132
    continuous, 85
Skin
    movements of, artifacts from, 46,47
    stimulation of, and seizure initiation, 284
Skull
    defects of
        and beta activity, 83
        and fast activity in sleep, 135
    thickness of, and voltage asymmetry, 82
Sleep deprivation, and activation of EEG, 258,291
Sleep recordings, 25,124–138,141,492,513–514
    and activation of EEG, 256–258,286–291
    all-night monitoring in, 291
    beta activity in, 82,84–86
    fast activity in, 132–135
        asymmetry in, 134–135
        sedation affecting, 133–134
    and induction of sleep, 511–512
    in infant, 162–163
    interpretation of, 290–291
    occipital transients in, 138
    perinatal, 159,161,164,165
    positive occipital sharp transients in, 135–138,289
        asymmetrical, 137
        characteristics of, 137–138
        in migraine, 389
    in premature infants, 155,157,162
    somnogram in, 465
    spike-and-sharp-waves in, 227,230
    spike-and-slow-wave complex in, 239
    spindles in, 127–132
        in infants, 163
        in newborn, 170
        spike activity with, 512
    in stage I sleep; *see* Drowsiness
    vertex sharp-wave transients in 124–127, 128,129
        asymmetry in, 124
        high voltage in, 126
    and waking record, 290–291
Slow waves

    anterior, 100–102
    in arousal reaction, 120–121
    delta, polymorphic, and arrhythmic, 344
    in diffuse cerebral dysfunction, 344
    in drowsiness
        monorhythmic activity, 112–117
        paroxysmal activity, 115–119
    and frequency/voltage ratio, 102
    and hyperventilation response
        in adults, 112
        in children, 112,142
    and ideal EEG, 102–103
    intermittent, rhythmic, bilaterally synchronous, 344,346
    occipital transient of sleep, 138
    posterior, 90–100
        age factor in, 91
        in behavior disorders, 90–91
        and index of abnormality, 95–96
        polyphasic waves, 91,92,104,105
        and posterior slow activity of youth, 91,92,104,105,142
        random, 93–94,503
        rhythmic, 100,503
    sharp-and-slow-wave complex, 248–250
    spike-and-slow-wave complex, 239–244
        multiple spikes in, 245–248
    and supernormal EEG, 102,104
    temporal, 103–109,110
        age incidence of, 105
Small sharp spikes, 417–418
Sodium depletion, affecting EEG, 359
Somnogram, 465
Spectral analysis, 460–465
    and area display of information, 467–469
Sphenoidal electrodes, 298
Spikes and sharp waves, 508
    and behavioral defects, 233
    differentiating criteria for, 512–513
    epileptiform, *see* Epileptiform discharge
    focal, 227–233,311
    in hypoglycemia, 349
    multifocal, 235–237
    neonatal, 166
    in occipital region, 231

Spikes and sharp waves *(contd.)*
  positive
    fourteen-and-six per second, 412–414
    occipital sharp transient of sleep, 135–138,289
    six-per-second, 414,415
  recognition in CSA technique, 469
  rolandic, 227,231
  and sensitivity control, 199,200
  in sleep, 227,230,513–514
  and slow-wave discharge, 239–244,511
    compared to slow spike-and-wave, 248–250
    multiple spikes in, 245–248
  small sharp spikes, 417–418,516
    in headache, 384,386
  in sylvian region, 227
  in temporal region, 227,231,233
  vertex sharp-wave transients in sleep, 124–129
  in waking state, 227
  and wave complex, from thalamic stimulation, 427,428
Spinal cord function, and evoked potential recordings, 445
Spindles
  and coma pattern in head injury, 373,375
  and delta bursts
    in perinatal EEG, 159
    in premature infants, 157,168
  drugs causing, 132
  in sleep patterns, 127–132
    in infants, 163
    in newborn, 170
  spike activity with, 512
Standards of practice in EEG, 1–4,484
  for equipment, 485
  for recording, 488–492
Startle-sensitivity triggers, and seizure discharge, 285
Status epilepticus, neonatal, 173
Status of patient, affecting EEG, 24,25,71,73,492
  and artifacts, 118
Stellate cells, in neocortex, 422

basket-type, 422
Succinimides, affecting EEG, 402,406
Succinylcholine, for artifact suppression, 52,55,212
Sulfonamides and derivatives, affecting EEG, 402,406
Supernormal EEG, 102,104
Suppression-burst pattern
  as artifact pattern, 212
  in premature infants, 501
Sweat, artifacts from, 43,46,48–51
Sylvian region
  spikes in, 227
  theta activity in, 105
Synapses
  in hippocampus, 425
  in neocortex, 422
Syncope, 262–264,349
  cyanotic, 264
  micturition, 509
  pallid, 262
  tussive, 509

Tay-Sachs disease, 368
Technical requirements, minimal, 7–25
Technologists, qualifications of, 2,485,486–487
Telephone ringing, artifacts from, 39,42
Telephone transmission of EEG, 3–4,209,473–479
  cost of, 519
  guidelines for, 496–498
Temporal lobe abnormalities, small triangle montage in, 190
Temporal region
  alpha rhythm in, 80
    asymmetry of, 82
  slow activity in, 103–109,110
  spikes in, 227,231,233
Tension, psychological, affecting EEG, 142–143
Thalamus
  and cortical EEG activity, 422,428–432
  and generation of spikes, 519

Theta activity
  in drug toxicity, 359
  emotional state affecting, 142–143
  in eye-open periods, 18
  frontal and frontocentral, 74,87–90
    age factor in, 87
    monomorphic high-voltage, in asymptomatic patients, 87–90
  in hypoxia, 349
  in infants, 163
  in metabolic disorders, 345–346
  in migraine, 388
  monomorphic
    frontal, in asymptomatic patients, 87–90
    in parietal regions, 253
  in newborn, 170
  in perinatal EEG, 159
  in premature infants, 157
  rhythmic temporal bursts of drowsiness, in headache, 384,388
  slowing of, 344
  sylvian, 105
Thiopental sodium injections, effects of, 252
Tics, artifacts from, 66
Time constants, effects of, 25
Tolbutamide test, and activation of EEG, 349
Tomography, computerized, transaxial, 316,319,331–339
Tongue movements, artifacts from, 63
Toxic states, affecting EEG, 359–364
Tracé alternant pattern
  perinatal, 159,501,502
  of sleep in premature infant, 157,162
Training programs in EEG, 1–4
Transients
  in neonatal EEG
    frontal sharp, 166,168,172,504–505
    slow, 166,168
  positive occipital sharp transients of sleep, 135–138,289
  vertex sharp-wave transients in sleep, 124–127,128,129
Trauma of head
  affecting EEG, 371–377

cortical, beta activity in, 84
and posttraumatic headache, 393
Tremors, artifacts from, 66
Trimethadione, affecting EEG, 359
Triphasic wave pattern, in hepatic coma, 353,356
Tumors, *see* Focal intracranial lesions
Tussive syncope, 509
Twin studies of EEG patterns, 140

Uremia, 357

Vacuum tubes, artifacts from, 44–199
Vascular headaches, affecting EEG, 387–393

Vertex sharp-wave transients in sleep, 124–127,128,129
Visual analysis of EEG
and electrical fields, 28–35
hypothetical problem in, 35–36
and polarity convention, 27–28
Visual assessment, evoked potentials in, 448
Voltage
alpha rhythm, 76–77
area display of contours, 469–473
high-voltage slow pattern, perinatal, 157, 159
low-voltage pattern
irregular, perinatal, 157,159
in newborn, 163,166–169

measurements of, 198
ratio to frequency, and slow activity in EEG, 102

Waking record, value of, 290–291
Water intoxication, affecting EEG, 345,359
Withdrawal
from alcohol, affecting EEG, 362
from drugs
affecting EEG, 361–362,365,366,383–384
and seizures in infants of addicted mothers, 503
Written date with EEG, 25,491
in electrocerebral inactivity, 213,215,220